D1737826

INTERNATIONAL TRENDS IN GENERAL THORACIC SURGERY

VOLUME 1

LUNG CANCER

N. C. Delarue, Toronto, Canada
H. Eschapasse, Toulouse, France

VOLUME 2

MAJOR CHALLENGES

H. Grillo, Boston, Massachusetts, U.S.A.
H. Eschapasse, Toulouse, France

VOLUME 3

BENIGN ESOPHAGEAL DISEASE

T. R. DeMeester, Omaha, Nebraska, U.S.A.
H. R. Matthews, Birmingham, United Kingdom

VOLUME 4

ESOPHAGEAL CANCER

N. C. Delarue, Toronto, Canada
E. W. Wilkins, Jr., Boston, Massachusetts, U.S.A.
J. Wong, Hong Kong

Forthcoming

VOLUME 5

FRONTIERS, MEDIASTINUM, UNCOMMON PROBLEMS

N. Martini, New York, New York, U.S.A.
I. Vogt-Moykopf, Heidelberg, F.R.G.

VOLUME 6

INFECTIVE LUNG DISEASE

B. T. LeRoux, Durban, South Africa
D. Skinner, Chicago, Illinois, U.S.A.

VOLUME 7

THE PLEURAL SPACE

J. Deslauriers, Quebec City, Canada
L. K. Lacquet, Nijmegen, Holland

VOLUME 8

PERIOPERATIVE MANAGEMENT IN THORACIC SURGERY

R. M. Peters, San Diego, California, U.S.A.
J. Toledo, Madrid, Spain

VOLUME 9

CHEST INJURIES

A. Besson, Lausanne, Switzerland
W. R. Webb, New Orleans, Louisiana, U.S.A.

VOLUME 10

GENERAL THORACIC SURGERY IN INFANTS AND CHILDREN

R. M. Filler, Toronto, Canada
G. Lemoine, Paris, France

VOLUME 11

CHEST PAIN

H. Urschel, Dallas, Texas, U.S.A.
F. París, Valencia, Spain

INTERNATIONAL TRENDS IN GENERAL THORACIC SURGERY

Editors-in-Chief

N. C. DELARUE
  Toronto, Canada

H. ESCHAPASSE
  Toulouse, France

INTERNATIONAL TRENDS IN GENERAL THORACIC SURGERY

VOLUME 4

ESOPHAGEAL CANCER

Edited by

NORMAN C. DELARUE, M.D.

Emeritus Professor of Surgery,
University of Toronto, Toronto, Canada

EARLE W. WILKINS, Jr., M.D.

Clinical Professor of Surgery,
Harvard Medical School; Visiting Surgeon,
Thoracic Surgical Unit, Surgical Services,
Massachusetts General Hospital,
Boston, Massachusetts

JOHN WONG, M.D., Ph.D.

Professor and Head, Department of Surgery,
University of Hong Kong;
Professor, Department of Surgery,
Queen Mary Hospital, Hong Kong

with 369 illustrations, including 6 four-color plates

The C. V. Mosby Company

ST. LOUIS • WASHINGTON, D.C. • TORONTO   1988

MOSBY

A TRADITION OF PUBLISHING EXCELLENCE

Editor: Thomas A. Manning
Developmental editor: Elaine Steinborn
Assistant editor: Laurel Fuller
Project manager: Mark Spann
Production editor: Stephen C. Hetager
Book design: Gail Morey Hudson

Volume 4

Copyright © 1988 by The C.V. Mosby Company

Printed in the United States of America

The C.V. Mosby Company
11830 Westline Industrial Drive, St. Louis, Missouri 63146

Library of Congress Cataloging in Publication Data

Esophageal cancer/edited by Norman C. Delarue, Earle W. Wilkins,
   Jr., John Wong.
       p.   cm.—(International trends in general thoracic surgery;
   v. 4)
     Includes bibliographies and index.
     ISBN 0-8016-2048-1
     1. Esophagus—Cancer. I. Delarue, Norman C.   II. Wilkins, Earle
   W., 1919-   . III. Wong, John. IV. Series.
     [DNLM: 1. Esophageal Neoplasms. WI IN914 v. 4/WI 250 E762]
   RC280.E8E76 1988
   616.99′432—dc19
   DNLM/DLC
   for Library of Congress   87-34952
                                                                CIP

GW/MV/MV   9 8 7 6 5 4 3 2 1

Contributors

SHICHISABURO ABO, M.D.

Professor, Second Department of Surgery, Akita University Hospital, Akita, Japan

Pulmonary complications

HIROSHI AKIYAMA, M.D.

Chief of Surgery, Department of Surgery, Toranomon Hospital; Professor of Surgery, Department of Surgery, Tokyo Medical College, Tokyo, Japan

Imaging techniques

ISRAEL BARNETT ANGORN,† M.D.

Professor, Department of Surgery, University of Natal, Faculty of Medicine; Senior Specialist Surgeon, King Edward VIII Hospital; Senior Lecturer, Addington Hospital, Durban, Republic of South Africa

Endoesophageal intubation for palliation in obstructing esophageal carcinoma

MANJIT S. BAINS, M.D.

Associate Professor of Clinical Surgery, Department of Surgery, Cornell University; Associate Attending Surgeon, Thoracic Service, Department of Surgery, Memorial Sloan-Kettering Cancer Center, New York, New York

Transabdominal esophagogastrectomy for the poor-risk patient
Discussion: Chapters 40 to 43

ATTILA BAJTAI, M.D., Ph.D.

Assistant Professor, Department of Pathological Anatomy, Postgraduate Medical School, Budapest, Hungary

Discussion: Cytologic screening for carcinoma and dysplasia of the esophagus in the People's Republic of China

JEAN BIAGINI, M.D.

Clinical Assistant Professor in Surgery, Department of Surgery, St. Joseph University; Clinical Assistant Professor in Surgery, Department of Surgery, Hôtel-Dieu de France Hospital, Beirut, Lebanon

Prophylactic operative techniques: 380 esophageal anastomoses using the stapler

ÁGNES BOHÁK, M.D.

Postgraduate Medical School, Budapest, Hungary

Submucography in the diagnosis of esophageal tumors

JUAN J. BORETTI, M.D.

Professor of Surgery, Rosario University School of Medicine, Rosario, Argentina

Median sternotomy in radical surgery for esophageal carcinoma involving cervical and upper thoracic segments

---

† Deceased.

J. R. BOUDERLIQUE, M.D.

Chief of Medicine, Centre Medical de Forgilles, Ferolles Attilly, France

Discussion: Perioperative management of carcinoma of the esophagus: the reduction of operative mortality

FRANK JAMES BRANICKI, M.B.B.S., D.M.F.R.C.S.

Senior Lecturer, Department of Surgery, University of Hong Kong; Honorary Consultant Surgeon, Department of Surgery, Queen Mary Hospital, Hong Kong

Esophagoscopy and bronchoscopy

MICHAEL BURT, M.D., Ph.D.

Assistant Professor of Surgery and Biochemistry, Departments of Surgery and Biochemistry, Cornell University Medical College; Assistant Attending Surgeon, Department of Surgery, Thoracic Service, Memorial Sloan-Kettering Cancer Center, New York, New York

Discussion: Chapters 40 to 43

ALAN JOHN CAMERON, M.B., M.R.C.P.

Associate Professor of Medicine, Department of Gastroenterology, Mayo Clinic, Rochester, Minnesota

Adenocarcinoma in the columnar epithelial–lined lower esophagus of Barrett

NOAH C. CHOI, M.D.

Assistant Professor, Department of Radiation Therapy, Harvard Medical School; Associate Radiation Oncologist, Department of Radiation Medicine, Massachusetts General Hospital, Boston, Massachusetts

The relative merits of definitive radiotherapy and palliative resection

PHILIPPE CLERC, M.D.

Assistant, Department of Surgery, University of Bordeaux II, Bordeaux, France; Assistant Surgeon, Department of Thoracic Surgery, Hôpital Xavier Arnozan, Pessac, France

The current role of partial esophagectomy in the surgical treatment of middle- and lower-third esophageal carcinoma
Use of tubular isoperistaltic gastroplasty after total or partial esophagectomy

ANDREW ALAN CONLAN, MB., B.Ch., F.R.C.S.(Eng.), F.A.C.S.

Senior Thoracic Surgeon and Lecturer, Department of Cardiothoracic Surgery, University of the Witwatersrand Medical School; Chief Cardiothoracic Surgeon, Department of Cardiothoracic Surgery, Rand Mutual Hospital, Johannesburg Academic Hospital, Johannesburg, South Africa

The malignant tracheoesophageal or bronchoesophageal fistula

LOUIS COURAUD, M.D.

Professor, Department of Thoracic Surgery, University of Bordeaux II, Bordeaux, France; Chief Thoracic Surgeon, Department of Thoracic Surgery, Hôpital Xavier Arnozan, Pessac, France

The current role of partial esophagectomy in the surgical treatment of middle- and lower-third esophageal carcinoma
Use of tubular isoperistaltic gastroplasty after total or partial esophagectomy

TOM R. DeMEESTER, M.D.

Professor and Chairman, Department of Surgery, Creighton University School of Medicine; Chief of Surgery, Department of Surgery, Saint Joseph Hospital, Omaha, Nebraska

Perioperative management of carcinoma of the esophagus: the reduction of operative mortality

ANDRÉ DURANCEAU, M.D., F.A.C.S., F.R.C.S.

Professor, Department of Surgery, University of Montreal; Division of Thoracic Surgery, Department of Surgery, Hôtel-Dieu de Montréal, Montreal, Quebec, Canada

Epidemiologic trends and etiologic factors of esophageal carcinoma

F. HENRY ELLIS, Jr., M.D., Ph.D.

Clinical Professor of Surgery, Harvard Medical School, Boston, Massachusetts; Senior Consultant, Section of Thoracic and Cardiovascular Surgery, Lahey Clinic Medical Center, Burlington, Massachusetts; Chief, Department of Thoracic and Cardiovascular Surgery, New England Deaconess Hospital, Boston, Massachusetts

Discussion: Surgical management of adenocarcinoma at the gastroesophageal junction
Surgical palliation: esophageal resection—a surgeon's opinion

A. ELMAN, M.D.

Service de Chirurgie Digestive, Hôpital Beaujon, Paris, France

Immediate complications following esophageal surgery

MITSUO ENDO, M.D.

Professor of Surgery and Chairman, First Department of Surgery, Tokyo Medical and Dental University, Yushima, Bunkyo-Ku, Tokyo, Japan

Special techniques in the endoscopic diagnosis of esophageal carcinoma

FRANÇOIS FEKETE, M.D.

Professor of Surgery, Department of Medicine, University of Paris VII, Paris, France; Chief, Department of Digestive Surgery, Hôpital Beaujon, Clichy, France

Prophylactic operative techniques: 380 esophageal anastomoses using the stapler
Prophylactic operative techniques: thoracic esophageal squamous cell cancer surgery, with special reference to lymph node removal

JACK FISHER, M.D.

Assistant Clinical Professor, Department of Plastic Surgery, Vanderbilt University; Department of Plastic Surgery, Parkview Medical Center, Nashville, Tennessee

Esophageal reconstruction: free jejunal transfer or circulatory augmentation of pedicled intestinal interpositions using microvascular surgery

ALBINO D. FLORES, M.D., F.R.C.P.C.

Clinical Associate Professor, Department of Surgery, University of British Columbia; Radiation Oncologist, Department of Radiation Oncology, Cancer Control Agency of British Columbia, Vancouver, British Columbia, Canada

Discussion: Brachytherapy for inoperable cancer of the esophagus and cardia

HIROMASA FUJITA

Lecturer, First Department of Surgery, Kurume University School of Medicine, Kurume, Fukuoka, Japan

Combined radical resection of adjacent organs involved by esophageal carcinoma

BRICE GAYET, M.D.

Maître de Conference, University of Paris VII; Department of Digestive Surgery, Hôpital Beaujon, Paris, France

Prophylactic operative techniques: 380 esophageal anastomoses using the stapler
Prophylactic operative techniques: thoracic esophageal squamous cell cancer surgery, with special reference to lymph node removal

ROBERT GIULI, M.D., F.A.C.S.

Professor of Surgery, Faculté Xavier-Bichat, Paris, France; Chirurgien des Hopitaux de Paris, Department of Digestive Surgery, Hôpital Beaujon, Clichy, France

Discussion: Perioperative management of carcinoma: the reduction of operative mortality
Discussion: Surgical management of adenocarcinoma at the gastroesophageal junction
Surgical involvement in cooperative study protocols: experience of the OESO international group
Immediate complications following esophageal surgery
Discussion: Chapters 37 to 39

XIAN-ZHI GU (KU HSIAN-CHIH) B.S., M.D.

Professor and Chairman, Chinese Society of Radiation Oncology, Department of Radiation Oncology, Cancer Institute and Hospital, Chinese Academy of Medical Sciences, Beijing, People's Republic of China

Definitive radiotherapy
Combined preoperative irradiation and surgery for esophageal carcinoma

ABDULLAH S. HAFEZ-ALQUDAH, M.D.

Assistant Professor, Department of Special Surgery, Cardiothoracic Section, Faculty of Medicine, University of Jordan; Cardiothoracic and Vascular Consultant, Department of Special Surgery, Cardiothoracic Section, Jordan University Hospital, Amman, Jordan

The current role of partial esophagectomy in the surgical treatment of middle- and lower-third esophageal carcinoma
Use of tubular isoperistaltic gastroplasty after total or partial esophagectomy

ARIFF AHMED HAFFEJEE, F.R.C.S.(Ed.)

Associate Professor, Department of Surgery, University of Natal, Faculty of Medicine; Senior Specialist Surgeon, Transplant Surgeon, King Edward VIII Hospital; Senior Lecturer, Head of Alimentation Unit, Addington Hospital, Durban, Republic of South Africa

Endoesophageal intubation for palliation in obstructing esophageal carcinoma

GUO JUN HUANG, B.S., M.D.

Professor of Surgery, Chinese Academy of Medical Sciences and China Union Medical University; Professor of Thoracic Surgery, Department of Thoracic Surgical Oncology, Cancer Institute and Hospital, Chinese Academy of Medical Sciences, Beijing, People's Republic of China

Natural progression of esophageal carcinoma
Recognition and treatment of the early lesion
Combined preoperative irradiation and surgery for esophageal carcinoma

KAICHI ISONO, Ph.D.

Professor, Second Department of Surgery, School of Medicine, Chiba University, Chiba, Japan

Postoperative long-term immunochemotherapy

HIDENOBU KAI, M.D.

Department of Surgery II, Faculty of Medicine, Kyushu University, Fukuoka, Japan

Combined preoperative irradiation and surgery for esophageal carcinoma
Hyperthermia treatment effective for patients with carcinoma of the esophagus

HIDEYUKI KAWAHARA, M.D.

Assistant Professor, Department of Thoracic and Cardiovascular Surgery, University of Occupational and Environmental Health, Japan, School of Medicine; Assistant Professor, Department of Thoracic and Cardiovascular Surgery, University Hospital of Occupational and Environmental Health, Japan, School of Medicine, Fukuoka, Japan

Combined radical resection of adjacent organs involved by esophageal carcinoma

MICHAEL ROBERT BURCH KEIGHLEY, M.D.

Professor of Surgery, The General Hospital, University of Birmingham, Birmingham, England

Assessment of intramural spread

DAVID KELSEN, M.D.

Associate Professor, Department of Medicine, Cornell University Medical College; Head, Gastrointestinal Section, Solid Tumor Service, Department of Medicine, Memorial Sloan-Kettering Cancer Center, New York, New York

Preoperative chemotherapy in epidermoid carcinoma of the esophagus

JANOS KISS, M.D., Ph.D.

Professor of Surgery, First Department of Surgery, Postgraduate Medical School, Budapest, Hungary

Discussion: Cytologic screening for carcinoma and dysplasia of the esophagus in the People's Republic of China
Submucography in the diagnosis of esophageal tumors
Anastomosis using wire sutures in one layer
Surgical palliation in obstructing lesions—intrathoracic bypass procedures

TAMOTSU KUDO, M.D.

Sub-professor, Second Department of Surgery, Akita University School of Medicine; Associate Professor, Second Department of Surgery, Akita University Hospital, Akita, Japan

Pulmonary complications

FRIGYES KULKA, M.D.

Professor of Surgery, First Surgical Clinic, Postgraduate Medical School; Chief of Department, Thoracic Surgical Clinic, National Institute for Pneumology, Budapest, Hungary

Discussion: Pulmonary complications
Surgical palliation in obstructing lesions—intrathoracic bypass procedures

KAM-HING LAM, M.S., F.R.C.S.E, F.R.A.C.S, F.A.C.S.

Professor, Department of Surgery, University of Hong Kong; Consultant in Surgery, Department of Surgery, Queen Mary Hospital, Hong Kong

Elective surgical techniques for cervical and postcricoid lesions

AYLWYN MANNELL, M.B., B.S., B.Sc. (Med.), M.S., F.R.A.C.S., F.R.C.S.(Eng.)

Senior Lecturer, Department of Surgery, University of the Witwatersrand, Johannesburg, South Africa; Principal Surgeon, Department of Surgery, Baragwanath Hospital, Soweto, South Africa

Update of experience with esophageal cancer: now and tomorrow

TOSHIHIDE MARUYAMA, M.D.

Department of Gastroenterology, School of Medicine, Juntendo University, Tokyo, Japan

Radiologic patterns of early esophageal carcinoma

HIDEMASA MATSUFUJI, M.D.

Research fellow, Department of Surgery II, Faculty of Medicine, Kyushu University, Fukuoka, Japan

Hyperthermia treatment effective for patients with carcinoma of the esophagus

HUGOE R. MATTHEWS, F.R.C.S.

Consultant Thoracic Surgeon, Regional Department of Thoracic Surgery, East Birmingham Hospital, Birmingham, England

Esophageal carcinoma as a complication of achalasia: the screening controversy

MOLLY K. McAFEE, M.D.

Mayo Clinic and Mayo Foundation, Rochester, Minnesota

Adenocarcinoma in the columnar epithelial–lined lower esophagus of Barrett

JAMES S. McCAUGHAN, Jr., M.D., F.A.C.S.

Assistant Clinical Professor, Department of Surgery, Ohio State University; Director, Grant Laser Center and Laser Medical Research Foundation, Grant Medical Center, Columbus, Ohio

Palliation of esophageal malignancy with photodynamic therapy

RICHARD B. McELVEIN, M.D.

Associate Professor, Department of Surgery, Division of Cardiothoracic Surgery, University of Alabama at Birmingham; Assistant Chief-of-Staff, Associate Professor, Department of Surgery, Division of Cardiothoracic Surgery, University Hospitals, Birmingham, Alabama

Laser therapy as palliation for advanced, nonresectable carcinoma

KENNETH CHARLES McKEOWN, C.B.E., D.L., M.Ch., F.R.C.S.(Eng.), F.R.C.S.(Ed.)

Associate Clinical Lecturer, University of Newcastle upon Tyne, Newcastle upon Tyne, England; lately Senior Consultant, Department of Surgery, Memorial Hospital, Darlington, England

Discussion: Recognition and treatment of the early lesion

SERGE MERIOT, M.D.

Attaché Chirurgical, Université de Bordeaux II; Service de Chirurgie Thoracique, Hôpital Xavier-Arnozan, Pessac, France

The current role of partial esophagectomy in the surgical treatment of middle- and lower-third esophageal carcinoma
Use of tubular isoperistaltic gastroplasty after total or partial esophagectomy

GEORGES J.M. MOLAS, M.D.

Maître de Conference des Universités, Department of Pathologic Anatomy, Faculté Xavier Bichat, Paris, France; Praticien Hospitalier, Department of Pathologic Anatomy, Hôpital Beaujon, Clichy, France

Prophylactic operative techniques: thoracic esophageal squamous cell cancer surgery, with special reference to lymph node removal

KEYVAN MOGHISSI, M.D., F.R.C.S.(Eng.), F.R.C.S.(Ed.)

Consultant Cardiothoracic Surgeon, Humberside Cardiothoracic Surgical Centre, Castle Hill Hospital, Cottingham, Hull, England

Discussion: Combined radical resection of adjacent organs involved by esophageal carcinoma

RYOICHI MOTOKI, M.D.

Professor of Surgery, First Department of Surgery, Fukushima Medical College, Fukushima, Japan

Critical postoperative care using the Swan-Ganz catheter

CLIFTON F. MOUNTAIN, M.D.

Professor of Surgery, Department of Thoracic Surgery, The University of Texas System Cancer Center, M.D. Anderson Hospital and Tumor Institute, Houston, Texas

Rationale in staging of cancer of the esophagus

GORDON FRANKLIN MURRAY, M.D.

Professor and Chairman, Department of Surgery, West Virginia University; Professor and Chairman, Department of Surgery, West Virginia University Hospitals, Morgantown, West Virginia

Discussion: Chapters 14 to 18

ERIC M. NANSON, O.B.E., M.B., Ch.B.(N.Z.), F.R.C.S.(Eng.), F.R.C.S.(C), F.A.C.S., F.R.A.C.S.
Emeritus Professor of Surgery, University of Auckland, Auckland, New Zealand
Synchronous combined abdominothoracocervical esophagectomy: the team approach

MAMORU NISHIZAWA, M.D., Ph.D.
President, Department of Gastroenterology, Tokyo Metropolitan Cancer Detection Center, Tokyo, Japan
Radiologic patterns of early esophageal carcinoma

C. NOIROT, M.D.
Hôpital Beaujon, Clichy, France
Discussion: Perioperative management of carcinoma of the esophagus: the reduction of operative mortality

TAKENORI OCHIAI, M.D.
Assistant Professor, Department of Surgery, School of Medicine, Chiba University, Chiba, Japan
Postoperative long-term immunochemotherapy

SHOICHI ONODA
Assistant Professor, Second Department of Surgery, School of Medicine, Chiba University, Chiba, Japan
Postoperative long-term immunochemotherapy

MARK B. ORRINGER, M.D.
Professor and Head, Division of Thoracic Surgery, Department of Surgery, University of Michigan Hospital, Ann Arbor, Michigan
Transhiatal esophagectomy without thoracotomy for esophageal carcinoma

KEITH MICHAEL PAGLIERO, M.B., B.S., F.R.C.S.
Honorary Research Fellow in Surgical Oncology, University of Exeter, Devon, England; Clinical Tutor, University of Bristol, Bristol, England; Consultant Thoracic Surgeon, Royal Devon and Exeter Hospital, Torbay Hospital, North Devon Hospital, Devon, England
Brachytherapy for inoperable cancer of the esophagus and cardia

FRANCISCO PARÍS
Titular Professor of Surgery, Valencia University; Head of Thoracic Service, Department of Surgery, Hospital General "La Fe" National Health Institute, Valencia, Spain
Use of tubular isoperistaltic gastroplasty after total or partial esophagectomy

EDWARD FROST PARKER, B.S., M.D., Sc.D.(Hon.)
Professor Emeritus, Department of Surgery, Medical University of South Carolina; Consultant in Cardiothoracic Surgery, Medical University Hospital, Charleston, South Carolina
Excisional, radiational, and chemotherapeutic methods and results

CHARLES WILLIAM PATTISON, M.B., Ch.B., F.R.C.S., F.R.C.S.(Ed.)
Registrar in Cardiothoracic Surgery, Department of Cardiothoracic Surgery, Harefield Hospital, Harefield, England
Esophageal carcinoma as a complication of achalasia: the screening controversy

W. SPENCER PAYNE, M.D.

James C. Masson Professor of Surgery, Department of Surgery, Mayo Medical School; Consultant in Thoracic Surgery, Department of Thoracic Surgery, Mayo Foundation, Rochester, Minnesota

Adenocarcinoma in the columnar epithelial–lined lower esophagus of Barrett
Esophageal reconstruction: free jejunal transfer or circulatory augmentation of pedicled intestinal interpositions using microvascular surgery

FREDERICK GRIFFITH PEARSON, M.D., B.Sc., F.R.C.S., F.A.C.S.

Professor, Department of Surgery, Faculty of Medicine; Surgeon in Chief, Department of Surgery, Toronto General Hospital, Toronto, Ontario, Canada

Discussion: Synchronous combined abdominothoracocervical esophagectomy: the team approach
Discussion: Transabdominal esophagogastrectomy for the poor-risk patient
Discussion: Median sternotomy in radical surgery for esophageal carcinoma involving cervical and upper thoracic segments
Discussion: Elective surgical techniques for cervical and postcricoid lesions

ISTVÁN PÉNZES, M.D.

Chief of Department, Associate Professor, Department of Anaesthesiology and Intensive Care Unit, National Institute for Pulmonology, Budapest, Hungary

Discussion: Pulmonary complications

ALBERTO PERACCHIA, F.A.C.S.

Professor of Surgery, Chairman, Department of Clinical Surgery I, University of Padua, Padua, Italy

Discussion: En bloc resection for esophageal carcinoma
Discussion: Transhiatal esophagectomy without thoracotomy for esophageal carcinoma

STÉPHANE PLACE, M.D.

Chief Clinical Assistant, Department of Surgery, Hôpital Beaujon, Chichy, France

Prophylactic operative techniques: 380 esophageal anastomoses using the stapler

R.W. POSTLETHWAIT, M.D.

Professor of Surgery Emeritus, Duke University, Durham, North Carolina

Complications of the anastomosis: leak and stricture

CHRISTOPHER GILES ROWLAND, B.Sc.(Ham.), M.B., B.S., D.M.R.D. & T., F.R.C.R.

Senior Lecturer in Oncology, Postgraduate Medical School, University of Exeter; Consultant in Oncology and Radiation Therapy, Department of Radiotherapy and Oncology Centre, Royal Devon and Exeter Hospital, Devon, England

Brachytherapy for inoperable cancer of the esophagus and cardia

AVIEL ROY, M.D.

Creighton University School of Medicine, Omaha, Nebraska

Perioperative management of carcinoma of the esophagus: the reduction of operative mortality

EIICHI SATO, M.D.

Professor, Department of Pathology, Faculty of Medicine, Kagoshima University, Kagoshima, Japan

Pathology of esophageal carcinoma in relation to dysplasia

QIONG SHEN, M.D.

Professor of Pathoanatomy, Chairman of Department of Precancerous Studies, University of Medicine, Zhengzhou, People's Republic of China

Cytologic screening for carcinoma and dysplasia of the esophagus in the People's Republic of China

HIKOO SHIRAKABE, M.D.

Honorary Professor, Juntendo University; Directing Chief, Central Clinic, Foundation for Detection of Early Gastric Carcinoma, Tokyo, Japan

Radiologic patterns of early esophageal carcinoma

KING FUN SIU, M.B., B.S., F.R.C.S.(Ed.)

Lecturer, Department of Surgery, University of Hong Kong, Hong Kong

Squamous cell carcinoma of the esophagus

DAVID B. SKINNER, M.D.

Dallas B. Phemister Professor of Surgery, Department of Surgery, University of Chicago Pritzger School of Medicine; Chairman, Department of Surgery, University of Chicago Hospitals and Clinics, Chicago, Illinois

En bloc resection for esophageal carcinoma

ZWI STEIGER, M.D.

Professor, Department of Surgery, Wayne State University School of Medicine, Detroit, Michigan; Chief, Division of Thoracic Surgery, Department of Surgery, Veterans Administration Medical Center, Allen Park, Michigan

Concurrent chemotherapy and radiation therapy for squamous cell cancer of the esophagus
Discussion: Chapters 46 to 48

JULIUS L. STOLLER, M.B., Ch.B., F.R.C.S.(E.), F.R.C.S.(C)., F.A.C.S.

Clinical Professor, Faculty of Medicine, Department of Surgery, University of British Columbia; Head, Division of General Surgery, Department of Surgery, Vancouver General Hospital, Vancouver, British Columbia, Canada

Discussion: The relative merits of definitive radiotherapy and palliative resection

KEIZO SUGIMACHI, M.B., F.A.C.S.

Professor and Chairman, Department of Surgery II, Faculty of Medicine, Kyushu University; Professor and Chairman, Department of Surgery II, Kyushu University Hospital, Fukuoka, Japan

Hyperthermia treatment effective for patients with carcinoma of the esophagus

IMRE SZÁNTÓ, M.D.

Assistant Professor of Surgery, First Department of Surgery, Postgraduate Medical School, Budapest, Hungary

Submucography in the diagnosis of esophageal tumors

ENDRE SZIRÁNYI, M.D.

Assistant Professor, First Department of Surgery, Postgraduate Medical School, Budapest, Hungary

Anastomosis using wire sutures in one layer

MANUEL TOMAS-RIDOCCI, M.D.

Associate Professor, Department of Medicine, University of Valencia; Head of Digestive Motility Unit, Division of Gastroenterology, University Hospital, Valencia, Spain

Use of tubular isoperistaltic gastroplasty after total or partial esophagectomy

VICTOR F. TRASTEK, M.D.

Assistant Professor of Surgery, Department of Thoracic and Cardiovascular Surgery, Mayo Medical School; Consultant, Department of Thoracic and Cardiovascular Surgery, Mayo Clinic, Rochester, Minnesota

Adenocarcinoma in the columnar epithelial–lined lower esophagus of Barrett

MASAHIKO TSURUMARU, M.D., F.A.C.S.

Deputy Chief, Department of Surgery, Toranomon Hospital, Tokyo, Japan

Imaging techniques

HARUSHI UDAGAWA, M.D.

Department of Surgery, Toranomon Hospital, Tokyo, Japan

Imaging techniques

K. KRISHNAN UNNI, M.B., B.S.

St. Marys and Rochester Methodist Hospitals; Department of Pathology, Mayo Clinic, Rochester, Minnesota

Adenocarcinoma in the columnar epithelial–lined lower esophagus of Barrett

ATTILA VÖRÖS, M.D.

Assistant Professor of Surgery, First Department of Surgery, Postgraduate Medical School, Budapest, Hungary

Submucography in the diagnosis of esophageal tumors
Anastomosis using wire sutures in one layer
Surgical palliation in obstructing lesions—intrathoracic bypass procedures

GUO QING WANG, M.D.

Department of Precancerous Studies, University of Medicine, Zhengzhou, People's Republic of China

Cytologic screening for carcinoma and dysplasia of the esophagus in the People's Republic of China

LIANG JUN WANG, M.D.

Associate Professor, Department of Surgical Oncology, Cancer Institute and Hospital, Chinese Academy of Medical Sciences, Beijing, People's Republic of China

Combined preoperative irradiation and surgery for esophageal carcinoma

ZHENG YAN WANG, M.D.

Professor, Department of Diagnostic Radiology, Cancer Institute and Hospital, Chinese Academy of Medical Sciences, Beijing, People's Republic of China

Combined preoperative irradiation and surgery for esophageal carcinoma

ANTHONY WATSON, M.D., F.R.C.S.

Associate Professor, Department of Surgery, Creighton University School of Medicine, Omaha, Nebraska; Consultant Surgeon, Department of Surgery, Royal Lancaster Infirmary, Lancaster, England

Pathologic changes affecting survival in esophageal cancer
Discussion: Endoesophageal intubation for palliation in obstructing esophageal carcinoma

WILLIAM IGNACE WEI, DLO, F.A.C.S.

Senior Lecturer in Surgery, Department of Surgery, University of Hong Kong; Honorary Consultant in Surgery, Department of Surgery, Queen Mary Hospital, Hong Kong

Elective surgical techniques for cervical and postcricoid lesions

EARLE W. WILKINS, Jr., M.D.

Clinical Professor, Department of Surgery, Harvard Medical School; Visiting Surgeon, Department of Thoracic Surgery, Massachusetts General Hospital, Boston, Massachusetts

Discussion: Chapters 21 to 23
Perspective

THOMAS E. WILLIAMS, Jr., M.D.

Director, Open Heart Program, Department of Open Heart Surgery, Grant Medical Center, Columbus, Ohio

Palliation of esophageal malignancy with photodynamic therapy

JEAN-PAUL WITZ, M.D.

Professor, Department of Thoracic Surgery, Faculty of Medicine, Université Louis Pasteur; Chirurgien des Hôpitaux, Chef de Service, Service de Chirurgie Thoracique, C.H.R.U., Strasbourg, France

Discussion: Complications of the anastomosis: leak and stricture

JOHN WONG, M.D., Ph.D., F.R.A.C.S., F.A.C.S., F.R.C.S.E.

Professor and Head, Department of Surgery, University of Hong Kong; Professor, Department of Surgery, Queen Mary Hospital, Hong Kong

Esophagoscopy and bronchoscopy
Squamous cell carcinoma of the esophagus

GORO YAMAKI, M.D.

Staff, Department of Internal Medicine, School of Medicine, Juntendo University; Department of Diagnostic Radiology, Toranomon Hospital, Tokyo, Japan

Radiologic patterns of early esophageal carcinoma

KAN YANG, M.D.

Associate Professor, Department of Pathology, Cancer Institute, Chinese Academy of Medical Sciences, Beijing, People's Republic of China

Combined preoperative irradiation and surgery for esophageal carcinoma

WEI-BO YIN, M.D.

Professor and Director, Department of Radiation Oncology, Cancer Institute and Hospital, Chinese Academy of Medical Sciences, Beijing, People's Republic of China

Definitive radiotherapy
Combined preoperative irradiation and surgery for esophageal carcinoma

DA WEI ZHANG (DAVID CHANG), M.D.

Professor and Chairman, Department of Thoracic Surgery, Cancer Institute and Hospital, Chinese Academy of Medical Sciences, Beijing, People's Republic of China

Surgical management of adenocarcinoma at the gastroesophageal junction
Combined preoperative irradiation and surgery for esophageal carcinoma

LI JUN ZHANG, M.D.

Associate Professor, Department of Laser Therapy; Departmental Director, Department of Radiation Oncology, Cancer Institute and Hospital, Chinese Academy of Medical Sciences, Beijing, People's Republic of China

Combined preoperative irradiation and surgery for esophageal carcinoma

RU GANG ZHANG, M.D.

Associate Professor and Deputy Chairman, Department of Thoracic Surgery, Cancer Institute and Hospital, Chinese Academy of Medical Sciences, Beijing, People's Republic of China

Combined preoperative irradiation and surgery for esophageal carcinoma

ZHI XIAN ZHANG, M.D.

Associate Professor, Department of Radiation Oncology, Cancer Institute and Hospital, Chinese Academy of Medical Sciences, Beijing, People's Republic of China

Combined preoperative irradiation and surgery for esophageal carcinoma

Foreword

General thoracic surgery already has a glorious past. It has given birth to the modern discipline of cardiovascular surgery and has seen the prodigious growth of that discipline. It has developed the fundamental techniques of intrathoracic operations. The time has come to recognize the specialty of general thoracic surgery as a full-fledged discipline that is in the process of becoming progressively more distinct and unique. In many teaching centers it is already separated from both general surgical service and cardiovascular disciplines. The separate status presently held honors the surgical pioneers who made this recognition inevitable. However, continuing advances will require effective exchange of new ideas and steady reinforcement of the sense of identity that must remain the cornerstone of the edifice that has earned these past accolades. By stimulating the dialogue necessary for these goals to be attained, the current series of books is designed to help in generating an equally bright future.

Although an enormous volume of information is available in textbooks, monographs, and journals concerning matters the practicing general thoracic surgeon may find of great interest, retrieval of information is not always simple. Textbooks may not contain the most up-to-date information because of their extended publication schedules. Relevant articles may be in journals that do not primarily relate to the individual specialty and therefore are overlooked. In addition, the language problem militates significantly against the ready transfer of information from one country to another. It was in an attempt to bridge these sorts of gaps that *International Trends in General Thoracic Surgery* was designed. We believe this forum will most effectively convey new information in relation to the practical aspects of actual patient care as well as emphasize the clinical application of the material.

This series of books was developed to deliberately foster international interplay on relevant topics as expeditiously as possible. Initially, biennial publication was planned, but the enthusiastic reception given the proposal led to an expansion of the horizons and an annual publication schedule. As the concept was refined, it was agreed that, as a general principle, an attempt should be made to cover major subjects in single-topic issues and provide a forum for discussion of other topics and diseases in multitopic volumes released in an alternating sequence. Editorial boards were chosen to ensure that attention would be drawn to new and important contributions from all geographic areas, thereby providing the broadest possible audience at the earliest possible moment. The contributors were asked to stress their personal concepts and proposals in order to engender a worthwhile exchange of opinions that would ultimately prove informative and stimulating for an international readership.

Coverage will be restricted to general thoracic surgical problems (including esophageal diseases), and no attempt will be made to include cardiovascular topics. Although emphasis will be placed on the practical aspects of patient care, an attempt will be made to review the relevant historical background whenever necessary for better understanding of complex issues. The application of new basic and clinical investigative studies will be discussed in their clinical contexts in order to maintain the emphasis on practical clinical issues.

We believe that by following the plan just outlined, this series of books will pay particular attention to the needs of the specific target groups for whom the books are intended: practicing general thoracic surgeons, general thoracic surgical trainees, referring physicians (including respirologists and gastroenterologists), and of course the reference resources housed in university, hospital, and inservice libraries. In most instances, the information presented will also be of particular interest to many other allied disciplines, notably oncologists, radiotherapists, otolaryngologists, emergency care physicians, and general internists.

North American and European editorial boards have been created to meet annually to select topics for consideration and choose knowledgeable authors who are best able to present the requested information from a broad base of clinical experience. An international advisory board has also been constituted to ensure an effective international approach to the process of topic selection and author choice. The editors-in-chief wish to acknowledge their indebtedness to the many members of these various boards, who have accepted their responsibilities conscientiously and effectively.

Undoubtedly, as time passes, the manner in which editorial policy is pursued in attempting to achieve these objectives may well change as part of a natural evolutionary process. Nonetheless, if the fundamental aim continues to represent the basis for future decisions, we feel that the developing series will serve a useful purpose—provided the books satisfy the requirements of the target audiences. The editorial boards are determined to make every effort to merit a continuing favorable reception, since it is clearly recognized that readership acceptance must be the final arbiter of the books' value.

The editors-in-chief would be remiss indeed were they not to express—on behalf of all the board members—their warm appreciation of the efforts made by the guest editors and those who have contributed in such willing fashion to ensure that the goals established for this ongoing series are met. Its eventual success will, assuredly, depend entirely on the dedicated fashion in which they have accepted their responsibilities.

The appearance of thoracic surgical units in teaching hospitals ensures the availability of consultative services that will provide knowledgeable advice regarding the indications for surgical investigation and treatment as well as experienced management of serious postoperative problems. It is to be hoped that the books in this series will support and strengthen the role of these units in clarifying those situations in which complex issues and unusual pathologic conditions require highly sophisticated—rather than routine or traditional—therapeutic approaches.

The W.B. Saunders Company published the first two volumes (*Lung Cancer* and *Major Challenges*). With the release of volume 3 *(Benign Esophageal Disease)*, The C.V. Mosby Company took on the responsibility for publication. The editors-in-chief join with the guest editors and their authors in expressing sincere appreciation to Thomas Manning and Elaine Steinborn for their enthusiastic support and knowledgeable guidance in the production of the current volume and for their sensible advice in the planning of future issues.

NORMAN C. DELARUE
HENRY ESCHAPASSE

Preface

Volume 4 of *International Trends in General Thoracic Surgery* pursues the single-topic format that had been utilized in volume 1. Just as the latter was devoted to one subject alone (lung cancer), volume 4 deals only with esophageal carcinoma. The intervening volumes had multitopic orientations: *Major Challenges* (volume 2) and *Benign Esophageal Disease* (volume 3). Because of its worldwide incidence pattern with specific geographic areas of extraordinary incidence—in which management may differ so dramatically and where scientific study is constantly producing new information—carcinoma of the esophagus is particularly well suited to the concept of *International Trends*. Fundamentally sound contributions from many countries are balanced by knowledgeable comments or viewpoints from those whose judgment is based on broad experience in other parts of the world.

Early in the planning for this volume, one of us structured its contents into some eleven parts. These cover various parameters—from the international scope of the problem, through consideration of diagnosis, staging, and the pathologic aspects, to the many facets of therapy, including the management of perioperative morbidity, surgical techniques, postoperative complications, adjuvant therapy, and palliative care. The volume concludes with a general overview reflecting current therapeutic trends based on this accumulated information. All in all, it is a rather neat arrangement of a complex subject matter.

Contributors come from some twelve nations representing six continents. Of the 52 chapters, 28 come from countries where English is not the primary language. The result is a presentation of the subject of esophageal carcinoma that is not only international in flavor but also broadly representative of differing attitudes and approaches.

An understanding of all these opinions is clearly essential in dealing with a problem which is so frustrating as far as its management is concerned and in which the statistical outcome still carries such dismal implications.

Maintenance of an acceptable book size has made it impossible to invite comments on each individual chapter. Nonetheless, an effort has been made to present another viewpoint, usually from a country or continent other than that of the original contributor, when the subject, or group of subjects, merits another opinion or when there is a particular authority whose contribution would be noteworthy. The 18 discussions cover some 33 primary chapter presentations—no less than one third of the authors have accepted the responsibility of discussing two thirds of the subject matter.

The editors recognize one potential deficiency in regard to the general subject of adjuvant therapy: chemotherapy and trials of its application are sufficiently new that some statistics may already be outdated by the time of publication.

Appreciation is in order: to The C. V. Mosby Company for taking on the project; to Elaine Steinborn, the developmental editor; to all the contributors, some of whom have waited so patiently for publication of their material; and especially to all the contributors' "unseen" assistants. We believe the result of their efforts is a volume that should be required reading for all those treating esophageal carcinoma and a book to be found on the reference shelves of all thoracic surgeons.

Norman C. Delarue
Earle W. Wilkins, Jr.
John Wong

Contents

PART XI
AN OVERVIEW OF THE PROBLEM OF ESOPHAGEAL CARCINOMA

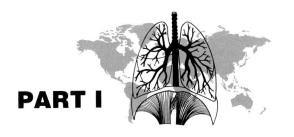

PART I

SCOPE OF THE PROBLEM

CHAPTER 1

Epidemiologic trends and etiologic factors of esophageal carcinoma

André Duranceau

The causes of esophageal carcinoma are unknown. Its incidence is low in most countries, affecting 3 to 10 persons per 100,000 population per year in these areas. In some parts of the world, however, the incidence reaches such a magnitude that it becomes the leading cause of death. When such a variation in incidence and mortality is observed, similarities and differences in geographic, sociologic, nutritional, and predisposing factors become evident. This chapter draws a perspective of esophageal carcinoma and its various etiologies as it is perceived around our globe.

GEOGRAPHIC CLUSTERING
Asia

The Asian esophageal carcinoma belt includes China and Japan, the southern part of Russia, Iran, India, the Middle East, and Singapore.

China

There are six areas within China showing very high rates of esophageal cancers: the Linxian County in Henan Province, Northern Sichuan, the Da-Bie mountainous region at the border of Hebei Province, southern Fukien, northern Jiangsu, and northern Xinjiang. Each of these areas may show variable rates within a given region. A mass survey in Linxian county of Henan Province has shown a prevalence of 0.9% in subjects over 30 years of age.[1] In early 1980 the survey of the Cheng Guan commune revealed that within 530 individuals with marked epithelial dysplasia, 90% of the subjects had evidence of chronic esophagitis. Over a period of 9 years of follow-up, 79 of these persons developed esophageal carcinoma (14.9%).[2] This represents a 140-fold increase in the chance of developing a cancer.

A fascinating observation was that this paralleled the incidence of esophageal cancers in the poultry population in the same areas. The domestic fowl population aged over 6 months showed development of cancers at the pharyngoesophageal junction in 27% of cases and in the upper end of the esophagus in 15% of the cases. Fifty-four percent of the poultry developing these cancers belonged either to the patients suffering from esophageal cancer or to their neighbors.[3]

With such findings, factors common to the diet of both birds and humans or other environmental agents may suggest a significant etiology. The staple diet in high-incidence areas of China is composed of cereals, corn meal, and pickled vegetables. Pickled vegetables are made by placing uncooked chopped Chinese cabbage, leaves of sweet potatoes, turnip leaves, and other vegetables in a large ceramic pot together with water. After several months and without adding salt or any seasoning, the pH reaches a level of 3 to 4.[4] These pickled vegetables are eaten daily; the mortality rate from esophageal cancer appears to be related to the time of consumption and the amount consumed.[2]

Maize and millet are the staple foods in Linxian County, and, like the pickled vegetables, they are frequently contaminated by fungi, most commonly *Geotrichum candidum* and yeast. The diet is low in animal products and fat. Salted fish is eaten from early childhood and might be an additional factor.

When tested, all these food items contained nitrosamines in 23% of the samples; in low-incidence areas, nitrosamines were found in only 1.2% of samplings. Deficiency in molybdenum in the soil as well as mold contaminations are suspected to be the major contributing factors to the elevated levels of nitrosamines in foods and the subsequent development of esophageal carcinoma. Moreover, the limited intake of fresh vegetables and fruits may result in riboflavin and vitamin C deficiencies.

Although a positive correlation between esophageal carcinoma and use of alcohol and tobacco has not been observed in Linxian County, a strong drink made of a distillate of *kaoliang* and containing 60% to 80% alcohol is used in Northern China.

In general, the presence of carcinogens and mutagens in moldy food shows transforming effects on cells. These effects may play an important role in the neoplastic evolution of the esophageal epithelium.

Iran

Iran is known as a country where incidence and mortality for esophageal cancer are among the highest. A majority of the patients are between 35 and 54, and nearly all come from the poorest stratum of rural society.[5] The lesions are found most frequently in the middle and lower thirds of the esophagus, although in the southern Fars Province an unusual proportion of these cases (32%) present with primary tumors in the upper third of the esophagus. Among most age groups the risk for males and females is nearly equal in the southern Fars province, but older females do have a higher incidence than older males.[6]

Up to 180 new cases per 100,000 population have been recorded each year in northeastern Iran, specifically the provinces of Gonbad, Maquandaran, and Gorgan.[7] This is the highest incidence area in the world, and esophageal cancer is the most common cause of death among adults here. A steep fall in incidence is observed as one moves westward along the littoral of the Caspian Sea.

Risk factors in Iran are different from those suspected in the Western world. Although no single food item is positively associated with a carcinogenic effect, as risk increases, bread and tea increasingly predominate in the diet. Within the high-incidence areas individuals developing carcinoma have the most restricted diet. Smoking and alcohol consumption are infrequent and play a negligible role.

The prevalence of the use of opium, with its pyrrolysates, and the frequent use of very hot tea have been proposed as mechanisms injurious to the esophageal mucosa, making it susceptible to cancer formation. The chewing of *sukhteh,* which is prepared from scrapings of tar from opium pipes, is considered a cause of esophageal cancer among Turkomans in the north. Dowlatshahi and Miller,[7] following their observation on opium usage and esophageal cancer, suggested that opium decreases esophageal peristalsis through the direct action of its 1% papaverine fraction on smooth muscle and inhibits the relaxation of the lower esophageal sphincter via its morphine con-

stituent. This results in a relative stasis that allows swallowed carcinogens to have a prolonged contact with the esophageal mucosa and to enhance neoplasia development in a mucosa made more susceptible by nutritional deficiencies.

Endoscopic surveys made in the high-risk population have revealed that 86% of the population screened was affected by significant esophagitis. An area of intact mucosa was nearly always present between the stomach and the most distal part of the esophagitis area, thus ruling out reflux damage.[1]

Russia

The Soviet Republics of Turkmenia, Kazakhstan, and Uzbekistan form the central portion of the Asian esophageal cancer belt, with the northern part of Iran. High rates of esophageal cancer are found in these areas, just as in Iran. The disease rate is found to be much higher in the indigenous Asian-Moslem population than in the immigrant Russians. In the Kazakhstan province, esophageal carcinoma is responsible for 30% of the morbidity caused by all cancers.

India, Pakistan, and Sri Lanka

Traditionally, the high incidence of esophageal cancer in India has been believed to be due to tobacco chewing, either alone or with betel nut, betel leaf, slaked lime, or *catechu,* a resin from the acacia.[8] Ranadive et al.[8] conducted experiments using the hamster cheek pouch, which is similar histologically to the esophagus, to confirm the potent carcinogenicity of the tannin-containing polyphenolic fraction of the betel nut and its combinations with lime and tobacco. They found a direct relationship between frequency of chewing and the induction of carcinoma. While untreated controls did not show any malignancy, animals exposed to tobacco and the various betel quid ingredient combinations developed lesions ranging from atypia of the mucosal cells to frank carcinomas.

The overall percentage of cancers related to smoking or chewing tobacco is only 50%; factors related to diet are considered of equal importance. Bhatia and Bhide[9] studied the risk factors for esophageal cancer in the state of Manipur, which is located in the northeastern part of India near Burma, and their observations show some similarities with risk factors found in other high-incidence areas. The male-female ratio for esophageal cancer in Manipuris is 1.36. The esophagus is the ninth commonest site of all cancers in this state. Dietary habits of these people include the ingestion of very hot rice, fermented foods, and highly pungent chilis. Fish is prepared by sun drying and putrification to obtain a foul-smelling *ngari*, which is fermented in earthen pots for 6 to 8 months to form *utongari*, an important part of the daily diet. Meat is also fermented, but the fat intake is very low. Local shrimps or *khajing* are usually fried without removing the spines, which is known to cause irritation in the gullet. *Bidi*, a locally grown tobacco, has been smoked for more than 25 years by over 80% of the patients afflicted with esophageal cancer. Betel nut chewing is common as well.

Mohan-Kumar and Ramachandran[10] reported a high number of esophageal cancers in north Kerala, with a higher prevalence among Muslims. Dietary risk factors included the ingestion of smoked fish, large amounts of hot tea, and decaying organic matter containing nitrosamines. Tobacco smoking and chewing are similarly involved as risk factors.

In Pakistan, among 163 malignant lesions of the head, neck, and esophagus, esophageal tumors are second in frequency. The true incidence is difficult to calculate, but esophageal carcinoma is found in high concentration among immigrants from India. The main risk factor identified was the chewing of *pan* (leaf of betel) and tobacco.[12]

In Sri Lanka (formerly Ceylon), as on the southern tip of the Indian mainland, the peak incidence of carcinoma of the esophagus is in the 40-to-60 age group. However, there is a strong female proponderance in this population, which might be related to the common female habit of chewing tobacco and betel quid.[11]

Other Asian countries

In Singapore 75% of the population is of Chinese origin. The incidence of esophageal carcinoma is higher in the Singapore Chinese, especially if the patient belongs to the Horrien or Toechew dialect groups. Other significant risk factors for this population are the consumption of beverages at temperatures stated to be "burning hot," the smoking of Chinese tobacco, and the consumption of *samsu*, a Chinese wine.[13]

Japan does not have a particularly high incidence of esophageal carcinoma, although a positive relationship between the incidence of mucosal dysplasia and alcohol intake and smoking is suggested in some prefectures. When this high dysplasia incidence is noted, it appears to correspond to the death rate for esophageal carcinoma. In the Miyagi prefecture, where a high risk for esophageal carcinoma has been observed, the population frequently eats pickled Chinese cabbage prepared with possible fungal contaminations, as in China. Hot tea and smoked fish may similarly be involved in the induction of dysplasia

in the esophageal mucosa. For the Japanese, the regular use of both *shoshu*, a distilled liquor made from sweet potato, and whiskey results in a higher incidence of esophageal cancer in males.[4,14]

The mean annual incidence of esophageal cancer in Israel is 2.3 per 100,000, with a male-female ratio of 1:6. The incidence is highest in Asian-born patients originating from Iran, Turkey, or Yemen.[15] A similar observation can be made in Lebanon, where 62% of the squamous carcinomas have been found to be in patients from the Arabian peninsula, who actually form only 2.5% of total hospital admissions. The lack of an epidemiologic survey in this area makes any relationship with dietary, sociologic, or other risk factors inconclusive.[16]

Africa

In the early 1960s, the observation of a significant increase in esophageal carcinomas in South African Bantus and Zulus prompted the formation of a "Transkei patrol" to complete a demographic survey of this condition and its resulting morbidity and mortality.[17,18] The incidence rates and constant pattern of variation indicated environmental influences in the causation of the disease. The strongest associations between environmental factors and the distribution of esophageal carcinoma were (1) the geological soil formation, with a high silica content that can result in chronic esophageal irritation, and (2) the poor farming conditions, with significant deficiencies in a number of trace elements; molybdenum, zinc, copper, iron, and magnesium were noted to be deficient in the gardens of cancer sufferers.[19,20] The absence of these trace elements leads to accumulation of nitrates and nitrites in the plants instead of the normal process of breakdown of these substances with the production of amino acids. This accumulation leads to nitrosamine formation. The presence of poor and thrifty plants leads to infestation by fungi, which in turn produces hyperkeratosis and basal cell hyperplasia in the esophageal mucosa. A home-grown tobacco is used for smoking and snuffing. *Injonga*, a pipe stem extract, and *dagga*, a locally grown marijuana, are known to be very mutagenic and contain high levels of nitrosamines. Similarly, wild plants used for medicinal purposes may cause significant esophageal irritation. Overall, soil conditions and farming practices produce poor-quality plants, which are consumed by the inhabitants and result in nutritional deficiency states. These cause an increased susceptibility to carcinogenic agents and further the development of esophageal cancer.

When habits and customs are examined, an

unvaried diet carries the most convincing association with development of esophageal cancer. Although the precise nature of the carcinogens cannot be determined at this point, nitrosamines and mycotoxins are possibly the involved agents. Experimentally it has been shown that the staple diet of the Transkeian contains toxic factors that can result in esophageal cancers. Sprouting maize is used to produce a home-brewed beer; dried beans provide the protein source. Storage of maize and the addition of molds to food and beer to improve flavor lead to a heavy contamination of fungi, especially from the *Fusarium* species. It is interesting to observe that *Fusarium* infestation can result in necrotic lesions within the esophagus and eventual chronic inflammation of the mucosa. Although there is a strong suspicion that molds can lead to the production and development of carcinogens, at present the correlation between the incidence of fungal infection and the incidence of esophageal cancer in Transkei does not provide sufficient evidence to support a causal relationship. However, *Fusarium verticilloides*, which is active in a common corn infestation, is the same agent affecting foodstuffs in the high-incidence areas of China. In addition, this same agent is known to produce nitrosamines in corn meals and mutagens in culture.

Besides the high incidence recorded in the Transkei districts,[17,19] cancer of the esophagus is reported infrequently in western Nigeria, Senegal, and Uganda. However, persons in Malawi, Mozambique, and Rhodesia seem to show a high preponderance of the disease.[21] After studying 26 consecutive cases of carcinoma of the esophagus, Wapnick et al.[21] found that these lesions occurred more among the Malawian Africans than among Rhodesians. Moreover they seemed to be most common among the Kore Kore tribe, which is exposed to *kachasu,* an alcohol known to be highly carcinogenic with a high concentration of nitrosamines. A significant association existed when alcohol consumption had been present for more than 14 years. A further strong association was present between esophageal cancer and cigarette smoking, with all patients being heavy smokers. Oettlé et al.[22] documented, in South African blacks in high-risk areas, the same high incidence (75%) of endoscopically identifiable, diffuse, and nonulcerative esophagitis as in the high-risk groups of China and Iran.

The rest of Africa has not been screened as thoroughly as south Africa for the true incidence of esophageal cancers. However, Boulos and El Nasri[23] in Khartoum reported 135 patients with esophageal carcinomas treated at the University Department of Surgery over a period of 10 years.

This represents 1.4% of all malignant tumors in Sudan. The true incidence, geographic distribution, and etiology remain to be assessed.

Ajao and Solanke[24] also reported that carcinoma of the esophagus was not as rare in west Africa as previously thought. During a little more than 3 years, 30 cases were evaluated in the University College hospital in Ibadan; the etiologic factors suggested are similar to those seen in other parts of Africa.

Europe

France shows high incidence and mortality rates for cancer of the esophagus, mainly in Normandy and Brittany. The mortality had increased until 1966, when it leveled off. This may be related to the leveling of alcohol consumption. In 1968, a cancer registry was established in the department of Ille-et-Vilaine and centralized in Rennes. In 6 years, 718 cases were registered, with male-female ratio of 23.9.[25] The data collected in this and a second study in Calvados analyzed the consumption of alcohol (calculated in grams of pure ethanol) and the consumption of tobacco.[26] There is a clear dose-response relationship between daily alcohol intake and tobacco consumption and the development of an esophageal carcinoma. For each level of tobacco consumption the risk increases with the amount of alcohol used. Likewise, for each level of alcohol consumption the risk increases with the amount of tobacco smoked. With this multiplication effect alcohol and tobacco prove to be the principal factors involved in France.

Pure ethanol as such is not considered a carcinogen. However, its role may be to facilitate diffusion of a very small amount of carcinogens and expose them to the basal layer of the esophageal mucosa. Histologically, the esophageal mucosa in heavy drinkers is altered, with a zone of hyperplasia, leukoplakia, keratosis, and acanthosis in nearly 50% of all patients.

The northern part of Italy shows a high concentration of esophageal cancer. Epidemiologic findings from a study in the Padua and Veneto populations[27] and from the province of Trieste[28] showed that alcohol and maize flour (*pollenta*) are the two factors significantly involved in the development of esophageal carcinoma. In Trieste, the incidence in men was found to be exceedingly high, predominantly in the young and middle-aged populations.

In Poland, Staszewski studied 88 patients with esophageal cancer and found that all except one of the 81 male patients were cigarette smokers. When comparing these patients with a control group of patients with stomach and bowel cancer, a statistically positive association with smoking was found.[29]

North America and Australia

Canada has a low mortality for esophageal cancer: 3.7 for males and 1.2 for females. The United States shows a mortality for black males of 12.4 per 100,000 population, while it is 4.1/100,000 for white males. Black females have a 2.6 mortality, while for white females it is 1.0. There is an inverse relationship between income level and this type of cancer. Alcohol use is a strong factor, as much as tobacco use.[30,31] It has been noted that inner city blacks are more frequently exposed to multifactorial agents that could be responsible for tumor development.[32,33] Demographic studies within the United States have shown similar pockets of high mortality from esophageal cancer, with similar risk factors. South Carolina, Washington, D.C., California, the northeastern United States, and midwestern cities all show high incidences in the same socioeconomic population.[34] In Alaskan Eskimos esophageal cancers are seen mainly in females, which may be related to the hide-chewing responsibility of these women.[35] Australians show the same association of alcohol and tobacco in their esophageal carcinoma patients.[36]

PREDISPOSING FACTORS
Caustic injury

The development of carcinoma in the site of an old caustic burn may possibly result from persisting chronic inflammatory reaction once the damage is done. Kiviranta,[37] who based his opinion on nine cases that developed among 381 cases of esophageal carcinoma, estimated the possibility of development of a carcinoma as being 1000 times greater in patients who have had a corrosive injury for more than 24 years. Appelquist and Salmo[38] published the largest series, 63 patients who developed carcinoma from among 2414 patients with caustic burns (2.6%). Lye stricture is always the site where the carcinoma develops, and all carcinomas are squamous. Esophageal carcinoma appears in the damaged area an average of 41 years later. The resectability rate is usually higher than for the standard lesion, and the overall survival is usually better than 25%. Hopkins and Postlethwait[39] had 12 patients with carcinoma following caustic injury. The lesion appeared an average of 40 years after the injury, and 2 of 4 patients with a curative resection lived over 5 years. The chronic inflammation from the caustic burn and repeated trauma from subsequent

dilatations always suggest the possibility of carcinoma developing at the site of a lye stricture.

Achalasia

Achalasia is associated with the development of an esophageal carcinoma in 1% to 7% of all cases. However, only long-term follow-up in properly diagnosed cohorts can establish the true prevalence and incidence. The tumor is located in the middle esophagus in the large majority of cases.[40,41] Aperistalsis and an unrelaxing lower sphincter result in retention of stagnant and eventually putrefying food. Rake[42] observed the pathologic changes in this setting. Mucosal inflammation from the chronic retention was found to be proportional to the duration of the disease. Attempts at healing are present, with ulcerations and irregular epithelial hyperplasia giving a verrucuous appearance to the mucosa. The motor abnormality has usually been present for more than 20 years when the diagnosis of carcinoma is established. This carcinoma occurs in younger individuals, usually becoming large before diagnosis, is frequently not resectable, and carries a poor prognosis.[43]

Gastroesophageal reflux and Barrett's esophagus

Adenocarcinomas developing in heterotopic gastric epithelium are reported with an increasing frequency. Naef et al.[44] found an occurrence of malignant change of 8.6% in their series. The sequence of events leading to adenocarcinoma is thought to be a pattern of development of a columnar mucosa, followed by multifocal dysplasia, carcinoma in situ, and then invasive carcinoma. Herlihy et al.[45] found dysplasia in 10% of patients with circumferential columnar metaplasia without adenocarcinoma. Columnar metaplasia of the esophagus represents end-stage reflux esophagitis disease, and it is accepted that this condition has a malignant potential. Spechler et al.[46] consider that most adenocarcinomas reported in association with a columnar-lined esophagus represent prevalence of the disease in a limited population. However, the analysis of the true incidence of the malignancy still shows a 42.5-fold increase in its occurrence when a patient has a columnar epithelium in the esophagus. When adenocarcinoma develops in a columnar epithelium, it behaves aggressively. Preventive programs with regular endoscopic and cytologic studies have been proposed. Although it seems reasonable to believe that a patient will benefit from a continuing surveillance program, benefit in the form of increased longevity or cancer-free survival remains to be proved.

Irradiation

Radiation-induced esophageal carcinoma appears in the irradiated area, with a long latent interval between the irradiation and the appearance of the malignancy. Although irradiation may be the sole etiologic factor, a synergistic effect may be present with the use of chemotherapy.[47] All groups of irradiated patients with a long life expectancy may be at risk for subsequent cancer development when the esophagus is included in the radiation portal.[48]

Other risk factors

Diverticula of the esophagus at the pharyngoesophageal junction, in the middle esophagus (parabronchial) or in the epiphrenic location favor local stasis or are associated with chronic inflammation. Carcinomas of the esophagus have been reported to develop in all forms of esophageal diverticula. Celiac disease and idiopathic steatorrhea have been implicated in the development of both primary intestinal lymphoma and carcinoma of the esophagus. It is of interest to observe that in the southern part of Iran both these conditions are diagnosed with a high frequency. Shearman et al.[49] observed the possible association between esophageal carcinoma and previous gastric surgery, suggesting nutritional deficiency or regurgitation as the involved mechanisms. MacDonald[50] and Stalsberg[51] failed to confirm this predisposition. Tylosis is an autosomal-dominant condition causing palmar and plantar keratosis and associated with a high incidence of esophageal carcinoma.

PATHOGENESIS

There is one common background to the formation of esophageal carcinoma: the chronic insult of inflammation on an esophageal mucosa weakened by poor defense mechanisms.

Irritations

Over 80% of the populations affected by esophageal cancer in Iran, Russia, and China show chronic esophagitis. The figure is 75% in South African blacks. The causes of such changes are numerous. Whether it is the daily thermal insult of hot rice or tea or the chronic changes induced by the use of alcohol or tobacco, the end result is the same. Chronic trauma from the diet may be similarly implicated. Flour containing asbestos-like fibers in Iran, the highly pungent chili or the uncut spines of shrimps in India, and the coarse mustard leaves or wild spinach or the fine

needles of silica found in the soil and plants of Africa, are all factors leading to similar repetitively irritant lesions of the esophageal mucosa and submucosa. Long-term ingestion of bracken fern has been shown to have radiomimetic effects on digestive tract histology and is associated with a high incidence of esophageal cancers in cattle. In areas of high human incidence of esophageal cancer, Chinese fowls have a high incidence of pharyngoesophageal cancers.

Nutritional deficiencies

Whether esophageal carcinoma patients are from Asia, Africa, Europe, or North America, a majority of them will be from the poorer classes of these societies. Among the nutritional factors that can result in an added insult or a poorer defense mechanism for the esophageal mucosa are the following.

Zinc deprivation is usually associated with an increased serum level of copper. Experimentally, a zinc-deficient diet leads to alterations of the esophageal mucosa that include parakeratosis, hyperkeratosis, and hyperplasia.[52] Zinc deficiency in the soil leads to zinc-deficient plants and accumulation of nitrates conducive to the formation of nitrosamines. Zinc deprivation may affect the primary antibody response by influencing the stability of the lymphocyte membrane. The incidence of esophageal tumors is higher and the lag time for induction of these tumors is shorter in zinc-deficient experimental animals. Globally, zinc deficiency seems to lead to abnormal cell differentiation and turnover through alteration of the normal nucleic acid metabolism. The basal layer of the esophageal mucosa responds to the various insults in this setting.

Zinc usually interacts with other trace elements. The absence of molybdenum in the soil contributes to an accumulation of nitrites and nitrates in plants and vegetables. These compounds lead to the accumulation of nitrosamines. Molybdenum fertilizers reduce this accumulation and increase the content of ascorbic acid in plants.

Vitamin levels seem to be important for the stability of the esophageal mucosa. Vitamin A is mobilized from the liver with appropriate zinc levels and helps to maintain normal integrity of the epithelium. When vitamin A depletion occurs, a decrease in the RNA and DNA of epithelial cells occurs and keratinization, mitosis, and metaplastic changes increase significantly. Riboflavin and other group B vitamins are also essential for maintaining the integrity of the squamous epithelium in the esophagus. However, such specific deficiencies and their role in the development of precancerous lesions of the esophagus remain to be established. Vitamin C seems to offer some protection, mainly by reacting with nitrites and nitrous acid. The observation that molybdenum fertilizers reduce the accumulation of nitrates and nitrites and increase the content of ascorbic acid in plants also leads to the conclusion that the presence of vitamin C offers protection by acting against the formation of carcinogenic nitrosamines.[4]

Nitrosamines are the principal compounds known to induce esophageal tumors. The main source of these compounds is the secondary amines with nitrites and nitrates found in food and water. Nitrosamines are also produced in vivo by synthesis of these precursors in the stomach. In addition, bacteria and fungi may provide favorable conditions for the synthesis of nitrosamines.

Summary

In summary, nutritional deprivation occurs from a soil with poor content of trace metals such as zinc, molybdenum, magnesium, and iron. Malnutrition and vitamin deficiencies also occur from alcohol and tobacco overuse. Such deprivation sets the stage for the development of esophageal cancer by creating an esophageal mucosa and submucosa with poor defense mechanisms and subject to chronic irritation and inflammation. The vulnerable mucosa has defective repair mechanisms; premalignant changes occur, with a chronologic evolution toward chronic esophagitis, atrophy, and then hyperplasia and dysplasia, culminating in carcinoma in situ. Mutagenic and carcinogenic agents promote cancer more easily in this setting.

REFERENCES

1. Crespi, M., Munoz, N., and Grassi, A.: Precursor lesions of esophageal cancer in high-risk populations in Iran and China. In Pfeiffer, C.J., editor: Cancer of the esophagus vol. 1, Boca Raton, Fla., 1982, CRC Press, pp. 111-123.
2. Li, Ming-Xin, and Cheng, Shu-Jun: Carcinogenesis of esophageal cancer in Linxian, China, Chin. Med. J. **97:**311, 1984.
3. Priester, W.A.: Esophageal cancer in North China: high rates in human and poultry populations in the same areas, Avian Dis. **19:**213, 1975.
4. Fong, L.Y.Y.: Environmental carcinogens and dietary deficiencies in esophageal cancer in Asia. In Pfeiffer, C.J., editor: Cancer of the esophagus, vol. 1, Boca Raton, Fla., 1982, C.R.C. Press, pp. 41-63.
5. Iran-International Agency for Research on Cancer (IARC) Study Group: Esophageal cancer studies in the Caspian littoral of Iran: results of population studies—a prodrome, J. Natl. Cancer Inst. **59:**1127, 1977.
6. Sadeghi, A., Behmard, S., Shafiepoor, H., and Zeighmani, E.: Cancer of the esophagus in southern Iran, Cancer **40:**841, 1977.
7. Dowlatshahi, K., and Miller, R.J.: Role of opium in esophageal cancer: a hypothesis, Cancer Res. **45:**1906, 1985.
8. Ranadive, K.J., Ranadive, S.N., Shivapurkar, N.M., and Gothoscar, S.V.: Betel quid chewing and oral cancer: experimental studies on hamsters, Int. J. Cancer **24:**835, 1979.
9. Bhatia, P.L., and Bhide, S.V.: Risk factors in oesophageal cancer, Indian J. Cancer **20:**43, 1983.
10. Mohan-Kumar, K., and Ramachandran, P.: Carcinoma of the oesophagus in North Kerala, Indian J. Cancer **10:**183, 1973.
11. Stephen, S.J., and Urogoda, C.G.: Some observations on esophageal carcinoma in Ceylon including its relationship to betel chewing, Br. J. Cancer **24:**11, 1970.
12. Beg, M.H.A., Amina Rehman, Malik, S., and Qayum, A.: Pattern of malignant tumours in otolaryngology in Karachi, J.P.M.A. **33:**110, 1983.
13. deJong, U.W., Breslow, N., Goh Ewe Hong, J., Sridharan, M., and Shanmugaratnam, K.: Aetiological factors in oesophageal cancer in Singapore Chinese, Int. J. Cancer **13:**291, 1974.
14. Sato, E., Mukuda, T., and Sasano, N.: Dysplasia as related to esophageal carcinoma in Japan. In Pfeiffer, C.J., editor: Cancer of the esophagus, vol. 1, Boca Raton, Fla. 1982, CRC Press.
15. Shani, M., and Modan, B.: Esophageal cancer in Israel: selected clinical and epidemiological aspects, Dig. Dis. Sci. **10:**951, 1975.
16. Abdul Razek, M.S., and Nassar, V.H.: Carcinoma of the esophagus in the Middle East, Leb. Med. J. **27:**149, 1974.
17. Burrell, J.W.: Distribution maps of esophageal cancer among Bantu in the Transkei, J. Natl. Cancer Inst. **43:**877, 1969.
18. Schonland, M., and Bradshaw, E.: Oesophageal cancer in Natal Bantu: a review of 516 cases, S. Afr. Med. J., p. 1028, 1969.
19. Rose, E. F.: Esophageal cancer in the Transkei: 1955-69, J. Natl. Cancer Inst. **51:**7, 1973.
20. Rose, E. F.: Esophageal cancer in Transkei: the pattern and associated risk factors. In Pfeiffer, C. J., editor: Cancer of the esophagus, vol. 1, Boca Raton, Fla., 1982, CRC Press, pp. 19-28.
21. Wapnick, S., Zanamwe, L.N.D., Chitiyo, M., and Mynors, J.M.: Cancer of the esophagus in Central Africa, Chest **61:**649, 1972.
22. Oettlé, G. J., Paterson, A.C., Leiman, G., and Segal, I.: Esophagitis in a population at high risk for esophageal carcinoma, Cancer **57:**2222, 1986.
23. Boulos, P.B., and El Nasri, S.H.: Carcinoma of the oesophagus in Sudan, Trop. Geogr. Med. **29:**150-54, 1977.
24. Ajao, O.G., and Solanke, T.F.: Carcinoma of the esophagus, J. Natl. Med. Assoc. **71:**703, 1979.
25. Tuyns, A.J., and Massé, G.: Cancer of the oesophagus in Brittany: an incidence study in Ille-et-Vilaine, Int. J. Epidemiol. **4:**55, 1975.
26. Tuyns, A.J.: Epidemiology of esophageal cancer in France. In Pfeiffer, C.J., editor: Cancer of the esophagus, vol. 1, Boca Raton, Fla., 1982, CRC Press, pp. 3-18.

27. Rossi, M., Ancona, E., Mastrangelo, G., Solimbergo, D., Paruzzolo, P., Azzarini, G., Sorrentino, P., and Peracchia, A.: Rilievi epidemiologici sul cancro esofageo nella regione Veneto, Minerva Med. **73:**1531, 1982.

28. Giarelli, L., Silvestri, F., Ferlito, A., Brollo, A., and Clocchiati, L.: Observations on the epidemiology of esophageal carcinoma in the province of Trieste, Clin. Otolaryngol. **5:**13, 1980.

29. Staszewski, J.: Smoking and cancer of the alimentary tract in Poland, Br. J. Cancer **23:**247, 1969.

30. Ernster, V.L., Selvin, S., Sacks, S.T., Merrill, D.W., and Holly, E.A.: Major histologic types of cancers of the gum and mouth, esophagus, larynx and lung by sex and by income level, J. Natl. Cancer Inst. **69:**773, 1982.

31. Lynch, H.T., Ewers, D.D., Krush, A.J., Sharp, E.A., and Swartz, M.J.: Esophageal cancer in a midwestern community, Am. J. Gastroenterol. **55:**437, 1971.

32. Rogers, E.L., Goldkind, L., and Goldkind, S.F.: Increasing frequency of esophageal cancer among black male veterans, Cancer **49:**610, 1982.

33. Mandal, A.K., Shaman, I.N., Bier, R.K., and Oparah, S.S.: Outcome of thoracic esophageal carcinoma in blacks in the inner city, Cancer **54:**924, 1984.

34. O'Brien, P.H., Parker, E.F., and Gregorie, H.B.: Epidemiology and treatment of carcinoma of the esophagus in South Carolina, a high risk area in the U.S. In Pfeiffer, C.J., editor: Cancer of the esophagus, vol. 1, Boca Raton, Fla., 1982, CRC Press.

35. Hurst, E.E., Jr.: Malignant tumors in Alaskan Eskimos: unique predominance of carcinoma of the esophagus in Alaskan Eskimo women, Cancer **17:**1187, 1964.

36. Kune, G.A., and McLaughlin, S.: Smoking, alcohol and squamous cell cancers of the oral cavity and gullet, Med. J. Aust. **1:**204, 1983.

37. Kiviranta, U.K.: Corrosion carcinoma of the esophagus: 381 cases of corrosion and 9 cases of corrosion carcinoma, Acta Otolaryngol. **42:**89, 1952.

38. Appelquist, P., and Salmo, M.: Lye corrosion carcinoma of the esophagus, Cancer **45:**2655, 1980.

39. Hopkins, R.A., and Postlethwait, R.W.: Caustic burns and carcinoma of the esophagus, Ann. Surg. **194:**146, 1981.

40. Pierce, W.S., MacVaughn, H., and Johnson, J.: Carcinoma of the esophagus arising in patients with achalasia of the cardia, J. Thorac. Cardiovasc. Surg. **59:**335, 1970.

41. Hankins, J.R., and McLaughlin, J.S.: The association of carcinoma of the esophagus with achalasia, J. Thorac. Cardiovasc. Surg. **69:**355, 1975.

42. Rake, G.: Epithelioma of the esophagus in association with achalasia of the cardia, Lancet **2:**682, 1931.

43. Carter, R., and Brewer, L.A.: Achalasia and esophageal carcinoma: studies in early diagnosis for improved surgical management, Am. J. Surg. **130:**114, 1975.

44. Naef, A.P., Savary, M., and Ozzello, L.: Columnar-lined lower esophagus: an acquired lesion with malignant predisposition, J. Thorac. Cardiovasc. Surg. **70:**826, 1975.

45. Herlihy, K.G., Orlando, R.C., Bryson, J.C., Bozymski, E.M., Carney, C.N., and Powell, D.W.: Barrett's esophagus: clinical, endoscopic, histologic, manometric and potential difference characteristics, Gastroenterology **86:**436, 1984.

46. Spechler, J.S., Robbins, A.H., Rubbins, H.B., Vincent, M.E., Heeren, T., Doos, W.G., Colton, W.G., and Schimmel, E.M.: Adenocarcinoma and Barrett's esophagus: an overrated risk? Gastroenterology **87:**927, 1984.

47. Sherrill, D.J., Grishkin, B.A., Galal, F.S., Zajtchuk, R., and Graeber, G.M.: Radiation associated malignancies of the esophagus, Cancer **54:**726, 1984.

48. Goffman, T.E., McKeen, E.A., Curtis, R.E., and Schein, P.S.: Esophageal carcinoma following irradiation for breast cancer, Cancer **53:**1808, 1983.

49. Shearman, D.J.C., Finlayson, N.D.C., Arnott, S.J., and Pearson, J.C.: Carcinoma of the oesophagus after gastric surgery, Lancet **647:**581, 1970.

50. MacDonald, J.B., Waissbluth, J.G., and Langman, M.J.S.: Carcinoma of the oesophagus and gastric surgery, Lancet **688:**19, 1971.

51. Stalsberg, H.: Carcinoma of the oesophagus after gastric surgery, Lancet **746:**381, 1972.

52. Fong, L.Y.Y., Sivak, A., and Newberne, P.M.: Zinc deficiency and methylbenzylnitrosamine-induced esophageal cancer in rats, J. Natl. Cancer Inst. **61:**145, 1978.

CHAPTER 2

Esophageal carcinoma as a complication of achalasia: the screening controversy

Hugoe R. Matthews and Charles William Pattison

The coincidence of achalasia and carcinoma of the esophagus has been recognized since 1872,[1] and it is now generally accepted that the one condition predisposes to the other. If we assume this to be the case, there are important implications for the long-term surveillance and management of patients with achalasia. Yet this aspect of their care is rarely debated in the literature, and no clear guidelines have been established. Perhaps the main reason for this is that the individual clinician is unlikely to see enough cases of achalasia with carcinoma to comprehend fully the nature of this association, which is undoubtedly rare. We were therefore prompted to analyze all previously reported cases to see if we could establish the answers to a number of pertinent questions:

1. Is there a genuine etiologic association between achalasia and carcinoma?
2. If so, is the risk of carcinoma high enough to justify routine screening?
3. If so, are the necessary procedures available and practicable?
4. If so, are they likely to yield a significant clinical benefit?
5. And finally, if they are, would they need to be applied to all patients with achalasia, or only to certain subgroups in which the risk is particularly high?

SURVEY OF PREVIOUSLY REPORTED CASES

To March 1983 a total of 281 patients with achalasia and carcinoma had been reported, from 81 different centers. Of these centers, 39 reported a single case, 39 reported between 2 and 10 cases, 2 reported 13 cases, and one reported 24 cases.[2]

There was therefore an average of 3.5 cases per center. A notable feature of these publications is the frequency with which confident assertions and recommendations have been made on the basis of limited clinical material.

The diagnosis of carcinoma in these patients is generally reliable, but objective evidence of achalasia (e.g., from radiologic, endoscopic, operative, or autopsy findings) was given in only 100 of the 281 cases. The typical histologic findings of achalasia were not apparently sought or recorded in any patient, and none had the diagnosis confirmed by esophageal manometry.

Presentation

Early in our analysis it became apparent that the literature referred to two main types of presentation. In one group, comprising 66 patients, achalasia has been diagnosed, and in most cases treated, some years before the development of a carcinoma; this we have called the "metachronous" group. In a second group, comprising 79 patients, the subjects presented because of a carcinoma and were incidentally found to have coexisting achalasia; these constitute the "synchronous" group. In 13 cases, which might be classed as intermediate, a carcinoma was diagnosed within 1 year of the diagnosis of achalasia; presumably these patients had tumors that were present but missed at the time of the original diagnosis. In 123 patients the type of presentation could not be deduced from information given in the report.

Population

Of the reported cases, 255 were Caucasians from 70 different centers in North America, England, France, Belgium, Germany, Italy, and Spain; 21 were Japanese from eight centers; and

5 were blacks from two centers in North America and one in South America. These figures, however, cannot be taken to indicate the true incidence of achalasia with carcinoma in different races, since neither the relative incidence of achalasia in different racial groups nor the frequency of reporting of malignant change is known. So far there have been no reports of this association in non-Japanese Asians—although achalasia does occur in this group, as we know from our own practice.

Sex was stated in 133 of the 281 cases: 105 patients were male and 28 female, a male-female ratio of 3.75 to 1. There was no difference in this ratio between the metachronous and the synchronous groups.

The evolution of tumors

The length of time that it takes for a tumor to develop in achalasia is obviously central to any assessment of the role of screening. We therefore calculated this interval, and the effect of treatment on it, for all cases in which the necessary information was available. The results for the metachronous group are shown in Fig. 2-1, and the metachronous and synchronous groups are compared in Fig. 2-2. The overall findings are shown in Fig. 2-3.

Metachronous group (66 patients)

The age at the time of onset of the symptoms of achalasia was available in 40 cases and ranged from 8 to 72 years, with a mean of 31.5 years. The distribution is shown in Fig. 2-1, *A*. The age at the time of first treatment for achalasia was available in 41 cases and ranged from 22 to 72 years, with a mean of 42.8 years (Fig. 2-1, *B*). The age at the time of presentation with tumor was available in 42 cases and ranged from 32 to 78 years, with a mean of 52.0 years (Fig. 2-1, *C*). There was therefore a mean interval of 11.3 years between the onset of symptoms and the time of treatment, and a mean interval of 9.2 years between the time of treatment and the development of a tumor. The total interval from symptoms to tumor could be calculated in 54 cases and ranged (excluding the first-year intermediate cases) from 1 to 42 years, with a mean of 20.5 years.

The type of treatment given for achalasia was stated in 62 cases: 21 were treated by myotomy, 1 by esophagectomy, 34 by dilatation, and 6 had medical or no treatment. The patients who received dilatation were treated rather earlier in their course, but there was no significant difference in the interval from symptoms to tumor between those treated by dilatation (20.3 years) and

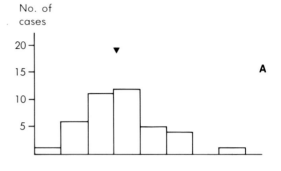
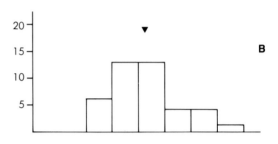
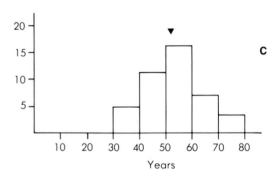

Fig. 2-1. Age distributions at various stages in patients with metachronous tumors. **A,** Age at onset of symptoms of achalasia (n = 40; mean = 31.5 years). **B,** Age at time of treatment for achalasia (n = 41; mean = 42.8 years). **C,** Age at time of presentation with tumor (n = 42; mean = 52.0 years).

those treated by myotomy (18.2) years (see Fig. 2-2, *A* and *B*).

Synchronous group (79 patients)

By definition, these patients had no treatment for achalasia, and they can therefore be regarded as a control group. The age at the onset of symptoms was available in 44 of the cases and ranged from 14 to 70 years, with a mean of 32.2 years. The age at the time of presentation with tumor was available in 44 cases and ranged from 14 to 84 years, with a mean of 52.0 years. The total interval from symptoms to tumor could be cal-

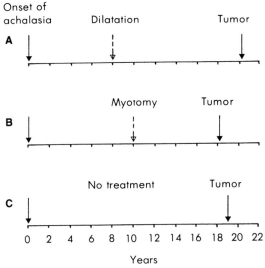

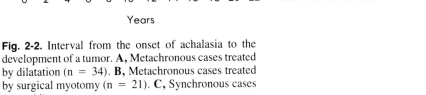

Fig. 2-2. Interval from the onset of achalasia to the development of a tumor. **A,** Metachronous cases treated by dilatation (n = 34). **B,** Metachronous cases treated by surgical myotomy (n = 21). **C,** Synchronous cases (n = 44).

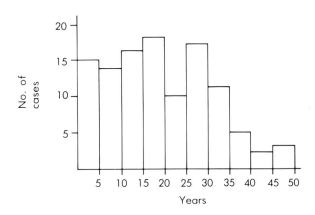

Fig. 2-3. Interval from onset of achalasia to the development of a tumor in 111 cases in which the necessary data were available.

culated in 44 cases and ranged from 0 to 50 years, with a mean of 19.1 years, which was not significantly different from the metachronous group (see Fig. 2-2, *C*).

All cases

The interval from symptoms to tumor for all 111 cases in which it could be calculated ranged from 0 to 50 years, with a mean of 19.1 years. The distribution of these cases with respect to time is shown in Fig. 2-3.

Pathology
Size of esophagus

An indication of the size of the esophagus at the time of occurrence of the tumor was given in 185 of the 281 cases. All had either gross or moderate dilatation of the esophagus, and there was no apparent difference in esophageal size between the metachronous and the synchronous groups.

Site of tumor

The site of the tumor was stated in 168 of the 281 cases: 14 were in the upper third, 113 were in the middle third, and 41 were in the lower third of the esophagus, giving a site ratio of 1 to 8 to 3, with no significant difference between the metachronous and the synchronous groups.

Histology

The tumor cell type was stated in 144 of the 281 cases. 136 had a squamous or epidermoid carcinoma, and only 8 had a tumor of other cell type: 1 anaplastic carcinoma, 1 "carcinosarcoma," and 6 adenocarcinomas. Although the high incidence of squamous tumors in this distribution gives some support to an etiologic connection between these tumors and achalasia, the extremely low incidence of nonsquamous tumors suggests that these may not be etiologically connected but may be due either to a genuine coincidence of two different diseases or to an incorrect diagnosis of achalasia. We therefore reviewed the evidence for the diagnosis of achalasia in these eight individual case reports.

The anaplastic tumor and the "carcinosarcoma" were both well-documented metachronous tumors, and their authenticity can be accepted, but the evidence for achalasia in the six adenocarcinomas is less satisfactory. Two cases were poorly reported and gave no further details. The remaining four were all synchronous tumors: three of these were in the lower third of the esophagus, where they could have caused obstructive dilatation that could have been misinterpreted as achalasia; the fourth was in the midesophagus, and the barium study was said to show a megaesophagus, but the report did not state whether there was any dilatation distal to the tumor. It is open to doubt, therefore, whether achalasia is ever etiologically associated with an adenocarcinoma.

Spread of tumor

The presence or absence of metastases at the time of presentation with tumor was stated in 78 of the 281 cases: 62 patients (79.5%) were reported to have metastases, while the remaining 16 (20.5%) did not. The synchronous and metachronous groups were similar. In order of frequency, the reported sites included the tracheobronchial tree, the mediastinum and recurrent laryngeal nerve, bone, the neck, and the liver.

Treatment of tumor and survival

Details of the treatment given for the tumor were reported in 132 of the 281 cases: 61 patients received no active treatment, and 39 were treated palliatively by radiotherapy and/or gastrostomy, but none were reported to have undergone endoscopic dilatation or intubation. All these 100 patients died within 9 months.

Surgical resection was performed in 24 metachronous and 8 synchronous cases, with 10 (31%) postoperative deaths. No follow-up was reported in 4 patients, and a further 7 died within 1 year of operation. Of the remaining 11 patients, 9 died at unspecified times within 2 years of resection and 2 were alive and well at 3 and 6 years respectively after operation. This last patient had undergone subtotal esophagectomy with colon interposition for a metachronous node-positive squamous carcinoma of the lower esophagus and is the only known patient to have survived 5 years after developing a carcinoma in association with achalasia.

TO SCREEN OR NOT TO SCREEN?

Screening for carcinoma in patients known to have achalasia has been recommended by a number of authors,[3-12] but is practiced in very few centers. So far there have been no reports of cures resulting from such a policy. The management of achalasia from this point of view is therefore uncertain, but the survey does at least provide partial answers to the questions posed at the start of the chapter.

1. Is there a genuine etiologic association between achalasia and carcinoma? To date there have been no studies in which a large group of patients with achalasia have been followed for long enough to determine how many subsequently develop a carcinoma. Absolute proof of an etiologic association is therefore lacking, but the fact that 281 cases have been reported does provide circumstantial evidence, particularly since achalasia is not a common disease. Further evidence comes from two findings in our survey, namely, (a) that the mean age of patients with carcinoma and achalasia is at least 10 years younger than that of patients with esophageal carcinoma alone and (b) that the site distribution, with 113 out of 168 tumors occurring in the middle third, is unlike that for carcinoma without achalasia. It is reasonable to accept, therefore, that achalasia is etiologically connected with esophageal carcinoma, even if not absolutely proven.

2. Is the risk of carcinoma high enough to justify routine screening? Estimates of the incidence of carcinoma in achalasia range from 0.3%[13] to 20%[14] with an average of 5.4%, but these have generally been arrived at by comparing the number of cases of achalasia with carcinoma with the number of cases of achalasia without carcinoma seen during a given period of time. These calculations, however, fail to take into account the number of unrecognized cases of achalasia in the population, and it is likely that they exaggerate the "true" incidence of malignant change in achalasia. Nevertheless, even if we accept a low estimate of the risk (say 1%), it is clear that this is much higher than for esophageal carcinoma alone in most populations. It is clear that undetected tumors carry a bad prognosis, with metastases at the time of presentation in 79.5% and only one 5-year survivor in 281 cases. We have recently reported a case in which a tumor was identified at the in situ stage,[15] and it is reasonable to suppose that treatment at this stage will result in improved survival. Screening is therefore both logical and desirable, but it remains to be determined whether it is feasible.

3. Are the necessary procedures available and practicable? Screening on the basis of symptoms alone would clearly not be adequate, since the esophagus is invariably dilated and tumors reach considerable size before causing recurrence of dysphagia. Indeed, this is one of the main causes of the bad prognosis at present. Techniques that can detect tumors at an early stage include the barium swallow, exfoliative cytology,[16] esophagoscopy,[3-7] and a combination of these.[8-12] The necessary techniques are therefore available, but it is less certain whether they are practicable. Compared to other screening procedures, these are all relatively labor intensive, and repeated cytology and endoscopy are uncomfortable for the patient, which may cause significant problems with long-term patient compliance. It is also clear that patients would have to be screened once or twice a year over long periods of time (e.g., up

to 50 years in young patients) if all were to be protected against the risk of near-certain death from delayed diagnosis of malignancy.

4. Is screening likely to yield a significant clinical benefit? This has never been determined by any prospective clinical study, and one can therefore only attempt an estimate. If we assume that 1% of cases of achalasia will develop a tumor, then to detect that case it would be necessary to do a minimum of one test a year for a period of 10 years (that being the mean time from treatment to tumor) in 100 patients—making a total of 1000 relatively complex investigations. It is also relevant that screening for malignancy is generally most productive when the treatment required is reasonably simple and effective. This is hardly the case with carcinoma in achalasia. Radiotherapy might be effective, but this has still to be proved, and surgical treatment would involve complete esophagectomy, an operation of great magnitude with a high postoperative mortality and a low success rate. The possible benefit from routine screening for carcinoma in achalasia is therefore small or nonexistent.

5. Would all patients need to be screened, or only certain subgroups in which the risk is particularly high? The results of this survey indicate that screening would have to be carried out in virtually all patients with achalasia if no tumors were to be missed. Although males may be particularly susceptible and elderly patients might be excluded on the grounds that they will not live long enough to develop a tumor, we have not been able to identify any groups that could be excluded completely on the grounds of age, sex, race, or the underlying stage of disease. It has been suggested that effective treatment for achalasia (e.g., myotomy) reduces the risk of carcinoma,[2,8,17] but our findings and those of others[18-20] do not confirm this. Tumors can develop for at least 30 years after treatment, and there is no group that can be excluded from screening simply because its members are "not yet eligible" or "no longer eligible" to develop a tumor.

CONCLUSION

In the light of these considerations, we can see no grounds for advocating a policy of routine screening for carcinoma in achalasia at the present time. The most that can be suggested is that a long-term prospective multicenter study might be mounted to see if there is any evidence of benefit from more active surveillance of these patients.

REFERENCES

1. Fagge, C.H.: A case of simple stenosis of the oesophagus, followed by epithelioma, Guy's Hosp. Rep. **17**:413, 1872.
2. Lortat-Jacob, J.L., et al.: Cardiospasm and carcinoma of the esophagus, Surgery **66**:969, 1969.
3. Bensaude, A., and Viguie, R.: Megaoesophage et cancer, Arch. Mal. Appar. Dig. **35**:544, 1946.
4. Gore, I., and Lam, C.R.: Carcinoma of the esophagus complicating cardiospasm: report of a case, J. Thorac. Surg. **24**:43, 1952.
5. Kastl, W.H.: Carcinoma of the esophagus as a complication of achalasia: case report, Surgery **34**:123, 1953.
6. Potter, S.E., Rasmussen, J.A., and Best, R.R.: The problem of carcinoma in achalasia, J. Thorac. Surg. **31**:543, 1956.
7. Peyman, M.A.: Achalasia of the cardia, carcinoma of the oesophagus and hypertrophic pulmonary osteoarthropathy, Br. Med. J. **1**:23, 1959.
8. Just-Viera, J.O., and Haight, C.: Achalasia and carcinoma of the esophagus, Ann. Thorac. Surg. **3**:526, 1967.
9. Bolivar, J.C., and Herendeen, T.L.: Carcinoma of the esophagus and achalasia, Ann. Thorac. Surg. **10**(1):81, 1970.
10. Wychulis, A.R., Woolam, G.L., Anderson, H.A., and Ellis, F.H., Jr.: Achalasia and carcinoma of the esophagus, JAMA **215**(10):1638, 1971.
11. Hankins, J.R., and McLaughlin, J.S.: The association of carcinoma of the esophagus with achalasia, J. Thorac. Cardiovasc. Surg. **69**(3):355, 1975.
12. Carter, R., and Brewer, L.A.: Achalasia and esophageal carcinoma, Am. J. Surg. **130**(2):114, 1975.
13. Matthews, E.C., and Vinson, P.P.: Carcinoma of the esophagus complicating cardiospasm: report of a case, Gastroenterology **15**:747, 1950.
14. Rake, G.W.: Epithelioma of the oesophagus in association with achalasia of the cardia, Lancet **2**:682, 1931.
15. Lamb, R.K., Edwards, C.W., Pattison, C.W., and Matthews, H.R.: Squamous carcinoma-in-situ of the oesophagus in a patient with achalasia, Thorax **40**:795, 1985.
16. Klayman, M.I.: The diagnosis of esophageal carcinoma by exfoliative cytology, including two cases of cardiospasm associated with carcinoma of the esophagus, Ann. Intern. Med. **43**:33, 1955.
17. Camara-Lopes, L.H.: Carcinoma of the esophagus as a complication of megaesophagus: an analysis of seven cases, Am. J. Dig. Dis. **6**:742, 1961.
18. Le Roux, B.T., and Wright, J. T.: Cardiospasm, Br. J. Surg. **48**:619, 1961.
19. Barrett, N.R.: Achalasia of the cardia: reflections upon a clinical study of over 100 cases, Br. Med. J. **1**:1135, 1964.
20. Pierce, W.S., MacVaugh, H., and Johnson, J.: Carcinoma of the esophagus arising in patients with achalasia of the cardia, J. Thorac. Cardiovasc. Surg. **59**:335, 1970.

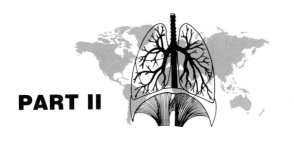

PART II

DIAGNOSTIC CONSIDERATIONS: METHODS OF EARLY DIAGNOSIS

CHAPTER **3** Radiologic patterns of early esophageal carcinoma

Hikoo Shirakabe, Goro Yamaki, Toshihide Maruyama, and Mamoru Nishizawa

In 1972 the Japanese Society for Esophageal Disease established guidelines for clinical and pathologic studies on carcinoma of the esophagus.[1] According to these guidelines, early esophageal carcinoma was defined as a lesion wherein invasion is confined to the mucosa and submucosa without metastasis to lymph nodes or other organs. Improved ability to detect and treat esophageal carcinoma in its early stage was expected to raise curability rates. However, nationwide statistics[2] show that the postoperative 5-year survival rate for 230 individuals with esophageal carcinomas including submucosal invasion (SM carcinoma) was 69.2% (Fig. 3-1). This is unexpectedly discouraging when compared with the rate for SM carcinomas of the stomach (96.96%).[3] Endo et al.[4] reported that lymph node metastasis and vessel invasion were each encountered in about half of those cases of SM carcinoma without clinical lymph node metastasis; these researchers suggested that both lymph node metastasis and vessel invasion were responsible for the high incidence of postoperative recurrence of SM carcinoma. In our series, lymph node metastasis was noted in 5 of 22 cases (22.7%) and vessel invasion in 8 of 17 cases (40.1%) of SM carcinoma without clinical evidence of lymph node metastasis.

For comparison, the postoperative 5-year survival rates for intraepithelial (EP) carcinomas and carcinomas in which the invasion is confined to the muscularis mucosae (MM carcinoma) are 100% and 85.3%, respectively (Fig. 3-1). Therefore EP and MM carcinomas carry a good prognosis, comparatively, but these forms are not found frequently,[2] with only 102 cases (17%) in 604 resections showing early or superficial carcinoma (invasion confined to the mucosa and submucosa without lymph node metastasis).

CLINICAL FEATURES

Over the past 14 years, 30 patients with 31 lesions (one with double lesions—one SM and one EP carcinoma) have been identified and operated on in our department. Of these lesions, 6 (19.4%) were EP carcinoma, 8 (25.8%) were MM carcinoma, and the remaining 17 (54.8%) were SM carcinoma. One SM carcinoma was found in the upper intrathoracic esophagus; 25 (80.8%), including 3 EP, 6 MM, and 16 SM carcinomas, were found in the middle intrathoracic esophagus; 3 (9.6%), including 2 EP and 1 MM carcinoma, were in the lower intrathoracic esophagus; and the remaining 2 (6.4%), 1 EP and 1 MM carcinoma, were in the abdominal esophagus. The male-female ratio was 6:1, with 26 males and 4 females.

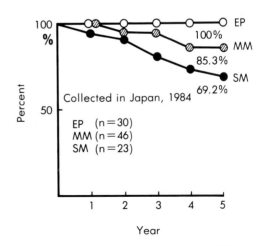

Fig. 3-1. Postoperative 5-year survival rates for early esophageal carcinoma according to nationwide statistics for Japan, 1984.

19

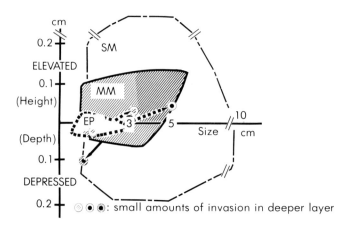

Fig. 3-2. Morphologic features of early esophageal carcinomas.

These early carcinomas were detected in patients who ranged in age from 25 to 75 years, but more than 90% of the patients were over age 40, with the peak incidence in the sixth decade. The symptoms recorded included chest pain on swallowing (7 patients, 23.3%) and sense of food sticking in the esophagus (4 patients, 13.3%). It should be noted that 18 patients (60%), including all 5 patients with EP carcinoma, 6 of 8 (75%) patients with MM carcinoma, and 7 of 17 (41%) patients with SM carcinoma, were asymptomatic. Therefore clinical symptoms do not serve well for early detection.

RADIOLOGIC PATTERNS

Fig. 3-2 shows the height of elevation and the depth of depression in resected early esophageal carcinomas as well as their sizes. With regard to size, EP carcinomas are all between 0.6 and 3.0 cm, and MM carcinomas are between 0.8 and 5.5 cm. Both the height of elevation and the depth of depression in EP and MM carcinomas are consistently less than 0.1 cm on measurement of histologic sections. As shown in Fig. 3-2, EP and MM carcinomas give rise only to very fine mucosal alterations and are often hardly recognizable even in the macroscopic examination of the resected specimens. Radiologic patterns of EP and MM carcinomas were reported by Yamada et al.,[5] Yamada and Laufer,[6] Katayama et al.,[7] and Yamamoto et al.,[8] but the macroscopic features of these carcinomas have not yet been defined because the total number of cases available for study in Japan is insufficient to completely define them. Therefore this chapter will present the radiologic patterns of EP and MM carcinomas that were clearly visualized by the double-contrast technique, and the radiologic manifestations of SM carcinomas.

Elevated EP and MM carcinoma

Fig. 3-3, *A,* shows a faintly outlined area of radiolucency on the prone left anterior oblique double-contrast view of the middle esophagus. Postoperatively, this lesion was superficial elevated EP carcinoma, 0.8 × 0.8 cm in size. Elevated MM carcinoma can be more clearly visualized than EP carcinoma, as shown in Fig. 3-3, *B,* where a well-circumscribed plaque-like elevated MM carcinoma is documented. Superficial elevated intramucosal carcinomas can be visualized by double-contrast technique with a moderate amount of air and good mucosal coating. Differentiation between EP and MM carcinoma may be possible by the sharply demarcated margin of MM carcinoma.

Depressed EP and MM carcinoma

A shallow (less than 0.2 mm in depth) superficial depression in EP and MM carcinomas found on measuring of the histologic sections is extremely difficult to visualize radiologically, even using double-contrast technique via intubation. The macroscopic features of this depression can be faithfully reflected only on postoperative roentgenogram of the resected specimen (Fig. 3-5, *D*). Radiologically, a depressed area is often visualized as a vaguely outlined area where the mucosal relief pattern disappears (Fig. 3-4, *A*), an area with mucosal granularity (Fig. 3-4, *B*), or a faintly outlined thin barium patch (Fig. 3-5, *A*) on the double-contrast view. The margin of mucosal depression in MM carcinomas can be more clearly outlined than that in EP carcinomas (Fig. 3-5, *A,* and Fig. 3-6, *A*). The radiologic manifestations of these shal-

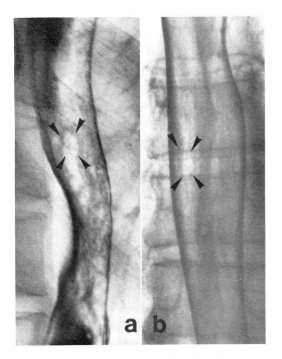

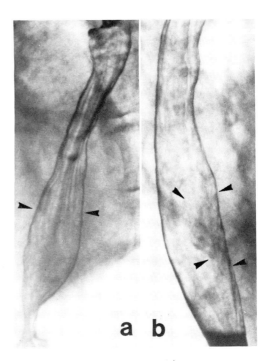

Fig. 3-3. A, Prone left anterior oblique double-contrast view showing a faintly outlined radiolucency (an elevated EP carcinoma 0.8 × 0.8 cm). **B,** Erect frontal double-contrast view showing a plaque-like MM carcinoma 1.0 × 1.0 cm.

Fig. 3-4. A, Erect left anterior oblique double-contrast view showing an area with disappearance of mucosal relief patterns (depressed EP carcinoma 3.0 × 4.5 cm). **B,** Erect right anterior oblique double-contrast view showing an area with mucosal granularity (depressed EP carcinoma 2.5 × 2.0 cm).

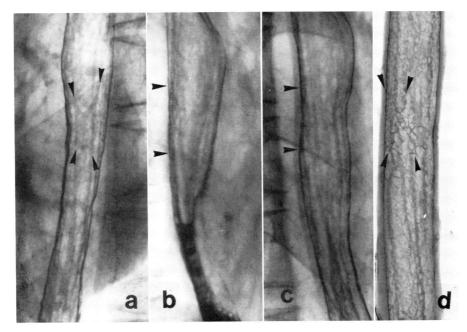

Fig. 3-5. Superficial depressed EP carcinoma 2.5 × 2.0 cm. **A,** Erect left anterior oblique double-contrast view showing a faintly outlined barium patch. **B** and **C,** Erect right anterior oblique double-contrast views. Wall irregularity is more clearly visible on the double-contrast view with the moderate amount of air **(B). D,** Postoperative roentgenogram of the resected specimen faithfully showing a depressed EP carcinoma.

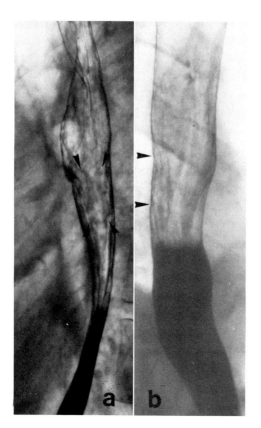

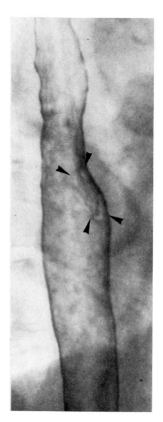

Fig. 3-6. A, Erect left anterior oblique double-contrast view showing a sharply outlined area of mucosal depression (depressed MM carcinoma 1.5 × 1.5 cm). **B,** Erect right anterior oblique double-contrast view showing diagnostic wall irregularity (depressed MM carcinoma 1.5 × 1.5 cm).

Fig. 3-7. Erect double-contrast view showing mixed SM carcinoma. Recognition of central depression is important.

low depressions are often inconclusive alone.

When a malignant focus lies across the lateral margin of the esophagogram, wall irregularity and stiffness are more diagnostic than the mucosal appearance; therefore, careful attention should be paid to the esophagogram margins to pick up EP and MM carcinomas. The wall irregularity in EP carcinoma (Fig. 3-5, *B* and *C*) is not so fixed that the degree of the irregularity may be altered by the amount of air. A moderate amount of air is best suited to the visualization of the irregularity in EP carcinoma, and the involved segment is seen to be obviously different from the smooth margin of the neighboring intact portion, as shown in Fig. 3-5, *B*. More diagnostic wall irregularities and stiffness are seen in MM carcinomas (Fig. 3-6, *B*); the irregularity in Fig. 3-6, *B,* is so evident that this sign alone suggests the presence of early carcinoma. Therefore the esophagus should be filmed in multiple projec-

tions to increase the opportunity of visualizing wall irregularity and stiffness seen when a focus of carcinoma lies across the lateral margin of the esophagogram.

To detect superficial depressed intramucosal carcinomas radiologically, wall irregularity and stiffness are carefully sought and then mucosal appearances adjacent to the abnormal margin are just as carefully interpreted.

SM carcinoma

Morphologically, the majority of SM carcinomas differ considerably from EP and MM carcinomas; some SM carcinomas are rather similar to advanced (invasive) carcinomas. Yet the radiologic recognition of SM carcinomas is difficult, even at a routine examination.

SM carcinomas are divided into the following three types: (1) elevated, with subdivisions of (a) tumorlike elevation, (b) wormlike broad-based elevation, and (c) nodular elevation; (2) depressed; and (3) mixed (elevation and depression). Double-contrast views with good mucosal coating obtained routinely allow SM carcinomas to be detected without difficulty.

After an analysis of SM carcinomas, Uematsu et al.[9] concluded that those with transverse diameter less than half of the transverse width of the esophagus or those with longitudinal diameter less than 3.0 cm cannot be detected by the barium filling technique; however, the double-contrast technique is always capable of visualizing both elevated and depressed SM carcinomas.

Occasionally a small SM carcinoma presents some problems in identification (Fig. 3-7). In this type of lesion, radiologic recognition of central depression is very important because in mixed types the cancerous invasion is always deeper than the submucosal layer, regardless of size.

DEVICES FOR EARLY DIAGNOSIS

Fig. 3-8 shows in graphic form the capability of routine radiologic examination to detect early elevated esophageal carcinomas, those less than 4.0 cm in longitudinal diameter. All but one of 9 carcinomas more than 1.0 cm (88.9%) could be visualized. Yamada et al.[10] pointed out that early elevated carcinomas more than 0.5 cm in longitudinal diameter are radiologically visible. Detection of early elevated types is easier than detection of depressed types.

One MM carcinoma in the distal third of the esophagus was overlooked because the double-contrast view of this portion was not obtained at the routine examination. In two other radiologic false-negative results, the elevation was less than 0.2 mm on measurement of the histologic sections, and staining with Lugol's solution was required in order to identify the lesion even on macroscopic examination of the resected specimens.

Fig. 3-9 shows in graphic form the capability of routine radiologic examination to detect early depressed esophageal carcinomas, those less than 4.0 cm in longitudinal diameter. Only 5 of 13 carcinomas (38.5%) were detected. The remaining 8 (61.5%) were later unexpectedly discovered at endoscopy for other abnormalities in the upper gastrointestinal tract. In 7 of 8 cases (87.5%) with a radiologic false-negative result, the diagnostic double-contrast views were not obtained. In these cases, the portion with carcinoma was always filled with or covered with a thick layer of barium. The remaining false-negative EP carcinoma, which was 0.6 × 0.5 cm and coexisted with two more striking submucosal tumors, was invisible on good-quality double-contrast view, even retrospectively.

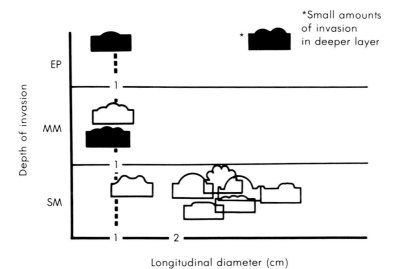

Fig. 3-8. Radiologic capability in detection of elevated early esophageal carcinomas (those less than 4.0 cm in longitudinal diameter) at routine examination. Black tumor outlines indicate missed diagnoses.

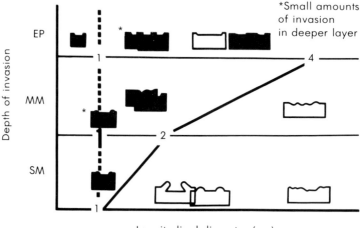

Fig. 3-9. Radiologic capability in detection of depressed early esophageal carcinomas (those less than 4.0 cm in longitudinal diameter) at routine examination. Black tumor outlines indicate missed diagnoses.

At the preoperative detailed radiologic examination using the double-contrast technique via intubation, 30 of the 31 lesions of early carcinoma (96.8%) could be visualized. Not only wall irregularities and stiffness but also fine mucosal abnormalities were well documented on the double-contrast view with a moderate amount of air and good mucosal coating. Katayama et al.[7] and Yamamoto et al.[8] also emphasized using a moderate amount of air for the diagnostic double-contrast technique.

False-negative radiologic errors most commonly occurred in cases in which the diagnostic double-contrast views were not routinely obtained. Therefore, if double-contrast views with good mucosal coating and an adequately distended esophagus are always obtained, the ability to detect such lesions on routine examination can be increased. Filming of the esophagus in multiple projection also improves the detectability of wall irregularities and stiffness that exist when a focus of carcinoma lies across the lateral margin of the esophagogram. Active use of the double-contrast technique via intubation is also important. When vague wall irregularities or mucosal abnormalities are visible under fluoroscopy, the nasogastric tube is inserted near the doubtful area and several double-contrast views are obtained by insufflation through the tube.

At present, better detection results can be obtained by endoscopy, but assessing the depth of cancerous invasion is not easy by this method. Therefore, the combined use of both modalities is advisable for early detection and accurate diagnosis of early, curable esophageal carcinomas.

REFERENCES

1. Japanese Society for Esophageal Diseases: Guide lines for the clinical and pathologic studies on carcinoma of the esophagus. I. Clinical classification, Japn. J. Surg. **6**:69, 1976.
2. Japanese Society for Esophageal Diseases: Treatment of so-called early esophageal carcinoma. A questionnaire at the 37th Annual Meeting of the Japanese Society for Esophageal Diseases, 1984.
3. Japanese Research Society for Gastric Cancer: The report of treatment results of resected stomach carcinoma cases without adjuvant chemotherapy **15**:62, 1984.
4. Endo, M., Yamada, A., Ide, H., Yoshida, M., and Hayashi, T.: Progress in the diagnosis of early esophageal carcinoma. In Nakayama, K.: Shokakigeka seminar 7, Tokyo, 1982, Herusu Shuppan Co., pp. 7-20.
5. Yamada, A., Kobayashi, S., Isobe, Y., Yoshida, M., Sugiyama, A., and Endo, M.: The screening for cancer of the esophagus from the viewpoint of x-ray diagnosis, Stomach and Intestine **19**(2):129, 1984.
6. Yamada, A., and Laufer, I.: Tumors of the esophagus. In Laufer, I.: Double contrast gastrointestinal radiology with endoscopic correlation, Philadelphia, 1979, W.B. Saunders Co., pp. 129-153.
7. Katayama, H., Nakai, A., Sakai, Y., and Matsuda, H.: A radiological study of esophageal carcinoma with special reference to the superficial lesions, Nippon Acta. Radiol. **41**:194, 1981.
8. Yamamoto, I., Nanami, K., and Nakajima, T.: The recent progress in x-ray diagnosis of early-stage esophageal cancer, Jpn. J. Clin. Radiol. **31**(2):239, 1986.
9. Uematsu, S., Isono, K., Ryu, M., Watanabe, Y., Furukawa, T., Kikuchi, T., Ozaki, M., and Sato, H.: Radiological study of SM-esophageal cancer, Jpn. J. Clin. Radiol. **26**(6):629, 1981.
10. Yamada, A., Kobayashi, S., Ogino, T., and Endo, M.: A study on x-ray diagnosis of esophageal diseases: what is the help from endoscopy? Stomach and Intestine, **14**(3):311, 1979.

CHAPTER 4 Cytologic screening for carcinoma and dysplasia of the esophagus in the People's Republic of China

Qiong Shen and Guo Qing Wang

The world's highest incidence of esophageal cancer occurs in parts of north central China, particularly in the Taiheng Mountain area, within which is located Linxian in Henan province. The Linxian county population is 800,000, and here the crude rates for esophageal cancer per 100,000 are 163 for males and 103 for females. The death rates were nearly constant from 1959 to 1984.

Since 1959, an anticancer team of Henan province has been working in Linxian in cooperation with members of the Chinese Academy of Medical Sciences, Beijing. The team investigated many aspects of this disease, but the results of treatment remain unsatisfactory because patients with severe dysphagia come for treatment when the disease is in its late stages, and about one third already have lymph node metastases.

Balloon cytologic technique was devised in 1961 for early diagnosis of this disorder. This technique has proven useful both in daily practice in the clinic and in surveys of this high-incidence area.[1-3]

The purpose of this chapter is to report the method and results in the detection of early carcinoma and dysplasia both in the past and in recent years in Linxian, including the results of the cooperative work with the U.S. National Cancer Institute. The feasibility and practicality of the technique used to detect and follow up dysplastic cases were evaluated by statistical analyses and by comparison with the results of epidemiologic survey.

COLLECTING THE CELL SPECIMEN

The apparatus used consists of a double-lumen tube and an abrasive balloon. The tube is made of rubber and plastic and is about 65 cm long and 0.25 cm in diameter; it is graduated every 5 cm.

At the distal end is an inflatable balloon about 5 cm long and 2.5 cm wide and covered with a mesh net. At the proximal end the apparatus is divided into two tubes, one for air injection and the other for suction. The apparatus is sterilized by soaking in alcohol solution for 1 hour after cleansing with soapy water and irrigating the suction lumen with a syringe (see Fig. 4-1).

The examination is usually done in the morning. The person to be examined is instructed to come with an empty stomach and is asked to swallow the tube, while the deflated balloon is being put on the back of the tongue. After each deglutition the mouth is opened slightly. The examiner pushes the tube down gently. In this way, the intubation is easily performed.

After the balloon passes through the cardia, it is inflated with 30 ml or more of air and then slightly deflated so that it can be pulled back past

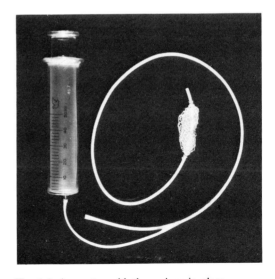

Fig. 4-1. Apparatus with the syringe in place.

25

the cardia. When the balloon enters the lower segment of the esophagus, it is redistended with sufficient air to obtain complete contact with the mucous surface, then again slightly deflated. The tube is retracted for 5 cm, and again the balloon is distended and deflated. The process is repeated until the 20-cm mark is reached, when the balloon should be deflated completely and withdrawn.

A direct smear is made onto four slides for each subject, and each slide is stained with Papanicolaou's method. Throughout the staining procedure the slides should be kept wet.

Contraindications to the balloon test include recent history of hematemesis, acute pharyngitis, severe liver cirrhosis, and heart failure.[4]

The technique is very safe. No severe complications occurred in a wide experience.

ACCURACY OF BALLOON CYTOLOGY

In the first year of cytologic examination in the outpatient department of Lin county hospital (1961 to 1962), a total of 256 subjects with esophageal symptoms were examined. The correct rate for diagnosis of carcinoma was 87.8%. The causes of error in false-negative and false-positive situations were carefully analyzed and the reasons for error determined. The cooperation between cytologist, roentgenologist, endoscopist, and pathologist has been emphasized. The correct rate of cytologic examination for diagnosis of carcinoma was 91.9% in 1969.[5,6]

For the inpatient population of Lin county hospital the rate was increased to 98.1% in 110 cancer cases in 1966 by repeated balloon testing when necessary. These results have been reproduced in many clinics in this country.

One method of testing the accuracy of cytologic diagnosis in a large-scale survey is by dividing the number of carcinomas found in the survey by that number plus those found in the same group during the next 2 years. For instance, in a 1977 epidemiologic survey in the suburban area of the city of Hebi, Henan province, among 5800 people examined, 121 cases of cancer were found at the time of survey and nine more in the following 2 years. The rate of correct diagnosis was therefore 93.1% (121 out of 121 + 9).

Steps in diagnosis

Step 1. Persons with positive smear but without frank symptoms should be considered as suspected early carcinoma cases.

Step 2. Roentgenologic examination of those suspected early cases should be carried out in time. In some of these patients the x-ray findings are indistinct, but the majority of them do show some mucosal changes:

a. Thickening, interruption, and tortuosity of the mucous folds, with rough and irregular margins
b. Small ulceration, single or multiple, frequently appearing on the thickened mucosa
c. Localized filling defect resulting from intraluminal tumor growth and usually with a diameter around 0.5 cm
d. Early carcinoma developed from esophageal glands may produce localized narrowing of the lumen or stiffness of the wall of the affected segment.[7,8]

Step 3. The uppermost location of the early cancerous lesion should be determined by balloon cytology. In the surgical treatment of early esophageal carcinoma, it is very important to determine by balloon cytology the uppermost limit in cases that are roentgenologically and endoscopically occult early carcinoma of the esophagus. This may be done as a routine test to detect the minute foci of early cancer above the main lesion before surgery is performed and thereby help ensure complete excision of the cancerous lesion at operation.[9,10]

The examination consists of successive balloon tests at different levels, starting from the upper part of the esophagus and descending as far as desired. For instance, in the first test, the tip of the balloon is 20 cm from the upper incisor, in the second test 25 cm, and in the third test 30 cm. X-ray studies may be helpful in deciding how far to go. The smears are made separately from the upper and lower halves of the balloon. The uppermost limit may be determined by mapping the positive and negative smears at different levels of the esophagus and finding the levels where the smear from the upper part of the balloon is negative and that from the lower part is positive.

To show the significance of this localization, in a series of 70 resected specimens with early esophageal carcinoma in Linxian Hospital from 1973 to 1980, when this examination was performed routinely, only one case with a minute cancerous focus in the upper resection margin of the specimen was found by pathologic examination. In Chun-Guan Hospital in Linxian, where this routine was not done before surgery in early cancer patients, 4 of 80 specimens had minute cancerous foci present in the surgical resection line.

Sun Shao-Chien and Wu Hsia[11] reported a pathologic study of 100 resected specimens of late esophageal carcinoma and found 22 cases with early foci not discernible by gross inspection along the line of surgical resection. These authors pointed out that it is quite possible for a new carcinoma to have developed from the minute early cancerous foci in the stump of the esophagus. In addition, we have had two cases of early esophageal carcinoma with postoperative recurrences 7 and 9 years after operation. Close cooperation between surgeon, cytologist, endoscopist, and pathologist in the preoperative diagnosis is a unique way to ensure a sufficiently radical resection and possible cure of the patient.

DETECTION OF EARLY CARCINOMA AND DYSPLASIA

Early esophageal carcinoma includes the following types:
1. Carcinoma in situ, in which cells of the whole thickness of the epithelium are similar to those of invasive carcinoma but the basement membrane is intact
2. Microinvasive carcinoma, in which the invasive lesion passes through the basement membrane but not the muscularis mucosae
3. Early invasive carcinoma, in which the cancerous tissue extends into the submucosa but not the muscular layers of the wall

None of these lesions bear evidence of lymph node metastasis.

In the surveys presented in Table 4-1, the prevalence of dysplasia was much higher in the 1983 data than that found in the data from 1974 to 1977. Possible reasons for this may be that the subjects examined were older and that the cytologic screening in the 1983 survey included the steps of collecting cell specimen, smear staining, microscopic examination of the slides, and adherence to the criteria for classification of dysplasia. A special team was charged with each step to ensure that it was carefully performed.

CLASSIFICATION OF ESOPHAGEAL DYSPLASIA

Dysplastic cells in the smear are classified into four grades (with the early carcinoma as grade V) according to the morphology of the cells, with emphasis on the structural changes of the nuclei.[12]

Grade I—normal. Cells in a smear from a normal subject are chiefly of intermediate type, 10% to 15% of superficial cells. Parabasal cells are rarely exfoliated, and basal cells usually not. (See Fig. 4-2, *A.*)

Grade II—hyperplasia. There is a mild degree of hyperplasia of the cells. The chromatin content of the nucleus is increased, and the nucleus is two or more but less than three times larger than in normal cells of the same layer. The chromatin granules are fine, and the nuclear membrane is not thickened. (See Fig. 4-2, *B.*)

Grade III—severe (marked) dysplasia. The size of the dysplastic nuclei of the intermediate cells is three to four times that of the normal intermediate cells. Hyperchromasia is more marked. The chromatin granules become coarse but are rather uniform in size and even in distribution. The nuclear membrane is slightly thickened but regular. A total number of three or more such cells is required to make this diagnosis. This type of dysplasia may be divided into two subgroups:

Group IIIa. The nuclear size of dysplastic cells is three times or more, but less than four times, that of the normal cells in the same layer (see Fig. 4-2, *C*).

Group IIIb. The nuclear size of dysplastic cells is four times or more that of normal cells of the same layer (see Fig. 4-2, *D*).

Grade IV—near carcinoma. The nuclei in near-carcinoma cells are five or more times

TABLE 4-1. Mass surveys of persons aged 30 or above and aged 40 to 65

Year	1974	1975	1977	1983*
Age	30 or above	30 or above	30 or above	40-65
Total number examined	14,002	19,250	5,800	17,388
Number of subjects with proven carcinoma	221 (1.57%)	232 (1.20%)	121 (2.08%)	395 (2.27%)
Number of subjects with early carcinoma	174 (78.73%)	198 (85.34%)	102 (84.29%)	—
Number of subjects with severe dysplasia	460 (3.28%)	547 (2.84%)	250 (4.31%)	4589 (26.39%)

*Cases of suspected early carcinoma in 1983 were confirmed by endoscopy and biopsy.

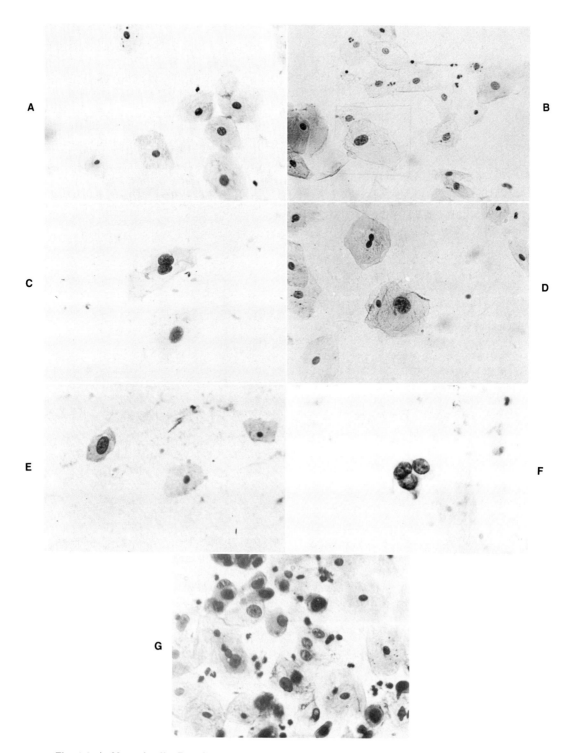

Fig. 4-2. A, Normal cells. **B,** Mild hyperplasia. **C,** Severe dysplasia, group I. **D,** Severe dysplasia, group II. **E,** Near carcinoma. **F,** Early carcinoma of small area. **G,** Early carcinoma of large area. (×264, Papanicolaou stain.)

greater in size than those in the normal cells of the same layer. The chromatin granules of the nuclei are not as coarse as those of typical cancer cells. Near-carcinoma cells always lie in the epithelium overlying carcinoma of the basal layers.[13] (See Fig. 4-2, *E*.)

Grade V—early carcinoma. Typical cancer cells are present in the smear. The diameter of the nucleus exceeds one third of the diameter of the cell. The malignant features of the cancer nuclei are very distinct. The chromatin granules are coarse, varied in size, and uneven in distribution. All these morphologic characteristics serve to distinguish carcinoma cells from near-carcinoma cells. (See Fig. 4-2, *F* and *G*.)

These morphologic criteria for classification of cells are established by visual estimation of the degree of enlargement of the nuclei. Reliability has been checked by measurement with a micrometer.[10]

FEASIBILITY OF CYTOLOGIC CLASSIFICATION OF DYSPLASIA
Cell grading

The preliminary results of prospective studies of dysplasia in Linxian and in the suburban area of Hebi city, Henan province, showed that the cell gradings represent a sequence of cell events in carcinogenesis of the esophagus. For instance, a number of patients in Linxian were not undergoing treatment. After periodic follow-up by cytology for 8 to 15 years, their dysplastic cells changed from group I to group II, to near carcinoma, and eventually to early carcinoma. In regression in response to therapy, the reversed changes in dysplastic cells may be seen in patients undergoing a program of malnutrition intervention for 8 years in Hebi city.

Shu et al.[14] reported a study of 530 cases of severe dysplasia of the esophagus. In a follow-up period of 1 to 12 years, 79 (14.91%) patients developed cancer. In another group of 530 with hyperplasia followed for the same length of time, 5 (0.94%) cases of cancer were found. In the normal group followed for 1 to 5 years no esophageal cancer was found.

In the 1983 survey covering four communes in the northern part of Linxian, 17,388 persons aged 40 to 65 were examined (see Table 4-1). As shown in Fig. 4-3, a striking similarity exists between the percentages of cell grades between these communes. Fig. 4-4 presents the curves of cell grades in age groups; it should be noted that the dysplastic curves of groups I and II are closely parallel. In addition, Fig. 4-5 shows that the curve of dysplasia in group II surpassed that of group I at age 45 and descended after reaching its peak around age 55. These curves are in positive cor-

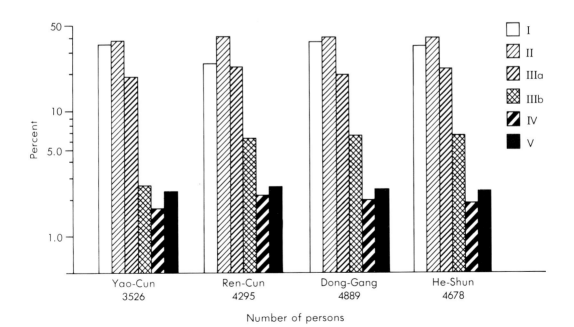

Fig. 4-3. Results of cytologic screening in four communes.

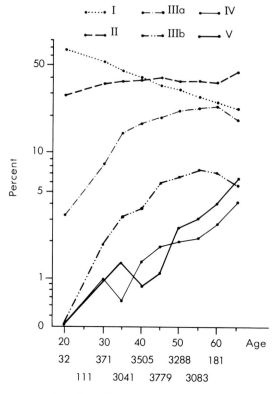

Number of persons in different age groups

Fig. 4-4. Curves of cell grades by age groups.

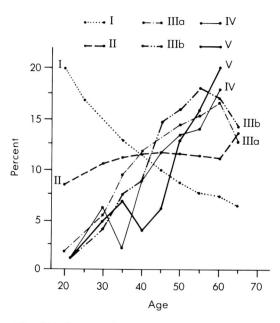

Fig. 4-5. Curves of percentages of cell grades in the age groups found in subjects in mass survey of 1983. The correlation of cell grades to carcinoma: I, r = −0.81; II, r = 0.484, p > 0.05; IIIa, r = 0.856, p < 0.05; IIIb, r = 0.88, p < 0.01; IV, r = 0.92, p < 0.01.

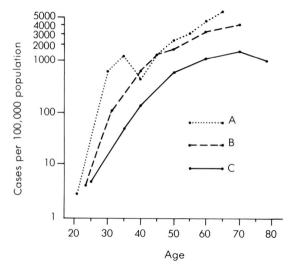

Fig. 4-6. Comparison of the prevalence of esophageal carcinoma in mass survey with its incidence by epidemiologic study. *A,* Cytology in mass survey of 1983 (393/17388). *B,* Cytology in mass survey before 1975 (646/54715). *C,* Epidemiologic survey.

relation with carcinoma, whereas the curves for grades I and II are negatively correlated.

The curve (Fig. 4-6) denoting carcinoma found in the 1983 survey and that for before 1975 are parallel to the curve obtained by epidemiologic study.

Cytologic examination

The effectiveness of medical management can be evaluated by the following criteria:

1. Stabilization. The follow-up smears show no significant change since the previous examination.
2. Progression. Dysplasia progressed by one or more grades.
3. Regression. Dysplasia regressed by one or more grades.
4. Cancerous change. Cancer cells are found for the first time.

These criteria were applied to a pilot study of nutritional intervention for dysplasia in Hebi over a period of 8 years. The follow-up smears were taken once every 1 to 2 years, and the tendency of cell changes became apparent when three successive results were taken into consideration.

REFERENCES

1. Li, B., and Li, J.Y.: National survey of cancer mortality in China, Chin. J. Oncol. **2**:1-10, 1980. (In Chinese.)
2. Shen, C., Qu, S.L., and Chao, N.T.: Cytologic diagnosis of carcinoma of the esophagus: a preliminary report, Chin. J. Pathol. **7**:19, 1964. (In Chinese.)
3. Shen, C., Qu, S.L., and Liu, F.Y.: Carcinoma in situ of the esophagus: report of one case, Chin. J. Pathol. (suppl.) **8**:403, 1964. (In Chinese.)
4. Department of Pathology, Henan Medical College: The use of exfoliative cytology in clinical diagnosis and mass survey for cancer of the esophagus, Chin. Med. J. **6**:479, 1967.
5. Medical Team of Henan Province for Preventive and Therapeutic Studies of Esophageal Carcinoma and Linxian Hospital: Early diagnosis of carcinoma of the esophagus, Beijing, 1973, People's Medical Publishing House, pp. 31-52.
6. Shen, C., and Qu, S.L.: Study on the exfoliative cytology, Henan Med. Coll. Bull. *1*:3, 1966. (In Chinese).
7. Su, J.H., Tian, Z.S., and Han, J.F.: X-ray studies of early esophageal carcinoma: an analysis of 100 cases, Chin. Med. J. **55**:573, 1975. (In Chinese.)
8. Wang, Z.Y.: Radiological appearance in early esophageal carcinoma, J. R . Soc. Med. **73**:849, 1980.
9. Huang, G.J., Wu, Y.K.: Carcinoma of the esophagus and gastric cardia, New York, 1984, Springer-Verlag, pp. 156-190.
10. Pfeiffer, C.J., editor: Cancer of the esophagus, vol. 2, Boca Raton, Fla., 1982, CRC Press, pp. 3-15.
11. Sun, S.C., and Wu, H.: Squamous carcinoma of the esophagus: carcinomatous changes of the epithelium adjacent to the principal lesion, Chin. Med. J. **81**:557, 1962.
12. Shabad, L.F.: Precancerous morphologic lesions, J. Natl. Cancer Inst. **50**:1421, 1973.
13. Ayre, J.E.: Cancer cytology of the uterus, London, 1951, Churchill Livingstone, p. 40.
14. Shu, Y.J., et al.: Further investigation of the relationship between dysplasia and cancer of the esophagus, Chin. Med. J. **1**:39, 1980. (In Chinese.)

Cytologic screening for carcinoma and dysplasia of the esophagus in the People's Republic of China

DISCUSSION

Attila Bajtai and Janos Kiss

In Hungary the mortality rates from malignant tumors have been increasing considerably from 1946 to the mid-1980s (1946: 111.3 per 100,000 population; 1984: 266.7 per 100,000 population).

Within those figures, of course, mortality from tumors of the digestive tract, including cancer of the esophagus, has also increased. Although cancer of the esophagus was once a disease of the elderly, recently more and more cases have occurred at a young age. Table 4-2 shows the changes in mortality caused by cancer of the esophagus in Hungary. Both the absolute figures and the number of cases calculated per 100,000 population have doubled. The rise is particularly obvious in the male population.

The data in Table 4-2 also reveal that the high incidence rate found in China is unlikely to occur in Hungary in the near future.

Table 4-3 shows the absolute figures and the rates per 100,000 population for mortality from cancer of the esophagus in a few major countries. The Hungarian figures are comparable to those reported from the United States, Spain, and the Federal Republic of Germany.

Especially since more cases are occurring in the young, it is absolutely paramount to strive for earlier diagnosis.

For well-known reasons the value of early diagnosis is unquestioned. Therefore, complex diagnostic procedures have to be given more attention. Directed biopsy and brush cytology, coupled with endoscopic examination, are highly important components.

The method described by Shen and Wang is essentially the second among the classical techniques for cytologic sampling and was reported in the early 1950s as the blind abrasive method.

Panico et al.[1,2] published their experience with the use of a balloon, by means of which spontaneously exfoliated cells could be collected. As early as 1952, Panico[3] described how this method could be used for the diagnosis of cancer of the esophagus.

An abrasive balloon technique for cytologic sampling from the esophagus was developed by Shu.[4] His results were reported in 1980 at the 28th Scientific Meeting of the American Society of Cytology, in Boston. To 1979 more than 500,000 patients had been examined by this method within the framework of mass screening in China, with 90% accuracy. Of the cancers detected in this way, 67% were in situ or minimally invasive.

Berry et al.[5] used an inflatable balloon catheter for cytologic sampling. The surface of the balloon was adsorbent. They examined 500 complaint-free patients and found 15 cases with positive cytologic findings, confirmed later without exception by endoscopically directed biopsies. Of the 15 cancers, 10 were early!

K. Nabeya[6] and Nabeya et al.[7] described an abrasive cytologic method utilizing a capsule. We have obtained by this method 100,000 cells with a single intervention. This cytologic method proved to be successful in 75% of the grade IV and V smears, and in 94% if we count the grade III smears.

The cancer precursor role of dysplasia is a confirmed fact in the carcinogenesis of other organs (uterine cervix, larynx). In Henan province of China follow-up studies revealed that in the course of 7 to 10 years, 30.3% of the cases of severe dysplasia changed into cancer, 27.3% persisted unchanged, and 42.4% regressed.

TABLE 4-2. Esophageal cancer deaths in Hungary

Year	No. of patients	Rate per 100,000 population
1964	210 (170 male, 40 female)	2.0
1974	242 (206 male, 36 female)	2.3
1984	411 (361 male, 50 female)	3.8

TABLE 4-3. World esophageal cancer deaths

Country	Deaths	Population	Incidence per 100,000 population
Federal Republic of Germany	2067	67 million	3.4
France	5520	53 million	10.7
Spain	1328	35 million	3.8
Japan	5241	115 million	4.6
United States	7224	215 million	3.4
Hungary	411	10.7 million	3.8

TABLE 4-4. Results of cytology and biopsy in 112 cases of esophageal changes

Findings	Patients	Percent
Positive cytologic findings	104	92.8
Negative cytologic findings	8	7.2
Positive biopsy	100	89.3
Negative biopsy	12	10.7
Both cytology and biopsy positive	93	83.0
Positive biopsy and negative cytology	7	6.3
Negative biopsy with positive cytology	11	9.8
Both cytology and biopsy negative	1	0.9

For the classification of dysplasia we use a formula valid also for other squamous epithelial tissues:

I. *Mild dysplasia:* changes in the lower third of the epithelium. Basal hyperplasia in which, however, the cells remain stratified. There are a few dark-stained, glycogen-negative cells.

II. *Moderately severe dysplasia:* basal hyperplasia in the lower and middle thirds. More extensive hyperchromasia, polymorphism. On the surface hyperkeratosis and parakeratosis and mitotic figures are visible.

III. *Severe dysplasia:* epithelial lesion involves the entire thickness of the epithelium. There is marked hyperchromasia and polymorphism; polarity has disintegrated. Bizarre and mitotic forms are common. Cell density is high.

In the classification suggested by Shen and Wang it is not difficult to recognize the influence of the classification recommended for dysplasias of the gastric mucosa by T. Nagayo.[8] In the Nagayo classification grade IV is "probable cancer," while here it is "near cancer." Grade V is true cancer in both classifications.

In our own study we have tested the efficacy of cytology and biopsy in 112 cases of esophageal changes proved to be malignant by histopathologic examination of biopsy or resected specimens. The results are presented in Table 4-4.

When both methods were used, positive results were obtained in 99.1% of all malignant esophageal tumors, by one or the other technique.

When the cytologic evidence is equivocal, further examinations should be carried out. In the course of upper digestive tract cytologic studies we employed image analysis by television (Vidimet-1 type apparatus, "VASKUT," Budapest, Hungary), which we believe to be more accurate than measurement by the micrometer. In doubtful cases the karyogram may decide the issue. In one of our cases the x-ray evidence and the clinical

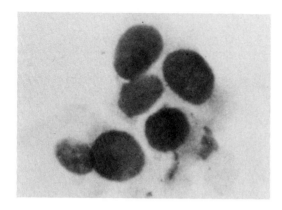

Fig. 4-7. Suspicious cells in the esophageal smear of grade III in Papanicolaou grading. (Giemsa staining, ×200.)

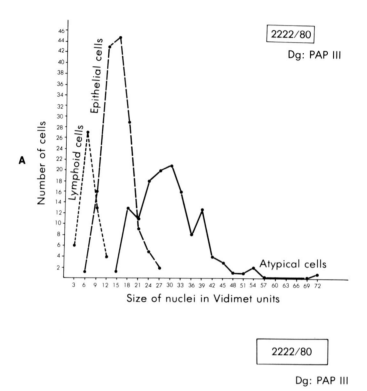

Fig. 4-8. The result of television-image analysis of esophageal smear. **A,** The distribution of three kinds of cells on karyogram. Each cell type can be found in different ranges. **B,** The average of each cell type differs significantly from the others.

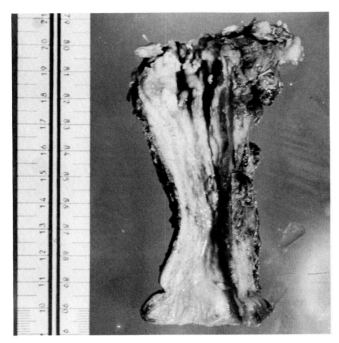

Fig. 4-9. The resected specimen showed diffuse tumor infiltration in the esophageal wall.

course suggested a benign stricture of the esophagus in a dysphagic patient. Repeated endoscopic examinations revealed only dysplasia, which later turned out to be a precancerous lesion. In the cytologic specimen there were several suspicious cell forms (Fig. 4-7). In the histogram obtained by the image analytical method, the presence of the atypical cell forms indicated unequivocally a malignant process (Fig. 4-8). The means were significantly different in the three kinds of cells examined (lymphoplasmacytoid cells, normal squamous epithelial cells, and tumor-suspect atypical cell forms). The data obtained from the investigations were evaluated by computer, on the basis of the University of California, Los Angeles, program pack BMDP9D. The accuracy of measurements and the correctness of diagnosis were confirmed by histologic examination of the resected specimen (Fig. 4-9).

REFERENCES

1. Panico, F.G., Papanicolaou, G.N., and Cooper, W.A.: Abrasive balloon for exfoliation of cancer cells, JAMA **143:**1308, 1950.
2. Cooper, W.A., and Papanicolaou, G.N.: Balloon technique in the cytological diagnosis of gastric cancer, JAMA **151:**10, 1953.
3. Panico, F.G.: Improved abrasive balloon for diagnosis of gastric cancer, JAMA **149:**1447, 1952.
4. Shu, Y.J.: Esophageal cytopathology in China. Abstracts of the Scientific Sessions of 28th Annual Scientific Meeting of the American Society of Cytology, Acta Cytol. **25:**454, 1981.
5. Berry, A.V., Baskind, A.F., and Hamilton, D.G.: Cytologic screening for esophageal cancer, Acta Cytol **25:**135, 1981.
6. Nabeya, K.: Early detection for esophageal cancer. In Proceedings of the 2nd International Congress of the International Society for Diseases of the Esophagus, Rome, October 3-6, 1983, p. 173.
7. Nabeya, K., Onozawa, L., Ri, S.: Brushing cytology with capsule for esophageal cancer, Chir. Gastroenterol. **13:**101, 1979.
8. Nagayo, T.: Histological diagnosis of biopsied gastric mucosae with special reference to that of borderline lesions. GANN Monograph on Cancer Research, no. 11, Early gastric cancer, Tokyo, 1972, University Park Press, p. 245.

5 Esophagoscopy and bronchoscopy

John Wong and Frank James Branicki

ESOPHAGOSCOPY

Attempts to view the esophagus were made by Semelder and Stoerk in 1868; their instrument, a pair of forceps with spoon-shaped blades, was designed in that year by Semelder, who had the courage to offer himself to Stoerk for experiment. In the same decade Desmoreaux and Berin and also Kussmaul employed scopes that could be passed down the esophagus in sword-swallowing fashion. These endeavors were eclipsed by the work of Mikulicz, who described in detail the appearances of the esophagus and stomach seen with an articulated, jointed gastroscope using electric light.[1,2,3] The modern flexible fiberoptic endoscope based on the phenomenon of total internal reflection of light was invented in 1958 by Hirschowitz et al.[4]

Important features of the variety of rigid instruments currently available are rounded edges at the tip to prevent trauma, a distal fiberoptic light source, and a choice of sizes to suit individual patients. Rigid esophagoscopy is still preferred by many surgeons undertaking esophageal surgery. Its main advantage is a wide lumen (6.0 to 9.0 mm), permitting adequate clearance of retained debris or blood in an obstructed esophagus so that the mucosa can be thoroughly inspected. Nevertheless, inspection of the mucosa via a fiberoptic endoscope is regarded as the best way to evaluate mucosal detail,[5] although magnifying telescopes such as the Storz-Hopkins system may be utilized through the rigid open esophagoscope. The larger lumen of the rigid scope does allow the introduction of biopsy forceps able to take much deeper biopsy specimens. This is of particular importance in the assessment of the extent of disease in patients in whom submucosal spread is extensive in the absence of corresponding mucosal abnormality.

There are, however, disadvantages to rigid esophagoscopy. In addition to usually mandatory general anesthesia, the rigid scope may cause more trauma; perforation is a significant, although infrequent, complication even if the examination is performed by an experienced surgeon. Mucosal laceration or bruising is occasionally encountered in the resected specimen when rigid endoscopy immediately precedes esophagectomy. In contrast, the fiberoptic instrument produces less trauma, is usually undertaken under local anesthesia, and in about three quarters of patients the endoscope can be maneuvered through a malignant stricture, permitting estimation of its length and a view of the distal esophagus, stomach, and duodenum. Since stomach is our first choice as esophageal substitute following resection, prior knowledge of any coexistent gastroduodenal pathology, or of previous gastric surgery, has an important bearing on the choice of organ used to restore continuity. Careful and gentle manipulation of the endoscope is particularly important in the presence of Zenker's diverticulum, large osteophytes of the cervical vertebrae, extreme kyphoscoliosis, or a large goiter.[6]

The incidence of perforation of the esophagus during fiberoptic endoscopy is low.[7] Serious complications occur in only 1 in 1000 examinations and death in 1 in 5000 endoscopies of the upper gastrointestinal tract.[8]

Normal appearances

The esophageal mucosa is arranged in four to six longitudinal folds, which are largely eliminated by air insufflation. The epithelium is white to pink-gray, with a network of longitudinally arranged blood vessels.[9,10] The ora serrata, or Z-line, permits a clear distinction between squamous and columnar cardiac mucosa; the latter has a slightly irregular pitted surface.[10]

Esophagoscopy for malignant esophageal disease

Esophagoscopy is the most reliable investigative procedure to diagnose cancer of the esophagus. It has been claimed that the fixation of the tumor to adjacent structures can be assessed by maneuvering the rigid scope after it has engaged the top of the tumor.[11] This is a subjective assessment, and we have found that it does not add to the decision in the selection of operative procedure. More than 50% of the esophageal circumference must be involved by tumor before obstruction is sufficient to cause dysphagia.[12] When the tumor is large and most of the esophageal circumference is involved, the rigid esophagoscope cannot be passed into the distal esophagus without prior esophageal dilatation. In practice, although the level of the tumor is a determining factor in the selection of the surgical approach, the barium swallow offers more decisive information, since the tumor can be seen in relation to other structures, eliminating any inaccuracies resulting from variations in patient stature.

Cancer of the esophagus has a tendency to spread submucosally and produce satellite lesions well away from the primary malignancy.[10] Carcinoma arising in a hiatal hernia is always an adenocarcinoma.[9] The macroscopic appearances of esophageal cancers are well known, although many combined or transitional forms exist.[10,12-15] The Japanese Society for Esophageal Diseases recognizes five gross types: superficial, elevated, depressed, stricture, and an unclassifiable group.[13] The most common is the circumferential apple-core lesion with mucosal replacement by visible tumor.[14] Diffusely infiltrating scirrhous cancers manifest obvious thickening and rigidity of the esophageal wall, of variable length, with fixation of the irregularly thickened, coarsely nodular, rarely ulcerated mucosa to the deeper layers.[10,15] These infiltrating lesions, producing what may appear to be a benign stricture with normal overlying mucosa, may be betrayed by nodularity of submucosally infiltrated esophageal mucosa. The appearances may be confused by the presence of an inflammatory esophagitis, identical in gross and histologic features to peptic or reflux esophagitis.[12] An exophytic-polypoid growth is rare[14]; such a growth is often bulky with a wide base and usually has a coarsely nodular hemorrhagic surface.[15] The tumor may also be soft, friable, firm, or irregular with a sarcomatous appearance.[14] Occasionally a primary ulcerative configuration, where most of the tumor has been replaced by an excavating ulcer, is encountered.[13] This is characterized by central meniscoid necrosis surrounded by heaped-up everted edges. Usually a major part of the circumference is involved, leading to early circular tortuous narrowing.[10,15] Necrotic tissue may cover the tumor extensively and give a false-negative biopsy result. This latter type must be differentiated from benign causes of ulceration, including reflux esophagitis.[12]

Esophageal stricture: benign or malignant?

Benign peptic stricture

Peptic strictures are smooth in appearance, with conical narrowing of the distal esophagus,[8,16] and occur in about 11% of patients with reflux.[17] Endoscopic features of benign strictures, which are usually 1 to 8 cm long, include the presence of mucosal inflammation, narrowing with failure of actual contraction of the involved segment, proximal dilatation, and a patulous gastroesophageal junction, indicating an incompetent lower esophageal sphincter.[16] Benign stricture formation may also occur secondary to candidiasis, granulomatous esophagitis (Crohn's disease), or corrosive ingestion, or as the result of drug therapy, particularly with nonsteroidal anti-inflammatory agents.[18] Although fistulae are usually associated with malignancy, multiple esophageal fistulae resulting from reflux esophagitis have been described.[19]

Malignant esophageal stricture

No difficulties are usually encountered in obtaining a histologic diagnosis for polypoid tumors and meniscoid lesions in which the proximal tumor edge is clearly visible.[15] Problematic, however, are stenotic lesions. It is often difficult, if not impossible, to make an exact endoscopic diagnosis,[15] particularly when these tumors extend proximally by undermining normal mucosa.[9] It is in such cases that flexible fiberoptic endoscopy with small-caliber endoscopes is particularly helpful[9,15] in negotiating the stricture for biopsies along the length of the lesion. In addition to the type of tumor, other important information to note during the examination include the location of the proximal limit of tumor, the extent and location of the lesion longitudinally and circumferentially, the location of the distal edge in relation to the cardia, the diameter of the existing lumen, and the mucosal appearance of the proximal esophagus.[20]

The length of the tumor is important, since it gives some indication of the stage of the disease. T_1, or stage I, is present when the primary lesion is less than 5 cm in length with incomplete circumferential involvement. T_2, or stage II, appearances are of a primary lesion more than 5 cm long or with complete circumferential esophageal involvement. The TNM stage of disease has been found to correlate well with response to treatment[21]; staging also permits valid comparison of various treatment modalities. Endoscopy also allows the identification of certain complications of malignancy. Bolus obstruction with retention of food may cause dysphagia. Fistulization into the mediastinum or bronchial tree with carcinoma arising in the midesophagus can occasionally be demonstrated by direct injection of contrast material.[9]

Endoscopic biopsy—histology and cytology in esophageal cancer

Biopsy and cytology are complementary techniques.[10,15] Unless contraindicated, it is recommended that multiple biopsies be obtained from nonnecrotic areas. Biopsies should be taken preferentially from junctional areas between proliferative growth and infiltration and not from ulcer bases or edematous adjoining areas.[15] If flexible fiberoptic endoscopy is performed, the central bayonet or spike type of biopsy forceps is preferred,[10,12] especially for tangential lesions.[15] It is vital to recognize that a nondiagnostic biopsy result does not give strong assurance that a tumor is not present.[12] Small nodular elevations with white-yellow discoloration and erosive changes or areas around fistulous openings should be biopsied. The diagnostic yield can be improved by introducing the biopsy forceps into the strictured area and by taking biopsies blindly from the more distal sites.[10,15]

An alternative maneuver is to gently dilate the stricture, so that a small-caliber endoscope can be passed to take biopsies and cytology brushings from within and below the stricture,[15] a procedure that has been shown to be both practical and safe.[22] The flexible fiberscope has been found extremely useful for obtaining cytology samples from visually selected areas, rather than blind nylon brushings.[12] Cytology brushings may be carried out before biopsy to avoid heavy bloodstaining,[10] while some authorities[12] prefer to obtain cytologic material last, believing that bleeding from the brushings may obscure the biopsy target.

Carcinoma of the esophagus is usually a squamous cell lesion, but unusual variants such as varicoid, oat cell, and adenoid cystic carcinoma have been described.[23] The appearance of an organic small stricture with an intact mucosa suggests the presence of extrinsic disease by direct extension from carcinoma of the stomach, lung, or hypopharynx, or by metastasis from carcinoma of the breast, pancreas, or prostate.[12]

Flexible or rigid endoscopy for esophageal malignancy?

It has been proposed that patients who are thought to have esophageal malignancy be examined initially with the flexible scope. Biopsies obtained by fiberscope may be of poor quality; although accurate for the diagnosis of squamous cell carcinoma, a significant false-negative rate is observed when this biopsy technique is applied to adenocarcinoma arising from the cardia and lower esophagus.[24] The open rigid esophagoscope is considered to provide a more satisfactory view and biopsy than flexible fiberoptic examination[12,20] for tumors in the high cervical esophagus.

A prospective comparison of flexible and rigid endoscopy in the evaluation of patients undergoing surgery for esophageal carcinoma has been undertaken in our department. Confirmation of diagnosis was obtained using a flexible fiberscope in all 71 patients studied, in 78% of whom additional information regarding tumor length, the distal esophagus, and gastroduodenal assessment was obtained. Rigid bronchoscopy and esophagoscopy, in that order, and before endotracheal intubation, were performed immediately prior to surgery; no attempt was made to pass the rigid scope beyond the tumor-bearing segment. Fixation of the tumor to the surrounding structures was also assessed by gauging the maneuverability by hand once the rigid scope had engaged the proximal extent of the tumor. Advantages of the fiberoptic scope are that the procedure may be performed under local anesthesia and is far less traumatic and hence less likely to give rise to complications. One patient underwent resection following esophageal rupture arising from rigid esophagoscopy. No other complication arose from endoscopic examination.

The rigid scope was found to detect the proximal extent of tumor at a level 2.4 cm more distal than that diagnosed by the fiberscope. This was believed to be due to a combination of the pulsion effect of the heavier rigid scope and gripping of this larger instrument by the cricopharyngeal sphincter. This difference in tumor level assessment is not of paramount importance for middle- and lower-third tumors, but when a tumor is located in the upper third of the esophagus, confident knowledge of the exact levels of the cricopharyngeus and the tumor is imperative in the selection of anastomotic site and in the decision as to whether laryngectomy is also required in order to obtain proximal tumor clearance. The assessment of pedunculated tumors, which make up 2% to 3% of all squamous cell lesions, with flexible and rigid scopes may occasionally be misleading. A falsely high tumor level may be doc-

PLATE 1. A small polypoid cancer, 9 mm in size, that infiltrated submucosa.

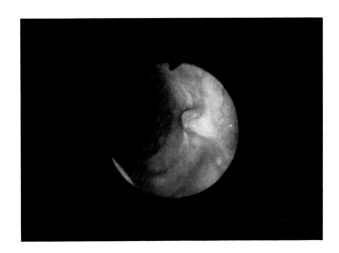

PLATE 2. An erosive cancer that invaded the lamina propria mucosae.

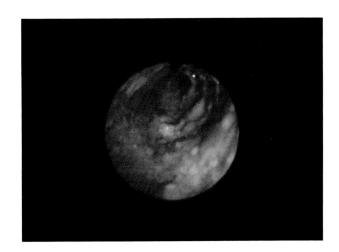

PLATE 3. A minute epithelial cancer, 8 mm in size, appears as a reddish flat lesion.

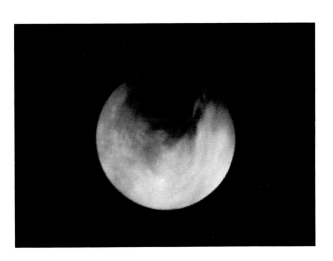

PLATE 4. An intraepithelial cancer 2.9 cm in size. On the right, the lesion is revealed as an unstained area by Lugol's staining.

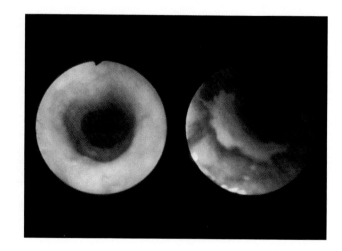

PLATE 5. Cancer tissue (mucosal cancer) is stained blue by toluidine blue.

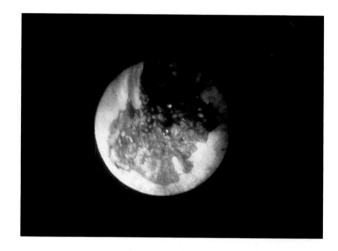

PLATE 6. With Lugol's staining, the normal mucosa turns dark brown while cancerous tissue remains unstained.

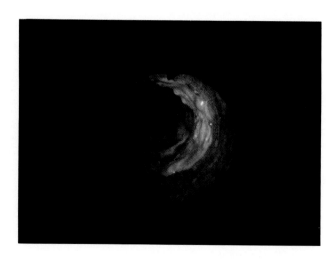

umented, which is perhaps of little consequence when such a lesion is encountered in the distal two thirds of the esophagus. If such a pedunculated lesion in the upper third of the esophagus is incorrectly evaluated at endoscopy, then a pharyngolaryngoesophagectomy may be performed inappropriately when esophagectomy alone might have sufficed.

Difficulty was occasionally encountered in obtaining an adequately large and deep biopsy for histologic examination. Five of the 71 patients required a second examination for confirmation of diagnosis. Certainly, confirmatory biopsies may be difficult to obtain in lesions around the cardioesophageal junction, especially in the presence of inflammatory disease of the distal esophagus resulting from gastroesophageal reflux. In these situations multiple biopsies on separate occasions may be necessary before a diagnosis of carcinoma—and in particular, adenocarcinoma—can be either confirmed or refuted. Flexible endoscopy in these circumstances may be less reliable than rigid esophagoscopy. If the tumor can be negotiated with the flexible scope, then retroflexion may provide a view of the cardia.[12]

We conclude that although endoscopy has limitations in the preoperative evaluation of patients, flexible endoscopy is accurate and in certain situations superior to examination with the rigid scope and, if available, is the examination of choice.

Endoscopy in the detection of early esophageal cancer

Early esophageal cancer is difficult to detect at endoscopy. It has been known for a decade that the early diagnosis of carcinoma in situ or limited to the mucosa (epithelium and lamina propria) is of considerable benefit to the patient in view of the high (90%) 5-year survival rate following surgery.[25] Although it is generally accepted that patients with known risk factors for esophageal cancer should undergo periodic fiberoptic endoscopy, with multiple biopsies and cytologic brushings, the optimum time interval between examinations remains to be established.[12] It has been proposed in China and Iran that esophagitis leads to mucosal atrophy, dysplasia, and subsequently invasive esophageal cancer.[26] In these countries esophagitis is characterized by an irregular friable mucosa with varying degrees of edema, hyperemia, and leukoplakia, but without ulceration. In contrast to reflux esophagitis, these findings occur principally in the middle and lower esophagus but spare the area just proximal to the cardia.[27] The risk of carcinoma has been estimated to be in-

creased 22 times for corrosive lye strictures, 9 times for esophageal webs, 7 times for achalasia, and 6 times for peptic stenosis; it is also thought to be increased in various types of esophageal diverticula.[28]

Barrett's esophagus and the development of adenocarcinoma

There is now good documentation that Barrett's esophagus is secondary to gastroesophageal reflux and that it occasionally leads to adenocarcinoma of the esophagus, with a reported incidence of malignancy of 3% to 9%.[16] A length of 3 cm of columnar lining above the cardia is required as a minimum for diagnosis of a fully developed Barrett's esophagus[29]; this criterion avoids inclusion of many borderline cases. Sequential follow-up studies with endoscopy and biopsy usually fail to identify columnar lining regression with therapy.[30] Nevertheless, the report of two presymptomatic patients who were diagnosed cytologically as developing adenocarcinoma in a Barrett's esophagus and who are now long-term survivors after resection does give some support to the case for continued surveillance.[31] Follow-up examinations may need to be more frequent than twice yearly if the columnar-lined esophagus extends above the aortic arch or dysplasia is evident.[32]

Endoscopic appearances of early lesions

The microscopic changes of early carcinoma are relatively easy to recognize in biopsy and cytology specimens.[27] Dissatisfaction, however, with the Japanese classification of early esophageal cancer, which is based solely on the surface irregularity of lesions, led Monnier et al. in 1985 to a more complete description of these early lesions.[33] This system takes into account mucosal color changes preceding surface irregularity, and also emphasizes the importance of mapping of the mucosal lesions (topographic distribution of the lesions and their relationships). Adequate air insufflation is important to flatten out mucosal folds.[12] In vivo techniques of dye scattering, spraying, or staining (i.e., chromoesophagoscopy) are currently advocated for the detection of early lesions.[10,15,33] The stains most often used are 1% to 2% Lugol's solution, 1% to 2% toluidine blue, and 1% to 2% methylene blue. The esophagus is cleaned with 1% acetic acid, and the segment to be studied is stained by introducing 10 ml of the dye into the lumen via a plastic tube. After 2 to 3 minutes the excess stain is washed away with water or another thorough rinse with 10 ml of 1% acetic acid.[10] The Lugol's iodine test shows that normal esophageal mucosa is iodine positive and that in situ and invasive squamous cell carcinomas are always represented by sharply defined iodine-negative zones.[34] Multicentricity has been defined as tumor sites separated by 5 cm or more of unstained normal mucosa.[35]

These staining techniques permit better targeting of biopsy forceps when diffuse lesions are present. Japanese authors have stressed the importance of discoloration, slight or subtle reddening, shallow depression, uneven grainy surface, and plateau-like elevation in the assessment for early carcinoma. In a report of 115 cases of early carcinoma, Chinese authorities have emphasized features of congestion and edema, superficial erosions, granular and coarse surface patterns, and the identification of polypoid protrusions.[36]

"Early" carcinoma has been classified by European authors into four types.[33] Type I consists of a white, single, localized, elevated lesion in which intraluminal growth and deep infiltration are prominent features, toluidine blue being of minimal help. Type II, the most common lesion, is characterized by diffuse erythroplasia or reddish discoloration. This depressed lesion is multicentric and is characterized by superficial spread, toluidine blue being particularly useful in mapping the extent of the disease. Type III, the mixed variety, consists of white elevated lesions together with red diffuse depressed areas. Type IV is the invisible or occult form of dysplasia and in situ carcinoma and can be detected only with the use of vital staining with toluidine blue. Since squamous cell carcinogenesis of the upper aerodigestive tract may be multicentric and multifocal, a thorough endoscopic screening of the whole mucosa exposed to the action of carcinogens (mouth, pharynx, esophagus, larynx, trachea, bronchi) should be undertaken in the evaluation of high-risk patients and in the investigation of patients awaiting therapy for early cancer at one of these sites, toluidine blue being used for examination of the digestive tract.[33] It has been claimed that rigid instruments allow better differentiation of small mucosal lesions in the esophagus than do fiberoptic ones, the optical resolution power as well as the color differentiation in blue being higher in optical instruments.[37]

Endoscopic ultrasound

An ultrasound transducer may, as an integral part of an endoscope, be introduced into the gastrointestinal tract. Within the esophagus deep penetration of the ultrasonic beam is unnecessary, allowing the use of higher sonographic frequencies to provide greater resolution. There is, however, a decrease in penetration as higher frequencies are employed.[38] The extent and depth of local malignant infiltration and adjacent metastases can be recognized by means of endoscopic ultrasound, which enables differentiation between intramural and extramural lesions in the esophagus.[39] With this technique lymph nodes can be identified along the aorta, in the mediastinum, and at the celiac axis. The technique can detect small lymph glands missed by CT scanning, these glands being more easily distinguished from blood vessels by means of endoscopic ultrasound. Further refinements and advances will depend on simplification of technique, a better understanding of ultrasound images obtained in this way, and improved technical characteristics of the instrumentation.[38]

Electronic endoscopy

The advent of the electronic video endoscope, or "endo TV camera,"[40] directly transmitting the image to monitor as an electronic signal, may finally change endoscopy to endography.[41] At its tip the video endoscope incorporates a small light-sensitive microprocessor chip that transmits signals to a videoprocessor for display on a television screen. Freeze-frame facilities and video replay may allow subsequent reviews of endoscopic examinations by the endoscopist and other members of the gastroenterologic team.[42] This system abolishes the need for fiberoptic light bundles, which are the source of recurring expenditure in endoscope maintenance. Parallel to these developments has been the introduction of microcomputers for analysis and storage of endoscopic data.[43] Endoscopic service data analysis will probably be improved by their application.

BRONCHOSCOPY

The first endoscopic examination of the upper airways was performed in 1880 by Zaufal, using a modified cystoscope.[44] Killian in 1896 began to devote his whole time to endoscopy and adapted the esophagoscope to the direct examination of the trachea. Chevalier Jackson in 1904 improved the direct lighting principle and designed a scope with a suction tube as well as a light carrier.[45]

The main advantage of the flexible bronchoscope, developed in 1968 by Ikeda et al.,[46] over rigid bronchoscopy is the ability to visualize and sample bronchial pathology much more peripherally than is possible with the rigid scope.[47] Fiberoptic bronchoscopy has much to offer in the diagnosis of bronchial and pulmonary disease, particularly tumors of the segmental divisions of the upper lobe bronchi.[48] Furthermore, under radiologic control flexible endoscopy permits biopsy sampling of lesions well beyond visibility.[47]

Tracheobronchial invasion in esophageal cancer

Carcinoma of the esophagus often extends through the esophageal wall to infiltrate neighboring structures, even before the tumor is large enough to cause dysphagia. The trachea or a main bronchus may be involved, often with the development of fistulas.[49] Involvement of the bronchial tree carries a grave prognosis,[50] for in general it precludes the possibility of curative resection. It has been known for more than 20 years that some esophageal cancers can grow to a large size without infiltration of surrounding structures. These tumors may carry a rather better prognosis than infiltrative lesions, which occasionally erode into blood vessels and/or the trachea early in the course of the disease.[51]

Autopsy studies in patients with esophageal cancer have shown the trachea to be infiltrated in about 30% and the bronchi in 18% of cases.[52,53] An esophagobronchial fistula developed in 13 (14.4%) of one reported series of 90 consecutive patients with squamous cell carcinoma of the esophagus.[54] In 1985 Postlethwait summarized 40 years of experience with tracheobronchial invasion by esophageal cancer.[49] Of 153 patients with a carcinoma in the cervical esophagus or thoracic inlet, 26 patients had tracheobronchial invasion on initial evaluation, 24 cases involved trachea, 2 cases involved the left main bronchus, and 4 patients had a tracheoesophageal fistula. Tracheobronchial invasion was identified in 82 of 487 patients with cancer of the upper thoracic esophagus. The trachea was invaded in 36 patients, the left main bronchus in 31, and the right main bronchus in 5; 31 had an established fistula. Bronchial invasion was evident in only 6 of 268 patients with distal thoracic esophageal malignancy, only 2 patients having fistula formation. In Angorn's series[55] tracheobronchial invasion was present in 184 of 1045 patients with carcinoma of the upper thoracic esophagus, a fistula being present in 75 cases. The trachea was invaded in 57%, a bronchus in 40%, and the lung in 3%.

Abnormal bronchoscopic findings in 33.9% of 525 patients with esophageal cancer undergoing evaluation have been previously described in reports from our department.[50,56] Three categories of bronchoscopic involvement are identified. In category I no discernible abnormalities are evi-

dent. Abnormalities observed and classified as impingement (category II) included a bulge at the posterior wall of the trachea or a major bronchus, widening of the carina, and deviation of the trachea or bronchus with or without narrowing. An esophagobronchial fistula was diagnosed when there was a persistent discharge of fluid or air bubbles from a bed of tumor or from the lumen of a bronchus involved by tumor.[56] Tumors invading the tracheobronchial wall or mucosa and/or the presence of a tracheoesophageal fistula were classified as category III.[50]

Normal bronchoscopic findings were seen in 66.1% of patients, impingement was observed in 91 patients (17.3%), and invasion was observed in 87 patients (16.6%). It is in category II that involvement of the tracheobronchial tree is rather uncertain. Impingement may be due only to the presence of an adjacent large tumor, and curative resection may still be seriously considered. Of patients in whom surgery was considered advisable, 48 of 63 patients with impingement and 7 of 51 patients with invasion were found to have resectable tumors.[50]

Tumors of the cervical esophagus and the upper thoracic esophagus tended to involve the trachea. The left main bronchus was most frequently involved in middle-third tumors, this finding being consistent with observations made over 20 years ago by Flavell, who regarded the posterior wall of the left main bronchus as being particularly at risk.[57] Bronchoscopic abnormalities were found in 47.4% of tumors greater than 10 cm in length and in 21.1% of tumors 1 to 3 cm in length evaluated in our department. Thus, even small tumors may occasionally be associated with impingement or invasion of the bronchial tree.[56] The incidence of abnormal appearances at bronchoscopy in esophageal carcinoma[56] were as follows: cervical esophagus and hypopharynx (51.3%), upper-third thoracic (61.1%), middle-third (37.3%), lower-third (12.5%), and abdominal esophagus (5%). These data confirm the belief that bronchoscopy is mandatory in the assessment of patients with esophageal cancer, regardless of the size and location of the tumor in the esophagus.[50,56]

Flexible or rigid bronchoscopy in esophageal carcinoma?

Rigid endoscopy and flexible fiberoptic endoscopy have been found to be equally good for the diagnosis of bronchial carcinoma.[58] The fiberscope can be introduced orally or via the nasal passages into the larynx, or even via an endotracheal or a tracheostomy tube if necessary, using topical anesthesia. For examination via an endotracheal tube, satisfactory conditions can also be obtained using light general anesthesia, muscle relaxants, and intermittent positive-pressure ventilation (IPPV) through a wide-bore (9-mm) tube to which a modified suction unit has been attached.[59] In earlier studies in our department, the results of arterial blood gas analyses confirmed that effective oxygenation and ventilation were maintained using this technique. Flexible bronchoscopy is said to be associated with a low incidence of complications, with the rigid scope sometimes being responsible for laryngeal trauma.[47] It is possible to obtain brush cytologic and transbronchial biopsies at even secondary or tertiary carinae during fiberoptic examination,[60] although the flexible scope is claimed to be less effective than the metal bronchoscope in the evaluation of the rigidity of the bronchus for assessment of operability.[58]

The rigid bronchoscope, a large-caliber, straight-axis instrument, allows detection of even minor degrees of deviation of the trachea by external compression. Only large bronchi can be entered, however, and since the examination is also carried out under general anesthesia the procedure cannot be prolonged unless intermittent jet ventilation is instituted. Although the use of large biopsy forceps may provide satisfactory biopsy specimens, such forceps may lead to brisk hemorrhage, and blood may be inhaled. Fiberoptic transbronchial biopsy may also result in brisk hemorrhage from a bronchial artery or pneumothorax from visceral pleural penetration.[48] Fiberoptic bronchoscopy offers the advantage of a local anesthetic procedure, which in most instances may be undertaken without the constraints of a rigid examination. Fiberoptic bronchoscopy also permits a more complete examination of the vocal cords and posterior walls of the bronchi, the latter being viewed only tangentially through the rigid scope.

The fiberoptic bronchoscope (unlike the rigid bronchoscope, which is an open tube) acts as a space-occupying lesion within the main airway and impairs respiratory function both in patients with obstructive airways disease and in patients with no history of respiratory symptoms.[61,62] Protracted examinations, especially if heavy sedation is used, can lead to a critical reduction in P_{O_2}, and it is recommended that patients with a history of dyspnea during exercise undergo simple respiratory function tests and arterial blood gas analysis prior to fiberoptic bronchoscopy.[48]

The 71 patients with esophageal carcinoma investigated with flexible bronchoscopy in our department subsequently underwent preoperative rigid bronchoscopy, the data obtained being correlated with operative findings. No complications were encountered with either method of bronchoscopic examination.

Flexible fiberoptic and rigid bronchoscopy detected no abnormality in 48 cases (category I), while 20 patients were found to have impingement (category II). In the three patients in category III the fiberscope demonstrated a definite fistulous opening, one in the trachea and two in the left main bronchus. With the rigid instrument a definite fistulous opening was observed only in the patient with a tracheal fistula; the remaining two fistulas were not visualized with certainty, although tumor infiltration into the left main bronchus was noted.

Carinal widening was found to be a very insensitive indicator of subcarinal lymphadenopathy. Unilateral vocal cord paralysis was seen in 5 of 71 patients examined by the fiberscope, with findings being confirmed by recurrent laryngeal nerve compression or encasement by tumor at operation. Seventeen of 48 patients with normal bronchoscopic findings during rigid or flexible examination were found to have advanced mediastinal disease at operation. Infiltration involving pleura, pericardium, lungs, aorta, or vertebrae may not result in impingement or bronchial invasion.

Virtually all patients who are fit for surgery, including those with extensive mediastinal disease, can undergo resection regardless of the presence of bronchoscopic abnormality. Resection would probably be contraindicated only in patients in whom infiltration of the membranous trachea or fistula formation could be demonstrated. We recommend the flexible bronchoscope as the instrument of choice for tracheobronchial evaluation in esophageal cancer.

Flexible esophagoscopy and bronchoscopy together with simple radiographic investigation are sufficient in the preoperative assessment of most patients with carcinoma of the esophagus.

REFERENCES

1. Bremner, C.G.: A joy to swallow: experiences with oesophageal disease (inaugural lecture) Johannesburg, 1984, Wittwatersrand University Press, pp. 1-21.
2. Franklin, R.H.: Oesophagoscopy. In Franklin, R.H., editor: Surgery of the oesophagus, London, 1952, Arnold, pp. 43-48.
3. McSherry, C.K., Cwern, M., Ferstenberg, H., et al: Interventional endoscopy, Curr. Probl. Surg. 22(7):3, 1985.
4. Hirschowitz, B.I., Curtiss, L.E., Peters, C.W., et al: Demonstration of a new gastroscope—the fiberscope, Gastroenterology 35:50, 1958.
5. Silverstein, B.D., and Pope, C.E., II: Role of diagnostic tests in esophageal evaluation, Am. J. Surg. **139**:744, 1980.

6. Demling, L., Elster, K., Koch, H., et al: Endoscopic instruments and techniques for endoscopy of the upper digestive tract. In Endoscopy and biopsy of esophagus, stomach and duodenum: a color atlas, Philadelphia, 1982, W.B. Saunders Co. pp. 3-16.

7. Skinner, D.B., and DeMeester, T.R.: Gastro-esophageal reflux, Curr. Probl. Surg. **13:**5, 1976.

8. Laurence, B.: Upper gastrointestinal endoscopy. In Readings in gastroenterology, 1982, pp. 15-20.

9. Demling, L., Elster, K., Koch, H., et al.: Histopathology of esophageal diseases. In Endoscopy and biopsy of the esophagus, stomach and duodenum: a color atlas, Philadelphia, 1982, W.B. Saunders Co., pp. 21-84.

10. Tytgat, G.N.: Non-radiological investigation of the oesophagus. In Watson, A., and Celestin, L.R., editors: Disorders of the oesophagus: advances and Controversies, London, 1984, Pitman, pp. 24-36.

11. McKeown, K.C.: Carcinoma of the esophagus. J. R. Coll. Surg. Edinb. **24:**253, 1979.

12. Vinayeh, R., and Levin, B.: Endoscopic diagnosis. In DeMeester, T.R., and Levin, B., editors: Cancer of the esophagus, New York, 1985, Grune & Stratton, pp. 43-55.

13. Japanese Society for Esophageal Diseases: Guidelines for the clinical and pathologic studies for carcinoma of the esophagus. I. Clinical classification, Jpn. J. Surg. 6(2):69, 1976.

14. Rubin, P.: Cancer of the gastrointestinal tract: esophagus: detection and diagnosis, JAMA **226:**1544, 1973.

15. Tytgat, G.N.: Diagnosis of malignant lesions in the oesophagus. In Postgraduate course: oesophagus, Stockholm, 1982, World Congress of Digestive Endoscopy, pp. 15-19.

16. Mukhopadhyay, A.K.: Idiopathic lower esophageal sphincter incompetence and esophageal stricture, Arch. Intern. Med. **140:**1493, 1980.

17. Palmer, E.D.: The hiatus–esophagitis–esophageal stricture complex: twenty year prospective study, Am. J. Med. **44:**566, 1968.

18. Wilkins, W.E., Ridley, M.G., and Pozniak, A.L.: Benign stricture of the oesophagus: role of non-steroidal anti-inflammatory drugs, Gut **25:**478, 1984.

19. Raymond, J.I., Khan, A.H., Cain, L.R., et al.: Multiple esophago-gastric fistulas resulting from reflux esophagitis, Am. J. Gastroenterol. **73**(5):430, 1980.

20. Savary, M., and Miller, G.: Der Ösophagus: Lehrbuch und endoskopischer Atlas, Solothurn, 1977, Gussman.

21. Beatty, J.D., DeBoer, G., and Rider, W.D.: Pretreatment assessment, correlation of radiation treatment parameters with survival, and identification and management of radiation treatment failure, Cancer **43:**2254, 1979.

22. Barkin, S., Tomb, S., and Rogers, A.I.: The safety of combined endoscopy, biopsy and dilatation in oesophageal strictures, Am. J. Gastroenterol. **76:**23, 1981.

23. Geboes, K.: Tumours of the oesophagus, Curr. Opin. G. **1**(4):573, 1985.

24. Lusink, L., Sali, A., and Chou, S.T.: Diagnostic accuracy of flexible endoscopic biopsy in carcinoma of the oesophagus and cardia, Aust. N.Z. J. Surg. **53:**545, 1983.

25. Coordinating group for research in oesophageal cancer under rural conditions, Chin. Med. J., 1975, p. 113.

26. Munoz, N., and Crespi, M.: Studies in the aetiology of oesophageal carcinoma. In Watson, A., and Celestin, L.R., editors: Disorders of the oesophagus: advances and controversies, London, 1984, Pitman, pp. 147-154.

27. Thompson, J.J.: Esophageal cancer and the premalignant changes of esophageal diseases. In Cohen, S., and Soloway, R.D., editors: Diseases of the esophagus, New York, 1982, Churchill Livingstone, pp. 239-276.

28. Joske, R.A., and Benedict, E.B.: The role of benign oesophageal obstruction in the development of carcinoma of the esophagus, Gastroenterology **36:**749, 1959.

29. Bremner, C.G., and Hamilton, D.G.: Barrett's esophagus: controversial aspects. In DeMeester, T.R., and Skinner, D.B., editors: Esophageal disorders: pathophysiology and therapy, New York, 1985, Raven Press, pp. 233-239.

30. Savary, M., Monnier, P., and Miller, G.: Diagnosis and pathophysiology of Barrett's oesophagus. Workshop. Diagnosis and treatment of pathological gastro-esophageal reflux, Noordwijk, Netherlands, 1982.

31. Skinner, D.B., Dowlatshahi, K.D., and DeMeester, T.R.: Potentially curable cancer of the esophagus, Cancer **50:**2571, 1982.

32. Harle, I.A., Finley, R.J., Belsheim, M., et al.: Management of adenocarcinoma in a columnar lined esophagus, Ann. Thorac. Surg. 40(4):330, 1985.

33. Monnier, P., Savary, M., and Anani, P.: Endoscopic morphology of "early" esophageal cancer. In DeMeester, T.R., and Skinner, D.B., editors: Esophageal disorders: pathophysiology and therapy, New York, 1985, Raven Press, pp. 333-346.

34. Mandard, A.M., Tourneux, J., Gignoux, M., et al.: In situ carcinoma of the oesophagus: macroscopic study with particular reference to the Lugol test, Endoscopy **12:**51, 1980.

35. Reboud, E., Pradoura, J.P., Fuentes, P., et al.: Multicentric esophageal carcinoma: yield of total endoscopy and vital staining. In DeMeester, T.R., and Skinner, D.B., editors: Esophageal disorders: pathophysiology and therapy, New York, 1985, Raven Press, pp. 347-353.

36. Yang Guanrei, Huang He, Qui Sungliang, and Chang Yuming: Endoscopic diagnosis of 115 cases of early esophageal carcinoma, Endoscopy **14:**157, 1982.

37. Hopkins, H.H.: Fibreoptics in medical endoscopy, Proc. S. M. I. E. R. Reims, 1977, p. 1.

38. Thatcher, B.S., Sivak, M.V., and George, C.: Endoscopic ultrasonography: a preliminary report, Gastrointest. Endosc. **31**(4):237, 1985.

39. Tio, T.L., and Tytgat, G.N.: Endoscopic ultrasonography in the assessment of intra- and transmural infiltration of tumors in the oesophagus, stomach and papilla of Vater and in the detection of extraoesophageal lesions, Endoscopy **16**(6):203, 1984.

40. Classen, M., and Phillip, J.: Electronic endoscopy of the gastrointestinal tract: initial experience with a new type of endoscope that has no fibreoptic bundle for imaging, Endoscopy **16:**16, 1984.

41. Vantrappen, G.: The oesophagus, Curr. Opin. G. **1**(4):547, 1985.

42. Rutgeerts, P.: Oesophagoscopy, Curr. Opin. G. **1**(4):567, 1985.

43. Rozen, P., and Levy, E.: Data management in a gastroenterology endoscopy service: initial experience using a microcomputer, Front. Gastrointest. Res. **7**:96, 1984.

44. Buiter, C.T. In Endoscopy of the upper airways, Amsterdam, 1976, Excerpta Medica, pp. 41-49.

45. Stevenson, S., and Guthrie, D. In History of otolaryngology, Edinburgh, 1976, Churchill Livingstone, pp. 79-109.

46. Ikeda, S.N., Yamai, S., and Ishikawa, K.: Flexible bronchoscope, Keio J. Med. **17**:16, 1968.

47. Stradling, P.: Broncho-fibreoscopy. In Diagnostic bronchoscopy: an introduction, Edinburgh, 1976, Churchill Livingstone, pp. 26-33.

48. Hazards of fibreoptic bronchscopy (editorial), Br. Med. J. **1**:212, 1979.

49. Postlethwait, R.W.: Tracheobronchial invasion by carcinoma of the esophagus. In DeMeester, T.R., and Skinner, D.B., editors: Esophageal disorders: pathophysiology and therapy, New York, 1985, Raven Press, pp. 389-391.

50. Choi, T.K., Siu, K.F., Lam, K.H., et al.: Bronchoscopy and carcinoma of the esophagus. II. Carcinoma of the esophagus with tracheobronchial involvement, Am. J. Surg. **147**:760, 1984.

51. Kay, S.: A ten year appraisal of the treatment of squamous cell carcinoma of the esophagus, Surg. Gynecol. Obstet. **117**:167, 1963.

52. Anderson, L.L., and Lad, T.E.: Autopsy findings in squamous cell carcinoma of the esophagus, Cancer **50**:1587, 1982.

53. Mandard, A.M., Chasle, J., Villediu, B., et al.: Autopsy findings in 111 cases of esophageal cancer, Cancer **48**:329, 1981.

54. Cassidy, D.C., Nord, H.J., Boyce, H.W., Jr., et al.: Malignant esophago-pulmonary fistula treated with and without peroral esophageal prosthesis, Am. J. Gastroenterol. **76**:173, 1981.

55. Angorn, I.B.: Intubation in the treatment of carcinoma of the esophagus, World J. Surg. **5**:535, 1981.

56. Choi, T.K., Siu, K.F., Lam, K.H., et al.: Bronchoscopy and carcinoma of the esophagus I. Findings of bronchoscopy in carcinoma of the esophagus, Am. J. Surg. **147**:757, 1984.

57. Flavell, G.: The investigation of oesophageal disease: oesophagoscopy. In The oesophagus, London, 1963, Butterworths, pp. 12-19.

58. Ashraf, M.H., Walesby, R.K., Shepherd, M.P., et al.: The surgeon's use of the rigid and flexible bronchoscopes in the diagnosis of bronchial carcinoma, Endoscopy **15**:1, 1983.

59. Lett, Z., and Ong, G.B.: Anaesthesia for flexible fibreoptic bronchoscopy, Anaesthesia **29**(5):623, 1974.

60. Webb, J., and Clare, S.W.: A comparison of biopsy results using rigid and fibreoptic bronchoscopes, Br. J. Dis. Chest **74**(1):81, 1980.

61. Albertini, R., Harrel, J.H., and Moser, K.M.: Hypoxemia during fibreoptic endoscopy, Chest **65**:117, 1974.

62. Salisbury, B.G., Metzger, L.F., Altose, M.D., et al.: Effect of fibreoptic bronchoscopy on respiratory performance in patients with chronic airways obstruction, Thorax **30**:441, 1975.

6 Special techniques in the endoscopic diagnosis of esophageal carcinoma

Mitsuo Endo

The operative mortality for esophageal cancer has been reduced by progress in the techniques of esophageal surgery, anesthesiology, and postoperative management. However, the long-term survival has not improved significantly, largely because 82% of the cases are already in stage III or IV at the time of detection.

DETECTION OF EARLY-STAGE CANCER

To improve the postoperative survival rate, the detection of early-stage cancer and adequate combined treatment are important. Of these two, the detection of early cancer is more essential.

What is the early stage of esophageal cancer? This can be considered in terms of depth of invasion and size of the cancer.

Depth of cancerous invasion

In terms of cancer infiltration, mucosal cancer and submucosal cancer are defined as superficial cancer of the esophagus.[1] The 5-year survival rate for patients with mucosal cancer is close to 100%, and that of submucosal cancer patients is 48%, when death from other disease is excluded.

Theoretically, metastasis is present in carcinoma invasive to the level of the lamina propria. In analysis of the depth of superficial cancer, nodal involvement, and vascular invasion, lymph node metastasis was not observed in 17 of 19 mucosal cancer cases. Of these 17 cases, there was no vascular invasion in 16 cases. Thus, 84% of mucosal cancer cases had neither nodal involvement nor vascular invasion.

In contrast, in 104 cases of submucosal cancer, lymph node metastasis was absent in 58 cases, and of these vascular invasion was not seen in 31 cases. Thus, in submucosal cancer cases only 30% of cases had neither nodal involvement nor vascular invasion (see Table 6-1).

From the point of view of cancerous infiltration, therefore, excellent long-term survival can be anticipated in mucosal cancer.[2]

Size of cancer

At the 38th Annual Meeting of the Japanese Society for Esophageal Diseases, held in May 1985, data concerning a total of 54 cases of minute esophageal cancer (1 cm or less in greatest dimension) were collected from 26 institutions in Japan. Of these cases, 53 were superficial cancers—38 (71%) mucosal and 15 (29%) submucosal. There was one case infiltrating as far as the outer wall.

One case of lymph node metastasis (2%) was seen in a submucosal cancer case. Vascular invasion was seen in 3 cases (6%).

Hence, long-term survival could be anticipated in 94% of 54 cases of minute cancer. From this point of view, excellent results could be anticipated in this limited stage of esophageal cancer.

ENDOSCOPIC DIAGNOSIS OF SUPERFICIAL ESOPHAGEAL CANCER

The conventional diagnostic methods for esophageal cancer are barium esophagography and endoscopy combined with biopsy and/or cytologic brushing. Of these methods, the role of endoscopy is the more important in the diagnosis of early-stage esophageal cancer. Because barium passes rapidly if no esophageal obstruction exists, small erosive lesions and flat lesions may be easily overlooked. An endoscopic diagnostic approach is more effective because the color of the lesion is generally distinct. Therefore, endoscopy

TABLE 6-1. Lymph node metastasis and vascular invasion in superficial esophageal cancer (123 cases)

	Epithelial cancer	Mucosal cancer	Submucosal cancer
With nodal involvement			
+ vascular invasion		2	43
− vascular invasion			3
Without nodal involvement			
+ vascular invasion		1	27
− vascular invasion	5	11	31
Total number of cases	5	14	104

should be performed even at the screening phase of esophageal cancer, to detect cancer of the erosive or flat type, or minute lesions.[3,4]

Endoscopic instruments

Forward-viewing fiberoptic endoscopes are usually employed for the diagnosis of the esophageal lesion. Both panendoscopes and shorter esophagofiberscopes are utilized. Most fiberscopes can be angulated to 210 degrees at the tip. This permits visualization of the gastric cardia from a retrograde direction (Fig. 6-1). At present a variety of fiberscopes with different diameters are employed in the ordinary clinic. These include narrow forward-viewing fiberscopes with a standard biopsy channel (e.g., the Olympus XQ-type), which are convenient for both observation and ancillary procedures.

Endoscopic findings of superficial cancer of the esophagus

Superficial cancer—that is, mucosal or submucosal cancer—can be detected by conventional endoscopic examination. Endoscopically, submucosal cancer appears as a small protruding or depressed lesion without esophageal obstruction. The surface is fragile and granular. Fibrin or white furlike material is sometimes attached to its surface (Plate 1).

Mucosal cancer is commonly observed as an erosive lesion with clearly demarcated reddening, shallow depression, faint granularity, and coarseness, a flat lesion, or, less commonly, a small sessile or low plateau-like lesion (Plate 2). Even in erosive lesions, when the surface is markedly granular, the cancerous invasion reaches the submucosa.

Furthermore, intraepithelial cancer (carcinoma in situ) is observed among the flat-type lesions, the surface of which is almost completely flat and frequently reddened. In addition, epithelial cancer can appear as white thickened or slightly irregular mucosa without discoloration (Plates 3 and 4).

Endoscopic classification of superficial esophageal cancer

Endoscopic findings of superficial cancer can be categorized as (1) polypoid, (2) plateau, (3) flat, (4) erosive, (5) ulcerative, (6) mixed, (7) multiple, or (8) unclassified. Furthermore, the flat type of superficial cancer can be categorized into three subtypes depending on the surface appearance: reddening, coarseness, and dirty white surface. In the mixed type, a mixture of two or more basic types can sometimes be seen in a single lesion.

One hundred twenty-three resected cases of superficial esophageal cancer, analyzed according to this categorization, showed mucosal cancer in only the erosive and the flat types. In the small polypoid, the flat, and the erosive types of superficial cancer, the incidence of nodal involvement was low (see Table 6-2).

ENDOSCOPIC STAINING

In addition to gross appearance, dye spraying during the endoscopic procedure can provide even more precise information for diagnosis of minute cancer and the flat type of esophageal cancer. In transendoscopic dyeing procedures two staining techniques are employed, separately or together—staining with 2% toluidine blue and with 3% iodine (Lugol's) solution.[5,6]

Toluidine blue staining

A thin catheter is inserted into the esophagus through the biopsy channel of the fiberscope, and 2% toluidine blue solution is sprayed gradually from the lower to the upper esophagus. One min-

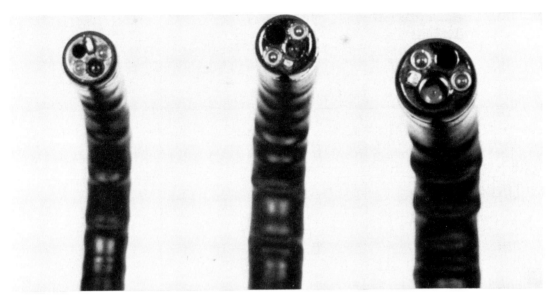

Fig. 6-1. Esophagofiberscopes. *Left,* Olympus P type. *Center,* Olympus XQ type. *Right,* Olympus B type.

ute after spraying, the esophagus is washed with water and suction is utilized to remove excess fluid.

Carcinomatous tissue appears blue. The normal mucosa is almost completely unstained (Plate 5). Necrotic tissue, fibrin, and ingested or refluxed foreign bodies stain dark blue. Cleansing of the esophageal lumen is therefore necessary before the staining process.

However, this staining method is not absolutely specific for cancer. Esophagitis and the esophageal ulcer also stain blue. The staining appearance of cancer differs from that of esophagitis. The former is stained blue in a meshlike appearance, but the latter is stained blue uniformly.

Much remains to be learned about the exact staining process. In the histologic examination of frozen sections, it can be seen that not only cancer cells absorb the dye pigment, but that the dye pigment is also taken up between cancer cells and also by necrotic material.[7]

Iodine (Lugol's) staining

The procedure for iodine staining is almost the same as that for toluidine blue staining, but it is unnecessary to wash the esophagus with water. Immediately after spraying of 3% iodine (Lugol's) solution, the normal mucosa turns dark brown while malignant tissue remains unstained (Plate 6).

Although it has been said that Lugol's solution turns intraepithelial glycogen particles dark brown in normal squamous epithelium, this phe-

nomenon is not yet completely understood.[5] Be that as it may, this procedure is very effective in obtaining precise information concerning intraepithelial invasion and small accessory lesions in esophageal cancer.[2,5]

Comparison of the two modes of staining

When the cancer appears on the surface of the esophagus, both modes of staining give positive results. When noncancerous epithelium covers cancerous tissue, only Lugol's staining is positive. Both modes of staining are negative when the cancerous tissue is under full-thickness normal mucosa. Of the two, iodine (Lugol's) staining is the more widely applied in screening examinations.

SYMPTOMS OF SUPERFICIAL ESOPHAGEAL CANCER

In the 123 cases, common symptoms of superficial esophageal cancer were mild esophageal pain at meals, slight dysphagia, and vague, undefined discomforts in the esophagus. In particular, the complaint of esophageal pain at meals or a tingling sensation was characteristic in erosive and ulcerative types of cancerous lesions. Asymptomatic cases (27%) were detected in routine gastric surveys, during follow-up for esophageal achalasia, and in cases accompanied by gastric cancer. (See Table 6-3.)

TABLE 6-2. Endoscopic classification and pathologic findings in superficial esophageal cancer (123 cases)

Endoscopic type	With lymph node metastasis			Without lymph node metastasis		
	Epithelial cancer	Mucosal cancer	Submucosal cancer	Epithelial cancer	Mucosal cancer	Submucosal cancer
Superficially elevated						
Polypoid	—	—	8	—	—	16
Plateau-like	—	—	7	2	1	11
Superficially flat	—	—	—	—	—	—
Superficially depressed						
Erosive	—	1	3	3	9	11
Ulcerative	—	—	6	—	—	9
Mixed						
Polypoid + flat	—	—	—	—	—	2
Polypoid + plateau-like	—	—	—	—	—	1
Superficially elevated + erosive	—	—	16	—	—	4
Erosive + ulcerative	—	—	1	—	—	2
Multiple						
Erosive	—	1	—	—	2	—
Superficially elevated erosive	—	—	4	—	—	2
Unclassified	—	—	1	—	—	—
TOTAL NUMBER OF CASES	—	2	46	5	12	58

TABLE 6-3. Chief complaints of superficial esophageal cancer patients (123 cases)

Chief complaints	Early cancer (75 cases)	Superficial cancer with metastasis (48 cases)
Slight esophageal or retrosternal pain in swallowing	15	9
Slight dysphagia	13	18
Foreign-body sensation in the throat	4	0
Pressure symptom in the lower esophagus	6	2
Epigastralgia	6	2
Chest pain	1	1
Nausea, hematemesis, anorexia	6	5
Supraclavicular lymph nodes involvement	0	2
No symptoms	24 (32%)	9 (19%)

Combined esophageal and gastric cancer is not uncommon. Eleven cases of gastric cancer among 123 cases of superficial esophageal cancer were encountered. Nine of the 11 cases were early gastric cancer. The necessity of careful examination of the esophagus and the stomach, if cancer has been detected in either of them, has been emphasized.

To detect asymptomatic cases, a semiannual mass survey program may be important in high-risk groups, such as men aged 50 or more.

CONCLUSION

The true early stage of esophageal cancer, in which long-term survival can be anticipated, is thought to be mucosal cancer, or minute cancer (1 cm or less in greatest dimension).

In the detection of these early cancers, the role of endoscopy is extremely important. For the diagnosis of small, flat, or erosive lesions, the endoscopic diagnostic approach is more effective than barium esophagography, because the color of the lesion is generally distinct. Moreover, endoscopic staining with iodine (Lugol) or toluidine blue can provide even more precise information for the diagnosis of small or superficial esophageal lesions.

REFERENCES

1. Japanese Society for Esophageal Disease: Guidelines for the clinical and pathologic studies on carcinoma of the esophagus, Jpn. J. Surg. **6:**69, 1976.
2. Endo, M., Kinoshita, Y., Yamada, A., Ide, H., and Nakayama, K.: Surgical treatment of thoracic esophageal cancer, including clinical evaluation of early esophageal cancer. In Pfeiffer, C.J., editor: Cancer of the esophagus, vol. 2, Boca Raton, Fla., 1982, CRC Press, Inc., pp. 57-69.
3. Endo, M., Yamada, A., Ide, H., Yoshida, M., Hayashi, T., and Nakayama, K.: Early cancer of the esophagus: diagnosis and clinical evaluation, Int. Adv. Surg. Oncol. **3:**49, 1980.
4. Monnier, P., Savary, M., and Anani, P.: Endoscopic morphology of "early" esophageal carcinoma. In DeMeester, T.R., and Skinner, D.B., editors: Esophageal disorders: pathophysiology and therapy, New York, 1985, Raven Press, pp. 333-346.
5. Voegeli, R.: Die Schillersche Jodprobe im Rahmen der Osophagus-Diagnostik (Vorlaufige Mitteilung), Pract. Oto-rhino-laryng. **28:**230, 1966.
6. Sano, M., Okuda, S., and Tamura, H.: Endoscopic diagnosis of esophageal cancer by staining with Lugol's solution. In Takemoto, T., et al., editors: Endoscopic dyeing, Tokyo, 1978, Igaku-Tosho-Shuppan, p. 13. (In Japanese.)
7. Endo, M., Sakakibara, N., Suzuki, H., et al.: Endoscopic observation of esophageal lesions by staining with methylene blue solution, Prog. Digest. Endoscopy **11:**34, 1972. (In Japanese.)

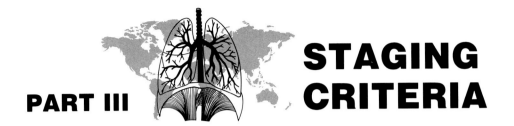

PART III

STAGING CRITERIA

Hiroshi Akiyama, Masahiko Tsurumaru, and Harushi Udagawa

There is no doubt that optimal patient management requires the most precise staging possible. From the surgical point of view, we expect imaging techniques to provide us with an accurate preoperative assessment of the following:

1. The extent of tumor invasion:
   a. The precise depth of superficial tumors that do not invade the muscularis propria
   b. The extent of extraesophageal invasion when present
2. The presence or absence of distant disease:
   a. Hematogenous metastases
   b. Lymph node metastases

In this chapter, modern imaging techniques are reviewed from this perspective.

DEPTH OF TUMOR INVASION
Diagnosing precise depth of superficial tumors that do not invade the muscularis propria

It is well known that esophageal carcinoma that has only invaded locally to the level of the submucosa may have widespread lymphatic metastases. However, in our experience, we have encountered only one case of lymphatic metastasis in a nonradiated tumor superficial to the submucosal layer. This patient demonstrated invasion only to the level of the muscularis mucosae, yet developed cervical lymph node metastases 3 years after resection of his primary tumor. Therefore, we believe that extended lymph node dissection may not be necessary if a preoperative diagnosis of carcinoma in situ or perhaps carcinoma invading only the lamina propria mucosae can be made with certainty. Although this degree of precision in staging is not generally available at present, endoscopic ultrasonography (EUS) is a promising new technique that may be available for this purpose in the future. Recently, several groups have been engaged in developing this technique,[1,2,3] but, at present, technical problems still limit its use to research programs.

Diagnosis of extraesophageal invasion of surrounding organs

Because contiguous extension into the aorta or tracheobronchial tree usually precludes a curative surgical resection, the extent of extraesophageal invasion is a critical area of preoperative evaluation. Formerly, this assessment could only be inferred from indirect evidence such as the esophageal axis deviation on barium esophagogram.[4] However, recent improvements in imaging techniques have made more direct information available.

Aortic invasion

In 1983, Picus et al.[5] reported abnormal findings on CT scan that could be used to make a preoperative diagnosis of direct aortic invasion by esophageal carcinoma. Their criteria are based on the extent of direct contact between the tumor and the aorta. If more than 90 degrees of the aortic circumference is in direct contact with the tumor, aortic invasion may be assumed. In general, this finding has been supported by other authors,[6-8] as well as by our own experience.

Since April, 1984, we have treated 33 patients with esophageal carcinoma who were evaluated by CT scan to rule out aortic invasion. In all cases the final assessment was made either intraoperatively or at autopsy.

Of these 33 patients, six had direct aortic invasion that could not be separated surgically. In all six of these cases, the preoperative scan showed greater than 90 degrees of the aortic surface to be in direct contact with the tumor. All of the other 27 patients had less than 90 degrees of contact.

This is compelling evidence in support of the criteria of Picus et al. for aortic invasion. However, it is not always easy to measure precisely the area of contact between the tumor and the aorta. Furthermore, the question remains: is the area of greatest contact the actual site of invasion?

Additional insight can be gained if we examine the aortic circular high-density layer. This is an area within the aortic wall that is slightly radi-opaque on plain CT scan (Fig. 7-1). Because calcified atheromatous plaque appears on its lu-minal surface, this is thought to represent the lamina media. If the quality of the CT scan is good enough to visualize the complete aortic cir-cular high-density layer above and below the tu-mor, the disruption of this layer at the level of the tumor may be direct evidence of invasion (Fig. 7-2).

Five out of six patients with confirmed aortic invasion demonstrated this sign. In one patient, direct aortic invasion was confirmed intraopera-tively despite good-quality CT scans that allowed the aortic circular high-density layer to be traced in all sections. Fig. 7-3 shows that this tumor had a marked tendency to infiltrate the periaortic fat. In this case, utilizing the criteria of Picus et al. would have allowed the correct diagnosis to be made.

We now regard disruption of the aortic circular high-density layer as direct evidence of aortic in-vasion, and greater than 90 degrees of tumor-aorta contact as being highly suggestive of aortic in-vasion.

Tumors in the area of the aortic arch pose a special problem in diagnosis. The oblique ori-entation of the aorta at this point obscures visu-alization of the circular high-density layer. In this situation, CT scan with contrast enhancement may provide additional information (Fig. 7-4).

Endoscopic ultrasonography is also useful in diagnosing aortic invasion, but only if the scope can be passed through the lesion.[2] Unfortunately, this is usually not possible. Fig. 7-5 is an example of the rare case in which it was. Here, we were able to examine the tumor invading the aorta di-rectly. The hypoechoic layer of the aortic wall is disrupted by direct invasion of the tumor, and the shape of the aorta is deformed.

The hypoechoic layer seems to be identical to the circular high-density layer visualized by CT scan. However, this correlation is not conclusive, because the number of cases we have examined is still small.

On the other hand, it is often easy to ascertain that there is no aortic invasion by using EUS (Fig. 7-6). Unlike CT scanning, which generates dis-continuous sections, EUS allows a complete, con-tinuous examination along the entire lesion. Hence EUS may yield more definitive results than CT scans in evaluating aortic invasion.

Direct invasion of the tracheo-bronchial tree

Although recently several reports have ap-peared that demonstrate the usefulness of CT scans in diagnosing direct invasion of the tra-cheobronchial tree by esophageal carcinoma,[5,7,8] this should not be accepted uncritically without further qualification. CT scanning is very useful in detecting advanced cases in which there is ei-ther polypoid intrusion into the tracheobronchial lumen or marked airway deformity (Fig. 7-7). However, at present, CT scans cannot resolve the membranous portion of the trachea or of the main stem bronchi as a distinct layer. Therefore, there is no way to distinguish with certainty between contiguous compression and direct invasion. This is shown clearly in Figs. 7-8 and 7-9. Similarly, because EUS is also unable to resolve this layer, it offers little hope for providing additional in-formation in this important area.

The most reliable examination at present, though still not completely satisfactory, seems to be flexible fiberoptic bronchoscopy.[9,10] Until ad-vancements in imaging techniques make it pos-sible to diagnose direct invasion of the tracheo-bronchial tree by esophageal cancer more accu-rately, flexible fiberoptic bronchoscopy should continue to be the essential part of the preoper-ative staging procedure.

METASTATIC LESIONS
Diagnosis of hematogenous metastases

The preoperative workup of esophageal car-cinoma should include a thorough evaluation of the three most common sites of hematogenous metastases: liver, lung, and bone.[11,12]

Abdominal ultrasound is the method of choice for detecting hepatic metastases. For this purpose, the convex, rather than the linear, probe should be used, since it has a smaller blind area.[13] The echographic characteristics of hepatic metastases have been reported elsewhere.[14,15] Although ab-dominal ultrasound is more sensitive, easier to perform, and less expensive than CT scanning, the differential diagnosis of metastatic tumor ver-sus hepatocellular carcinoma, hemangioma, or other hepatic tumor may occasionally require ad-ditional studies such as dynamic CT scanning or angiography.[16]

Bone scintigraphy using technetium 99m phos-phate compounds is the most sensitive imaging technique for detecting abnormalities in the skel-etal system. However, because it is nonspecific, all abnormalities should be further investigated to rule out benign inflammatory lesions before a di-agnosis of metastasis is made.

To detect pulmonary metastases, routine pos-terior-anterior and lateral chest x-ray films are still

Text continued on p. 59.

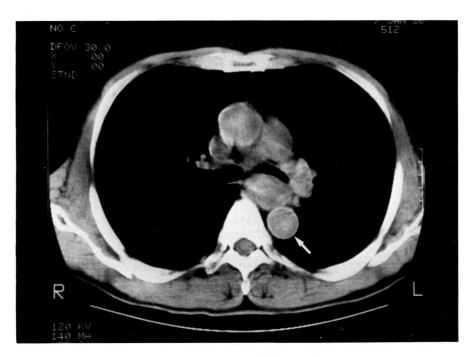

Fig. 7-1. Aortic circular high-density layer *(white arrow).*

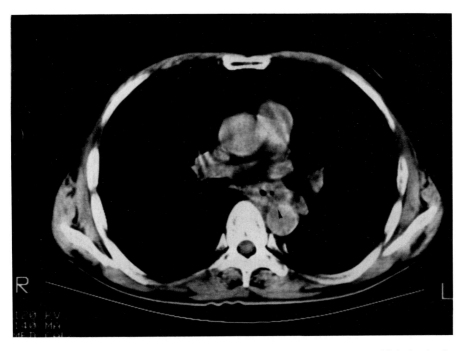

Fig. 7-2. Direct tumor invasion of the aorta with disruption of aortic circular high-density layer *(black arrowhead).*

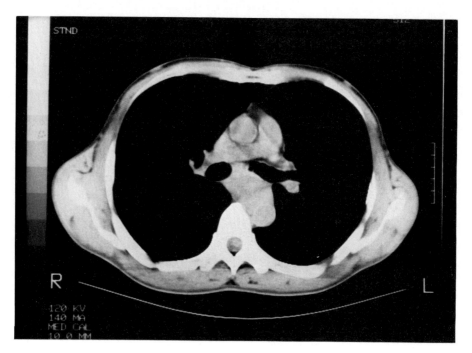

Fig. 7-3. Direct tumor invasion of the aorta without disruption of aortic circular high-density layer.

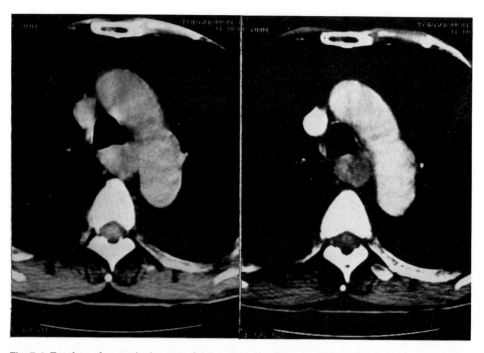

Fig. 7-4. Esophageal tumor in the area of the aortic arch. CT scan with contrast enhancement *(right)* provides more convincing evidence of lack of tumor invasion of the aortic arch than plain CT scan *(left)*.

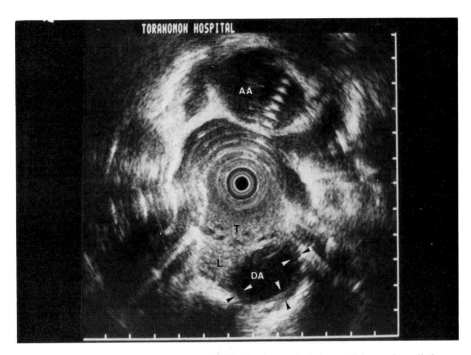

Fig. 7-5. Direct tumor invasion of the aorta (EUS). The hypoechoic layer of the aortic wall *(between arrowheads)* is disrupted. The shape of the aorta is apparently deformed. *AA,* Ascending aorta; *DA,* descending aorta; *T,* tumor; *L,* lymph node metastasis.

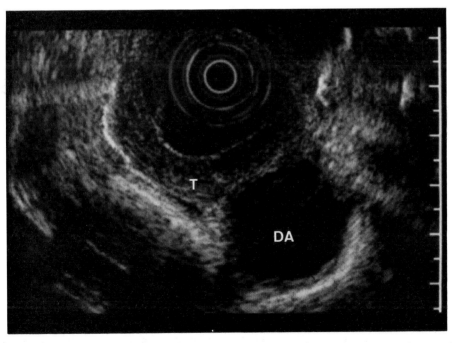

Fig. 7-6. Esophageal tumor without direct invasion of the aorta (EUS). The structure of the aortic wall is preserved, and there is a hyperechoic line between the tumor and the aortic wall. *DA,* Descending aorta; *T,* tumor.

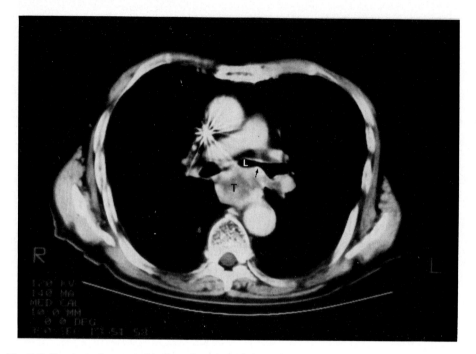

Fig. 7-7. Esophageal tumor with direct invasion of the main stem bronchus. The deformity of the left main bronchus *(L, black arrow)* is evident. *T,* Tumor.

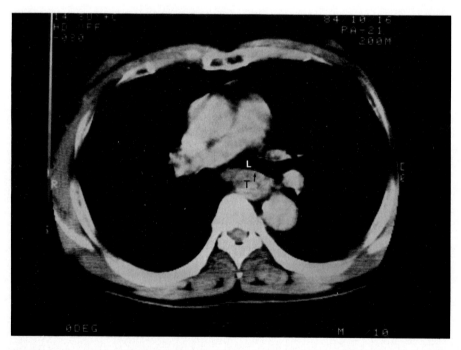

Fig. 7-8. Posterior wall of the left main bronchus is compressed by the tumor *(L, black arrow),* but there is no direct invasion. *T,* Tumor.

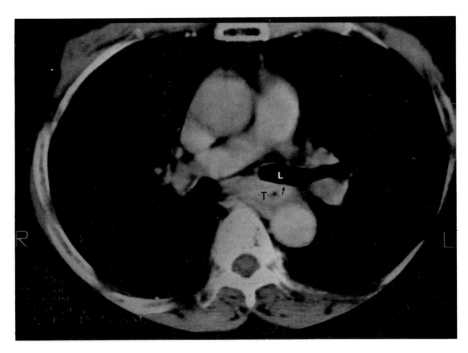

Fig. 7-9. Esophageal tumor with direct invasion of the left main bronchus *(L, black arrow).* One can point out no difference between this and Fig. 7-8. *T,* Tumor.

the most convenient and useful procedure. Gallium citrate scintigraphy is an ancillary procedure that is occasionally useful in evaluating any abnormalities. Chest linear tomography and CT scanning provide the most definitive noninvasive methods for evaluating suspicious lesions.

Diagnosis of lymph node metastases

The presence of hematogenous metastases greatly limits what a surgeon can offer a patient with esophageal cancer. On the other hand, metastasis to the regional lymph nodes is the very frontier where aggressive surgical intervention may cure a patient with a disseminating tumor. Therefore, preoperative detection of lymph node metastases, especially at the margins of the planned resection, is critically important. For this reason, abdominal ultrasound, cervical ultrasound, and endoscopic ultrasound have come to play an increasingly important role in the staging and preoperative evaluation of patients with esophageal carcinoma.

Detection of enlarged intraabdominal lymph nodes by transabdominal ultrasonography has been reported by many investigators.[17-19] Because lymph node metastases from esophageal cancer are usually limited to the region around the celiac axis and the upper paragastric area, these metastases are relatively easy to detect (Fig. 7-10), although EUS is superior when available. Most

detectable enlarged nodes (Fig. 7-11) contain tumor metastases, especially when they are hypoechoic overall and show coarse internal echoes.[19] More distant lymph node metastases usually indicate that the cancer has advanced beyond the limits of curative surgical resection (Figs. 7-12 and 7-13).

Cervical ultrasonography is another indispensable preoperative examination.[20-22] Scanning should not be limited to the neck proper (Figs. 7-14 and 7-15) but should also include the superior mediastinum, especially on the right side where there is a large acoustic window (Figs. 7-16 to 7-20). In other words, lymph nodes detected by this method include the very nodes located at the margin of the thoracic dissection.[23]

From April, 1984, to November, 1985, we performed preoperative cervical ultrasonography on 70 patients with esophageal carcinoma. This included 8 patients with hypopharyngeal or cervical esophageal tumors. Lymph nodes detected by ultrasound that were larger than 5 mm × 10 mm, or were spherical, clearly demarcated, hypoechoic, and larger than 5 mm, were diagnosed as metastases. Lymph nodes smaller than 5 mm or poorly demarcated nodes with fine homogeneous internal echoes that did not displace surrounding structures were diagnosed as nonmalignant.

Among these 70 patients examined by cervical ultrasound, 66 lymph nodes were identified; 50

Text continued on p. 65.

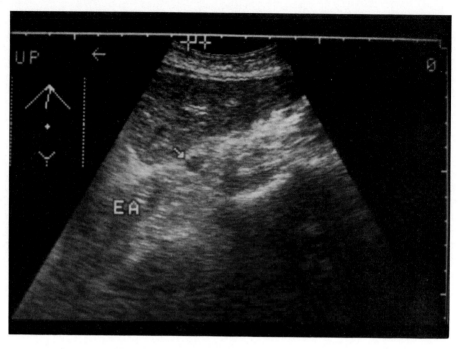

Fig. 7-10. Enlarged paracardiac lymph node. This node *(white arrow)* was proven to contain metastasis. *EA*, abdominal esophagus.

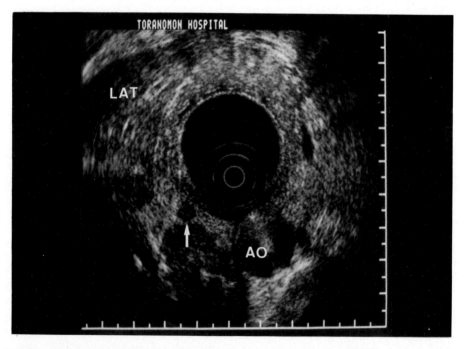

Fig. 7-11. Enlarged paracardiac lymph node on EUS. This *(white arrow)* is the same node shown in Fig. 7-10. *LAT*, Lateral segment of the liver; *AO*, aorta.

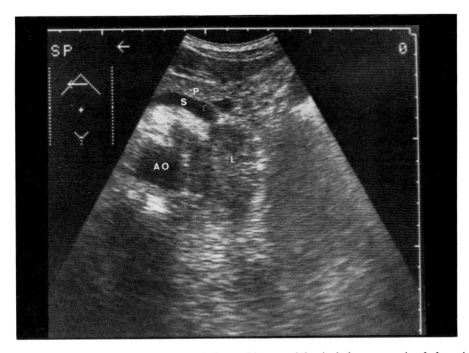

Fig. 7-12. Paraaortic lymph node metastasis detected by transabdominal ultrasonography. *L,* Lymph node metastasis; *P,* pancreas; *S,* splenic vein; *AO,* aorta.

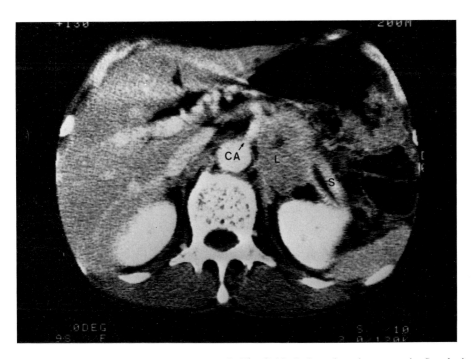

Fig. 7-13. CT scan of the same patient shown in Fig. 7-12. *L,* Lymph node metastasis; *S,* splenic vein; *CA,* celiac axis.

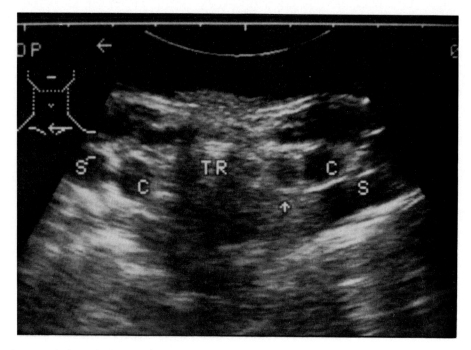

Fig. 7-14. Left cervical paraesophageal lymph node metastasis detected by cervical ultrasonography *(white arrow). C,* Common carotid arteries; *S,* subclavian arteries; *TR,* trachea.

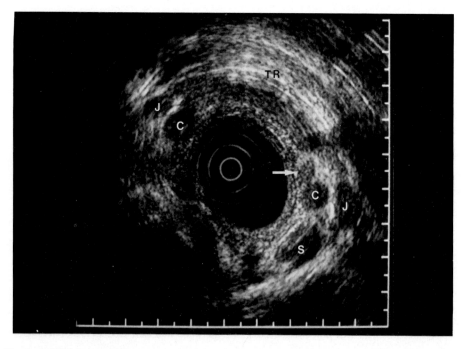

Fig. 7-15. EUS image of the same node shown in Fig. 7-14. *White arrow,* Lymph node metastasis; *C,* common carotid arteries; *S,* subclavian artery; *J,* internal jugular veins; *TR,* trachea.

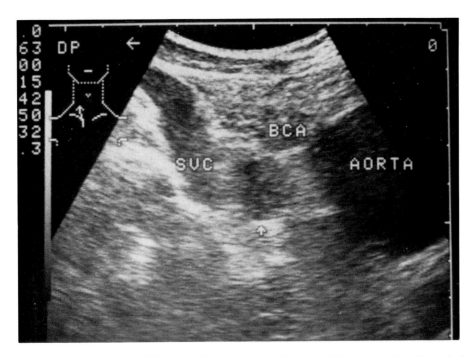

Fig. 7-16. Right paratracheal lymph node metastasis *(white arrow)* between the brachiocephalic artery *(BCA)* and the superior vena cava *(SVC)*.

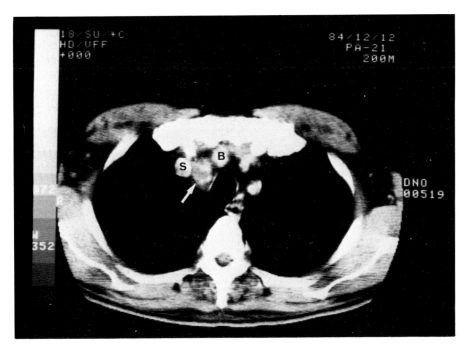

Fig. 7-17. CT scan of the same node shown in Fig. 7-16. *White arrow,* Lymph node metastasis; *B,* brachiocephalic artery; *S,* superior vena cava.

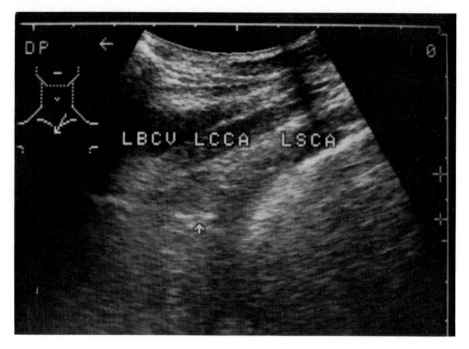

Fig. 7-18. Deep left superior mediastinal lymph node metastasis *(white arrow)* detected by cervical ultrasonography. *LBCV*, Left brachiocephalic vein; *LCCA*, left common carotid artery; *LSCA*, left subclavian artery. Such good visualization of the left superior mediastinum is rather rare.

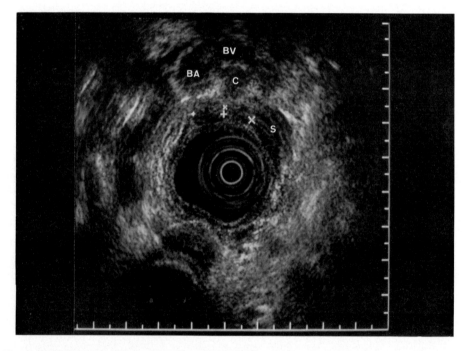

Fig. 7-19. EUS image of the same patient shown in Fig. 7-18. + +, *xx*, Lymph node metastases. Node indicated by *xx* is identical to the one in Fig. 7-18. *C*, Left common carotid artery; *S*, left subclavian artery; *BA*, brachiocephalic artery; *BV*, left brachiocephalic vein.

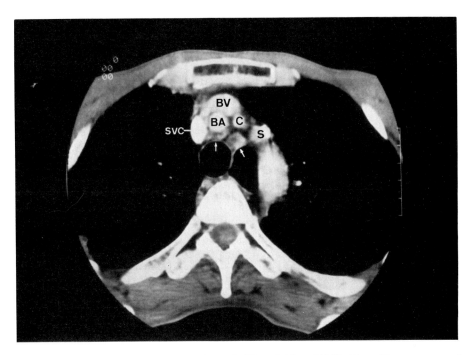

Fig. 7-20. CT scan of the same patient shown in Figs. 7-18 and 7-19. The white arrows are the same nodes indicated by + + and *xx* in Fig. 7-19. *SVC,* Superior vena cava. For other symbols, see legend to Fig. 7-19.

of these were diagnosed as metastases. Of these 50 lymph nodes, 38 (76%) contained cancer on histopathologic examination. Only one out of 16 nodes diagnosed as nonmalignant preoperatively contained metastases. (See Table 7-1.)

From another perspective, of these 70 patients 63 had histopathologically proven lymph node metastases within the area examined by cervical ultrasonography. Only 38 (60%) of these were correctly identified preoperatively. In the sub-group of nodes larger than 5 mm, 38 out of 43 nodes (88%) were correctly identified, including 23 of 25 cervical and superior mediastinal metastases from thoracic or abdominal esophageal tumors. (See Table 7-2.)

From these data, it is clear that at present there are limits to the accuracy of cervical ultrasonography. The rate of false-positive examinations was rather high, 24%, and ultrasonography failed to identify metastases smaller than 5 mm. Nevertheless, ultrasonography is still the best means available for identifying lymph node metastases in the superior mediastinal and cervical areas. Because this information is essential in selecting candidates for extended superior mediastinal and cervical lymph node dissection, we recommend that this examination be a routine part of the preoperative evaluation.

Endoscopic ultrasonography is another effective means of detecting lymph node metastases[1,2]

(see Figs. 7-15 and 7-19). EUS can often detect pathologic nodes that are missed by conventional ultrasonography (Fig. 7-21). Metastatic lesions around the celiac axis and in the upper paragastric area in particular are more easily and more accurately detected by EUS than by transabdominal ultrasonography (see Fig. 7-11).

The disadvantages of this examination are that (1) it is highly effective only in the regions near to the esophagus and the stomach (approximately 4 cm from the center of the shaft when a 7.5-MHz probe is used), (2) there cannot be any intermediate structures causing acoustic interference, and (3) it is often impossible to observe lymph nodes aboral to the tumor, because of esophageal stenosis. The second point is important to remember, because clear visualization of the right recurrent lymph node chain along the brachiocephalic artery and its bifurcation is obscured by the trachea. This region is more completely visualized by conventional cervical ultrasonography (see Figs. 7-16 and 7-17). Conversely, lymph nodes in the left superior mediastinum are more readily examined by EUS (see Figs. 7-18 to 7-20).

Finally, although EUS can detect very small lymph nodes that may be overlooked by ultrasonographic scanners using lower frequencies, it does not differentiate well between metastatic and nonmetastatic lymph nodes. This is a problem

TABLE 7-1. Pathologic diagnosis of lymph nodes detected by cervical ultrasonography

Ultrasound diagnosis	Pathologic diagnosis	
	Malignant	Nonmalignant
Positive 50 (29*)	38 (23)	12 (6)
Negative 16 (6)	1 (0)	15 (6)

*Carcinoma in thoracic or abdominal esophagus only.

TABLE 7-2. Detectability of histopathologically positive lymph nodes by cervical ultrasonography

Ultrasound diagnosis	Number of lymph nodes	
	All cases (n = 63)	Carcinoma in thoracic or abdominal esophagus only (n = 31)
Positive	38 (60%)	23 (72%)
Negative	1 (2%)	0 (0%)
Not detected	24 (38%)	9 (28%)
Nodes larger than 5 mm		
Positive	38/43 (88%)	23/25 (92%)

shared by all forms of ultrasonography and is a direct function of the frequency used. We can only hope that further technical improvements in the apparatus itself will yield better resolution and consequently more definitive diagnosis.

Computed tomography is also used to detect lymph node metastases as part of the preoperative evaluation[5-8,24] (see Figs. 7-13, 7-17, and 7-20). However, CT offers no definitive advantages over ultrasonography[19-21] as long as the ultrasound apparatus is applicable and an acoustic window is present. Moreover, it is impractical to take sections every 5 mm from the neck to the celiac axis, and this is the degree of definition required for CT effectiveness. Now that there are three separate ultrasonographic approaches—transabdominal, transcervical, and EUS—CT will probably play a subsidiary role in this area.

and the examiner can arbitrarily define the axis of orientation according to the requirements of each situation. Thus, anatomic abnormalities may be resolved as being malignant or not, and their precise structural relationships can be defined noninvasively. This would be true for both primary lesions and secondary lesions. At present MRI is still inferior to CT in spatial resolution, but this problem should be overcome in time.

It is true that the greater the number of perspectives we have, the more complete our understanding will be. The important question is: which perspectives do we need to make the best choice of therapy? Because MRI is still under development, and our experience is limited, we feel it is too early to pass final judgment on the relative merits of MRI and CT.

MAGNETIC RESONANCE IMAGING OF THE ESOPHAGEAL CANCER

Magnetic resonance imaging (MRI) is a technique that promises to offer advances in almost every area of preoperative evaluation.[25-28] Unlike other radiographic methods, which rely on radiopacity to create images, and which can visualize anatomic structures only in limited orientations, MRI is capable of detecting tissue characteristics,

CONCLUSION

Rapid developments in imaging techniques have led to highly accurate clinical staging of esophageal cancer. This in turn has allowed better therapeutic decisions for the individual patient. What is expected in coming imaging techniques is greater sensitivity and more precise specificity. This should be accomplished utilizing radiologic, physical, chemical, immunologic, and biologic

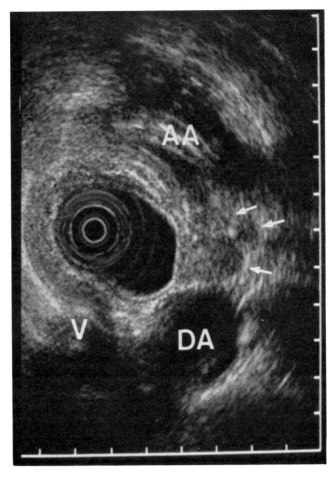

Fig. 7-21. Subaortic lymph node metastases detected by EUS *(white arrows). AA,* ascending aorta; *DA,* descending aorta; *V,* vertebra.

methods—in short, knowledge gained from every applicable field of science. As advances in imaging techniques become available, therapy for esophageal carcinoma should continue to improve.

REFERENCES

1. Ogino, Y., Kouzu, T., Maruyama, M., and Sato, H.: Usefulness of linear array ultrasonic fiberendoscope for diagnosis of esophageal cancer, Gastrointest. Endosc. **25:**1688, 1983.

2. Kumegawa, H., Murata, Y., Akimoto, S., Yoshida, M., and Endo, M.: Study of endoscopic ultrasonography for esophageal carcinoma, Jpn. J. Med. Ultrasonics **12:**207, 1985.

3. Aibe, T., Ootani, T., Yoshida, T., Noguchi, T., Harima, K., Kawahara, K., Fuji, T., Takemoto, T., and Kawa-mura, S.: Diagnosis of the depth of invasion of gastrointestinal cancer by endoscopic ultrasonography, Jpn. J. Med. Ultrasonics **12:**187, 1985.

4. Akiyama, H., Kogure, T., and Itai, Y.: The esophageal axis and its relationship to the resectability of carcinoma of the esophagus, Ann. Surg. **176:**30, 1972.

5. Picus, D., Balfe, D.M., Koehler, R.E., Roper, C.L., and Owen, J.W.: Computed tomography in the staging of esophageal carcinoma, Radiology **146:**433, 1983.

6. Samuelsson, L., Hambraeus, G.M., Mercke, C.E., and Tylen, U.: CT staging of oesophageal carcinoma, Acta Radiol. [Diagn.] **25:**7, 1984.

7. Thompson, W.M., Halvorsen, R.A., Foster, W.L., Jr., Williford, M.E., Postlethwait, R.W., and Korobkin, M.: Computed tomography for staging esophageal and gastroesophageal cancer: reevaluation, AJR **141:**951, 1983.

8. Halvorsen, R.A., and Thompson, W.M.: Computed tomographic evaluation of esophageal carcinoma, Semin. Oncol. **11:**113, 1984.

9. Choi, T.K., Siu, K.F., Lam, K.H., and Wong, J.: Broncoscopy and carcinoma of the esopagus, Part 2, Am. J. Surg. **147**:760, 1984.

10. Tanimura, S., Tomoyasu, H., Banba, J., and Masaki, M.: Fiberoptic bronchoscopy in cases of advanced esophageal carcinoma, J. Jpn. Soc. Bronchology **8**:26, 1986.

11. Postlethwait, R.W.: Surgery of esophagus, New York, 1979, Appleton-Century-Crofts, p. 357.

12. Sugimachi, K., Inokuchi, K., Kuwano, H., Kai, H., Okamura, T., and Okudaira, Y.: Patterns of recurrence after curative resection for carcinoma of the thoracic part of the esophagus, Surg. Gynecol. Obstet. **157**:537, 1983.

13. Nakanishi, T., Nakao, S., and Ogawa, H.: Comparison between linear probe and convex probe about the visualization of the liver, spleen and the pancreas. In Proceedings of the 44th meeting of the Japanese Society for Ultrasonic Medicine, 1984, pp. 613-614.

14. Wong, K.L., Lai, C.L., Wu, P.C., Hui, W.M., Wong, K.P., and Lok, A.S.F.: Ultrasonographic studies in hepatic neoplasm: patterns and comparisons with radiological contrast studies, Clin. Radiol. **36**:511, 1985.

15. Sugiura, N., Ebara, M., Ohto, M., and Okuda, K.: Differential diagnosis for small liver tumors including hepatocellular carcinoma, metastatic cancer and hemangeoma by echography. In Proceedings of the 43rd meeting of the Japanese Society for Ultrasonic Medicine, 1983, pp. 41-42.

16. Thompson, J.N., Gibson, R., Czerniak, A., and Blumgart, L.H.: focal liver lesions: a plan for management, Br. Med. J. **290**:1643, 1985.

17. Hillman, B.J., and Haber, K.: Echographic characteristics of malignant lymph nodes, J. Clin. Ultrasound **8**:213, 1980.

18. Antonmattei, S.R.: Echographic diagnosis of lymph nodes, Radiol. Diagn. **21**:437, 1980.

19. Yoshinaka, H., Nishi, M., Kajisa, T., Kuroshima, K., and Morifuji, H.: Ultrasonic detection of lymph node metastasis in the region around the celiac axis in esophageal and gastric cancer, J. Clin. Ultrasound **13**:153, 1985.

20. Udagawa, H., Watanabe, G., Tsurumaru, M., Suzuki, M., Ono, Y., and Akiyama, H.: Ultrasonic diagnosis of cervical and upper mediastinal lymphnode metastasis of esophageal cancer. In Proceedings of the 46th meeting of the Japanese Society for Ultrasonic Medicine, 1985, pp. 375-376.

21. Udagawa, H., Watanabe, G., Tsurumaru, M., Suzuki, M., Ono, Y., and Akiyama, H.: Ultrasonic diagnosis of cervical and upper mediastinal lymphnode metastasis of esophageal cancer, with special remarks on misdiagnosed nodes. In Proceedings of the 46th meeting of the Japanese Society for Ultrasonic Medicine, 1985, pp. 431-432.

22. Hajek, P.C., Salomonowitz, E., Turk, R., Tscholakoff, D., Kumpan, W., and Czembirek, H.: Lymph nodes of the neck: evaluation with US, Radiology **158**:739, 1986.

23. Akiyama, H., Tsurumaru, M., Kawamura, T., and Ono, Y.: Principles of surgical treatment for carcinoma of the esophagus: analysis of lymph node involvement, Ann. Surg. **194**:438, 1981.

24. Schneekloth, G., Terrier, F., and Fuchs, W.A.: Computed tomography in carcinoma of esophagus and cardia, Gastrointest. Radiol. **8**:193, 1983.

25. Smith, F.W., Hutchison, J.M.S., Mallard, J.R., Johnson, G., Redpath, T.W., Selbie, R.D., Reid, A., and Smith, C.C.: Oesophageal carcinoma demonstrated by nuclear magnetic resonance imaging, Br. Med. J. **282**:510, 1981.

26. Quint, L.E., Glazer, G.M., and Orringer, M.B.: Esophageal imaging by MR and CT: study of normal anatomy and neoplasms, Radiology **156**:727, 1985.

27. von Schulthess, G.K., McMurdo, K., Tscholakoff, D., de Geer, G., Gamsu, G., and Higgins, C.B.: Mediastinal masses: MR imaging, Radiology **158**:289, 1986.

28. Steiner, R.E.: Magnetic resonance imaging: its impact on diagnostic radiology, AJR **145**:883, 1985.

8 Submucography in the diagnosis of esophageal tumors

Ágnes Bohák, Imre Szántó, Attila Vörös, and Janos Kiss

When an operation is being planned, the surgeon feels it imperative to obtain information regarding the precise extent of an esophageal tumor. It is known from the literature[1] that the chances of postoperative survival in cases of esophageal tumor are determined decisively by two factors: metastases to lymph nodes and the extent of neoplastic invasion of the esophageal wall. We have introduced submucography for the more precise determination of the latter.

MATERIAL AND METHODS

In the period between January 21, 1984, and December 31, 1985, submucographic examinations were done in 52 patients. All of them had been subjected to the usual investigations (double-contrast radiography of the esophagus and stomach, and esophagogastrofiberoscopy combined with biopsy and cytologic sampling). The submucographic studies were carried out after that, by the method of Saito.[2]

By means of a GIF-D3 (Olympus) endoscope and an MN-1 K (Olympus) endoscopic injector, a total of 3 ml of Myodil (Glaxo, Ltd.) was injected at four to six sites 3 to 4 cm orally from the visible upper margin of the tumor, in an area confirmedly free from blood vessels. The movements of the contrast medium were followed radiologically. The first radiographs were taken immediately after the injection (within 30 minutes): posterior-anterior, right and left obliques, and during fluoroscopic visualization. The same radiographs were taken again on the fifth day, when the examination was supplemented by the conventional barium meal radiographic methods.

RESULTS

In the intact esophageal wall the contrast medium moves evenly in both the submucosal and the adventitial layers, downward and upward alike. A primary esophageal tumor, or a tumor of the gastroesophageal junction extending into the esophagus, may infiltrate the esophageal wall more or less extensively.

When mural neoplastic involvement affects the wall as a whole, or when the wall has been transgressed by tumorous proliferation, the spreading of the contrast medium will be blocked both in the submucosal and in the adventitial layers (Fig. 8-1). It may occur that the contrast medium moves freely in the submucosa, while its movement in the adventitia is restricted. Then the tumor is spreading intramurally or adventitially (Fig. 8-2.), not affecting the mucosa yet.

On the fifth day the investigations are supplemented with conventional barium meal radiographic methods. This is a modification of the method described by the Japanese authors,[2,3] and makes it possible to judge mural thickness above a tumor in an area that seems to be intact by classical x-ray and endoscopic techniques. This mural thickness is determined from the distance between the contrast medium swallowed or spreading submucosally and that in the adventitial layer. When mural thickness is found to have increased, it suggests intramural spreading of the tumor (Fig. 8-3.).

Immediately before surgery the upper margin of tumor invasion is marked by means of a tube inserted into the esophagus and provided with a sentinel line (Fig. 8-4).

Of the 52 patients involved in the study, 49 were males (mean age 58 years) and 3 were females (aged 50, 55, and 69 years).

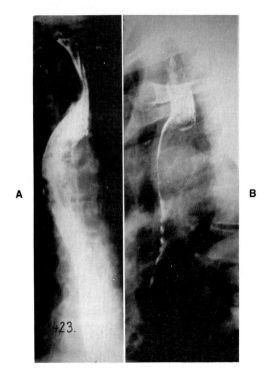

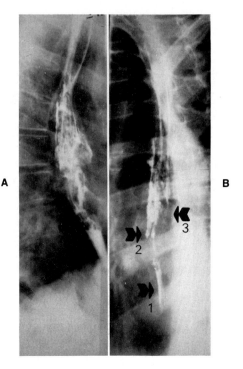

Fig. 8-1. Extensive tumor in the upper third of the esophagus. **A,** Conventional barium meal x-ray examination. **B,** Submucography. The anterior esophageal wall is not invaded by the tumor, and here the adventitial flow of the contrast medium is free.

Fig. 8-2. A, Conventional radiologic examination of an esophageal tumor in the middle portion. **B,** Submucography. On the left side the entire esophageal wall is involved by the tumor; on the right side the contrast medium spreads intramurally and adventitially, leaving the mucosa unaffected. On the right side contrast medium flows freely in the submucosal layer *(1)* while it is blocked in the adventitial layer *(2)*. On the left side flow is blocked in both layers *(3)*.

In six cases the complaints were due to benign disease (benign tumor of the esophagus in three cases and strictures resulting from esophagitis in three others).

In 46 cases the investigations and treatment were carried out because of malignant changes, with the tumor in the cardiac area in 27.

In the neoplastic group the results could not be evaluated for technical reasons in two cases and in three others because no operation had been performed. Thus, out of 41 cases, changes resulting from esophageal tumor were found in the superior portion in one case, in the middle portion in five cases, and in the lower portion in nine cases, while in 26 patients the tumor was at the gastroesophageal junction.

On the basis of additional information supplied by the new method of examination, the resection line had to be marked and carried higher than anticipated in nine patients (one case of lower-third tumor and eight cases of tumor at the gastroesophageal junction).

No tumor cells were found in the resection line by histologic examination in any of the cases.

DISCUSSION

Submucosal esophagography, developed by Saito,[2] makes it possible to ascertain more precisely the extent of tumor invasion. Osugi et al.[3] have examined 43 patients and reported favorable results.

However, the method alone cannot be used for an accurate assessment of mural thickness and intramural invasion. We have therefore combined the method of the Japanese authors with conventional barium meal x-ray techniques. In this way it has been possible to demonstrate better evidence of intramural invasion not yet shown by the classical x-ray and endoscopic methods.

Submucography has been performed in 52 patients. No complications have been observed. On the day of contrast medium administration three patients complained of a retrosternal burning sensation lasting a short time, and one had low-grade fever.

Detailed histologic investigations of the surgical specimens disclosed moderate changes of inflammatory character as a function of the duration of the interval between the diagnostic intervention and the operation. In the surgical specimens studied, neutrophilic and sometimes eosinophilic granulocytic infiltrations were found. In one case microabscesses and proliferative endangiitis were visible.

In 41 malignant cases the submucographic findings were confirmed by operation and by histologic studies. The mode of contrast medium flow (submucosal and adventitial) was in accord with the findings at operation. In the cases of early cancer, no block of flow was shown by submucography. When contrast medium flow was blocked in the adventitial layer, the tumor had broken through the external wall of the esophagus and invasion of surrounding tissue was visible.

In cases of tumor at the gastroesophageal junction, no extension toward the esophagus was observed when both the submucosal and the adventitial layers were free and there was no increase in wall thickness.

By demonstrating the increase in wall thickness, submucography combined with barium meal radiography supplied additional information

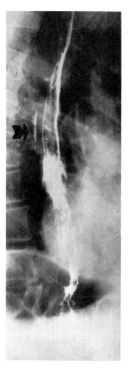

Fig. 8-3. Barium meal plus submucography. Note increased thickness of esophageal wall *(arrow)*.

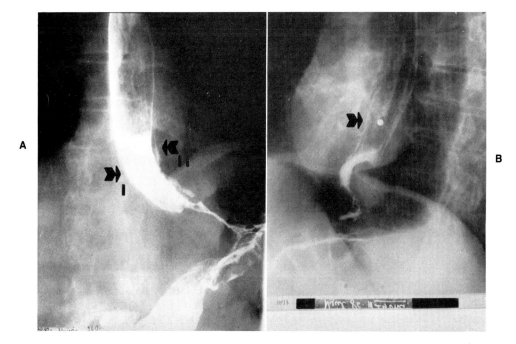

Fig. 8-4. A, Invasion of esophagus by tumor of the gastroesophageal junction. *I,* Normal mural thickness; *II,* intramural spread. **B,** Marking the site of the planned resection line by means of a tube with a radiopaque marker *(arrow)*.

influencing the surgical procedures in 19% (9 of 46) of the tumorous cases examined.

We think that our method is especially useful in assessing invasion of the esophagus by tumors of the gastroesophageal junction and in identifying the correct level for resection. We perform subtotal esophagectomy with anastomosis in the neck in cases in which the tumor is in the lower or middle part of the esophagus. Then a more precise assessment of intramural invasion is less important.

CONCLUSION

Submucography seems to be useful for ascertaining more accurately the extent of tumorous invasion of the esophageal wall; in this way, one of the factors fundamentally influencing prognosis can be determined preoperatively.

REFERENCES

1. Skinner, D.B., Dowlatshaki, K.D., and DeMeester, T.R.: Potentially curable cancer of the esophagus, Cancer **50:**2571, 1982.
2. Saito, J.: Submucosal esophagography: a new method for demonstrating the depth of invasion of esophageal cancer, Jpn. J. Surg. **9:**37, 1979.
3. Osugi, M., Hamanaka, Y., and Sakai, K.: Submucosal esophagography for esophageal cancer, World J. Surg. **5:**703, 1981.

CHAPTER 9 Rationale in staging of cancer of the esophagus

Clifton F. Mountain

The new international system for staging carcinoma of the esophagus represents a simplification of earlier recommendations of the Union Internationale Contre Cancer (UICC)[1] and the American Joint Committee on Cancer (AJCC).[2] These classifications have been modified to provide a single, consistent set of definitions that are applicable to clinical as well as pathologic staging and to carcinomas of both the cervical and the thoracic esophagus. Refinements in imaging technology, including techniques such as the sonography and submucography described in Chapters 7 and 8, magnetic resonance imaging,[3] and computed tomography,[4] have enhanced our ability to assess clinically the extent of the primary tumor and the status of the regional lymph nodes.

The new recommendations for staging this disease are supported by retrospective studies of carcinoma of the esophagus conducted by the National Tumor Registry of Japan under the direction of Dr. Toshifumi Iizuka of the National Cancer Hospital in Tokyo, Japan. The extensive data base consisted of the records of 3987 patients with carcinoma of the esophagus who underwent resection from 1969 to 1978 in Japanese institutes and hospitals. The data confirm that the depth of invasion of the tumor, the presence or absence of lymph node metastasis, the level of lymph node metastasis, and the presence or absence of distant metastasis are the primary determinants of survival. Selection of patients for definitive treatment also is influenced by these elements. The need for accurate, reproducible staging that can be readily remembered and applied is emphasized now that investigational treatment programs, particularly those involving preoperative chemotherapy, are showing encouraging results.[5]

ANATOMIC REGIONS OF THE ESOPHAGUS

The four anatomic regions of the esophagus are defined as follows and are shown in Fig. 9-1.

Cervical: from the pharyngoesophageal junction (the inferior border of the cricoid cartilage) to the suprasternal notch

Upper thoracic: from the suprasternal notch to the bifurcation of the trachea

Middle thoracic: from the tracheal bifurcation to a point midway between it and the gastroesophageal junction

Lower thoracic: from that midpoint to the gastroesophageal junction

PRIMARY TUMOR (T)

Earlier studies of the results of treatment of esophageal carcinoma in Japan from 1969 through 1973 did not support the prior definitions for T_1 and T_2 categories.[6] As shown in Fig. 9-2, the length of esophageal involvement, more or less than 5 cm, or the extent of circumferential involvement had no significant effect on the outcome; however, the presence of extra-esophageal spread had a markedly deleterious effect on the survival rate. Extraesophageal spread is interpreted as any one of the following[7]:

1. Recurrent laryngeal, phrenic, or sympathetic nerve involvement
2. Fistula formation
3. Involvement of tracheal or bronchial tree
4. Vena cava or azygos vein obstruction
5. Malignant effusion

Mediastinal widening by itself is not considered evidence of extraesophageal spread.

The effect of the depth of invasion of the primary tumor on survival is shown in Table 9-1. These end results clearly show the prognostic implications of this element and support the recommendations for definitions of the primary tumor descriptor.

Based on these studies, the definitions for the primary tumor categories are as follows:

T_X: minimum requirements to assess the primary tumor cannot be met

73

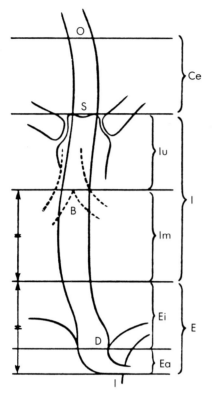

Fig. 9-1. Anatomic regions of the esophagus for recording precise locations of lesions—diagrammatic representation. *Ce,* Cervical region; *Iu,* upper thoracic region; *Im,* middle thoracic region; *Ei,* lower thoracic region; *Ea,* abdominal esophagus; *O,* oropharynx; *S,* suprasternal notch; *B,* tracheal bifurcation; *D,* distal esophagus. (From Japanese Society for Esophageal Diseases, K. Nakayama, president: Guidelines for the clinical and pathological studies on carcinoma of the esophagus, Jpn. J. Surg. **6:**70-78, 1976. With permission).

T_0: no evidence of primary tumor

T_{is}: preinvasive carcinoma (carcinoma in situ)

T_1: tumor invades into but not beyond the submucosa

T_2: tumor invades into but not beyond the muscularis propria

T_3: tumor invades into the adventitia

T_4: tumor invades contiguous structures

Classification of the primary tumor according to the depth of invasion is consistent with the recommendations for the T category in other gastrointestinal sites, such as the stomach and the colon-rectum. The end results when these definitions are applied to the primary tumor are shown in Table 9-2.

REGIONAL LYMPH NODES (N)

My own studies, as well as the end results of the Japanese Cancer Committee (JCC)[8] and the work of others,[9] support the opinion that regional

lymph node metastasis is an ominous prognostic sign in patients with carcinoma of the esophagus. The lymph node mapping schema and nomenclature recommended by the JCC for classification of surgical dissection of the regional lymph nodes in patients with esophageal cancer are shown in Fig. 9-3, and the accompanying nomenclature and nodal grouping according to primary site appear in Tables 9-3 and 9-4. By means of this schema, which relates the nodal groups to the primary tumor site, end results were generated for 1490 resected patients treated from 1969 to 1973. These end results are based on microscopic examination of the nodes. Forty percent of the patients with no involvement of the regional lymph nodes survived 5 years. In the group designated as N_1, which includes only metastasis to paraesophageal lymph nodes adjacent to the primary tumor segment, the survival was reduced to 21%. Progressive erosion of survival expectations as the disease involves nodes more distant from the primary tumor is shown—14.64% of the N_2, 5.12% of the N_3, and 0.00% of the N_4 groups achieved long-term survival.

On the basis of this work the following recommendations for classifying regional lymph nodes in esophageal cancer are made. Any other involved nodes, including nodes of the celiac axis, are considered distant metastasis (M_1).

Nodal stations

Cervical esophagus: cervical and supraclavicular nodes

Upper and middle thoracic esophagus: mediastinal nodes

Lower thoracic esophagus: mediastinal and perigastric nodes.

Categories

N_X: lymph nodes cannot be assessed

N_0: no demonstrable metastasis to regional lymph nodes

N_{1-4}: regional lymph nodes contain metastatic tumor (The higher the subscript number, the more distant the nodal involvement.)

The relationship of lymph node involvement to survival when these definitions are applied is shown in Table 9-5. Forty percent of 1439 patients treated from 1969 to 1978 who had no evidence of metastasis to the regional lymph nodes survived 5 years, which was significantly higher than the 17% (of 1211 patients) surviving with the N_1 classification.

DISTANT METASTASIS (M)

The presence of distant metastasis, whether to distant lymph nodes or to other organs, is synonymous with very poor 5-year survival; how-

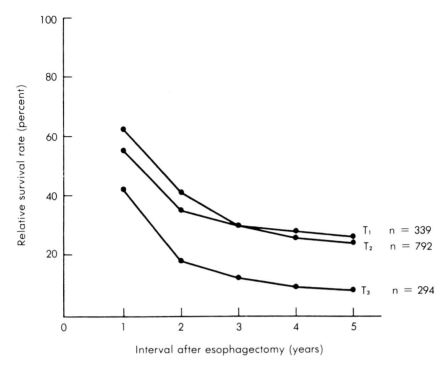

Fig. 9-2. Survival curve of patients with esophageal carcinoma according to T Classification (UICC). (From Japanese Research Society for Esophageal Diseases: The report of treatment results of esophageal carcinoma in Japan [1969-1973], Tokyo, National Cancer Center. With permission).

TABLE 9-1. Survival after esophagectomy, by depth of invasion of primary tumor, 1969 to 1973

Histologic depth of invasion	Total cases	Percentage surviving after esophagectomy				
		1 Yr	2 Yr	3 Yr	4 Yr	5 Yr
Submucosa	62	73.1	66.4	55.9	53.8	46.1
Muscularis propria	242	60.2	41.4	34.1	31.3	28.8
Reaching the adventitia	198	67.2	42.5	30.6	27.5	23.7
Invasion of the adventitia	519	56.4	34.1	26.3	21.3	21.4
Invasion of neighboring structures	254	34.9	13.4	9.0	9.2	9.0

From Japanese Research Society for Esophageal Diseases: The report of treatment results of esophageal carcinoma in Japan (1969–1973), Tokyo, National Cancer Center. (With permission.)

TABLE 9-2. Survival after esophagectomy by primary tumor category, 1969 to 1978

Primary tumor category	Total cases	Percentage surviving after esophagectomy				
		1 Yr	2 Yr	3 Yr	4 Yr	5 Yr*
T_1	228	75.9	59.5	51.0	46.4	46.1
T_2	669	65.7	45.6	37.5	33.8	29.5
T_3	1,949	59.1	35.6	27.2	23.0	21.7
T_4	486	32.7	12.8	9.2	7.3	7.0

Courtesy Dr. Toshifumi Iizuka, National Cancer Center Hospital, Tokyo, Japan, April 24, 1984.
*Standard error of 5-year survival rate (2 sigma): T_1 (7.24); T_2 (3.83); T_3 (2.07); T_4 (2.24).

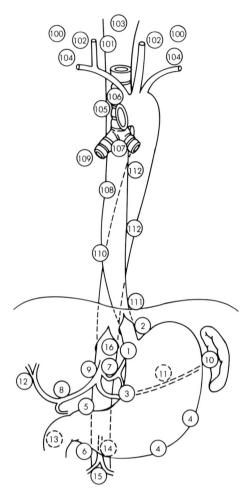

Fig. 9-3. Schema for surgical dissection and mapping of lymph nodes—carcinoma of the esophagus. Numbers are defined in Table 9-3. (From Japanese Society for Esophageal Diseases, K. Nakayama, president: Guidelines for the clinical and pathological studies on carcinoma of the esophagus, Jpn. J. Surg. **6:**70-78, 1976. With permission).

ever, as shown in Table 9-6, at 1 and 2 years following resection the survival for patients with metastasis to distant lymph nodes was substantially better than the outcome for those patients with involvement of distant organ sites. The definitions for the M categories are as follows:

M_x: distant metastasis cannot be assessed
M_0: no evidence of distant metastasis
M_1: distant metastasis present

STAGE GROUPING
Survival by TNM subset

The survival characteristics for patients in each of the TNM subsets is shown in Table 9-7. The

outcome for those with $T_1 N_0 M_0$ tumors is markedly superior to the outcomes for the other subsets, with 60% surviving 5 years. There is a progressive erosion of survival expectations with advancing depth of invasion and lymph node involvement. In the T_2 and T_3 patients, the primary tumor characteristics had less influence on survival than the involvement of regional lymph nodes. There is a marked drop in the survival rate in the $T_4 N_0 M_0$ patients, and if the regional lymph nodes are involved, less than 10% achieve 5-year survival.

Proceeding from this information, the Japanese Cancer Committee made the following recommendations for stage grouping of the TNM subsets (Table 9-8). These recommendations were accepted by the UICC and the AJCC. The TNM combinations provide for classification of four stages of disease, each having a unique survival experience, which is significant and which reflects an increasing burden of mortality as the disease progresses from stage I to stage IV.

Appropriate requirements for assessment of the T, N, and M categories

The following examinations are recommended as the appropriate requirements for assessment of the T, N, and M categories. If the T, N, or M characteristics cannot be assessed, then the symbol T_x, N_x, or M_x will be used.

T categories: clinical examination, radiography, endoscopy (including bronchoscopy for lesions proximal to the carina), and, where available, ultrasonography

N categories: clinical examination, radiography (including conventional or computed tomography), endoscopy, and, where available, ultrasonography

M categories: clinical examination and biochemical profile; where indicated, special studies including radionuclide scans, computed tomography, and/or ultrasound of the liver should be utilized

CONCLUSION

This new international staging system for carcinoma of the esophagus fulfills the need for a classification system for this disease that is simple, easily remembered, and readily applicable to both clinical and pathologic staging. The recommendations were derived from careful analysis

TABLE 9-3. Nomenclature of lymph nodes for surgical dissection

Numeric designator	Lymph nodes	Numeric designator	Lymph nodes
100	Lateral cervical lymph nodes	1	Right cardia lymph nodes
101	Cervical paraesophageal lymph nodes	2	Left cardia lymph nodes
102	Deep cervical lymph nodes	3	Lesser curvature lymph nodes
103	Retropharyngeal lymph nodes	4	Greater curvature lymph nodes
104	Supraclavicular lymph nodes	5	Suprapyloric lymph nodes
105	Upper thoracic paraesophageal lymph nodes	6	Subpyloric lymph nodes
106	Thoracic paratracheal lymph nodes	7	Left gastric artery lymph nodes
107	Bifurcation lymph nodes	8	Common hepatic artery lymph nodes
108	Middle thoracic paraesophageal lymph nodes	9	Celiac axis lymph nodes (lymph nodes at the root of the left gastric artery)
109	Pulmonal hilar lymph nodes		(lymph nodes at the root of common hepatic artery)
110	Lower thoracic paraesophageal lymph nodes		(lymph nodes at the root of the splenic artery)
111	Diaphragmatic lymph nodes	10	Splenic hilar lymph nodes
112	Posterior mediastinal lymph nodes	11	Splenic artery lymph nodes
		12	Hepatoduodenal ligament lymph nodes
		13	Retropancreatic lymph nodes
		14	Mesenteric lymph nodes
		15	Middle colic artery lymph nodes
		16	Paraaortic lymph nodes (abdominal)

From Japanese Research Society for Esophageal Diseases: The report of treatment results of esophageal carcinoma in Japan (1969–1973), Tokyo, National Cancer Center. (With permission.)

TABLE 9-4. Classification of lymph nodes by group according to primary tumor location

Primary tumor location	Group 1	Group 2	Group 3	Group 4
Cervical	101	102, 104	100, 103, 105, 106, 107, 108	109, 110, 111, 112 1, 2, 3
Upper intrathoracic	105	106, 107, 108, 112	101, 110, 111 1, 2	100, 102, 103 3, 4, 5, 6, 7 8, 9
Middle intrathoracic	108	105, 106, 107, 110, 111, 112 1, 2	3, 7 104, 109	100, 101, 102, 103 4, 5, 6
Lower intrathoracic	110	108, 111, 112 1, 2, 3, 7	105, 106, 107 109	100, 101, 102, 103, 104 4, 5, 6, 8

From Japanese Research Society for Esophageal Diseases: The report of treatment results of esophageal carcinoma in Japan (1969–1973), Tokyo, National Cancer Center. (With permission.)

TABLE 9-5. Survival after esophagectomy, by regional lymph node groups, 1969 to 1973

Lymph nodes positive	Total cases	Percentage surviving after esophagectomy				
		1 Yr	2 Yr	3 Yr	4 Yr	5 Yr
N_0*	483	71.2	54.0	45.3	42.9	39.6
N_1	137	59.1	37.0	26.2	22.1	21.0
N_2	363	51.1	27.7	18.9	15.2	14.6
N_3	177	38.1	12.4	7.9	6.9	5.1
N_4	72	28.0	5.2	3.5	0.0	0.0

From Japanese Research Society for Esophageal Diseases: The report of treatment results of esophageal carcinoma in Japan (1969–1973), Tokyo, National Cancer Center. (With permission.)
*N_0, No lymph node metastasis; N_1, metastasis to nodes of group 1; N_2, metastasis to nodes of group 2; N_3, metastasis to lymph nodes of group 3; N_4, metastasis to lymph nodes of group 4.

TABLE 9-6. Survival after esophagectomy, by regional lymph node category, 1969 to 1978

N category	Number	Percentage surviving after esophagectomy				
		1 Yr	2 Yr	3 Yr	4 Yr	5 Yr*
N_0	1242	73.8	55.7	47.2	42.8	39.9
N_1	1211	55.6	30.2	21.9	18.1	16.8

Courtesy Dr. Toshifumi Iizuka, National Cancer Center Hospital, Tokyo, April 24, 1985.
*Standard error of 5-year survival rate (2 sigma): N_0, 3.04; N_1, 2.31.

TABLE 9-7. Survival after esophagectomy, by TNM subset, 1969 to 1978

TNM subset	Number	Percentage surviving after esophagectomy				
		1 Yr	2 Yr	3 Yr	4 Yr	5 Yr*
Total	3073	58.3	36.1	28.6	25.0	23.1
$T_1N_0M_0$	134	89.7	74.2	67.2	63.1	60.4
$T_1N_1M_0$	52	62.2	43.2	29.6	30.5	29.2
$T_2N_0M_0$	323	77.8	63.6	53.5	47.8	42.6
$T_2N_1M_0$	190	57.3	32.5	28.0	26.4	22.1
$T_3N_0M_0$	612	73.6	53.8	45.5	40.9	38.6
$T_3N_1M_0$	695	60.8	33.5	22.7	18.0	17.1
$T_4N_0M_0$	117	53.6	26.3	19.5	18.1	15.6
$T_4N_1M_0$	200	36.7	14.5	11.7	8.1	8.3
M_1 lymph nodes	658	37.3	13.2	8.4	6.3	5.2
M_1 organ sites	92	21.5	5.6	2.9	3.0	3.0

Courtesy Dr. Toshifumi Iizuka, Tokyo, April 24, 1985.
*Standard error of 5-year survival rate (2 sigma): $T_1N_0M_0$, 9.50; $T_1N_1M_0$, 13.89; $T_2N_0M_0$, 6.03; $T_2N_1M_0$, 6.51; T_3N_0, 4.31; $T_3N_1M_0$, 3.08; $T_4N_0M_0$, 7.21; $T_4N_1M_0$, 4.12; M_1 lymph nodes, 1.87; M_1 organ sites, 4.09.

TABLE 9-8. Five-year survival data by stage

Stage	Subset	Percent surviving 5 years
Stage I	$T_1N_0M_0$	60.4
Stage II	$T_2N_0M_0$	31.3
	$T_1N_1M_0$	
	$T_2N_1M_0$	
Stage III	$T_3N_0M_0$	19.9
	$T_3N_1M_0$	
	$T_4N_0M_0$	
	$T_4N_1M_0$	
Stage IV	Any T, Any N, M_1	4.14

of prior UICC and AJCC staging systems' implications for survival. This work showed that the much-desired simplification and subsequent modification of the definitions were rational. When the new definitions for TNM categories and rules for stage grouping are applied to a large contemporary data base, reasonable estimates of long-term survival are reflected in each of the elements in the classification system. Stage I disease includes patients with the best prognosis—those with limited invasion and no lymph node metastasis. In the stage II and stage III categories, lymph node involvement has a more deleterious effect on the outcome than the advancing depth of invasion of the primary tumor in the T_2 and T_3 patients; however, extension of the primary tumor to involve contiguous structures (T_4 disease) carries a heavy burden of mortality; lymph node involvement in this group approaches that associated with distant metastasis.

Carcinoma of the esophagus is a far more prevalent malignancy in Japan than in the United States, and we are indebted to our Japanese colleagues for their extensive studies of this disease, studies that provided the rationale for the new international staging system for carcinoma of the esophagus.

ACKNOWLEDGMENT

I wish to acknowledge the partial support of National Cancer Institute Contract no. CA34503 and the assistance of Kay E. Hermes in the preparation of this chapter.

REFERENCES

1. Union Internationale Contre le Cancer: Oesophagus. In Spiessl, B., Scheibe, O., and Wagner, G., editors: TNM: atlas, illustrated guide to the classification of malignant tumors, Berlin, 1982, Springer-Verlag, pp. 60-69.
2. American Joint Committee on Cancer, Task Force on the Esophagus, Mountain, C.F., Chairman: Carcinoma of the esophagus. In Beahrs, O.H., and Meyers, M., editors: Manual for staging of cancer, ed. 2, Philadelphia, 1983, J.B. Lippincott Co., pp. 61-69.
3. Smith, F.W., Hutchison, J.M., Mallard, J.R., Johnson, G., Redpath, T.W., Selbie, R.D., Reid, A., and Smith, C.C.: Oesophageal carcinoma demonstrated by whole body nuclear magnetic resonance imaging, Br. Med. J. **282:**510, 1981.
4. Alessi, G., Gualdi, C.F., Zerilli, M., Biasi, C., Schillaci, A., Moraldi, A., and Stipa, S.: Computerized tomography in the study of cancer of the esophagus and cardia, Minerva Chir. **39:**191, 1984.
5. Kelsen, D., Bains, M., Hilaris, B., and Martini, N.: Combined modality therapy of esophageal cancer, Semin. Oncol. **11:**169, 1984.
6. Japanese Research Society for Esophageal Diseases: The report of treatment results of esophageal carcinoma in Japan (1969-1973), Tokyo, National Cancer Center.
7. Mountain, C.F., and Hermes, K.E.: The meaning of lymph node metastases and their treatment: squamous cell carcinoma of the esophagus. In Weiss, L., Gilbert, H.A., and Ballon, S.C., editors: Lymphatic system metastasis, Boston, 1980, G.K. Hall, pp. 250-261.
8. Kinoshita, Y., Endo, M., and Nakayoma, K.: Surgical treatment and combined radiotherapy for thoracic oesophageal carcinoma following the survival rate. In Silber, W., editor: Carcinoma of the oesophagus, Capetown, South Africa, 1978, A. A. Balkema, pp. 417-427.
9. Huang, G., Dawei, Z., Guoqing, W., Hua, L., Liangjun, W., Jiasui, L., Guiyu, C., and Xingjiang, W.: Surgical treatment of carcinoma of the esophagus: report of 1,647 cases, Chin. Med. J. **94:**305, 1981.

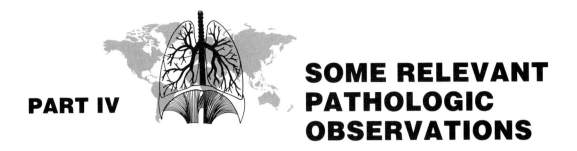

PART IV

SOME RELEVANT PATHOLOGIC OBSERVATIONS

10 Pathology of esophageal carcinoma in relation to dysplasia

Eiichi Sato

RELATIONSHIP OF DYSPLASIA TO CARCINOMA

Although it is not yet completely elucidated whether most carcinomas of the esophagus originate from a precursor lesion such as dysplasia or de novo, some of the recent follow-up studies have clearly implicated dysplasia as an important precancerous change in the esophageal epithelium. For example, a follow-up study by cytology in China disclosed that 21 (26.6%) of 79 patients with severe dysplasia progressed to carcinoma, 26 (32.9%) patients remained in the same grade or showed moderate change, and 32 (40.3%) returned to normal cytology or mild atypia.[1] Munoz and Crepsi[2] reported that in 4 of 20 individuals reexamined 1 year after the first endoscopic examination, esophagitis with atrophy or dysplasia had progressed to cancer. However, there is no general agreement about the histologic criteria for dysplasia, so the definition or grading differs among investigators. In general, mild, moderate, and severe dysplasia have been characterized. In autopsies dysplasia was found even in a 2-year-old child at the site of physiologic stenosis. On the other hand, dysplasia associated with carcinoma is far more advanced and extensive than is found incidentally in autopsies. In our histologic examination whole-step sections of surgically resected specimens showed varying degrees of epithelial atypia in almost all cases in the grossly normal-appearing mucosa around invasive carcinoma. In some early carcinomas confined to the mucosa or carcinoma in situ (CIS), the carcinomatous lesion surrounded by dysplastic epithelium generally showed a gradual transition to normal squamous epithelium.[3] Thus, in the incipient stage of cancer formation one can often recognize a close relationship between carcinoma and dysplasia.

OBSERVATIONS ON SURGICAL MATERIAL

The histologic findings of dysplasia are as follows:

1. Irregular arrangement of cells in the basal layer and appearance of nuclei of varying size and shape replacing normal oval nuclei

2. Increased population and disorderly arrangement of cells, with nuclear swelling in the second to fourth alignments from the base

3. Loss of transparency in cytoplasm located near the surface of the mucosa and migration of enlarged nuclei toward the surface

4. Variable staining density of nuclei in the lesion

The distinction between severe dysplasia and CIS is not always easy (see Fig. 10-1). When the mucosa is replaced in full thickness by highly atypical cells, we call the lesion CIS. However, when a lesion is not totally occupied by such atypical cells but invades only the lower part of the epithelial layer, the evaluation is occasionally very difficult. Therefore we need objective markers other than nuclear morphology. Our criteria for grading are as follows: In *mild* dysplasia, slightly atypical cells with somewhat larger and hyperchromatic nuclei are found in the basal half or less of the epithelium, preserving cellular alignment. In *moderate* dysplasia, atypical cells associated with occasional mitotic figures are prominent in the basal two thirds or less of the epithelium and are in a somewhat disorderly arrangement. In *severe* dysplasia, disarrangement of epithelial cells is marked, in addition to moderate cellular atypism with nuclear pleomorphism observable in the basal two thirds or more of the epithelium. In CIS, cellular atypism is extensive; each finding is compatible with carcinoma except for the absence of invasive growth.

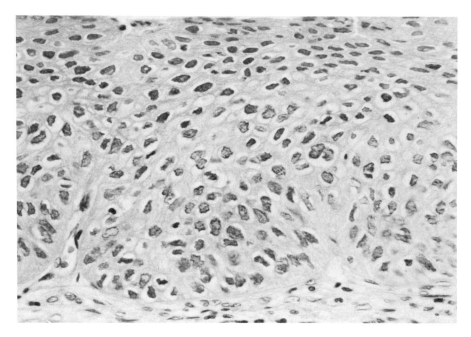

Fig. 10-1. Borderline lesion between dysplasia and CIS, showing marked nuclear atypia and disorderly arrangement occupying basal two thirds with gradual transition toward the surface of the mucosa.

TABLE 10-1. A comparison of the prevalence of dysplasia and death rates for esophageal carcinoma, according to prefecture

Prefecture	Prevalence of dysplasia (%)		Death rate*	
	Male	Female	Male	Female
Aomori	13.6	5.6	17.6	4.0
Akita	26.5	14.0	26.8	4.7
Miyagi	8.7	18.4	33.8	11.6
Nara	8.3	18.6	29.2	15.1
Wakayama	12.1	0	34.9	14.8
Kagoshima	36.2	7.8	37.2	8.4

*Per 100,000 population over 40 years of age.

In our observation of 50 cases of esophageal carcinoma that received no pretreatment before surgery, mild or moderate dysplasia was found in 44 cases (88%), severe dysplasia was found in 32 (64%), and independent foci of CIS, which were at least 5 mm apart from each other, were discerned in 12 (24%). And in 76 instances in which radiation was used as a preoperative therapy, moderate dysplasia was seen in 72 (95%) and severe in 57 (75%). Consequently, the evaluation of dysplasia should be interpreted with caution in cases in which preoperative radiotherapy or chemotherapy has been utilized.

DYSPLASIA IN AUTOPSY SPECIMENS

In autopsy study of subjects who had died from diseases other than esophageal carcinoma, the grade and incidence of dysplasia were lower than in the surgical specimens, but the prevalence rates varied widely among the six prefectures examined in Japan.[3] Only in one prefecture was the prevalence rate for moderate or severe dysplasia related to the death rate for esophageal carcinoma, as shown in Table 10-1. Akita and Kagoshima prefectures are areas of high consumption of al-

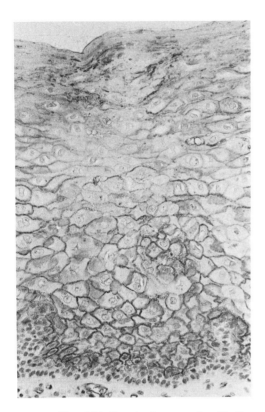

Fig. 10-2. Ulex-I binding in the normal epithelium. Note negative binding in the basal layer.

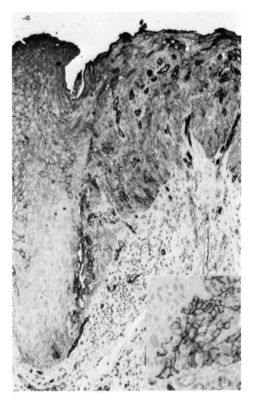

Fig. 10-3. Ulex-I binding in dysplasia *(left)* and CIS *(right)*. Note loss of the binding in dysplasia and positive binding also in the basal cell of CIS. *Inset,* Higher magnification of basal cells.

cohol, and a higher grade of dysplasia is prevalent there. Histologically, dysplasia in Kagoshima prefecture showed prominent downgrowth of the basal cells such as the rete ridge of the epidermis. Takubo et al.[4] reported that in Saitama prefecture, one of the high-risk areas in Japan, hyperplasia and atypia of ducts of esophageal glands were characteristic. These findings suggest that etiologic factors differ even within a country and in its high-risk areas. Alcohol and smoking seemed to be somewhat related to the incidence of dysplasia and CIS.

NUCLEAR DNA CONTENT

When the nuclear DNA content of carcinoma cells was compared with that in dysplasia, the histogram pattern of dysplasia appeared to closely resemble that of carcinoma cells, in proportion to increases in atypia. Occasionally, severe dysplasia showed an increased population of cells exceeding the 4c DNA content in comparison with carcinoma. The result of the DNA measurement underlines the significance of dysplasia as a pre-

cancerous lesion, but is not always helpful in the objective evaluation of CIS. The DNA study also showed that high ploidy cells were present more frequently in the second alignment of normal and dysplastic mucosa than in the basal layer. Therefore, it is possible that the cells in the second alignment are susceptible to carcinogens.

LECTIN-BINDING AND IMMUNOHISTOCHEMICAL STUDY OF BLOOD GROUP ANTIGEN

In order to find an objective marker for the evaluation of dysplasia and CIS, we have been seeking information about cytoplasmic differentiation to localize blood group antigens. By using lectin Ulex europaeus-I specific to Fuc1-2 Gal linkage, which is also a determinant of blood group O (H) substance, we have shown that there is antigen loss in dysplasia and granular appearance of antigen in the cytoplasm of CIS. In the latter, basal cells were also positive for the antigen differing from normal basal cells (Fig. 10-2 and 10-3). All the basal cells of normal epithelium were entirely negative for the patient's own antigen. Dysplasia was also negative, but some basal cells in severe dysplasia were positive, possibly indicating a carcinomatous transformation of some cytoplasmic character in part. Immunohistochemical study using monoclonal antibodies against blood groups H, A, and B indicated that these isoantigens were lost in dysplastic epithelia of the esophagus, whereas in CIS there was irregular and aberrant expression of the antigens. For example, the patients with blood group A were positive for B in two thirds of the cases examined, and the blood group B patients were all negative for A, B, and H antigens in their dysplastic epithelia. Thus, immunohistochemical study using lectins or antibodies against blood group substance is a potent method for the objective evaluation of the lesion in question.

REFERENCES

1. The coordinating group for research on etiology of esophageal cancer in North China: Chinese Med. J. **1:**167, 1975.
2. Munoz, N., and Crepsi, M.: Monograph on cancer research, Gann **31:**27, 1986.
3. Sato, E., Mukada, T., and Sasano, N.: In Pfeiffer, C.J., editor: Cancer of the esophagus, Boca Raton, Fla., 1982, CRC Press, Inc., pp. 125-138.
4. Takubo, K., Tsuchiya, S., Fukushi, K., Shirota, A., and Mitomo, Y.: Acta Pathol. Jpn. **31:**999, 1981.

CHAPTER 11 Natural progression of esophageal carcinoma

Guo Jun Huang

The natural progression of early esophageal carcinoma remains more or less a mystery. However, a review of the entire natural history of this disease may disclose some of the facts that may add to our understanding of this matter. Huang and Wu,[1] on the basis of correlated studies in the epidemiology, pathogenesis, pathology, and clinical course of esophageal carcinoma, proposed dividing the natural history of this malignancy into four phases—namely, initial, developing, overt, and terminal—which are described in the following paragraphs.

INITIAL PHASE

The initial phase of esophageal carcinoma covers a long period of time, possibly 20 years or more. The first changes are mild to moderate hyperplasia of the basal epithelial cells of the esophageal mucosa. As the pathologic process progresses, more marked hyperplasia and dysplasia of the epithelial cells are seen, involving not only the basal layer but also the intermediate layer of the mucosa. Hyperchromatism and dyskaryosis are evident in these cells.

Studies performed on the basis of mass screening by abrasive cytology in various parts of China have revealed a close correlation between the incidence of esophageal carcinoma and that of esophageal dysplasia.[2] In fact, dysplastic cells are almost always found on cytologic smears in cases of early esophageal carcinoma. Follow-up cytologic studies in high-incidence areas for esophageal carcinoma showed that severe dysplasia of esophageal epithelium, on the one hand, may regress to mild dysplasia or normal epithelium but, on the other hand, may progress to carcinoma in a relatively high percentage of cases.[2] Shu and associates,[3] in a follow-up study of 530 cases with marked dysplasia and another 530 cases with mild hyperplasia, each group being followed for 1 to 12 years, found 79 cases (14.9%) of carcinoma in the former group and only 5 (0.9%) in the latter group. In their control group of 477 subjects with normal cytology whose cases were followed for 1 to 5 years, however, no carcinoma was found. Their study also showed that the incidence of carcinoma increased with age and years of marked dysplasia; in a mass screening of 14,002 subjects, there were 460 cases of marked dysplasia, with an average age of 52 years, and 221 cases of esophageal carcinoma, with an average age of 57 years. It is therefore likely that it takes 5 years for severe dysplasia to develop into carcinoma.

It is clear that severe dysplasia of esophageal epithelium is precancerous in nature but may still be reversible, and preventive measures or intervention treatment may be effective in this phase.

DEVELOPING PHASE

One step further is the development of cancer in situ, which is clinically latent and may remain so for a long time. But eventually the growth breaks through the basal layer of the epithelium and becomes an infiltrative cancer, which may present itself as a granular plaque, protruding nodule, or depressed shallow ulcer. These changes are definitely cancerous and are irreversible, but the lesion remains within the confines of the mucosa and submucosa as an early, or stage I, lesion for a relatively long time.

In a series of 253 cases of stage I esophageal carcinoma treated surgically, as reported by Shao et al.,[4] the lesion was carcinoma in situ in 99 (39.1%) and early infiltrative carcinoma in 154 (60.9%). Pei and associates[5] reported that in a group of 23 untreated patients with early esophageal carcinoma diagnosed by cytology, the av-

TABLE 11-1. Natural survival period of 23 cases of untreated early esophageal carcinoma

| | Survival period (mo) | | |
Course	Shortest	Longest	Average
Developing phase	12	55	33.9
Overt and terminal phases	3	24	9.7
Entire course	20	78	43.6

Data from Pei, Y.H., Zhang, Y.D., Hou, J., et al.: Cancer Res. Prev. Treat. **9**:75.

erage duration of the developing phase was 33.9 months (range, 12 to 55 months) and the average survival period from the time of cytologic diagnosis to death was 43.6 months (range, 20 to 78 months) (see Table 11-1). Miao and associates[6] independently reported another 23 cases of untreated early esophageal carcinoma diagnosed by balloon cytology and further confirmed by barium esophagography and/or fiberesophagoscopy, in which 11 cases developed into late carcinoma in a mean duration of 55.5 ± 29.0 months, and 12 remained in the early stage of disease for a mean of 74.4 ± 27.3 months without developing into late carcinoma. In six of their patients who died with known dates, the average survival period from first diagnosis to death was 49.2 months.

It can be seen from the above observations that the developing stage of esophageal carcinoma may take a long time. During the early part of this stage the disease may be "preclinical" in that the patient may have no symptoms whatsoever and the lesions can be detected only by cytology or endoscopy. But as the lesion progresses, mild but definite symptoms related to swallowing of food will occur in most of the patients. It is because of the relatively long duration of the developing stage of esophageal carcinoma that there is ample potential for early diagnosis and treatment at this stage. Surgical treatment at this stage may produce 90% survival at 5 years and 60% at 10 years.[4]

OVERT PHASE

The overt phase is the main clinical phase including all stage II and III esophageal carcinomas that invade a part or the whole thickness of the muscular coat with or without extraesophageal invasion and lymph node metastasis. There are obvious symptoms and signs, such as progressive dysphagia, loss of weight, and retrosternal pain, and characteristic roentgenologic findings of filling defects and obstruction. Once the cancer comes to this phase it progresses with increasing

rapidity. In some cases the primary cancer may gradually enlarge from an originally small, localized, early lesion that in the process of development invades the deep layers of the esophageal wall, and in other cases it may develop from a superficial but extensive stage I lesion and rapidly attain great size as it invades the deeper layers of the esophagus. The average survival period without effective treatment in two series as reported by Wu[7] and Pei and associates[5] was only 9.4 to 9.7 months from the first appearance of obvious symptoms. The operability and prognosis after surgical treatment are good for stage II lesions but much less favorable for stage III lesions, although a 25% 5-year survival or a reasonable degree of palliation may still be expected in a goodly number of cases.

TERMINAL PHASE

The final phase of esophageal carcinoma is usually short. The cancer is extensive, with extraesophageal invasion into adjacent vital organs and regional or distant metastases. This is stage IV in clinical classification. Dysphagia may or may not be severe, but there is usually pain in the chest or the back. There may be hoarseness of the voice because of recurrent nerve involvement. Esophagotracheal or esophagobronchial fistulas may develop with severe pulmonary infection. Cachexia is common. The average life expectancy of a patient in this stage is only 3 months without treatment.[7]

COMMENT

Carcinoma of the esophagus remains a deadly disease because most of the patients today are seen at the rapidly progressing, short, late stages of this malignancy, when there is not much that medical science can offer to the patient. However, esophageal cancer can be prevented during its long initial, or precancerous, phase and can be detected and treated with excellent results during its relatively long developing, or early, phase. Efforts are being aimed at these goals, and there is good reason to believe that the prospects are bright in our fight against this disease.

REFERENCES

1. Huang, G.J., and Wu, Y.K.: Natural history of esophageal carcinoma. In Huang, G.J., and Wu, Y.K., editors: Carcinoma of the esophagus and gastric cardia, Berlin, 1984, Springer-Verlag, pp. 244-246.
2. The Coordinating Groups for the Research of Esophageal carcinoma, Henan Province and Chinese Academy of Medical Sciences: Studies on relationship between epithelial dysplasia and carcinoma of the esophagus, Chin. Med. J. **1:**110, 1975 (In Chinese.)
3. Shu, Y.J., Yang, X.Q., and Jin, S.P.: Further investigation of the relationship between dysplasia and cancer of the esophagus, Chin. Med. J. **60:**39, 1980.
4. Shao, L.F., Huang, G.J., Zhang, D.W., et al.: Detection and surgical treatment of early esophageal carcinoma. In Proceedings of the Beijing Symposium on Cardiothoracic Surgery, Beijing, 1981, China Academic Publishing and John Wiley & Sons, Inc., pp. 168-71.
5. Pei, Y.H., Zhang, Y.D., Hou, J., et al.: Natural evolution and follow-up study of early esophageal carcinoma in 23 cases, Cancer Res. Prev. Treat. **9:**75, 1982.
6. Miao, Y.J., Li, G.Y., Gu, X.Z., and Chen, W.H.: Detection and natural progression of early esophageal carcinoma: preliminary communication, J. R. Soc. Med. **74:**884, 1981.
7. Wu, Y.K.: Neoplasm of the esophagus. In Wu, Y.K., editor: Disease of the chest, Beijing, 1959, People's Medical Publishing House.

CHAPTER 12 Pathologic changes affecting survival in esophageal cancer

Anthony Watson

In the Western world, survival figures following treatment for esophageal cancer are particularly depressing, in relation both to other, more favorable tumors such as breast or colorectal lesions and to the early esophageal lesions detected by screening programs in areas of high incidence in China and the Far East. Five-year survival rates of 10% to 20% reflect the advanced stage of the disease at the time of presentation in the West, where the incidence of around six cases per 100,000 population militates against the logistics involved in the provision of screening programs. By the time persistent dysphagia is observed, tumors have encircled approximately two thirds of the circumference of the esophagus[1] and have been growing for some 34 months.[2] Of those amenable to resection, 72% have metastasized to lymph nodes.[3]

Although the overall outlook is gloomy, not all esophageal tumors have the same biologic behavior, and certain pathologic factors have been shown to have a bearing on survival. These relate to the histologic cell type, the status of contiguous and distant lymph nodes, and the characteristics of the primary tumor. It is important that the attending physician be aware of these factors so as to direct those therapeutic modalities most appropriate to the individual circumstances.

HISTOLOGIC CELL TYPE

The majority of esophageal carcinomas are of squamous cell type, but adenocarcinomas arising from mucosal or submucosal glands, heterotopic gastric mucosa, or Barrett's columnar-lined esophagus account for approximately 10% of esophageal cancers. If tumors of the cardia are included, the proportion rises to around 40%. Most esophageal adenocarcinomas occur in the lower third, but in a pooled series of 705 cases of esophageal carcinoma, 8% of adenocarcinomas occurred in the upper and middle thirds.[4]

Analysis of resected specimens from our institution has shown that adenocarcinomas are more advanced at the time of surgery than squamous lesions[5] (see Table 12-1). No adenocarcinomas were localized to the esophageal wall, and lymph node metastases were present in 85% of adenocarcinomas as compared with 54% of squamous carcinomas. A similar trend was shown by Gardiol et al.,[6] although squamous lesions had a higher incidence of vascular invasion.

Survival following resection appears to relate more to the staging of the tumor rather than to the cell type per se, but in view of the fact that adenocarcinomas are usually more advanced at the time of resection, differences in survival do exist. Borst et al.[7] showed that although survival for palliative resection of advanced lesions was similar for squamous carcinomas and adenocarcinomas, those patients undergoing "curative" resection for squamous lesions fared better than the small group with relatively favorable adenocarcinoma. Although overall quoted 5-year survival rates for esophageal cancer following resection range from 10% to 20% in the Western world,[8-10] this figure is largely supported by the better survival for squamous carcinoma, with 5-year survival of 2% for adenocarcinoma being reported by Turnbull and Goodner.[11]

In a series of 197 cases of esophageal carcinoma reported from our institution,[12] the overall 5-year survival of 11% following resection reflected figures of 26% for squamous lesions and 3% for adenocarcinomas. The mean survival was 32.4 months for squamous lesions and 15.1 months for adenocarcinomas. However, if the subset of patients without lymph node involvement were isolated, the 5-year survival was 55% for squamous carcinomas and 40% for adenocarcinomas, the mean survival being 4.5 years and

TABLE 12-1. Tumor staging and histologic cell type

	Squamous carcinoma	Adenocarcinoma	Overall
Localized to esophageal wall (%)	23	0	9
Transgressed esophageal wall (%)	23	15	19
Lymph node involvement (%)	54	85	72

3.3 years, respectively. Thus, there would appear to be a small advantage in favor of squamous lesions when compared stage for stage with adenocarcinomas, but since only 15% of adenocarcinomas had negative nodes, compared with 46% of squamous carcinomas, this relative unfavorability of adenocarcinomas is magnified in overall results.

Other factors related to histologic cell type that may have a bearing on survival are the degree of differentiation of squamous lesions and the relative radiosensitivity of this cell type compared with adenocarcinoma. The consensus of opinion regarding degree of differentiation appears to be that in isolation it has little influence on survival,[13] although since lymph node metastases are more frequently associated with poorly differentiated lesions,[14] their overall prognosis is less favorable than that for well-differentiated lesions. It is well recognized that squamous tumors are collectively more radiosensitive than adenocarcinomas, which may have a bearing on prognosis, but a discussion of radiotherapy is outside the scope of this chapter and considered fully in chapter 37.

Although squamous cell carcinoma and adenocarcinoma constitute the majority of esophageal tumors, there are less common variants of each cell type that may have a bearing on survival.

Variants of squamous cell carcinoma

The principal variants are verrucous carcinoma, spindle-cell carcinoma, and small-cell carcinoma. Verrucous carcinoma is an unusual variant, being an exophytic, papillary growth sometimes seen in association with achalasia and esophageal diverticula.[15] It is a slow-growing lesion of low metastasizing potential and therefore is associated with a relatively favorable prognosis. Spindle-cell carcinomas are polypoid, often pedunculated tumors occurring predominantly in the middle and lower esophagus, where they may attain considerable size. A spectrum of histologic appearances exists, depending on the relative proportions of squamous and spindle-cell components, ranging from the "carcinosarcoma," in which there is intermingling of the two components, to the "pseudosarcoma," in which the spindle-cell component dominates. These tumors, especially at the pseudosarcoma end of the spectrum, rarely invade deeply into the esophageal wall and consequently carry a better prognosis, with 5-year survival reaching 60%.[16] Small-cell carcinomas, on the other hand, resemble and behave like oat-cell bronchial tumors. They arise from the argyrophil cells found in the basal layers of the mucosa and may rarely secrete calcitonin or adrenocorticotropic hormone (ACTH). These tumors are characterized by their invasive nature and tendency to metastasize widely, and consequently are associated with a very poor prognosis.

Variants of adenocarcinoma

The rare variants of adenocarcinoma are adenosquamous carcinoma, adenoacanthoma, and choriocarcinoma. Adenosquamous lesions comprise coexisting adenocarcinoma and squamous carcinomas and are felt to represent areas of squamous metaplasia within adenocarcinomas arising from esophageal mucous glands, a pathologic process similar to that occurring in carcinoma of the stomach, pancreas, and colon, although very rarely carcinomatous change in both epithelial components may coexist.[17] In adenoacanthoma, the squamous component comprises mature squamous epithelium, and the likely origin is from areas of ectopic gastric epithelium.[18] These tumors spread extensively via the lymphatics in the submucosa and within the perineural spaces and are consequently associated with a poor prognosis. Choriocarcinoma of the esophagus is extremely rare, representing trophoblastic-like differentiation in adenocarcinoma, resulting in atypical giant cells that have been found to contain human chorionic gonadotropin.[19]

NODAL STATUS

In the Western world, the majority of esophageal tumors exhibit lymph node involvement at the time of presentation, this being more a characteristic of adenocarcinomas than squamous lesions (see Table 12-1). The pattern of lymph node

TABLE 12-2. Five-year survival according to tumor staging and histologic cell type

	Squamous carcinoma	Adenocarcinoma	Overall
Localized to esophageal wall (%)	80	—*	—*
Node-negative cases (%)	55	40	50
Node-positive cases (%)	11	0	6
All cases (%)	23	6	13
Mean duration of survival (mo)	37	15	24

*All adenocarcinomas transgressed the esophageal wall.

involvement has been recently documented by Akiyama et al.,[20] who have shown that lymph node involvement may exist in nodal groups at a considerable distance from the primary tumor. Tumors of the upper and middle thirds exhibit nodal metastases in celiac glands in over 30% of cases, and in lower-third tumors nodal metastases occur in about 10% in both the common hepatic artery and the superior mediastinal groups of nodes. Of practical relevance to treatment is the influence of nodal involvement on survival, and thus on the nature of the therapeutic approach in patients suspected of having lymph node involvement.

There is virtually universal consensus that in general terms, patients with positive lymph nodes fare worse prognostically than those without nodal involvement. If contiguous nodes are taken to include groups extending from the superior mediastinum to the hepatic and splenic arterial nodes, node-positive cases are associated with 5-year survival of 7% to 15% as compared with 12% to 54% for node-negative cases.[20-23] In our own series,[12] 5-year survival for node-positive cases was 6% and for node-negative 50%, the stratification according to cell type being shown in Table 12-2. Distant lymph node involvement is invariably associated with incurable disease, Postlethwait[21] and Lam et al.[22] reporting no 5-year survivors when scalene or supraclavicular nodes were involved.

The fact that 5-year survival can occur in the presence of contiguous node involvement, albeit in a relatively small percentage of patients, militates against the value of preoperative assessment of nodal status by mediastinoscopy[23-27] or computed tomography (CT) scanning[24] in order to determine the therapeutic approach. Not only does CT have a failure rate up to 40% in the detection of contiguous nodes,[25] but many of those detected will be the seat of reactive hyperplasia only, and even if they are involved, cure may still result from appropriate surgical intervention.

There is still controversy surrounding the most appropriate action regarding involved nodes dur-

ing resection of esophageal tumors. Although Akiyama et al.[20] and Skinner[26] advocate radical lymph node dissection, Orringer[27] claims similar 2-year survival using blunt esophagectomy without nodal dissection, placing greater emphasis on the biologic tumor characteristics than on extent of lymph node dissection as a determinant of survival. No controlled trial has been completed to elucidate this point, and since we have 5-year survivors with nodal involvement but no easy determinants of which patients will follow this course, it is our practice to dissect involved and contiguous lymph node groups in all cases.

TUMOR EXTENT

Several important factors in regard to the primary tumor have an important bearing on resectability, prognosis, and survival. These relate to tumor size, depth of invasion and extraesophageal spread, and longitudinal invasion.

Tumor size

In general, larger tumors tend to be more advanced in terms of local invasion and lymph node metastases than small tumors, and hence tumor length has a significant, if indirect, bearing on survival. Lesions less than 3 cm in length rarely have lymph node metastases[28] and only infrequently extend beyond the confines of the esophageal wall.[28,29] Conversely, longer lesions tend to be associated with greater degrees of lymph node involvement and extraesophageal spread, which is reflected in the proportion of curative resections.

The collective review by Rosenberg et al.[30] showed that for tumors 5 cm or less, 40% were localized to the esophagus, 25% extended beyond the esophagus, and 35% were unresectable or had distant metastases. For tumors longer than 5 cm, only 10% were localized to the esophageal wall, 15% extended beyond the esophagus, and 75% were unresectable or had distant metastases. In a series of 241 resected patients reported by

Postlethwait,[21] a curative resection was feasible in almost 50% of patients with tumors 4 cm or less in length, whereas for tumors greater than 8 cm, this rate fell to around 8%, largely because of lateral extension into adjacent structures. The relative distribution of various tumor lengths and curative resection rates is shown in Table 12-3.

As regards survival, Huang,[23] quoting a series of 976 patients with an overall 5-year survival of 30.3%, found that the 8% with tumors less than 3 cm in length had a 5-year survival rate of 43.3%, as compared with the 92% with tumors greater than 3 cm, in whom the corresponding figure was 28.9%. DeMeester and Lafontaine[31] have clearly shown the relationship between tumor length, staging, and 3-year survival (Fig. 12-1). In our own series,[12] we did not have 5-year survivors among patients with tumors greater than 6 cm in length, but survival between 1 and 2 years occurred in some patients with tumors 8 to 10 cm in length (Fig. 12-2). We therefore base our criteria for "curative" resection on other discriminants of tumor staging, principally degree of nodal involvement and fixation to adjacent structures rather than tumor length per se, and indeed in a multivariant analysis performed on 238 patients by Galandiuk et al.,[10] tumor length itself did not correlate with survival, although greater tumor length was more frequently associated with greater depth of invasion and nodal involvement.

Depth of invasion

The expression of depth of invasion varies depending on the staging system used, but the principal determinant is whether the lesion is confined to the mucosa (T_{1a}, T_m), to the muscularis propria (T_{1b}, T_{mp}), to the adventia (T_2, Ta_1), or extends beyond the confines of the esophagus (T_3, Ta_{2-3}). There is a progressive relationship between depth of invasion and incidence of nodal metastases, and an inverse relationship to survival. Two independent studies have alluded to this prognostic significance.[10,32]

In a multicenter prospective study conducted by OESO,* involving over 700 reported cases,[4] the incidence of nodal metastases rose progressively from 14% in T_{1a} lesions to 72% in T_3 lesions. The respective figures and distribution of the various degrees of invasion throughout the esophagus are shown in Table 12-4. If these data are extrapolated to survival statistics, 2-year survival after resection ranges from 69% to 29% for T_2 and T_3 tumors without nodal involvement, and

---

*Organisation Internationale d'Etudes Statistiques pour les Maladies de l'Oesophage.

TABLE 12-3. Rate of curative resection and tumor length

Length (cm)	Rate of curative resection (percent)
4	46
5-6	38
7-8	16
9-10	7
10	1

Data from Postlethwait, R.W.: Surgery of the esophagus, New York, 1979, Appleton-Century-Crofts, pp. 341-414.

from 33% to 4.5% with nodal involvement.[31] In T_1 lesions without nodal involvement, 5-year survival of 83% is reported.[23]

The spread of tumors outside the confines of the esophagus to involve adjacent structures has a profound effect on survival, 5-year survival rarely exceeding 5%.[23,33] In these circumstances, which can be accurately detected preoperatively by CT scanning,[24,25] resectional surgery is rarely feasible, hardly ever curative, and best avoided in favor of a palliative procedure such as fiberoptic endoscopic intubation.[34]

Longitudinal invasion

It is well recognized that both squamous carcinoma and adenocarcinoma can extend mucosally and submucosally for considerable distances from the apparent macroscopic tumor limits.[9,20,33] Miller[13] studied 72 resected esophageal cancers and, allowing for shrinkage during fixation, found proximal microscopic spread to be 3 cm in 64% of cases, 6 cm in 22%, 9 cm in 11%, and 10.5 cm in 3%. It is for this reason that resection series report incidences of residual tumor at the resection margins that can be as high as 46%,[35] being 12% in the multicenter OESO study.[4]

Not surprisingly, the presence of microscopic tumor at the resected margins has an influence both on the development of local recurrence and on survival. Miller[13] reported local recurrence in 77% of patients whose tumors had been inadequately excised according to histologic criteria, as opposed to 5% in whom excision was complete. In the OESO study,[4] early local recurrence developed in 37% of patients with microscopic tumor at the resected margins and in 6% of patients with microscopically healthy margins. Interestingly, local recurrence occurred in 18% of patients who had evidence of dysplasia but no microscopic tumor at the resected margins.

In terms of survival, the presence of residual tumor at the resected margins can influence re-

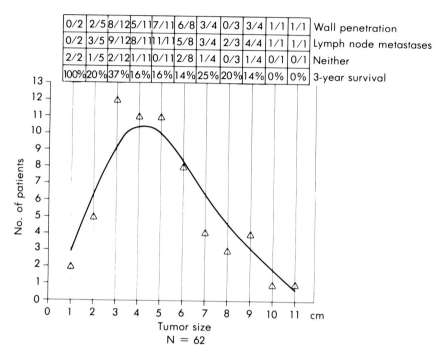

0/2	2/5	8/12	5/11	7/11	6/8	3/4	0/3	3/4	1/1	1/1	Wall penetration
0/2	3/5	9/12	8/11	11/11	5/8	3/4	2/3	4/4	1/1	1/1	Lymph node metastases
2/2	1/5	2/12	1/11	0/11	2/8	1/4	0/3	1/4	0/1	0/1	Neither
100%	20%	37%	16%	16%	14%	25%	20%	14%	0%	0%	3-year survival

Fig. 12-1. Incidence of tumor size and the relationship of tumor size to prognostic factors of depth of invasion and nodal metastases. (Modified from DeMeester, T.R., and Lafontaine, E.R.: Surgical therapy. In DeMeester, T.R., and Levin, B., editors: Cancer of the esophagus, Orlando, Fla., 1985, Grune & Stratton, pp. 141-197.)

covery from resection, since this is associated with an increased incidence of anastomotic dehiscence, which is one of the significant causes of perioperative mortality.[36,37] Adequate clearance is important in long-term survival also, as shown by Miller's series[13] in which the 5-year survival in 32 patients with an "inadequate" excision and a local recurrence rate of 75% was 2%, as compared with 20% in 76 patients with an "adequate" excision, in whom local recurrence occurred in 8%. Guili[38] expressed this same principle, reporting on a multicenter series of patients with carcinoma of the middle third of the esophagus in which the 5-year survival progressively increased in accordance with the level of the anastomosis, from 8% for a subaortic anastomosis to 13% for a supraaortic anastomosis and 24% when a cervical anastomosis was performed. The same author reported similar improvement in survival for cases of adenocarcinoma in which 10 cm of unfixed esophagus was resected.

Microscopic tumor involvement in a caudal direction is less extensive, but does occur, although rarely to a distance greater than 5 cm.[21] Another form of microscopic tumor extension, which may occur in either direction, is the embolization of tumor cells into submucosal lymphatics, producing skip or satellite nodules and thus the effect of dual carcinomas separated by intact epithelium.[39] This submucosal lymphatic embolization can easily be missed by the pathologist, which probably explains the rate of anastomotic recurrence of up to 27%[38] after resection with apparently healthy margins, and the failure of frozen-section biopsy to give a truly accurate indication of resection margin involvement.[33]

Esophagotomy, intraoperative frozen-section analysis, and subtotal esophagectomy have all been proposed as ways to overcome the problem of residual tumor at the resected margins. Esophagotomy alone is unreliable, since a healthy mucosal appearance does not exclude microscopic invasion.[40] Frozen-section analysis is time consuming and has a false-negative rate, principally related to failure of detection of submucosal lymphatic emboli.[33] We have preferred the principle of resecting at least 10 cm proximal and 5 cm distal to the apparent macroscopic tumor limits, performing a subtotal or total esophagectomy as necessary depending on the site of the tumor. This is likely to obtain total clearance in about 97% of cases,[13] and in a consecutive series of 82 resections we have had only one instance of residual microscopic tumor at the resection margin.[12]

The definition of distance from the macroscopic tumor limit has been addressed by Wong,[41]

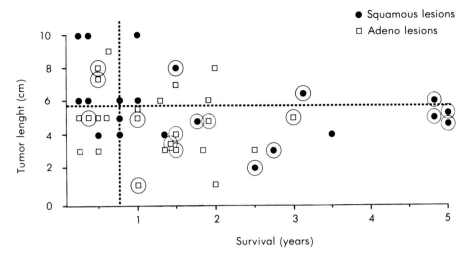

Fig. 12-2. Survival related to tumor length. The horizontal line indicates tumor length of 6 cm, above which tumors are considered to be incurable.[21] The vertical line indicates the mean survival of nonresected tumors in our series. Circles indicate patients still surviving. (Modified from Watson, A.: Ann. R. Coll. Surg. Engl. [In press.])

TABLE 12-4. Depth of invasion, nodal involvement, and tumor site

	Tumor stage			
	T_{1a}	T_{1b}	T_2	T_3
Tumor site (%)				
Upper third	0	4	30	66
Middle third	2	8	27	62
Lower third	2	7	29	62
Cardia	10	10	25	55
Total	0	6	12	81
Nodal metastases (%)				
Node positive	14	31	52	72
Node negative	86	69	48	28

Data from Giuli, R.: Proceedings, First Polydisciplinary International Congress, O.E.S.O., Paris, 1984, Maloine, S.A., Editeur, pp. 391-414.

who has shown that fixation results in a shrinkage of 50% of normal esophagus from the in situ length and that a 5-cm clearance in a fixed specimen rarely results in residual microscopic tumor.

CONCLUSION

Although overall 5-year survival rates for treated esophageal cancer are depressing, certain pathologic characteristics have been clearly shown to influence survival and to act as pointers to the most profitable direction for our therapeutic endeavors. The most important determinants are depth of invasion, involvement of contiguous organs, and the presence of lymph node and distant metastases, all of which adversely affect survival. Tumor length, degree of differentiation, and histologic cell type do not directly have a significant influence on survival, although long tumors, poorly differentiated tumors, and small-cell carcinomas and adenocarcinomas tend to be associated with greater degrees of local invasion and nodal metastases.

The two determinants reflecting virtually incurable disease are the presence of significant invasion of adjacent organs and of distant metastases, each of which should be predictable by accurate preoperative staging employing computed tomography or magnetic resonance imaging; in such cases a palliative approach can be planned. In other cases, even with long tumors, adenocarcinomas, poorly differentiated lesions, and the presence of local lymphatic metastases, cure is possible by resection that includes 10 cm proximal and 5 cm distal to the apparent tumor margins and by dissection of involved and contiguous lymph nodes.

Probably the most significant data in relation to pathologic changes affecting survival are that 5-year survival rates of over 50% for node-negative cases and over 80% for mucosal lesions have been achieved in many institutions, including our own. However, at the present time, such cases constitute but a small minority of the large spectrum of esophageal cancer, and our quest for the future must be to seek means of increasing this proportion.

REFERENCES

1. Edwards, D.A.W.: Carcinoma of the oesophagus and fundus, Postgrad. Med. J. **50:**223, 1974.
2. Huang, G.T., quoted by Wong, J.: Esophageal resection for cancer: the rationale of current practice. In Proceedings, 27th Annual Meeting of Society of Surgery of the Alimentary Tract, Am. J. Surg., **153:**18, 1987.
3. Watson, A.: A study of the quality and duration of survival following resection, endoscopic intubation and surgical intubation in oesophageal carcinoma, Br. J. Surg. **69:**585, 1982.
4. Giuli, R., editor: Proceedings, First Polydisciplinary International Congress, O.E.S.O., Paris, 1984, Maloine, S.A., Editeur, pp. 391-414.
5. Watson, A.: Therapeutic options and patient selection in the management of oesophageal carcinoma. In Watson, A., and Celestin, L.R., editors: Disorders of the oesophagus, London, 1984, Pitman, pp. 167-186.
6. Gardiol, D., Anani, P., and Fontolliet, C.: Should the histological type be taken into consideration in terms of the type of resection? In Giuli, R., editor: Proceedings, First Polydisciplinary International Congress, O.E.S.O., Paris, 1984, Maloine, S.A., Editeur, pp. 193-195.
7. Borst, H.G., Dragojevic, D., and Peck, W.: Carcinoma of the esophagus: results of resection and reconstruction. In Stipa, S., Belsey, R.H.R., and Moraldi, A., editors: Medical and surgical problems of the esophagus, New York, 1981, Academic Press, pp. 345-352.
8. Ellis, F.H.: Esophago-gastrectomy for carcinoma of the esophagus and cardia: current risks and results. In Watson, A., and Celestin, L.R., editors: Disorders of the oesophagus, London, 1984, Pitman, pp. 187-195.
9. McKeown, K.C.: Carcinoma of the oesophagus, J. R. Coll. Surg. Edinb. **24:**253, 1979.
10. Galandiuk, S., Hermann, R.E., Gassman, J.J., et al.: Cancer of the esophagus, Ann. Surg. **203:**101, 1986.
11. Turnbull, A.D.M., and Goodner, J.T.: Primary adenocarcinoma of the esophagus, Cancer **22:**915, 1968.
12. Watson, A.: The current status of resection in the management of oesophageal carcinoma, Ann. R. Coll. Surg. Engl. (In press.)
13. Miller, C.: Carcinoma of the thoracic oesophagus and cardia: a review of 405 cases, Br. J. Surg. **49:**507, 1962.
14. Mandard, A.M., Chasle, J., Marna, B., et al.: Autopsy findings in cases of esophageal cancer, Cancer **48:**329, 1981.
15. Minielly, J.A., Harrison, E.T., Fontana, R.S., et al.: Verrucous squamous cell carcinoma of the esophagus, Cancer **20:**2078, 1967.
16. Osamura, R.Y., Shimamura, K., Hata, J., et al.: Polypoid carcinoma of the esophagus: a unifying term for "carcinosarcoma" and "pseudosarcoma," Am. J. Surg. Pathol. **2:**201, 1978.
17. Troncoso, P., and Riddell, R.H.: Pathology. In DeMeester, T.R., and Levin, B., editors: Cancer of the esophagus, Orlando, Fla., 1985, Grune & Stratton, pp. 89-118.
18. Raphael, K.A., Ellis, F.H., and Dockerty, M.B.: Primary adenocarcinoma of the esophagus: 18 year review and review of literature, Ann. Surg. **164:**785, 1966.
19. McKechnie, J.C., and Fechner, R.E.: Choriocarcinoma and adenocarcinoma of the esophagus with gonadotropic secretion, Cancer **27:**694, 1971.
20. Akiyama, H., Tsuruamaru, M., Kawamura, T., et al.: Principles of surgical treatment of carcinoma of the esophagus: analysis of lymph node involvement, Ann. Surg. **194:**438, 1981.
21. Postlethwait, R.W.: Surgery of the esophagus, New York, 1979, Appleton-Century-Crofts, pp. 341-414.
22. Lam, K.H., Wong, J., Lim, S.T.K., et al.: Results of esophagectomy. In Stipa, S., Belsey, R.H.R., and Moraldi, A., editors: Medical and surgical problems of the esophagus, New York, 1981, Academic Press, pp. 353-359.
23. Huang, K.C.: Surgical treatment of carcinoma of the esophagus: results in 1647 patients. In Stipa, S., Belsey, R.H.R., and Moraldi, A., editors: Medical and surgical problems of the esophagus, New York, 1981, Academic Press, pp. 335-338.
24. Picus, D., Balfe, D.M., Koehler, R.E., et al.: Computed tomography in the staging of esophageal carcinoma, Radiology **146:**433, 1983.
25. Lebas, J.F., Sarrazin, R., Coulomb, B., et al.: Can the scanner supply sufficient elements to specify the state of the detected lymph nodes? In Guili, R., editor: Proceedings, First Polydisciplinary International Congress, O.E.S.O., Paris, 1984, Maloine, S.A., Editeur, pp. 92-93.
26. Skinner, D.B.: En bloc resection for neoplasms of the esophagus and cardia, J. Thorac. Cardiovasc. Surg. **85:**59-71, 1983.
27. Orringer, M.B.: Is it illusory to envisage extended lymph node dissection? In Guili, R., editor: Proceedings, First Polydisciplinary International Congress, O.E.S.O., Paris, 1984, Maloine, S.A., Editeur, pp. 138-140.
28. Yamada, A.: Radiologic assessment of resectability and prognosis in esophageal carcinoma, Gastrointest. Radiol. **4:**213, 1979.
29. Mori, S., Kasai, M., Watanabe, T., et al.: Pre-operative assessment of resectability for carcinoma of the thoracic esophagus. I. Esophagogram and azygogram, Ann. Surg. **199:**100, 1979.

30. Rosenberg, J.C., Franklin, R., and Steiger, Z.: Squamous cell carcinoma of the thoracic esophagus: an interdisciplinary approach, Curr. Probl. Cancer **5:**1, 1981.

31. DeMeester, T.R., and Lafontaine, E.R.: Surgical therapy. In DeMeester, T.R., and Levin, B., editors: Cancer of the esophagus, Orlando, Fla., 1985, Grune & Stratton, pp. 141-197.

32. Skinner, D.B., Dowlatshahi, K.B., and DeMeester, T.R.: Potentially curable carcinoma of the esophagus, Cancer **50:**2571, 1982.

33. Mannell, A.: Carcinoma of the esophagus, Curr. Probl. Surg. **19:**557, 1982.

34. Watson, A.: Palliative intubation in inoperable esophageal neoplasms, Ann. Thorac. Surg. **39:**501, 1985.

35. Scanlon, E.F., Morton, D.R., Walker, J.M., et al.: The case against segmental resection for esophageal carcinoma, Surg. Gynecol. Obstet. **101:**290, 1955.

36. Inberg, M.V., Linna, M.I., Scheinin, T.M., et al.: Anastomotic leakage after excision of esophageal and high gastric carcinoma, Am. J. Surg. **122:**540, 1971.

37. Chassin, J.L.: Esophago-gastrectomy: data favoring end to side anastomosis, Ann. Surg. **188:**22, 1978.

38. Giuli, R.: Surgical complications and reasons for failure. In DeMeester, T.R., and Levin, B., editors: Cancer of the esophagus, Orlando, Fla., 1985, Grune & Stratton, pp. 199-208.

39. Solomon, A., and Hunt, J.: Multiple squamous carcinomas and the oesophagus, S. Afr. Med. J. **55:**1028, 1979.

40. Giuli, R., and Gignoux, M.: Treatment of carcinoma of the esophagus: a retrospective study of 2400 patients, Ann. Surg. **192:**44, 1980.

41. Wong, J.: Methods available to assess the quality of surgical resection. In Guili, R., editor: Proceedings, First Polydisciplinary International Congress, O.E.S.O., Paris, 1984, Maloine, S.A., Editeur, p. 198.

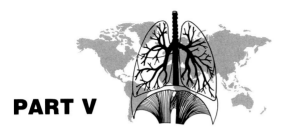

PART V

REDUCTION OF PERIOPERATIVE MORTALITY

CHAPTER 13 Perioperative management of carcinoma of the esophagus: the reduction of operative mortality

Aviel Roy and Tom R. DeMeester

Proper perioperative management of the patient with carcinoma of the esophagus is as important to the reduction of operative mortality as technical expertise. Intelligent perioperative care includes a rational choice of the operative procedure, careful selection of the operative candidate, and judicious use of supportive measures.

SELECTING THE OPERATIVE PROCEDURE

Diagnosis of esophageal carcinoma at an early stage, before distant metastases or local spread has occurred, is rare. There are four reasons for this: (1) the usual warning signs of malignancy, such as pain or hemorrhage, are uncommon in carcinoma of the esophagus; (2) the esophagus can adapt to a considerable degree of stenosis before any subjective dysphagia is evident; (3) an obvious decline in the patient's general condition does not occur until late in the course of the disease; and (4) mass screening tests, as used in China,[1] may result in early detection, but are not economically feasible in the Occident, because of the lower incidence of the disease.

In view of the inability to detect patients with early disease, it is not surprising that many surgeons believe that any surgical treatment of esophageal carcinoma is essentially palliative. This attitude explains the popularity of such conservative operations as the blunt esophagectomy without thoracotomy.[2] While this palliative approach is applicable to the majority of patients, it denies a possible cure in some.

The current TNM staging system for carcinoma of the esophagus was introduced in 1978 by the American Joint Committee for Cancer Staging and End Result Reporting. Staging of this disease is difficult because the organ is inaccessible and its lymphatic drainage is widespread.[3] Even with modern imaging techniques, such as computed tomography and magnetic resonance imaging, preoperative staging remains imprecise. When the data of the American Joint Committee for Cancer Staging and End Result Reporting are analyzed for the whole esophagus, the survival rates for stages I, II, and III are 15%, 5%, and 3%, respectively. This represents a minor difference in survival between the stages. As a consequence, this staging system is not generally useful in clinical practice.

Although the use of the TNM system has shown it to be imprecise, it has identified several characteristics of esophageal cancer that are associated with improved survival. Among them are tumors that are less than 5 cm in length, do not extend beyond the esophageal wall, or do not have lymph node metastasis. We endeavored to sharpen these observations by analyzing 58 patients in whom one or more of these favorable predictors were present.[4] This analysis showed that in patients who had favorable tumors, only metastasis to lymph nodes and tumor penetration of the esophageal wall had a significant and independent influence on prognosis. That is, the beneficial effects of the absence of one factor persisted even when the others were present. Other factors important in the survival of patients with advanced disease, such as tumor size, cell type, degree of cellular differentiation, and location of the tumor in the esophagus, had no effect on survival of patients who had resection of their disease at an early stage. Our analysis also in-

101

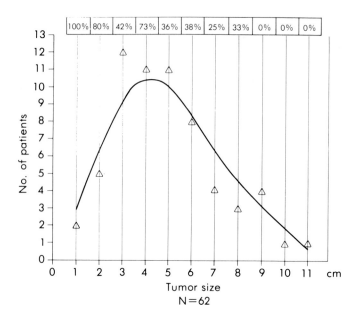

| 100% | 80% | 42% | 73% | 36% | 38% | 25% | 33% | 0% | 0% | 0% |

No. of patients

Tumor size
N=62

Fig. 13-1. Incidences of tumor sizes and the relationship of tumor size to the incidence of potentially curable tumors.

TABLE 13-1. Classification of esophageal carcinoma

Wall penetration
 W_0 = Tumor limited to mucosa
 W_1 = Tumor penetration through submucosa and into but not through muscle layers
 W_2 = Tumor penetration through muscle layers
Lymph node involvement
 N_0 = No lymph node involvement
 N_1 = One to four lymph nodes involved
 N_2 = Five or more lymph nodes involved
Systemic metastasis
 M_0 = No metastasis
 M_1 = Distant metastasis

dicated that esophageal tumors that met the criteria of no wall penetration or lymph node metastasis could be defined as potentially curable regardless of size, histologic grade, cell type, or location. Based on this analysis, Skinner et al. proposed a new staging system, which classifies the depth of wall penetration (W), the presence of lymph node involvement (N), and the presence of systemic metastases (M).[5] Table 13-1 shows the definitions for the various W, N, and M classifications. Skinner has shown a significant difference in survival curves between patients with favorable ($W_{0-1}N_{0-1}$ or W_2N_{0-1} or $W_{0-1}N_2$) and patients with unfavorable (W_2N_2) stages. A recent study by DeMeester et al.[6] showed that for cancer of the distal esophagus and cardia, patients with a favorable stage of disease could be selected out by preoperative and intraoperative assessment,

and had survival rates after a curative en bloc resection similar to those reported by Skinner et al. for the same stage of disease.

Armed with the knowledge of criteria favorable for survival, our approach to the patient with an esophageal tumor is structured by the answers to four clinical questions:

1. Is the tumor curable?
2. If it is not curable, does the patient have enough dysphagia to require palliation?
3. If palliation is indicated, can the tumor be resected?
4. If the tumor is not resectable, what other method of palliation is available?

Carcinoma of the esophagus is potentially curable in the absence of wall penetration or if there are four or fewer lymph node metastases, or both. Lymph node involvement can be detected by histologic examination of palpable nodes in the neck, with cervical mediastinoscopy, with laparoscopy, or at the time of surgery. Extension of the tumor through the esophageal wall is recognized by recurrent laryngeal or phrenic nerve paralysis, by the finding of an abnormal esophageal axis on barium swallow, or by intraoperative inspection of the tumor.[7] If both paralysis and an abnormal axis are present, the tumor should be considered incurable.

Fig. 13-1 shows the relationship of the endoscopically measured tumor size to the presence of favorable staging—that is, no wall penetration and four or fewer metastatic lymph nodes. There is a high incidence of favorable parameters in tumors shorter than 4 cm, but favorable criteria are found in tumors up to 8 cm long. As a con-

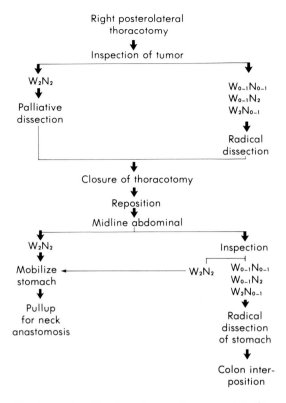

Fig. 13-2. Algorithm for a therapeutic approach to the patient with a potentially curable lesion. See Table 13-1 for explanation of staging symbols.

TABLE 13-2. Functional grades of dysphagia

Grade	Definition
I	Eating normally
II	Requires liquids with meals
III	Able to take semisolids but unable to take any solid food
IV	Able to take liquids only
V	Unable to take liquids but able to swallow saliva
VI	Unable to swallow saliva

sequence, length per se does not exclude the possibility of curative resection, but the finding of a small tumor should encourage an aggressive approach.

While blunt esophagectomy may be curative in patients with neither lymph node metastases nor wall penetration, it is clearly insufficient when one or the other is present. It is particularly disadvantageous for patients who have lymph node involvement without wall penetration. In this situation, simply fishing out the esophagus leaves tumor behind. Frequently, lymph node status and depth of invasion are determined only by thoracotomy. As a result, we believe that unless preoperative staging clearly demonstrates an incurable situation, an extensive operation with en bloc lymph node dissection should be planned. If in the course of the operation an incurable situation is identified, the surgeon should change to a limited procedure. Fig. 13-2 is an algorithm of our operative approach to the patient whose preoperative evaluation did not preclude a curable lesion. This approach allows operative adjustments to the extent of the dissection, based on the operative findings.

When the tumor is incurable, the goal of therapy is palliation. Palliative procedures are indicated in the presence of severe dysphagia or other incapacitating symptoms. Table 13-2 is a functional classification of the degrees of dysphagia, which we have found useful. We consider dysphagia of grade IV or higher an indication for a palliative procedure. Resection and reconstruction offer the best palliation, allowing the patient to eat normally and preventing the local complications of the tumor such as perforation, hemorrhage, fistula formulation, and incapacitating pain. Therefore, in the symptomatic patient, resection should be attempted. The presence of a malignant pleural effusion or metastatic disease other than to lymph nodes usually discourages a palliative resection.

A definitely unresectable tumor is identified by the presence of a tracheoesophageal fistula, obstruction of the vena cava, or vertebral spine erosion. Special studies that are helpful in detecting an unresectable tumor are azygograms showing azygos vein obstruction and CT scans showing evidence of cervical or thoracic spine erosion. If the tumor is unresectable, a variety of other palliative procedures should be considered, including surgical bypass, intubation, or an external artificial esophagus.

PREOPERATIVE PHYSIOLOGIC ASSESSMENT

Before proceeding with surgical therapy for carcinoma of the esophagus, the surgeon must confirm that the patient is able to withstand the planned operation. Physiologic assessment of the patient also affects the extent of the operation. It is futile to select an operation that is aimed at increasing the long-term survival for a patient whose physiologic life expectancy is short.

Carcinoma of the esophagus is predominantly a disease of men between the ages of 50 and 70.[8] Smoking and alcohol abuse are very common in patients with this disease. As a result, the pres-

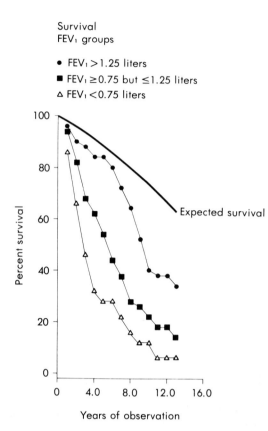

Survival
FEV₁ groups

- FEV₁ > 1.25 liters
- FEV₁ ≥ 0.75 but ≤ 1.25 liters
- Δ FEV₁ < 0.75 liters

Fig. 13-3. Survival of groups distinguished on the basis of FEV₁ at the time of enrollment in the study. There were 52 subjects with an initial FEV₁ greater than 1.25 liter, 90 in the middle group, and 58 with an initial FEV₁ less than 0.75 liter.

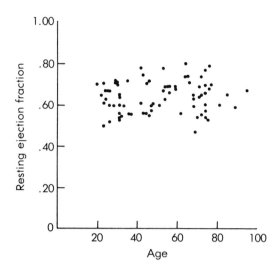

Fig. 13-4. Left-ventricular ejection fraction at rest plotted against age in 77 healthy subjects. There is no statistically significant change in resting ejection fraction with age (r = 0.10).

ence of additional chronic illnesses, such as chronic obstructive lung disease or ischemic heart disease, is the rule rather than the exception in these patients. Since the predominant symptom of esophageal carcinoma is dysphagia, many of the patients have, in addition, a poor nutritional status and low serum albumin level.

Following en bloc resection of the esophagus for cure, the lymphatic clearance of both lungs is compromised.[9] The lungs are supplied with a rich network of lymphatics that drain centrally toward the hili. The direction of the flow is maintained by a series of strategically placed valves.[10] The disruption of these lymphatic channels, as occurs when the middle mediastinal nodes are resected, leads to accumulation of interstitial lung water, which reduces alveolar volume and increases airway resistance. This phenomenon is manifested clinically by tachypnea, increased work of breathing, and eventually respiratory failure. *Rales may or may not be present,* because the edema is mainly interstitial.

Poor nutritional status may potentiate the problem. Guyton and Lindsey demonstrated experimentally that if the serum protein levels are normal, the left atrial pressure has to exceed 24 mm Hg before transudation into the alveoli develops. The critical left atrial pressure drops to 11 mm Hg when the serum protein levels are low.[11]

As a consequence, the patient must have sufficient cardiopulmonary reserve to tolerate the operation. The respiratory function is best assessed by means of the FEV₁, which should be 2 liters or more. Any patient with an FEV₁ of less than 1 liter is not a surgical candidate; first, he is unlikely to survive the operation, and second, if he does, his life expectancy is short because of lung disease (see Fig. 13-3).[12] Clinical evaluation and electrocardiography are not sufficient indicators of the cardiac status. The gated radionuclide pool scan is noninvasive and provides accurate information on wall motion and ejection fraction. If the latter is below .40 or does not increase on exercise, a coronary arteriogram and ventriculogram may be indicated. The use of the scan as a preoperative screening tool allows significant reduction of operative mortality in patients undergoing major vascular reconstructions.[13] In this regard, it is interesting to note that the ejection fraction at rest remains relatively constant with advancing age (see Fig. 13-4).[14] Therefore, a resting ejection fraction of less than .40 is an ominous sign. We do not advocate extensive en bloc resections for such patients.

A substantial number of esophagectomies are performed on elderly patients, and an important factor in the evaluation of the patient's physiology is age. It is therefore pertinent to assess the effect of age on surgical risk.

Advancing age is associated with decreased overall performance, regardless of the presence or absence of disease; in a study of marathon runners, who obviously have a high cardiopulmonary reserve, Stones and Kozma found rapidly decreasing performance after the age of 70.[15] The decreased physical performance is also manifested in increased operative mortality. Fig. 13-5 is adapted from a study of 15,930 surgical cases in Wisconsin. Both elective and emergency operations are included.[16] The graph demonstrates the effect of age on procedure-adjusted mortality. There is a steady increase in mortality with advancing age. The mortality climbs precipitously after the age of 75. The risk at age 90 to 94 is twice that at 75 to 84, and at 80 to 84 years it is nearly twice that at 0 to 69 years. There is a slight increase in risk in the 70-to-74 group over the 65-to-69 group.

Increased risks may be justified if they are outweighed by the expected benefits. Thus it is necessary to consider the overall life expectancy of this group of patients. Since the turn of the century, the average life expectancy from birth has almost doubled, going from 47 years in 1900, to almost 75 in the 1980s. Although these figures are impressive, they are largely due to the elimination of acute disease and infant mortality. The maximum life span has not changed much.[17] The life expectancy at 65 years was 76 in 1900 and improved only to 81 in 1975. There has been no increase in the number of centagenerians or in the maximum age at which death occurred in the last 150 years. From actuarial data of the federal government, one can calculate a maximum average life span of somewhat less than 85 years. This number corresponds with the experimental results of Heyflick,[18] who calculated a theoretical maximum life span of less than 90 years based on the observation that human fibroblasts are capable of a finite number of divisions in tissue culture.

Excluding trauma, suicide, and miscellaneous uncommon conditions, the majority of deaths over the age of 75 are due to cancer, stroke, or heart disease. Since humans must die, reducing the number of cancer deaths will only increase the mortality from heart disease or stroke, and will not affect life expectancy at birth. This is a theorem of the theory of competing risks, which states: "In a developed society where the exponentials describing the cumulative rates with age for the more common causes of death have similar intercepts, the elimination of one cause of death

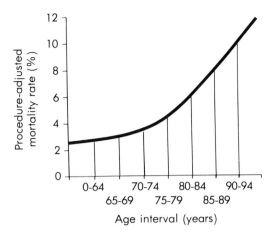

Fig. 13-5. The procedure-adjusted mortality rate increases with age. Note the steepness of the curve after 75 years. (Adapted from Sikes, E.D., Jr., and Detmer, D.E.: Wisc. Med. J. 78:27, 1979.)

does not significantly affect life expectancy."[19] In other words, curing an octogenarian of cancer will only change the cause of death but not the eventual life expectancy. As a result, the goal of surgical intervention in advanced age is to palliate: "add life to years, not years to life."

It is clear from this discussion that after the age of 75 a radical operation for cure of carcinoma of the esophagus is unwise, because of the additional risk and reduced benefits. A palliative resection, however, besides having a small chance of cure, does provide better palliation than radiotherapy or intubation. This is because there are fewer problems with dysphagia, hemorrhage, perforation, fistula formation, and incapacitating pain after the tumor is resected.[20] Thus we advocate a palliative resection, if possible, even in older patients. After the age of 80, however, the risks of resection become formidable, and it is prudent to resort to other means of palliation.

SUPPORTIVE MEASURES

Supportive measures are performed to improve the ability of the patient to tolerate the operation, and to sustain him in the postoperative period. Patients with mild congestive failure can be improved to some extent with vigorous medical management. Likewise, cessation of smoking, aggressive bronchopulmonary toilet, and bronchodilators may improve the FEV_1 of some patients. Patients with chronic lung disease do better if their operations are scheduled for the afternoon. This allows them to ambulate and cough up the secretions that have accumulated in the lung dur-

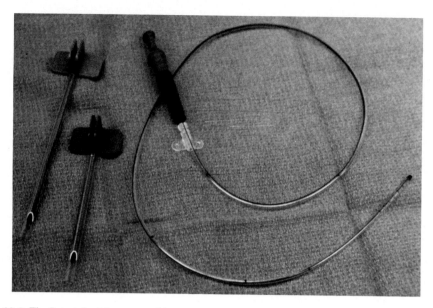

Fig. 13-6. The Intestofix jejunostomy kit (Intestofix, Braun Melsungen AG, West Germany). Note the two breakaway needles and the large plastic cannula.

ing the night. Patients undergoing esophageal resection are prone to develop postoperative respiratory failure, mainly because of the development of interstitial pulmonary edema; as discussed above, rales may be absent. As a consequence, it is necessary to maintain low left-atrial pressures (estimated by the pulmonary artery wedge pressure or by the central venous pressure) during the postoperative period. This goal is achieved by restricting the amount of parenteral fluids administered during the operation and in the postoperative period. The surgeon must discuss this with the anesthesiologist to ensure that excessive fluids are not given. If the serum albumin level is low, colloids should be employed, because low serum protein levels lower the critical left-atrial pressure—a situation in which transudation into the lung occurs.[11]

The nutritional status of the patient is of paramount importance to the outcome. Low serum protein levels have a deleterious effect on the cardiovascular system, and a poor nutritional status affects the host resistance to infection and the rate of healing of anastomoses and wounds.[21] The simplest way to assess the nutritional status of the patient is to measure the serum albumin level prior to any hydration. A value below 3.4 g/dl indicates poor caloric intake and an increased risk of surgical complications, including anastomotic breakdowns.[22]

Nutritional support can be provided in several ways. Oral intake is usually inadequate for the majority of esophageal carcinoma patients, and passage of a nasogastric tube can be difficult. The use of the gut for alimentation has several advantages over the intravenous route, including better utilization of nutrients and lower caloric requirement,[23] decreased incidence of metabolic, septic, and thrombotic complications, a tenfold decrease in cost per patient,[24] and ease of performance in outpatients. In our experience, a feeding jejunostomy tube provides the most reliable and safest method for nutritional support in patients with esophageal carcinoma who cannot consume an oral diet, and who have a functionally normal small bowel. A gastrostomy is inadvisable for these patients, because it may interfere with the use of the stomach for reconstruction. The jejunostomy permits nutritional support early in the postoperative period, and minimizes the danger of regurgitation into the esophagus with possible aspiration when a gastrostomy is used.

The so-called Witzel jejunostomy, which employs a 12-mm tube placed through a serosal tunnel, was never very popular, because of serious and frequent complications, most notably intraperitoneal leaks, kinking of the bowel, and intestinal obstruction. These complications were eliminated with the development of the intramural needle catheter technique described by Delaney

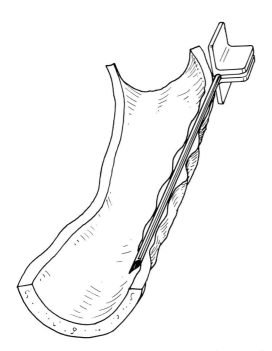

Fig. 13-7. The technique of developing an intramural tunnel for a jejunostomy tube.

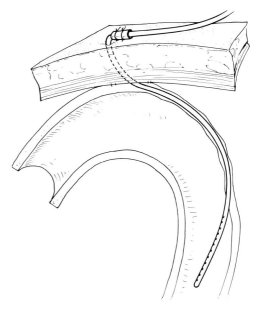

Fig. 13-8. Method of securing the feeding jejunostomy catheter to the parietal peritoneum and the skin of the abdominal wall.

et al.,[25] who used a 14-gauge needle and a catheter from a central vein catheterization set. The only problem with this technique is the small diameter of the tube, which frequently leads to clogging and sluggish flow; therefore, the choice of diet is restricted to a low-viscosity elemental diet (Vivonex), which is very hypertonic and relatively expensive.

We prefer a different commercial kit (Intestofix, Braun Melsungen AG, West Germany), which contains two breakaway needles and a flexible no. 12 French catheter (Fig. 13-6). The larger lumen allows the use of more viscous formulas at a faster rate, and clogging is less frequent. The tube is somewhat stiffer, which makes possible easy replacement through the established tract should the tube become dislodged. Maintenance is simple, and patients can easily take care of the catheter and the apparatus at home.

In severely malnourished patients, the catheter is placed as a separate procedure, to allow preoperative nutritional support. The latter is continued while the patient is investigated, thus saving valuable time. In this case, the abdomen is entered through a small supraumbilical midline incision, and the ligament of Treitz is exposed by applying traction to the transverse colon. Otherwise, the jejunostomy is placed at the time of the esophageal resection.

The kit includes two breakaway needles. The shorter one is used to pass the catheter through the skin and the longer to create the intramural tunnel. The surgeon selects a loop of jejunum, about 25 cm from the ligament of Treitz or from the most distal small bowel anastomosis, and places a purse-string suture on the antimesenteric side. To create the intramural antireflux tunnel, the serosa is pierced, the needle is held steady, and the wall of the bowel is secured over it. The tip of the needle should be visualized through the translucent serosa as the wall of the gut is pulled over the shaft. The length of the tunnel should be 12 to 15 cm, at which point the needle is angled in to pierce the mucosa (see Fig. 13-7). The catheter is threaded through the needle into the lumen for a distance of 25 to 30 cm. The needle is split and removed, and the purse string is tied down. We make it a point to verify the intraluminal position of the catheter by occluding the distal bowel and irrigating the catheter with saline. Next, the loop of jejunum is anchored to the parietal peritoneum and the transversalis fascia with four silk sutures placed circumferentially around the catheter. Finally, the catheter is secured to the skin with 3-0 stainless steel wire (see Fig. 13-8). We prefer wire for this purpose because it is nonreactive, and these sutures stay in for as long as the catheter is in place.

If the commercial kit has not been available, we have used a small gallbladder trocar to create the intramural tunnel. A no. 10 French infant feeding tube can be passed easily through the lumen of the trocar. We have found this an entirely satisfactory, if less elegant, alternative. The only caveat is that the feeding tube should be passed once through the trocar before the latter

TABLE 13-3. Feeding schedule for the use of the jejunostomy tube*

Postoperative day	Solution	Rate
3	D$_5$W	25 ml/hr
4	Half-strength Vital HN	25 ml/hr
5	Half-strength Vital HN	50 ml/hr
6	Half-strength Vital HN	100 ml/hr
7	Full-strength Vital HN	75 ml/hr
8	Full-strength Vital HN	100 ml/hr

*This is our routine schedule for gradual increase in concentration and rate of administration. We use elemental diet early on. If diarrhea occurs, we switch to an isotonic solution (Osmolite, Ross Laboratories, Inc.). Note the decrease in rate on day 5.

is inserted, because the proximal flared end may require trimming to allow the removal of the trocar after the tube is in place.

Feeding is begun on the third postoperative day. We start with 5% dextrose in water, and gradually advance, using a continuous drip infusion technique, to full-strength formula at a rate of 2400 to 3000 calories per day. Table 13-3 shows the feeding schedule that we use. Early in the postoperative period, elemental diet is used (Vital HN, Ross Laboratories, Inc.). However, the size of the catheter permits the use of any type of balanced formula, including Ensure, Pulmocare, Osmolite, and even a blenderized diet. As the patient resumes oral intake, the amount of nutritional support is tapered off. If oral intake is sufficient, the catheter is used to provide intermittent nutritional support at the convenience of the patient.

Patients who require nutritional support after discharge from the hospital are issued a portable pump (Ross Laboratories, Inc.) that can be carried on a shoulder strap while the patient goes about his daily activities (see Fig. 13-9). None of our patients had any difficulty with the use of the pump at home over prolonged periods of time.

We have used this technique in 24 consecutive patients undergoing surgery for esophageal disease. The catheters were used as an adjuvant at the time of the resection in 14 patients, as part of a staged operation in five, as a stand-alone for palliation in two, and as an interim preresection procedure in three. The catheters stayed in place as long as 7 months. Depending on the patient's weight and oral intake, the pump delivered up to 3000 calories daily. Patients who were totally supported were usually maintained on 1800 to 2400 calories per day.

Complications were few. Clogging is prevented by routine irrigation of the catheter with 30 ml of vinegar, cranberry juice, or Coca-Cola. Diar-

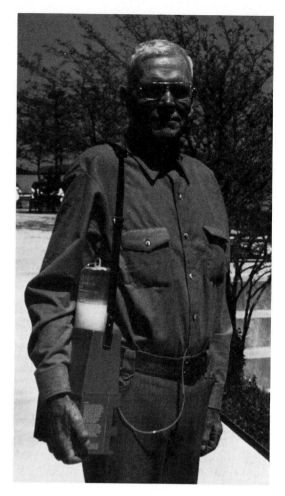

Fig. 13-9. This patient is 1 month after en bloc resection of the esophagus with colon interposition. The jejunostomy tube was removed after this photograph was taken.

rhea can occur, especially early on. This is easily controlled by adding Kaopectate or paregoric to the formula, by slowing the rate temporarily, or by switching to an isotonic formula. In our experience, diarrhea was not a reason for interruption of the feedings. The catheter dislodged or became kinked in five patients. In four, a new catheter was threaded through the established tract, and feeding was resumed without incident. Intraluminal positioning of the tube was verified by injecting a small amount of water-soluble contrast material and obtaining a single abdominal roentgenogram. One patient required operative replacement of the catheter. There was one case of infection along the catheter tract. This cleared by incision of the skin on top of the catheter, and did not require removal.

Using this technique, we were able to avoid the use of total parenteral nutrition with its attendant mechanical, thrombotic, and septic complications.[26] All our patients gained weight or maintained their weight while receiving nutritional support; excessive weight gain occurred in several patients and required reduction of the administration rate. One extremely obese patient, who had a failed colonic interposition, was placed on a 1500-calorie regimen for 4 months. Reconstruction was successfully carried out when he achieved ideal weight.

We found that intramural jejunostomy by the technique described is a safe and effective method for providing nutritional support. It is particularly suitable for esophageal cancer patients because it bypasses the obstruction and avoids violating the stomach. This way the stomach remains available for reconstruction, if needed. Although the standard needle-catheter jejunostomy is acceptable, the larger tube we use is easier to maintain, and prolonged nutritional support at home is well accepted by the patients and their families.

CONCLUSION

We have defined a group of patients with potentially curable carcinoma: the absence of either deep penetration or lymph node metastasis. For other patients the objective of surgical treatment is palliation. For selected groups, extended surgery is indicated, provided the patients are judged to be able to withstand the operation.

The major parameters of patient physiology are age, cardiopulmonary function, and nutritional status. In advanced age, curative surgery is not indicated, since cure does not affect survival rate, and the goal of surgery is palliation.

Supportive measures are most successful in managing nutrition. The preferred method of nutritional support is by an operative feeding jejunostomy, which can also be used for long-term management at home.

REFERENCES

1. Wu, Y.K., Chen, P.T., Fang, J.P., and Lin, S.S.: Surgical treatment of esophageal carcinoma, Am. J. Surg. **139:**805, 1980.
2. Orringer, M.B.: Technical aids in performing transhiatal esophagectomy without thoracotomy, Ann. Thorac. Surg. **18:**1, 1974.
3. Akiyama, H., Tsurumaru, M., Kawamura, T., and Ono, Y.: Principles of surgical treatment for carcinoma of the esophagus: analysis of lymph node involvement, Ann. Surg. **194:**438, 1981.
4. Skinner, D.B., Dowlatshahi, K.D., and DeMeester, T.R.: Potentially curable carcinoma of the esophagus, Cancer **50:**2571, 1982.
5. Skinner, D.B., Ferguson, M.K., Soriano, A., Little, A.G., and Staszak, V.M.: Selection of operation for esophageal cancer based on staging, Ann. Surg. **204:** 291, 1986.
6. DeMeester, T.R., Zaninotto, G., and Johansson, K.-E.: Selective therapeutic approach to cancer of lower esophagus and cardia, J. Thorac. Cardiovasc. Surg. **95:**42, 1988.
7. Akiyama, H., Kogure, T., and Itai, Y.: The esophageal axis and its relationship to the resectability of carcinoma of the esophagus, Ann. Surg. **176:**30, 1971.
8. Garfinkel, L., Poindexter, C.E., and Silverberg, E.: Cancer in black Americans, Cancer **30:**39, 1980.
9. Thomas, P.A.: Physiologic sufficiency of regenerated lung lymphatics, Ann. Surg. **192:**162, 1980.
10. Trapnell, D.H.: The peripheral lymphatics of the lungs, Br. J. Radiol. **36:**660, 1963.
11. Guyton, A.C., and Lindsey, A.W.: Effect of elevated left atrial pressure and decreased plasma protein concentration on the development of pulmonary edema, Circ. Res. **7:**649, 1959.
12. Diener, C.F., and Burrows, B.: Further observations on the course and prognosis of chronic obstructive lung disease, Am. Rev. Respir. Dis. **111:**719, 1975.
13. Boucher, C.A., Brewster, D.C., Darling, R.C., Okada, R.D., Straus, H.W., and Pohost, G.M.: Determination of cardiac risk by dipyridamole-thalium imaging before peripheral vascular surgery, N. Engl. J. Med. **312:**389, 1985.
14. Port, S., Cobb, F.R., Coleman, E., and Jones, R.H.: Effect of age on the response of the left ventricular response to exercise, N. Engl. J. Med. **303:**1133, 1980.
15. Stones, M.J., and Kozma, A.: Adult age trends in record running performances, Exp. Aging Res. **6:**407, 1980.
16. Sikes, E.D., Jr., and Detmer, D.E.: Aging and surgical risk in older citizens of Wisconsin, Wis. Med. J. **78:**27, 1979.
17. Fries, J.F.: Aging, natural death and the compression of senescence, N. Engl. J. Med. **303:**130, 1980.
18. Heyflick, L.: Aging under glass, Exp. Gerontol. **5:**291, 1970.
19. Maloney, J.V.: The limits of medicine, Ann. Surg. **194:**247, 1981.
20. Belsey, R.H.R.: Palliative management of esophageal carcinoma, Am. J. Surg. **139:**789, 1980.
21. Heatly, R.V., Lewis, M.H., and Williams, R.H.P.: Preoperative intravenous feeding: a controlled trial, Postgrad. Med. J. **55:**541, 1979.
22. Piccone, V.A., Ahmed, N., Grosberg, S., and Leveen, H.H.: Esophagogastrectomy for carcinoma of the esophagus, Ann. Thorac. Surg. **28:**369, 1979.
23. Allardyce, D., and Groves, A.: A comparison of nutritional responses from intravenous and enteral feedings, Surg. Gynecol. Obstet. **139:**179, 1974.
24. Lim, S.T.K., Choa, R.G., Lam, K.H., et al.: Total parenteral nutrition versus gastrostomy in preoperative preparation of patients with cancer of the esophagus, Br. J. Surg. **68:**69, 1981.
25. Delaney, H.M., Carnevale, N., and Garvey, J.W.: Jejunostomy by a needle catheter technique, Surgery **73:**786, 1973.
26. Ryan, J.A., Abel, R.M., Abbott, W.M., et al.: Catheter complications in total parenteral nutrition: a prospective study in 200 consecutive patients, N. Engl. J. Med. **290:**757, 1974.

Perioperative management of carcinoma of the esophagus: the reduction of operative mortality

DISCUSSION

C. Noirot, J.R. Bouderlique, and Robert Giuli

This discussion is limited to the supportive measures described by Roy and DeMeester—in particular, nutrition. In the OESO (Organisation Internationale d'Etudes Statistiques pour les Maladies de l'Oesophage, or International Organization for Statistical Studies on Diseases of the Esophagus) multicentric international prospective study, several important points emerge relative to nutritional status and methods and immunologic status.

NUTRITIONAL STATUS

Malnutrition is classically found in more than 50% of patients with esophageal cancer. However, as Table 13-4 shows, a weight loss in excess of 10% was found in only 37% of patients. These data show the importance of defining reliable indicators of nutritional assessment. The OESO prospective randomized trial (see Chapter 33) attempts to assess the most reliable indicators of malnutrition through investigation of biologic markers, anthropometric criteria, and immunologic state of the patients undergoing operation.

The reasons for malnutrition in esophageal cancer are anorexia related to alcohol use and smoking, decreased dietary intake with distaste for food, and metabolic disturbances resulting from the interaction between host and tumor, which include (1) increase in basal metabolism, (2) disturbances of hepatic gluconeogenesis with excessive protein catabolism, and (3) disturbances of lipid metabolism, electrolyte imbalances, and vitamin deficiencies.

In all patients with esophageal cancer, nutritional support is obligatory and should be begun as early as possible.

Is preoperative nutritional support effective? Numerous clinical studies indicate that preoperative replacement of nutritional losses is advisable. Today, this point is disputed. Because of the presence of the tumor, the increased metabolic disturbances, and malnutrition, it may be difficult to reverse the nutritional depletion. Thus, Table 13-5[1] shows a nonsignificant weight gain in patients receiving enteral or parenteral nutritional support. Nevertheless, in our opinion, nutritional support is indicated when there is a rapid (less than 2 months) and significant (more than 20% of usual weight) malnutrition, and when the caloric intake is very poor.

The aim of preoperative nutritional support is to compensate for fasting resulting from dysphagia and to increase the caloric intake and permit a positive nutritional balance after tumor depletion.

Effects of different treatments on nutritional status

The various treatments (chemotherapy followed by surgery, or surgery and radiotherapy, or surgery and chemotherapy) may themselves induce malnutrition.

Surgery. The catabolism that occurs after surgery persists for at least 20 days. Moreover, during that period, because of the anorexia and dysphagia involved, caloric intake is always decreased. Finally, functional sequelae following esophageal cancer surgery, such as those secondary to vagotomy, can disrupt the return of an anabolic state.

Radiotherapy. Radiotherapy induces, in doses of 15 to 20 cGy upward, some degree of radiotherapeutic esophagitis, resulting in anorexia, nausea, vomiting, and sometimes dysphagia. In all cases, food intake is decreased.

Chemotherapy. Whatever drugs and protocols are used, chemotherapy causes important nutritional disturbances. These include decreased intake with nausea and vomiting from cisplatin, diarrhea from 5-fluorouracil, anorexia in general,

TABLE 13-4. Weight loss

0	Average rate: 6.3 kg ± 11		<10%	>10%
107	551		63%	37%
	Circumference of the arm (51)	Triceps skin thickness (52)		
Time of admission nutritional support = 60%	25.8 ± 18	10.9 ± 17		
Preoperative state	25.9 ± 18	9.8 ± 11		

From First Polydisciplinary International Congress of OESO: Cancer of the esophagus in 1984: 135 questions, answers compiled by R. Giuli, Paris, 1984, Editions Maloine.

TABLE 13-5. Nutritional support

0 154 Average weight loss 6 kg I.D.—69%	+ 159 Average weight loss 9 kg I.D.—63%				
	Enteral 83%		*Parenteral* 74%		
	<3000 cal	3000-4000 cal	<20-40 cal/kg	20-40 cal/kg	>20-40 cal/kg
	85%	15%	20%	63%	13%
	Enteral + parenteral 57%				
	Average weight				
	Before nutritional support 60.8 kg		*NS* 5.5 days ± 4	After nutritional support 62.2 kg	

From First Polydisciplinary International Congress of OESO: Cancer of the esophagus in 1984: 135 questions, answers compiled by R. Giuli, Paris, 1984, Editions Maloine.

and, sometimes, dysphagia resulting from stomatitis with methotrexate.

• • •

In summary, no matter which treatment is chosen, nutritional support should be, in almost all cases, mandatory to permit a successful result.

Nutritional support also plays an important part in the maintenance of immunologic status. Immune depression may be due to the presence of the cancer itself, or to the various aggressive treatments given to the patient.

Choice of nutritional technique

The importance of a randomized prospective study to demonstrate the best method for restoring nutrition is stressed in Chapter 33.

In straightforward cases, oral caloric support is used. The aim is to achieve an intake of 35 to 40 cal/kg/day, including a protein intake of 1 to 1.5 g/kg/day, for all of the patients in this trial. In actual fact, oral nutritional support will be sufficient only in a small percentage of cases, and artificial support will be needed in all other patients, by either enteral or parenteral techniques.

The choice of nutritional technique will depend upon (1) the degree of stenosis (parenteral nutrition via a central line is necessary in the case of complete esophageal stenosis), (2) the degree of weight loss, and (3) the tolerance for enteral or parenteral nutrition.

For enteral nutrition, a small flexible Silastic feeding tube with a weighted end is inserted through a naris and directed into the stomach. For

TABLE 13-6. Skin tests (82 patients)*

Tuberculin 64	Candidin 53	Varidase 30	Others 46
+ 62%	51%	47%	65%

No. of tests
1:36%
2:62%
3:36%
4:35%

I.D.† − 82 (42%)
I.D. + 111

From First Polydisciplinary International Congress of OESO: Cancer of the esophagus in 1984: 135 questions, answers compiled by R. Giuli, Paris, 1984, Editions Maloine.
*Despite alimentation techniques, no negative tests ever became positive.
†*I.D.*, Immune defense.

TABLE 13-7. Complications

	42 I.D. +	19 I.D. −	WEIGHT LOSS	
			Average (kg)	% normal weight
OPERATION				
Palliative	21	6	8.4%	12%
			$p = 0.003$	
Curative	21	13 (68%)	7	10%
Postoperative complications	127 (49%)	33%	7.3	10
			NS	
No complication	159 (51%)	66%	8.2	11

From First Polydisciplinary International Congress of OESO: Cancer of the esophagus in 1984: 135 questions, answers compiled by R. Giuli, Paris, 1984, Editions Maloine.

the nutrition to be well tolerated, the solution needs to be administered slowly with the tube placed in the duodenum and a pump used. A sufficient volume of commercially prepared formula (1 cal/ml) is given by slow drip delivery to achieve a total daily caloric intake of 45 cal/kg/day.

In the field of oral nutrition, some investigations have indicated the anabolic and anticatabolic properties of ornithine-ketoglutarate. This formula acts by stimulation of insulin secretion and secretion of growth hormones, which oppose the effects of hyperglycemia-producing hormones. A recent study[2] has made it possible to specify that ornithine-ketoglutarate, at a dose of 20 mg/day, increases the potential of nitrogen anabolism of the liver, and is accompanied by effects favorable to enteral alimentation of malnourished patients, weight gain, and nitrogen retention. At present,

its newest form is a monohydrate, absorbable orally (Cetornan, Logeais Laboratories). It now may be considered for inclusion in the OESO protocol. A parallel "crossover" trial on the patients in the chemotherapeutic arm of the study will be carried out to verify not only its nutritional effects on the reduction of hypercatabolism and the decrease of anorexia but also its antiemetic effect. One might then anticipate a better tolerance of chemotherapy drugs.

In short, the OESO randomized prospective study will try to demonstrate the best nutritional support (parenteral versus enteral supplementation), especially when weight loss is less than 10% and oral intake is still sufficient. In this international trial, one aim is to appreciate the influence of parenteral feeding on the outcome of the 500 patients in the study. A specific hypothesis is that total parenteral nutrition, both preoperative and postoperative, improves tolerance to treatments of the three arms (surgery, chemotherapy, radiotherapy), and perhaps also improves response to treatments. In addition, it may reduce overall morbidity by reducing respiratory complications.

Results of the total parenteral nutrition group of patients will be compared with those of a low feeding regimen (700 cal/day) and, if possible, with those of normal enteral feeding (providing 30 cal/kg/day).

IMMUNOLOGIC ASSESSMENT

Noirot and Bernard have previously shown that skin tests of delayed hypersensitivity that investigate cell-mediated immunity do not have absolute prognostic value in esophageal cancer.[3] Tables 13-6 and 13-7,[1] from the OESO prospective study, also demonstrate the poor prognostic value of skin testing. In fact, skin tests only reflect the state of immune defense at a given moment, and it is impossible to predict what they will be like several months later.

To determine solid neoplastic activity, repeated assays of histamine blood levels seem to be a reliable indicator.[4-7] Blood histamine levels that fall progressively signify the presence of an advanced primary cancer and/or metastasis. This decrease in histamine levels precedes clinical relapse, recurrence, or metastasis by a minimum period of 1 month. This indicator also seems to have a prognostic value: increasing mortality is observed in patients with the lowest blood his-

tamine levels. Moreover, increasing blood histamine level is observed after successful resection of cancer.

Thus, repeated assays of blood histamine levels may provide a reliable indicator for the follow-up of neoplastic activity and for the surveillance of patients with esophageal cancer.

REFERENCES

1. First Polydisciplinary International Congress of OESO: Cancer of the esophagus in 1984: 135 questions, answers compiled by R. Giuli, Paris, 1984, Editions Maloine, p. 426.
2. Lepetitcorps, A.M., and Bernard, P.F.: Alpha-cétoglutarate d'ornithine en nutrition entérale exclusive, Med. Chir. Dig. 15(5):441, 1985.
3. Noirot, C., and Bernard, P.F.: Can immune depression be altered by renutrition of the patient? In First Polydisciplinary International Congress of OESO: Cancers of the esophagus in 1984: 135 questions, answers compiled by R. Giuli, Paris, 1984, Editions Maloine, p. 69.
4. Burtin, C., Noirot, C., Paupe, J., and Scheinmann, P.: Decreased blood histamine levels in patients with solid malignant tumours, Br. J. Cancer 47:367, 1983.
5. Burtin, C., Noirot, C., Giroux, C., and Scheinmann, P.: Decreased skin response to intradermal histamine in cancer patients, Allergy Clin. Immunol., 1986. (In press.)
6. Noirot, C., Scheinmann, P., and Burtin, C.: What can be expected from new markers of progression in carcinoma of the esophagus? In First Polydisciplinary International Congress of OESO: Cancer of the esophagus in 1984: 135 questions, answers compiled by R. Giuli, Paris, Editions Maloine, p. 377.
7. Burtin, C., Noirot, C., and Scheinmann, P.: What is the role of tumour markers in excision surgery? In First Polydisciplinary International Congress of OESO: Cancer of the esophagus in 1984: 135 questions, compiled by R. Giuli, Paris, 1984, Editions Maloine, p. 179.

14 Assessment of intramural spread

Michael Robert Burch Keighley

PREOPERATIVE ASSESSMENT OF TUMOR SPREAD

Gastroesophageal carcinoma may be associated with widespread metastases to the lungs, liver, bone, or brain. Hepatic metastases are usually easily recognized during a thoracoabdominal approach to the esophagus. It is preferable if these disseminated deposits can be detected preoperatively, and hepatic metastases can now usually be identified by preoperative ultrasound, isotope scans, or computed tomography. If metastatic disease is discovered at operation by the presence of ascites, nodules in the lung fields, or deposits in the liver parenchyma, they can be easily confirmed, either by cytology using fluid aspiration or by fine-needle aspiration biopsy with cytology. Furthermore, if there are widespread metastases, these can also be identified by true-cut needle biopsy with subsequent histologic examination. However, in most instances it is unnecessary to await the results of on-table cytology or frozen sections taken from true-cut needle biopsy, since the nature of the disseminated cancer is obvious at thoracolaparotomy.

Tumors of the esophagus and cardia may be associated with fixity to the surrounding structures. Fixity to retroperitoneal structures other than lymph nodes usually signifies nonresectability. Fixity to the diaphragm, however, does not necessarily indicate that the tumor is nonresectable, and local infiltration to the pericardium may also be amenable to surgical excision. However, fixation to right or left main bronchus, the arch of the aorta, or the great veins of the neck usually signifies nonresectability. Fine-needle aspiration cytology has, in our experience, often helped in determining whether a tumor is adherent because of an inflammatory reaction or because of malignant infiltration. Fine-needle aspirates are obtained during operation, and an immediate smear is prepared on a glass slide, which is fixed and stained with the Papanicolaou technique. Results are usually available and may be telephoned to

the operating room within 10 minutes of aspiration.

Gastroesophageal carcinoma commonly spreads widely through lymphatic channels. Enlarged lymph nodes may appear in the neck, in the superior mediastinum, behind the arch of the aorta, or around the descending aorta, and, in lower esophageal tumors, widespread lymphatic dissemination may be found in the nodes surrounding the bifurcation of the hepatic artery. The presence of widespread lymphatic metastases is associated with an appalling prognosis, and if these distant metastatic nodes can be identified before or during operation, a radical resection might not be undertaken. For this reason we advise fine-needle aspiration cytology of any palpable lymph nodes in the neck preoperatively, and we have also developed a technique for immediate harvesting of lymph nodes from the preaortic region in gastroesophageal tumors. When distant lymphatic metastases are involved, we do not usually proceed with a radical excision.

Perhaps the most important route of dissemination of malignancy is along the submucosal plane. Widespread involvement of the submucosal plexus may be present at a considerable distance from the primary tumor. Indeed, one of the most common reasons for inadequate resection of gastroesophageal carcinoma is the extent of submucosal spread.[1,2] Furthermore, if resection is performed in the presence of microscopic submucosal infiltration, there is a greater risk of anastomotic dehiscence, which is potentially fatal.[3] It is therefore particularly important during partial esophageal resection to assess whether there is submucosal infiltration at the line of resection or not.

STRATEGY OF TREATMENT

Most surgeons would take the view that if there are widespread metastatic deposits, resection is not advised. Tumors with local fixation to surrounding structures are not necessarily nonresectable, and long-term survival has occasionally been reported, even after excision of surrounding structures. However, if residual disease persists after excision of the tumor, local radiotherapy would be advised in order to attempt to prevent local recurrence and secondary obstruction of the superior vena cava or of the anastomosis, or infiltration into surrounding structures. For this reason, evidence of residual disease is of some importance in planning whether adjuvant radiotherapy is advisable.

It is now our policy to avoid resection in patients with gastroesophageal carcinoma when there is widespread lymphatic involvement.[4] We have studied the survival in 136 patients with gastroesophageal carcinoma in relation to whether or not preaortic or hepatic hilar lymph nodes were involved at the time of surgical treatment. Distant lymphatic involvement was recorded in 64% of patients with inoperable tumors, in 25% of patients with tumors associated with metastatic deposits, and in 39% of patients with locally fixed tumors, but widespread lymphatic involvement was also recorded in 18% of entirely mobile lesions that, at first glance, seemed localized and suitable for radical excision. The median survival in patients with inoperable tumors or those associated with distant metastases was only 3.5 months. Similarly, the median survival, despite radical excision of the primary tumor, in patients with mobile primary carcinomas and distant lymphatic involvement was only 4.5 months. Hence the presence of preaortic or hepatic hilar lymph node involvement was associated with a prognosis that was no better than the prognosis for patients with widespread metastatic disease to the lungs or liver. As a consequence of this survey we no longer perform radical excision, despite an apparently mobile primary lesion, if there are widespread metastatic deposits in preaortic lymph nodes or in lymph nodes at the hilum of the liver.

If tumor is discovered in the submucosal plane at a distance from the primary lesion, a strong case could be made for total esophagectomy. Indeed, it is because of this finding that many surgeons today favor total esophagectomy rather than partial esophagectomy for the treatment of gastroesophageal carcinoma.[5] Despite the increasing interest in total esophagectomy, there are certain circumstances, particularly in patients with distal esophageal lesions, in which total esophagectomy is not necessarily indicated. Under such circumstances it is very important to be sure that there has been adequate clearance of the tumor and that the site of anastomosis is not infiltrated by tumor in the submucosal plane.

RESIDUAL TUMOR

We have examined the presence of residual tumor after radical excision during operation by multiple biopsies and on-table brush cytology. Thirty-seven tumor beds have been examined, seven of which contained residual tumor, as judged by cytology or biopsy. All seven lesions contained obvious malignant cells on brush cytology, but biopsy identified only five of the seven patients with residual tumor at the resection site. It is our view that cytology is preferable to multiple biopsies for identifying residual disease after resection. Biopsies are frequently traumatic, and many areas require assessment. Conversely, by stroking a small swab over the tumor bed it is possible to assess residual malignant disease from a wide field. Certainly in the field of rectal cancer this technique has been superior to multiple biopsies.[6]

RELIABILITY OF ON-TABLE CYTOLOGY TO ASSESS DISSEMINATED LYMPHATIC DEPOSITS

We have analyzed the accuracy of imprint cytology from 182 lymph nodes harvested during resections for gastroesophageal cancer (see Table 14-1). Seventy-eight nodes were positive on histology and on cytology. In addition, 92 nodes were negative on histology and on cytology (overall accuracy, 93%). There were nine lymph nodes that on cytology were clearly involved with malignant cells even though histologic sections of the nodes failed to identify metastases. We believe that these were false-negative histologic reports, since all of the patients died within 6 months of operation and at postmortem in five of the nine cases extensive lymphatic deposits were identified. There were three imprint cytology reports which were negative on cytology but in which tumor replacement was clearly demonstrated on paraffin histology. These false-negative cytologic findings were due to technical errors in two of the three patients studied.

TABLE 14-1. Accuracy of imprint cytology of lymph nodes

	Cytology	
	Positive	Negative
Histology		
Positive	78	3
Negative	9	92

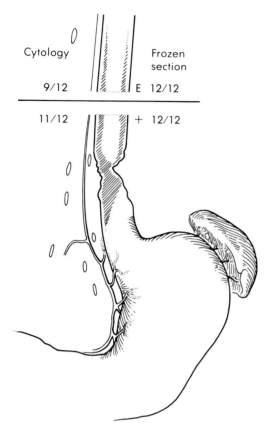

Fig. 14-1. Twelve inadequate resections (tumor involving the line of proximal resection). Comparison between cytology and frozen section. Results in patients with residual malignancy in the esophagus. *E*, Remaining esophagus; +, resected tumor. Shading indicates presence of tumor.

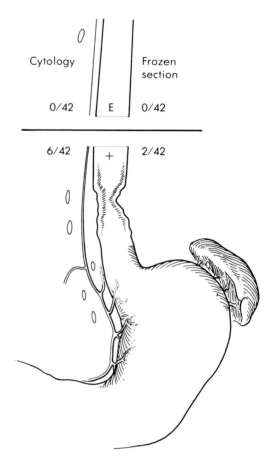

Fig. 14-2. Forty-two adequate resections (tumor clear at the line of proximal resection). Comparison between cytology and frozen section. Results in patients without residual malignancy in the esophagus. *E*, Remaining esophagus; +, resected tumor.

INTRAMURAL SPREAD

Involvement of resection margins has now been assessed in 54 patients undergoing gastroesophageal resection for malignant disease (see Figs. 14-1 and 14-2). We have analyzed the results from two sites: the proximal resection line and the free margin of the distal esophagus to be used for the subsequent anastomosis. Examination of the free margin of the distal esophagus to be used for the subsequent anastomosis. Examination of the free margin of the esophagus revealed that cytology and frozen-section histology provided an extremely reliable assessment of submucosal infiltration, frozen section being correct in all 54 specimens examined. There were no false-positive or false-negative frozen-section results. Cytology provided no false-positive results from the free margin of the lower esophagus but failed to identify submucosal infiltration in three of 12 pa-

tients undergoing an inadequate resection. These three false-negative cytologic findings were identified early in our series and were possibly due to lack of experience. By contrast, examination of the proximal margin of the resected specimen was less reliable. There were two false-positive frozen-section results in the 42 having an adequate resection and six false-positive cytology results. These false-positive cytology findings were almost certainly due to spillage of tumor cells from the malignant obstruction during mobilization of the gastroesophageal junction. By contrast, frozen section was invariably correct when the proximal margin of the specimen was examined, and 11 of 12 cytologic examinations from the proximal resection line of the specimen in patients with submucosal infiltration identified the presence of malignant cells. These findings led us to two conclusions. The first is that exami-

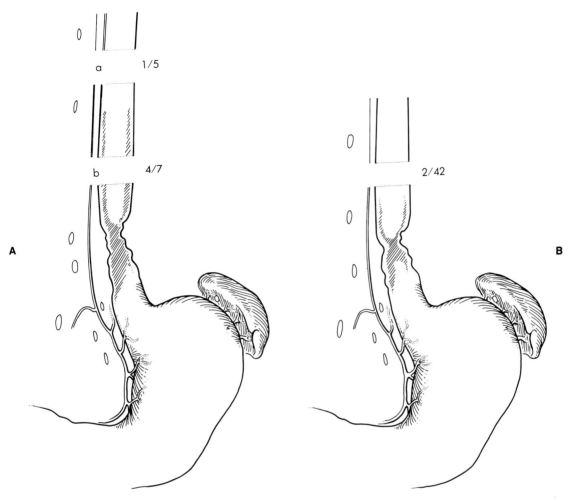

Fig. 14-3. A, Anastomotic leaks in patients in whom there was tumor involvement in the remaining esophagus. *a,* Where a more proximal resection was performed; *b,* where the surgeon ignored the results of intraoperative frozen section or cytology. **B,** Anastomotic leaks in patients in whom there was no tumor involvement of the remaining esophagus.

nation of the distal cut margin of the esophagus is much more reliable, particularly when cytology is used to assess submucosal infiltration, than examination of the proximal margin of the tumor. The second observation concerns the logistics of frozen section and cytology. Cytology results are usually available within 10 or 15 minutes of obtaining a smear from the cut edge of the esophagus, whereas frozen sections are often not available for at least half an hour to three quarters of an hour, since the entire circumference of the esophagus must be carefully examined.

When we examined the influence of our intraoperative technique for assessing submucosal infiltration, we found that the technique had a direct bearing on the rate of postoperative anastomotic dehiscence. Fatal anastomotic dehiscence was re-corded in only two of 42 patients having anastomosis performed in the absence of submucosal infiltration (see Fig. 14-3, *B*). However, fatal anastomotic dehiscence was recorded in four of seven patients in whom an esophageal anastomosis was performed in the presence of intraoperative evidence of submucosal infiltration (see Fig. 14-3, *A*). However, when the surgeon decided to act upon the results of intraoperative cytology or frozen section and perform a more proximal resection of the esophagus, only one of five patients having a second section of the proximal esophagus developed a fatal anastomotic breakdown. We accept that dehiscence of an esophageal anastomosis may be due to a variety of factors, including the blood supply to the site of anastomosis,[7] perianastomotic infection,[8] and inadequate suture or stapling techniques. Nevertheless, this survey seems to indicate that presence of submucosal infiltration in the cut edge of the esophagus is associated with a high incidence of fatal anastomotic dehiscence unless a further, more proximal esophageal resection is undertaken.

CONCLUSIONS

As a result of our studies on intraoperative staging of gastroesophageal carcinoma we advise avoidance of resection if there are obvious widespread metastatic deposits or if preaortic lymph nodes are involved by tumor infiltration. We tend to use postoperative radiotherapy only in cases in which cytologic examination of the tumor bed revealed residual malignant disease. The cut edge of the esophagus that is to be used for anastomosis is now always examined for malignant cells by stroking a glass microscope slide over the divided esophagus. If malignant cells are identified, a more extensive proximal resection is undertaken and serious consideration is given to performing a total esophagectomy with anastomosis of the cardia to the esophagus in the neck. We have now almost entirely abandoned the use of frozen section, since it is more time-consuming and may damage the lower cut edge of the esophagus. Cytology is now rarely associated with false-negative findings.

REFERENCES

1. McKeown, K.C.: Carcinoma of the oesophagus, Ann. R. Coll. Surg. Engl. **60:**301, 1978.
2. Groves, L.K.: Carcinoma of the esophagus; evaluation of treatment, Ann. Thorac. Surg. **1:**416, 1965.
3. Hermreck, A.S., and Crawford, D.G.: The esophageal anastomotic leak, Am. J. Surg. **132:**794, 1976.
4. Keighley, M.R.B., Moore, J., Roginski, C., Powell, J., and Thompson, H.: Incidence and prognosis of N_4 node involvement in gastric cancer, Br. J. Surg. **71:**863, 1984.
5. Earlam, R., and Cunha-Melo, J.R.: Oesophageal squamous cell carcinoma. I. A critical review of surgery, Br. J. Surg. **67:**381, 1980.
6. Silverman, S.H., Moore, J., Thompson, H., and Keighley, M.R.B.: Per-operative detection of patients with rectal cancer at high risk of local recurrence, Ann. R. Coll. Surg. **65:**164, 1985.
7. Maillard, J.N., Launois, B., de Lagausie, P., et al.: Cause of leakage at the site of anastomosis after esophageal gastric resection for carcinoma, Surg. Gynecol. Obstet. **129:**1014, 1969.
8. Hares, M.M., Hagerty, M.A., Warlow, J., Malins, D., Youngs, D., Bentley, S., Burdon, D.W., and Keighley, M.R.B.: A controlled trial to compare systemic and intraincisional cefuroxime prophylaxis in high risk gastric surgery, Br. J. Surg. **68:**276, 1981.

15 **Prophylactic operative techniques: 380 esophageal anastomoses using the stapler**

François Fekete, Brice Gayet, Stéphane Place, and Jean Biagini

Anastomotic leak remains a major complication of esophageal surgery, and it is still responsible for many deaths. If routine radiographic swallow examination or autopsy is done, many deaths reported to be due to pneumonia, septicemia, or cardiorespiratory insufficiency appear to be in fact due to fistulas. Chassin[1] recently reported a mortality over 10% from fistulas in 2156 anastomoses collected from 13 papers.

In recent series, leaks from sutured anastomoses have decreased. Apparently, the end-to-end stapling instruments extensively developed by Steichen and Ravitch[2] offer hope for a further decrease in the incidence of this complication. In 1984 Hopkins et al.[3] reported a rate of 6.3% for 239 collected stapled anastomoses.

In the Department of Digestive Surgery of Beaujon Hospital in Paris, 380 esophageal anastomoses were performed with the stapler technique from February 1, 1979, to December 31, 1984, using the EEA* 140 times and the ILS† 240 times. Our initial experience with 45 esophagogastric anastomoses has previously been reported.[4]

MATERIALS AND METHODS

In most cases the diseases were carcinomas of the esophagus, the gastroesophageal junction, or the stomach (see Table 15-1). Also, 37 anastomoses were performed for benign diseases with or without resection (see Table 15-2). This series includes 250 esophagogastrostomies, 83 esophagojejunostomies, and 47 esophagocolostomies.

There were 85 anastomoses located in the neck, 245 in the thorax, and 50 in the abdomen (see Table 15-3).

The mean age of the patients was 55 ± 9 for esophageal carcinoma, 63 ± 13 for carcinoma of the cardia, and 66 ± 5 for gastric carcinoma. The mean weight loss was 7 ± 5 kg. Seventeen patients had alcoholic cirrhosis proved by biopsy, and six had previous radiation therapy involving the mediastinal esophagus—three with Hodgkin's disease and three with carcinoma of the breast. Five of these developed esophageal carcinomas and one a benign stricture. Twelve additional patients submitted to radiation therapy for esophageal carcinomas and six for head and neck cancers; these individuals were referred to us secondarily for operation.

TECHNIQUES
Esophagogastric anastomoses

The esophagogastric anastomosis in the thorax was usually done for esophageal carcinomas below the aortic arch, through a combined abdominal and right thoracic approach. At the abdominal stage, colo-omental detachment was done.

TABLE 15-1. Disease distribution in 380 anastomoses

Disease	No. of patients
Esophageal squamous cell cancer	204
Adenocarcinoma of the cardia (including 12 carcinomas in Barrett's esophagus)	80
Carcinoma of the stomach	59
Benign diseases	37

*End to End Anastomosis, USCC.
†Intra Luminal Stapler, Ethicon.

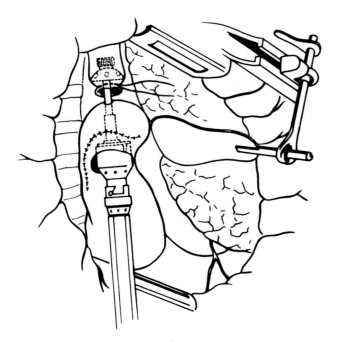

Fig. 15-1. Intrathoracic esophagogastric anastomosis.

TABLE 15-2. Distribution of benign diseases

Disease	No. of patients
Caustic strictures (including 4 acutely burned)	18
Peptic strictures or ulcers	9
Perforations	2
Stenosis following irradiation	1
Bronchogenic cyst	1
Megaesophagus	1
Benign gastric tumors	5

TABLE 15-3. Distribution of procedures

Site of anastomosis	Procedure	No. of patients
Cervical (85)	Esophagogastrostomies	43
	Esophagocolostomies*	42
Intrathoracic (245)	Esophagogastrostomies	207
	Esophagocolostomies*	5
	Esophagojejunostomies	33
Abdominal (50)	Esophagojejunostomies	50
TOTAL		380

*The cologastric anastomoses were also performed with the stapler.

Omental mobilization made it possible to wrap the anastomosis thoroughly with a large omental graft. The left gastric artery was severed at the celiac axis. The beginning of the gastric tube was created by application of a GIA stapler from the junction between the pyloric and left gastric arteries in order to resect all the lymph nodes along the left gastric vessels. A Kocher maneuver and a pyloroplasty were performed routinely.

At the thoracic stage a complete posterior "mediastinectomy" was performed. The esophageal resection was done as high as possible if a curative resection was attempted; the anastomosis was done at least at the superior edge of the azygos arch and most often at the thorax apex. The esophagus was progressively severed with scissors. A stay-suture was placed on the anterior wall, as soon as the lumen was opened, and three other markers were placed at the cardinal points. A purse-string suture of the transected end of the esophagus was a key stage, care being taken to include the entire mucosa. The esophagus was dilated with lubricated bougies of increasing sizes; the largest was left in place during the gastric preparation. The stomach was pulled up into the mediastinum, with care being taken to avoid any twisting. The transection of the gastric tube was achieved with several applications of the GIA stapler. The stapled line was inverted with a continuous Dexon suture.

The anastomosis

An end-to-side esophagogastric anastomosis (Fig. 15-1) was done on the posterior wall of the gastric tube. The size of the stapler was chosen according to the largest inserted bougie. Usually EEA 25 or 28 or ILS 25 or 29 fit. Most of the time, the stapler was inserted through a vertical anterior gastrotomy, 3 to 4 cm from the top of the stomach. A stab wound was done to place the central rod, and the posterior gastric wall was carefully pushed to the cartridge. The anvil was secured to the central rod. The bougie was withdrawn from the esophagus; the four esophageal stay-sutures provided a degree of contertraction during stapler introduction.

As a result of the previous dilatation, the anvil was easily inserted into the esophagus under direct vision, with the surgeon making sure that the posterior edge of the esophagus was free. The purse-string suture was tied while the assistant removed the four stay-sutures.

The stapler cartridge and anvil were approximated, with care being taken to avoid any interposition between the two organs. The appropriate degree of tightening is shown on the EEA stapler by the alignment of two markers. If the ILS is used, it is essential to observe the protrusion of the black button on the shaft of the device. The degree of tightening was measured with the specific instrument, with the surgeon taking into account the esophageal and gastric thickness. Upon firing of the instrument, the cartridge and anvil were separated from one another. Once again, the previous dilatation made the instrument easy to remove.

Checking the anastomosis

The external aspect is easy to appreciate. The endoluminal aspect can sometimes be seen by pushing back the edges of the gastrotomy. If not, the finger introduced through the gastrotomy allows insurance of the complete and regular contour of the anastomosis. Liquid may be injected through a nasogastric tube, but we do not consider this necessary. Resection of two "doughnuts" of tissue must be complete. These should be removed from the cartridge and inspected. When an incomplete ring of tissue is found, an anastomotic defect may be anticipated. In this case, the anastomosis should be done again.

In this study, closure of the gastrotomy was secured by manual suture. The omentum, brought up into the mediastinum with the stomach, was wrapped around the anastomosis and covered the gastrotomy. To relieve tension, the edges of the stomach were sutured to the adjacent pleura and to the prevertebral fascia. (Fig. 15-2 shows the intact anastomosis on postoperative barium esophagogram.)

Variations

Two variants of esophagogastric anastomosis were sometimes performed:

1. Esophagogastric resection through the left

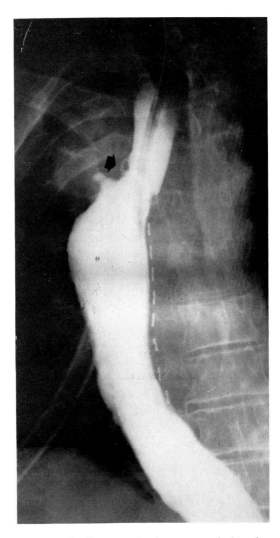

Fig. 15-2. Swallow examination on seventh day after intrathoracic anastomosis. Arrow indicates staple line.

thoracic or thoracoabdominal approach (Fig. 15-3) was reserved for elderly patients or for palliative procedures in cases of carcinomas of the lower third of the esophagus or of the cardia. The use of the stapler was identical.

2. Cervical esophagogastric anastomoses (Fig. 15-4) were performed in 45 cases, usually for cancer above the aortic arch or as a bypass. A long gastric tube (anteperistaltic two times, isoperistaltic 43 times) was fashioned by several applications of the GIA stapler. The tube was elevated behind the sternum if a palliative procedure was done, or into the mediastinum in the esophageal bed after esophagectomy through thoracic approach or after esophagectomy without thoracotomy. For cervical anastomosis, the stapler was better inserted via the top of the tube to preserve its blood supply. We have no experience with oral insertion of the stapler.

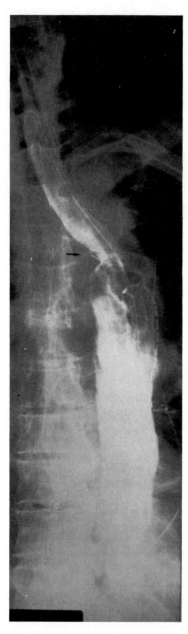

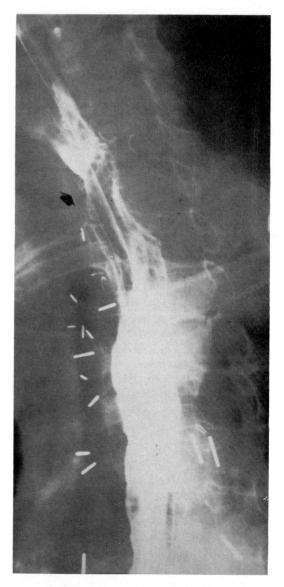

Fig. 15-4. Esophagogram of cervical esophagogastric anastomosis. Arrow points to staple line.

Fig. 15-3. Esophagogram of intrathoracic anastomosis through left thoracic approach. Arrow points to staple line.

Esophagojejunal anastomoses

Of the 83 esophagojejunostomies (Fig. 15-5) performed, three were done as palliative procedures, without gastrectomy. Eighty were performed after total gastrectomy. As far as carcinoma of the cardia or of the stomach (except antrum) is concerned, we use an extended total gastrectomy including omental detachment, splenopancreatic mobilization to the right side of the aorta, and dissection of the celiac axis. Celiac area nodes can be removed. The left gastric artery is severed at its emergence from the celiac axis. Lymph nodes of the splenic vessels are removed with splenectomy. The distal pancreas is resected only if it is invaded; in this way pancreatic fistulas and subdiaphragmatic abscesses are avoided. The lymph nodes along the hepatic artery are removed along with tissue around the portal vein and the common bile duct.

An abdominal approach was sufficient for carcinomas of the stomach. As far as carcinoma of the cardia with esophageal involvement was con-

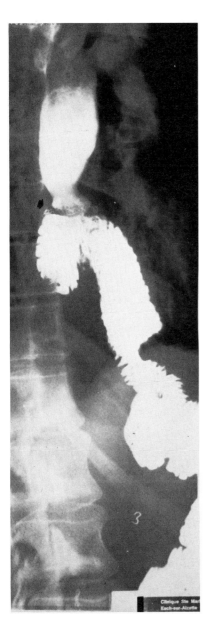

Fig. 15-5. Esophagogram showing esophagojejunal anastomosis. Arrow points to staple line.

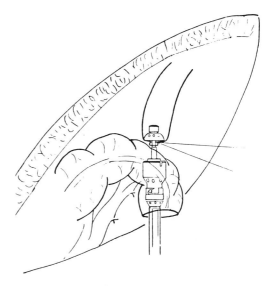

Fig. 15-6. Esophagocolic anastomosis: placement of stapler.

cerned, a thoracic stage was necessary. Posterior "mediastinectomy" includes intertracheobronchial node removal. Esophageal transsection was done 10 cm above the upper pole of the tumor to avoid esophageal spread to the resection margin (8% in this series).

In performing such an extended esophageal resection, two technical points must be considered: (1) the organ for gastroesophageal substitution and (2) the surgical approach.

As far as intestinal restoration is concerned,

colonic interposition appears to be a long, complex, and potentially septic procedure. We only recommend this procedure when the jejunum cannot be used, for a very high supraaortic anastomosis, or in the obese patient. A Roux-en-Y anastomosis is usually performed, but to achieve greater mobility of the loop, a special technique is necessary. After mobilization of the right colon and the Kocher procedure, the root of the mesentery can be divided from the posterior abdominal wall, to the level of the pancreas.

The fetal condition of the mesenterium commune is restored, which allows one to transpose the jejunal loop up to the aortic or azygos arch, thereby gaining about 6 cm in length.

The second point is the surgical approach. This procedure requires complete abdominal and high thoracic exposure. Left thoracolaparotomy allows both abdominal and thoracic dissection; however, this approach is traumatic, and does not allow as high a thoracic anastomosis. A double approach—laparotomy followed by right thoracotomy—can sometimes be recommended.

Finally, a 70-cm-long Roux-en-Y loop is prepared. The stapler is introduced through the open cut end of jejunum and the anastomosis done end-to-side. Dilatation with bougies is done on the jejunum as well as on the esophagus. The excess end of jejunum is then excised with the TA 55 stapler.

Esophagocolic anastomoses

Esophagocolic anastomoses (Fig. 15-6) were used primarily for benign conditions. The transverse colon was used in 45 cases and right ileo-

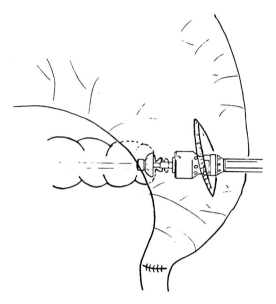

Fig. 15-7. Cologastric anastomosis: placement of stapler.

colon isoperistaltically in two cases. The esophagocolic or esophagoileal anastomosis was placed in the neck after restrosternal bypass, particularly for caustic stricture, or within the thorax after resection for peptic stenosis or occasionally for esophageal carcinoma in gastrectomized patients. The cologastric anastomosis (Fig. 15-7) was located on the posterior wall of the stomach, and the stapler was introduced through an anterior gastrotomy. An anterior antireflux partial valve could be developed. We took care that the plasty (Fig. 15-8) was as straight as possible in case endoscopic dilatation became necessary. Five esophagocolostomies were placed in the chest without morbidity, and 42 were carried out in the neck with a 9.5% leakage rate.

Hazards and pitfalls

1. The instrument. The plastic ring of the cartridge of the EEA failed once; the circular knife was unusable.

2. The purse string. Wide interval placement or tearing of sutures may lead to an incomplete anastomosis. The purse-string instruments provided by two manufacturers are inadequate relative to thickness of the esophagus. In several instances the purse-string suture had to be manually redone, because the mucosa was not included or the opposite mucosa was caught in it. Since 1985, the purse-string and stay-sutures have been replaced by a single ligature of the esophagus on the device's center rod.

3. The degree of tightening. The degree of tightening is critical. The proper amount is indicated on the EEA by the alignment of the mark-

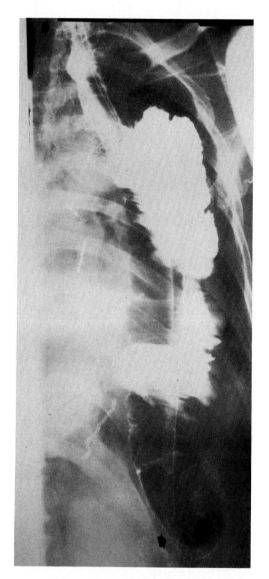

Fig. 15-8. Barium swallow showing esophagocoloplasty.

ers. On the ILS, there is the hazard of insufficient tightening; one must remember that the black button must jut out of the shaft. On the other hand, an excessive tightening is possible, and then the stapler becomes folded, shaping an "8" instead of a "3."

4. The interposition between the anvil and the cartridge. A purse string that carries too much tissue or a cartridge that is too small results in an interposition of esophageal tissue. It is necessary to release the instrument and sever the excess tissue, then to try again. Occasionally the purse string itself must be redone and a larger cartridge chosen.

If the jejunum is used, a fold of bowel may

appear on the mesenteric side (Fig. 15-9, *A*). To avoid this, one must spread the jejunal wall on the cartridge with two fingers and stretch the extremity of the loop with atraumatic forceps (Fig. 15-9, *B*). Otherwise the anastomosis may involve a double thickness of bowel. On two occasions the anastomosis had to be redone for this reason.

5. Introduction or removal of the anvil. Problems are avoided by prior dilatation. The dilatation should be gentle and gradual, with care being taken not to overdistend the organ. Otherwise, the muscular layer may split, requiring remaking of the anastomoses.

POSTOPERATIVE COURSE AND RESULTS

In this series of 380 esophageal anastomoses using a stapler, the overall mortality was 9.2%, with 3.2% resulting from leaks; this drops to 7.2% and 2.8%, respectively, if cirrhotic patients and patients with ruptured tumors perforated at endoscopy or following prosthesis insertion are excluded.

The average incidence of leakage was 6.8%, dropping to 5.1% if cervical anastomoses are excluded. (See Tables 15-4 to 15-8.) The anastomotic leakage may or may not be symptomatic. The leaks that are symptomatic are esophagocutaneous in the neck, and esophagopleural, esophagomediastinal, or esophagoaortic within the chest. The cervical anastomotic leaks were more frequent (12.9%), but all healed spontaneously. This high rate was due to poor blood supply and/or some degree of traction if the gastric tube was rather short. The incidence of stenosis was 8.1% (see Tables 15-6 and 15-9).

Thanks to better technique in the construction of the tube, including resection of the lesser curvature from the pyloric vessels to the apex of the stomach, a decrease in the incidence of cervical leakage has been observed (see Fig. 15-10). However, although they are less serious, these leaks increase the hospital stay and the incidence of stenosis.

TABLE 15-4. Morbidity

No. of patients	Frank leakage	Blind fistula	Stenosis
Overall series results			
380	6.8%	3.7%	8.1% (28/345)
Excluding cervical anastomosis			
295	5.1%	4.4%	7.5% (20/266)

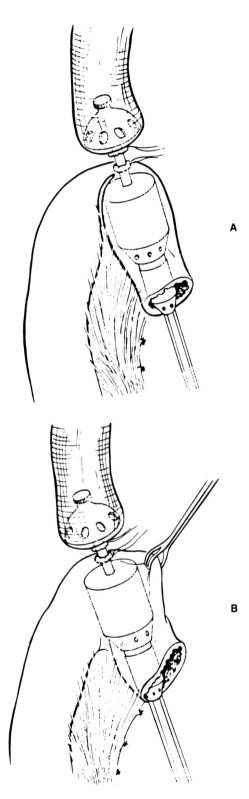

Fig. 15-9. A, Bowel fold in esophagojejunal anastomosis. **B,** How to avoid bowel fold.

TABLE 15-5. Fistula rate related to anastomosis level (n = 380)

Level	No. of patients	Symptomatic fistulas	Percent	Blind fistulas
Cervical	85	11	12.9	1
Thoracic	245	14	5.7	12
Abdominal	50	1	2	1
TOTAL	380	26	6.8	14

Fistulas (cervical anastomosis excluded)	15/295:5.1%
Death related to fistula	12/380:3.2%

TABLE 15-6. Morbidity correlated with level of anastomosis and viscus used

Type	No. of patients	Leakage	Stenosis	Death
Cervical				
Esophagocolostomy	42	9.5%	2.4%	4.7% (2)
Esophagogastrostomy	43	16%	16%	9.3% (4)
Thoracic				
Esophagogastrostomy	207	5%	8.7%	12.0% (25)
Esophagocolostomy	5	0	0	0
Esophagojejunostomy	33	6%	3%	6.0% (2)
Abdominal				
Esophagojejunostomy	50	2%	2%	4.0% (2)
TOTAL	380	6.8%	8.1%	9.2% (35)

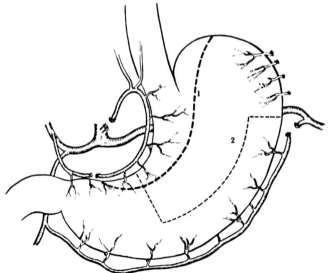

Fig. 15-10. Construction of the long gastric tube. *1*, Gastric tube along the lesser curvature (actually used). *2*, Gastric tube along the greater curvature (old style).

TABLE 15-7. Morbidity relative to the anastomosed organ (n = 380)

Organ	Site	No. of patients	Symptomatic fistulas
Stomach	Cervical	43	16%
(250)	Thoracic	207	6%
Colon	Cervical	42	10%
(47)	Thoracic	5	0%
Jejunum	Thoracic	33	6%
(83)	Abdominal	50	2%
	TOTAL	380	7%

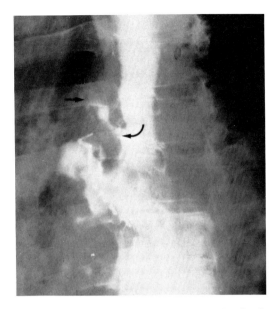

Fig. 15-11. Esophagogram demonstrating blind fistula (*arrows*), usually asymptomatic.

TABLE 15-8. Results of 37 stapler anastomoses for benign diseases

Site	Procedure	No. of patients	Fistula	Death
Cervical	Esophagocolostomy	23	1	1 (4.3%)
	Esophagogastrostomy	2	1	
Thoracic	Esophagogastrostomy	7	0	
	Esophagocolostomy	4	0	
Abdominal	Esophagojejunostomy	1	0	

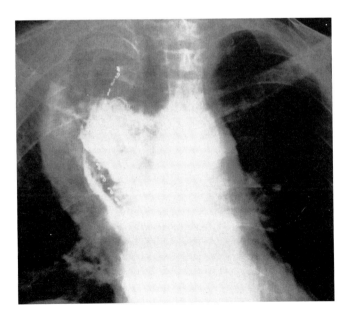

Fig. 15-12. Intraomental abscess resulting from fistula formation.

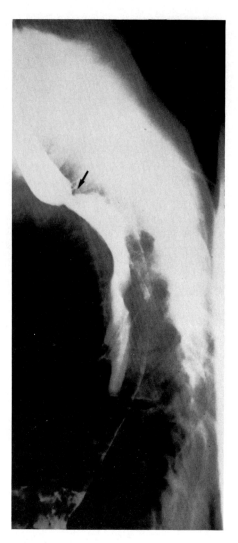

Fig. 15-13. Anastomotic stenosis (*arrow*) demonstrated in barium swallow.

TABLE 15-9. Anastomotic stenosis rate (8.1%) (n = 28/345)

	Occurrence
After symptomatic fistula	4
After blind fistula	3
After x-ray treatment	4
Cartridge size versus stenosis	
No. 21	3/14
No. 25	20/256
No. 28-29	5/71
No. 31-33	0/4

The intramediastinal leaks were less frequent (5.7%) but severe, responsible for pneumonia, requiring prolonged respiratory assistance, and contributing to mortality in 3% of the patients. The "blind" intramediastinal fistulas were asymptomatic or suspected only by persistent fever. They were recognized by a routine radiographic examination, using a water-soluble contrast medium, carried out on the seventh day (see Fig. 15-11).

The omental graft seems to prevent widespread mediastinal infection and aortic rupture: eight lethal fistulas occurred in the esophagogastric or esophagojejunal anastomoses without omental graft. Only four fistulas have been observed since intrathoracic anastomoses were wrapped with omentum. Two fistulas with intraomental ab-

scesses were cured by external drainage (see Fig. 15-12).

In esophageal carcinoma, the mortality and the incidence of fistulas were both higher after palliative surgery (12% and 16%) than after radical surgery (8% and 5%) (p: N.S.). No death resulting from leak occurred after resection for benign disease (one death for 37 resections, which was due to intracerebral hemorrhage) (see Table 15-8).

The stenosis rate (see Table 15-9 and Fig. 15-13) has been pointed out[5-7] in both sutured and stapled anastomoses. Stenosis results after delayed mucosal healing, especially in the stapled inverted anastomosis. The rate is generally about 10%.[3] We have observed 28 stenoses among 345 patients (8.1%), occurring within the two first postoperative months. No statistically significant difference was found relative to the size of the cartridge. Stenosis may be enhanced by fistulas and/or postoperative radiotherapy. The management of stenoses with bougienage was easily and efficiently accomplished in all cases but one. In addition, in all but one case of stenosis occurring more than 6 months postoperatively, the stenosis indicated recurrent carcinoma.

When the leakage and stenosis rates with the EEA and ILS staplers were compared, a statistically significant difference was not observed (see Table 15-10).

CONCLUSIONS

Evaluation of a consecutive series over 6 years yielded 380 stapled esophageal anastomoses and permitted evaluation of the advantages and disadvantages of these procedures. The anastomoses were performed by 11 surgeons, whose experience in esophageal surgery ranged between 0 and 25 years. To learn staple surgery is easier and

TABLE 15-10. Morbidity correlated with type of stapler

	No. of patients	Leakage	Blind fistula	Stenosis	Death
EEA	140	5.7%	4.3%	14/121 (11.6%)	13.6%
ILS	240	7.5%	3.3%	14/224 (6.2%)	6.7%

quicker than to learn hand-made esophageal anastomoses.

Reliability allows broadening of the indication for and extent of resectional surgery:

1. The anatomosis for subaortic esophageal cancer is now always done at the thoracic apex.
2. Resection can be planned for "borderline" cases, such as in the elderly, in patients with uncomplicated cirrhosis, and in cases of cancer after mediastinal irradiation.

The disadvantages of the stapler include stenosis in areas not reachable by endoscopic dilatation and the cost, which is higher than that of a hand-made anastomosis. One must remember, however, that a disposable stapler is cheaper than a long stay in an intensive care unit to repair anastomotic leakage.*

EDITOR'S NOTE: This chapter is included in the section on reduction of perioperative mortality because its technology has resulted in a decrease in fatal anastomotic leakage. It is not to be inferred, however, that manual anastomoses cannot achieve the same end. In our (F.W.W.) hands a near-zero leakage rate has been recorded in meticulous two-layer sutured anastomoses.

REFERENCES

1. Chassin, J.L.: Stapling technique for esophago-gastrotomy after esophago-gastric resection, Am. J. Surg. **136**:399, 1978.
2. Steichen, F.M., and Ravitch, M.M.: Mechanical sutures in esophageal surgery, Ann. Surg. **131**:373, 1980.
3. Hopkins, R.A., Alexander, J.C., and Postelthwait, R.W.: Stapler esophago-gastric anastomosis, Am. J. Surg. **147**:283, 1984.
4. Fekete, F., Breil, P., Ronsse, H., et al.: EEA stapler and omental graft in esophagogastrectomy, Ann. Surg. **193**:825, 1981.
5. West, P., Marbarger, J.P., Martz, M.N., and Roper, C.L.: Esophagogastrectomy with the EEA stapler, Ann. Surg. **193**:76, 1981.
6. Johnston, G.W.: Treatment of bleeding varices by esophageal transection with STPU gun, Ann. R. Coll. Surg. Engl. **59**:404, 1977.
7. Wu, W.C., Chen, F.T., Chou, H. K., et al.: Esophago-gastrotomic anastomosis instrument, Chin. Med. J. **4**:204, 1978.

16 Prophylactic operative techniques: thoracic esophageal squamous cell cancer surgery, with special reference to lymph node removal

François Fekete, Brice Gayet, and Georges J.M. Molas

Regardless of the method chosen, the overall results of treatment of esophageal carcinomas are unsatisfactory. The prognosis for esophageal squamous cell carcinoma following resection does not seem to have improved even with various combined treatments. Except for some Japanese series, which report a 34.6% rate,[1] the usual 5-year survival rates are less than 15%.[2] Factors influencing survival rates after curative surgery include lymph node involvement and wall penetration by the cancer. Anatomic lymphatic drainage of the esophagus accounts for wide tumor dissemination regardless of the location of the primary. In thoracic esophageal cancers, lymph node involvement is possible from the supraclavicular area to the abdomen, sometimes by "skipping" without intrathoracic nodal involvement.

The principles of surgical treatment call for a complete resection and appropriate reconstruction. Current mortality and morbidity of surgery, clearly decreasing these last years, permit this more extensive radical operation because an incomplete resection negates the primary aim of curative procedures.

This study reports the staging and long-term results after curative surgery of *thoracic esophageal squamous cell carcinoma* as judged by status of lymph node metastases.

MATERIAL AND METHOD

Between January, 1979, and December, 1984, 568 patients with carcinoma of the esophagus were admitted to the Department of Digestive Surgery, Beaujon Hospital, Clichy, France. To assess the prognostic histologic factors and the significance of staging, this study included only the 170 patients who *survived* "curative" surgery for thoracic squamous cell carcinoma. One hundred thirty-five adenocarcinomas have been excluded insofar as they started from the cardia as

TABLE 16-1. Groups of lymph nodes

1, 2	Right and left cardial
3	Lesser curvature
7	Left gastric artery
8	Common hepatic artery
9	Celiac artery
11	Splenic artery
5	Suprapyloric
6	Subpyloric
4	Greater curvature
10, 13	Splenic hilar and retropancreatic
12	Hepatoduodenal ligament
14, 15	Mesenteric and middle colic artery
101	Cervical paraesophageal
105	Upper thoracic paraesophageal
108	Middle thoracic paraesophageal
110	Lower thoracic paraesophageal
111	Diaphragmatic
112	Posterior mediastinal
109	Pulmonary hilar
107	Subcarinal
106	Thoracic paratracheal
113, 114	Along left and right recurrent laryngeal nerves
104	Supraclavicular
102	Deep cervical
100	Lateral cervical

TABLE 16-2. Thoracic N classification according to the JSED

Location of tumor	N_1	N_2	N_3	N_4
Upper third	105*	106, 107, 108, 112, 113, 114	101, 109, 110, 111, 1, 2, 104	$>N_3$
Middle third	108	105, 106, 107, 110, 111, 112, 113, 114, 1, 2	104, 109, 3, 7	$>N_3$
Lower third	110	108, 111, 112, 3, 7, 9, 10, 11	105, 106, 107, 109, 113 4, 5, 8	$>N_3$

*The numbers identify the specific lymph node groups listed in Table 16-1.

gastric cancers involving the distal esophagus. Twelve cases of primary esophageal adenocarcinomas originated from abnormal Barrett's epithelium lining the esophagus without involvement of the gastroesophageal junction. In the same way 79 squamous cell carcinomas of the hypopharynx and cervical esophagus have been excluded because their lymphatic drainage (1) is limited to the cervical areas and/or to the groups of recurrent laryngeal nerve nodes, (2) is more systematized, and (3) is independent of thoracic esophageal drainage. For these tumors a radical neck resection, including total esophagectomy, laryngectomy, and bilateral neck dissection, was indicated.

Surgery was called "curative" when the surgeon estimated that he had accomplished a total resection of the tumor and when the specimen margins were histologically free of disease. In squamous cell carcinomas of the thoracic esophagus, the operability rate was 70%, the resectability rate was 76.5%, and, as defined, the surgical curability was 78.5%. The follow-up of patients was 100%, to the time of death or to March, 1986.

Of the 170 patients included in this study there were 154 men and 16 women, a ratio of 9.6 to 1. The patients ranged in age from 35 to 82 years (median age, 55 years). For analysis, the thoracic esophagus was divided into three parts: upper third, above the aortic arch (28 cases, 16.5%); middle third, above the inferior pulmonary veins (96 cases, 56.5%); and lower third, above the gastroesophageal junction (46 cases, 27%).

This study used the JSED staging.[3] The American Joint Committee for Cancer Staging and the Union Internationale Contre le Cancer classifications were not used, because they are imprecise as far as regional lymph nodes are concerned; the presence or the absence of metastatic nodes alone determined the N classification for the thoracic esophagus. The staging of the primary tumor was exclusively histologic. The wall penetration was

TABLE 16-3. Thoracic esophageal carcinoma classification according to the JSED*

Stage 0	A_0 (<MP)	N_0	M_0	Pl_0†
Stage I	A_0 (MP)	N_0	M_0	Pl_0
Stage II	A_1	N_1	M_0	Pl_0
Stage III	A_2	N_2	M_0	Pl_0
Stage IV	A_3	N_3-N_4	M_1	Pl_1

* Stage determined by the most advanced part of the lesion.
† *Pl*, Pleura.

assessed according to degrees. It was noted A_0 when so-called adventitia was not involved. For these cases, the depth of invasion was precise: EP, intraepithelium; MM, to muscularis mucosae; SM, to submucosa; and MP, to muscularis propria. Other degrees were as follows: when invasion reached the "adventitia," A_1; when adventitia was invaded, A_2; and with invasion into neighboring structures, A_3. Dissected lymph nodes were grouped according to the 29 areas shown in Table 16-1. Removal of distant lymph nodes, including paraaortic, retropancreatic, splenic or mesenteric, was performed only when they were macroscopically involved and/or, for the cervical nodes, when the cancer was cervical. The figures thus must be interpreted with care.

According to the Japanese classification and thus depending also on the level of the tumor, the nodes were classified as N_0, N_1, N_2, N_3, or N_4 (see Table 16-2). Both left and right recurrent laryngeal nerve groups have been added because they were removed separately and might be responsible for direct cervical spread.

In terms of wall penetration, lymph node involvement, and the presence or absence of metastases, the patients were grouped in the five stages shown in Table 16-3. Finally, the location of involved nodes was assessed according to abdominal, thoracic, or cervical sites.

The histologic study was prospective, always regarding the totality of resected specimens. Sur-

TABLE 16-4. Rates of negative and positive lymph nodes

Reference	No. of patients	Percentage*				
		N_0	N_1	N_2	N_3	N_4
Postlethwait[5]	2440	23.1		76.9		
Akiyama[1]	205	41		59		
Skinner et al.[6]	81	28.4		71.6		
Younghusband[7]	77	48		52		
Sannohe et al.[8]	36	47.2		52.8		
Present series	170	34.7	13.5	30.6	16.5	4.7

*Those percentages not listed under a specific N category were not reported as N subtypes, but rather were listed as N only according to the American Joint Committee for Cancer Staging classifications.

TABLE 16-5. Lymph node metastases in 170 patients with thoracic esophageal squamous cell carcinoma

	Lymph node group																
	1, 2	3	7	8	9	11	101	102	104	105	106	107	108	109	110	112	113
Upper third	5*		4					2	2	8	5	3	3		2	2	3
Middle third	30	1	17	1	3	1	1			5	4	5	32	3	10	4	6
Lower third	13	2	15	—	5	4	—	—	1	—	1	2	5	2	20	—	1
TOTAL	48	3	36	1	8	5	1	2	3	13	10	10	40	5	32	6	10

*Number of patients with lymph node metastases.

vival rates were calculated by computer according to the method of Kaplan and Meyer,[4] with a log-rank test for the comparison of curves.

RESULTS
Surgical technique (see also Chapter 15)

Radical resection for middle- and lower-third neoplasms included, through a laparotomy and a right thoracotomy in all patients, total thoracic and abdominal esophageal removal with all lymphatic tissue within the posterior mediastinum including the left pulmonary hilar nodes, gastrohepatic and gastrosplenic ligaments, retroperitoneal tissue and left gastric pedicle from the superior pancreatic margin to the hiatus, and the proximal part of the stomach. When invaded, the thoracic duct, azygos vein, both pleurae, pericardium, and a cuff of diaphragm were resected. Retrocaval pretracheal space was dissected for patients later in the series. Distant lymph nodes were removed only when they were enlarged. The stomach was severed, using a gastrointenstinal anastomosis stapler,* with removal of all the branches of the left gastric vessels on the lesser curvature across to the greater curvature at the level of the left gastroepiploic vessels. Pyloroplasty was performed. Anastomoses were done at the apex of the thorax by advancing the stomach. The colon was used in case of prior gastrectomy. For upper-third carcinomas, radical resection included a cervical incision for total esophagectomy and periesophageal lymph node dissection. A neck dissection was added if a node seemed macroscopically involved. The esophagogastric anastomosis was cervical in these cases. The route for esophageal replacement was via either the posterior mediastinum or the retrosternal space. Operations were always carried out in one stage.

A nasogastric tube was inserted during surgery, for constant suction postoperatively to keep the thoracic stomach empty. This tube was very important in avoiding dilatation with stress at the suture line, interference with gastric vascularity, and vomiting with possible aspiration. It was not removed until a favorable barium contrast swallow had been obtained on the seventh postoperative day.

Respiratory assistance by means of a nasotracheal tube for 24 hours permitted better ventilation and removal of secretions. Bronchoscopic aspiration was used when necessary.

*GIA, Merlin Medical.

TABLE 16-6. Number of patients in relation to N classification and A classification

	N_0	N_1	N_2	N_3-N_4
A_0 (<MP)	26	4	1	1
A_0 (MP)	8	2	5	8
A_1	12	7	17	13
A_2	6	8	21	8
A_3	7	2	8	6

TABLE 16-7. Mapping of lymph node involvement

N classification	No. of patients	Percent of series
N_1	23	13.5
N_1N_2	26	15.3
$N_1N_2N_3$	7	4.1
$N_1N_2N_3N_4$	2	1.2
N_2	26	15.3
N_2N_3	13	7.6
$N_2N_3N_4$	0	
N_1N_3	3	1.8
$N_1N_2N_4$	0	
$N_1N_3N_4$	1	0.6
N_2N_4	2	1.2
N_3	5	2.9
N_3N_4	1	0.6
N_1N_4	0	
N_4	2	1.2

TABLE 16-8. Lymph node involvement in relation to anatomic regions and sites of cancer

Anatomic regions	Upper third	Middle third	Lower third	Total
Cervical	3*	1	1	5
Thoracic				
Superior	12	13	1	26
Middle	5	37	7	49
Inferior	3	14	20	37
Abdominal				
Paragastric	7	38	21	63
Celiac-aorta	4	17	15	36
Splenopan-creatic	0	1	4	5
Hepatopyloric	0	1	3	4

*Number of patients having a positive lymph node at this site.

Histologic staging and results

All 170 patients had radical resection. No patient in this group received preoperative radiotherapy or chemotherapy. Postoperative radiation was used for 45 patients in a prospective randomized trial, and 21 patients had postoperative chemotherapy by choice of the referring physician.

The percentage of spread by way of lymphatics was high. Table 16-4 summarizes the gross results reported in the literature. There was little difference in the percentage of positive lymph nodes according to location of the tumor: upper third, 60.8%; middle third, 64.6%; and lower third, 69.6%.

Table 16-5 shows the ratio of lymph node involvement per dissected area. No histologically involved nodes were found along the greater curvature, in the pyloric group, or in the splenic or hepatic hilar areas, although these regions were not systematically dissected. However, in 21 cases nodes were removed because the surgeon found macroscopic enlargement. Few distant

nodes were involved, because this series reported only the results of radical curative surgery, which was rarely proposed for patients having positive nodes in those areas.

Table 16-6 reports the A and N classifications in this series, according to the Japanese ANM classification described above. There was a tendency for lymph node involvement and depth of wall penetration to be related, although parietal spread does not predict nodal status. Another very important point was the possibility of lymph node involvement in a superficial tumor, a well-known phenomenon in gastric cancer. Of patients without muscularis propria invasion, 3.1% had an N_3 or N_4 metastasis, 3.1% an N_2, and as high as 12.5% an N_1. This provides a strong argument against esophagectomy without thoracotomy.

In order to appreciate the directions of lymphatic extension, a mapping was prepared for each patient with the distribution of positive lymph nodes. Results for the series are compiled in Table 16-7. Normal spreading of lymphatic involvement occurred in 52.2% of cases (58 of 111), while metastases jumped one "normal" relay in 40.5% of cases, two relays in 5.4% and three relays in 1.8%. These figures confirm anatomic data showing a nonsegmental drainage of lymph and a major intramural longitudinal drainage within the submucosa.

At the present time, a number of surgeons interested in esophageal diseases advocate extensive resection for esophageal carcinomas.[1,6] It was observed in a short Japanese series that lymph nodes were involved in the abdomen and in the neck without thoracic metastases in 27.8%.[8] Table 16-8 shows the percentage of positive

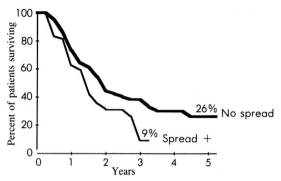

Fig. 16-1. Long-term actuarial survival according to intravascular tumor spread.

TABLE 16-9. Anatomic involvement according to lymph node metastases

	No. of patients
Mediastinum	43
Mediastinum + abdomen	37
Mediastinum + neck	3
Abdomen	26
Abdomen + neck	1
Neck	1
TOTAL	111

lymph nodes according to location of the gross extent of the tumor. The paragastric group included the nodes of the left and right paracardial areas, the lesser curvature groups, and the nodes along the left gastric artery. Lymphatic spread normally was most extensive in the immediate vicinity of the tumor.

Among 111 patients with positive lymph nodes, there were 83 with mediastinal metastases, 64 with abdominal metastases, and 5 with cervical metastases (see Table 16-9). The low percentage of cervical spread was due to the fact that we did not resect tumors in patients with proved positive supraclavicular nodes. Suggestive CT scanning or ultrasonography was followed by a preoperative open or transcutaneous needle biopsy.

Staging versus survival

There were 26 patients in JSED stage 0, 8 in stage I, 25 in stage II, 54 in stage III, and 57 in stage IV. Long-term results reported in the literature are variable. Values for 5-year survival rates ranged from 7% for Lam et al.[9] and for Cutler in a program of the National Cancer Institute[10] to 88% for Huang in a Chinese series of 220 superficial cancers.[11]

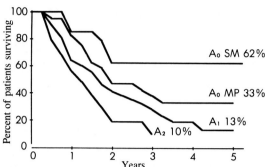

Fig. 16-2. Long-term actuarial survival according to tumor stage, Japanese classification.

Superficial cancers accounted for 18.8% (32 cases) in our series. They were noteworthy in that 18.7% had lymph node metastases and 59.4% had multicentric tumors with or without associated severe dysplasia. In this group of patients the 5-year survival rate was 62%.

Intravascular tumor spread is usually not considered in studies on survival. Fig. 16-1 shows the results of the entire series according to such involvement. Nevertheless, intravascular tumor spread was not an independent factor influencing survival; it was linked with lymph node metastases.

Finally, the JSED system seemed effective in determining the prognostic value of each element of staging. Survival curves are accurately discriminative for A (Fig. 16-2), for N (Fig. 16-3), two independent factors, and for the histologic stages (Fig. 16-4).

In our series, radiation therapy and chemotherapy were not systematically utilized with surgery. To date no prospective randomized trial has demonstrated any improvement in long-term results with these adjuvant treatments.

When curative surgery alone was considered, survival was 19% among patients who had apparently complete tumor removal. Thus we preferred to use the term "curative" to refer to radical operations realizing a complete gross removal of a stage 0, I, or II specimen. In these cases the 5-year survival rate was 29%, whatever the cause of death. Patients with a noncurative resection as defined above had only a 6% survival rate (see Fig. 16-5).

CONCLUSIONS

Surgical resection of esophageal cancer is the best treatment for possible cure in operable patients, and perhaps for all resectable patients. The

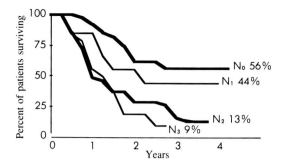

Fig. 16-3. Long-term actuarial survival according to adenopathy, Japanese classification.

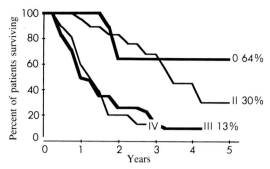

Fig. 16-4. Long-term actuarial survival according to histologic stages, Japanese classification.

mortality has been reduced to less than 10%, with an acceptable morbidity. The end results are still disappointing; combined radiation and chemotherapy may increase the duration of remission.

The generally poor results of currently available methods of treatment lead us to hope for early endoscopic detection of esophageal carcinoma. Systematic examination of high-risk patients by brush cytologic method and vital staining appears to be the only way to detect cancers in a curable stage.

However, at present, resection of regional lymph nodes with complete removal of the primary lesion provides the best prophylaxis against tumor recurrence.

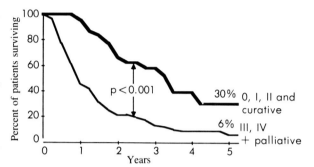

Fig. 16-5. Long-term actuarial survival according to Japanese staging *and* surgical classification of curative versus palliative resection.

REFERENCES

1. Akiyama, H., Tsurumaru, M., Kawamura, T., and Ono, Y.: Principles of surgical treatment for carcinoma of the esophagus: analysis of lymph node involvement, Ann. Surg. **194**:438, 1981.
2. American Cancer Society: Cancer facts and figures, New York, 1982: American Cancer Society.
3. Japanese Society for Esophageal Diseases: Guide lines for the clinical and pathologic studies on carcinoma of the esophagus, parts I and II, Jpn. J. Surg. **6**:69, 1976.
4. Kaplan, E.L., and Meyer, P.: Nonparametric estimation from incomplete observations, J. Am. Stat. Assoc. **53**:457, 1958.
5. Postlethwait, R.W.: Squamous cell carcinoma of the esophagus. In Surgery of the esophagus, New York, 1979, Appleton-Century-Crofts, p. 357.
6. Skinner, D.B., Dowlatshahi, K.D., and Demeester, T.R.: Potentially curable cancer of the esophagus, Cancer **50**:2571, 1982.
7. Younghusband, J.D., and Aluwihare, A.P.: Carcinoma of the oesophagus: factors influencing survival, Br. J. Surg. **57**:422, 1970.
8. Sannohe, Y., Hiratsuka, R., and Doki, K.: Lymph node metastases in cancer of the thoracic esophagus, Am. J. Surg. **141**:216, 1981.
9. Lam, K., Wong, J., Lim, S., and Ong, G.: Results of esophagectomy. In Stipa, S., Belsey, R., and Moraldi, A., editors: Medical and surgical problems of the esophagus, New York, 1981, Academic Press, pp. 324-326.
10. Cutler, S.J.: Trends in cancers of the digestive tracts, Surgery **65**:740, 1969.
11. Huang, K.C.: Surgical treatment of carcinoma of the esophagus: results in 1647 patients. In Stipa, S., Belsey, R., and Moraldi, A., editors: Medical and surgical problems of the esophagus, New York, 1981, Academic Press, pp. 335-338.

17 Anastomosis using wire sutures in one layer

Janos Kiss, Attila Vörös, and Endre Szirányi

The double-layer technique of suturing had dominated surgery for nearly 100 years when in 1887 Halsted[1] and a few followers began using intestinal suture in one layer. However, only during the past few decades have increasing attempts been made to use a one-layer anastomosis along the entire length of the digestive tract, esophagus, stomach, and small and large intestine.

Also during the last few decades metallic sutures have gained ground in surgery of the alimentary tract. Metallic stitches, specifically gold, were used by the ancient Greeks. In twentieth-century applications, gold and silver have been replaced by the stainless steel wire. This metal is so strong and resistant to chemical and thermal effects that it is called the "new precious metal." This material causes no tissue reaction, its tensile strength is enormous, and yet it is flexible and easy to tie into knots.

The use of wire sutures has a long tradition in Hungary. In a paper published in 1906 Verebely wrote: "Materials which do not absorb water, for instance the wire . . . caused infection much less frequently than the silk and catgut which do. . . . "

The introduction of staplers into surgery brought with it the suture technique employing metallic staples and clips in operations on the gastrointestinal tract.

These two advances—one-layer technique and stainless steel suture—have been unified in gastrointestinal surgery by Belsey.[2] He achieved excellent results by using single-layer wire sutures in esophagogastric and esophagocolonic anastomoses.[2]

Since 1965, innumerable reports have been published on the use of single-layer sutures (with wire or synthetic threads) in different parts of the gastrointestinal tract. Postlethwait et al.[3] subjected to histologic investigation the tissue reactions produced by different suture materials in 666 cases in which death ensued for any reason 1 day to 23 years after operation. It was demonstrated that wire produced no tissue reaction. Goligher[4] prefered its use mainly in those parts of the alimentary canal where there is no serosal layer (esophagus or rectum). Overall, though, this method has been slowly introduced into operating rooms without reports by the majority of the surgeons who use it.

MATERIAL AND METHODS

Anastomosis is made most frequently between the esophagus and the stomach or jejunum, and less frequently, between the esophagus and the colon or ileum. When making esophageal anastomoses, we prefer the end-to-side method, because it is easier technically to create the orifice this way. The esophagocolonic anastomosis can also be done end to end.

To illustrate the technique of an anastomosis we will describe the method used to anastomose the esophagus with a Roux-en-Y loop of intestine.

The oral stump of the esophagus is grasped with an instrument and is lifted forward (Fig. 17-1, *A*). A coapting stitch is placed in the esophageal wall 7 to 8 mm above the planned anastomosis site and also in the middle of the antimesenteric side near the closed tip of the Roux-en-Y loop. At the planned anastomotic level, in the posterior wall, the esophageal muscular wall and mucosa are cut transversally. The assistant keeps the esophagus grasped in the instrument pulled upward, so that the elevated anterior wall keeps the esophageal lumen patent. In the intestinal wall an opening is cut parallel to the longitudinal axis of the jejunum, on the antimesenteric side corresponding to the size of the esophageal lumen.

From 5 to 6 mm of esophageal wall is taken up by atraumatic wire stitches,* including the

---

*Surgicraft, 100 cm, 36 s.s.w., 22 mm, ½ circle round body—A.W. Showell, Ltd., Redditch, England.

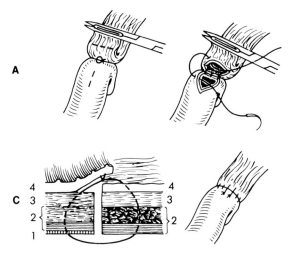

Fig. 17-1. Steps (**A** to **D**) in making the esophagojejunal anastomosis. *1,* Serosa; *2* and *3,* muscular layers; *4,* mucosa.

tough mucosa. A similar amount of jejunal tissue is taken, but only seromusculosubmucosal stitches are placed (Fig. 17-1, *B* and *C*). The wire knots are tied with a needle holder, inside the lumen. It suffices to have one true knot (two intertwining counterdirectional loops), but the four-throw surgeon's knots (four loops around a straight wire) will not hold. After it has been tied, the wire can be cut rather short.

Starting from the middle, the stiches are alternated right and left. The stitches may be 4 to 5 mm apart when the mentioned quantities of tissue are taken up. The knots of the last two or three stitches are on the outside, and stitches are placed over them to prevent trauma to adjacent structures by the wire sticking out 1 or 2 mm (Fig. 17-1, *D*).

Even when we surgically create an anastomosis of excellent quality, free of tension, and with a good blood supply, the row of sutures must be protected against stress to achieve undisturbed healing. The anastomosed organs must be protected against dilatation, accumulation of digestive enzymes, and major displacement. Tension causes disorders of blood flow, which may lead to tissue necrosis near the stitches. To protect the esophageal anastomosis, no peroral feeding is allowed for 8 to 10 days after surgery, intestinal contents are evacuated by tube, and the organ used for replacement of the esophagus is allowed to remain quiescent postoperatively.

To drain intestinal contents and gases, tubes passed down through the nose or mouth are used extensively. The nasogastric or, following total gastrectomy, the nasojejunal tube functions excellently in the majority of cases, but in some

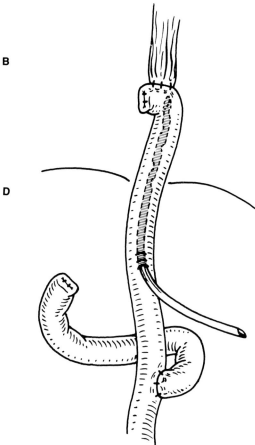

Fig. 17-2. Preventing distention by catheter-jejunostomy.

cases it has disadvantages:

1. The tube irritates the nose of the patient, increases bronchial secretions, and interferes with expectoration.
2. The tube may traumatize the anastomosis, interfering with healing.
3. Reliable placement of the tube is possible during surgery only, and if it is pulled out by the patient inadvertently or willfully, there is no way to evacuate accumulating fluids.

These disadvantages can be avoided by inserting a catheter into the jejunum distal to an esophagojejunal anastomosis (according to Marwedel) and leading it out through the abdominal wall. The catheter is not passed through the anastomosis (see Fig. 17-2). From under the anastomosis, swallowed saliva, intestinal juices, and accumulated gases pass through the catheter, and subsequent dilatation of the anastomosis occurs.

We cover the organ replacing the esophagus with mediastinal pleura or with a pleural flap detached from the chest wall. It then is prevented

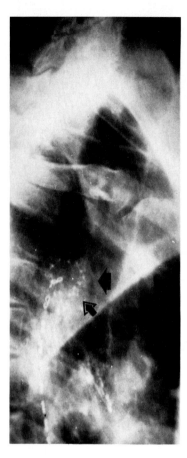

Fig. 17-3. Esophageal anastomosis *(arrow)* easily visible on postoperative oblique x-ray view.

from moving after the operation, and the position of the mesenteric artery, and therefore the blood supply of the organ, will not change.

In Fig. 17-3, the postoperative x-ray film shows clearly the wire *(arrow)* at the level of an esophagogastric anastomosis.

We have performed 562 esophageal anastomosis operations utilizing this technique between January 1, 1973 and December 31, 1985 (see Table 17-1).

DISCUSSION

During the past 13 years, we have made more than 2000 anastomoses by the single-layer wire suture method and have gained extensive experience with it throughout the alimentary tract, including esophageal surgery. As early as 1887, Halsted[1] recognized that the most important anchoring layer of the intestine is the submucosa.

Matheson and Irving[5] pointed out that this has particular significance when a single row of sutures is used. Correspondingly, we have employed the seromusculosubmucosal technique (on the gastric or intestinal side) when placing single stitches. When making esophageal and rectal anastomoses, we have sutured the walls through and through, because their mucosae are tough. This toughness plays an important role in keeping the sutures in place.

Certain advantages are evident with a single row of stitches. Tissues are less damaged. Microcirculation is interfered with to a lesser degree than with two rows of stitches. When submucosal apposition is correct, primary healing may be anticipated. Endoscopic studies conducted in the early postoperative period show the site of esophageal anastomosis merely as a sharp borderline where the two different mucosal layers are joined. There is histologic evidence that in such cases mucosal continuity is restored rapidly and the anastomotic line is covered by it.

A disadvantage of wire is the need to learn how to handle it. Care should be taken to avoid looping, and two or three true knots have to be tied with a needle holder.

CONCLUSIONS

"In end-to-end anastomosis of the intestine only one row of sutures should be taken. I should regard a second row as a factor of danger rather than security."[1] This statement was made by Halsted in 1887, but despite this, a century later, most surgeons still employ the double-layer technique. Some surgeons even add a third layer to reinforce the anastomosis, which merely reflects their lack of confidence and sense of insecurity rather than any supporting scientific data.[6]*

REFERENCES

1. Halsted, W.S.: Circular sutures of intestine, Am. J. Med. Sci. **94**:436, 1887.
2. Belsey, R.: Reconstruction of the esophagus with left colon, J. Thorac. Cardiovasc. Surg. **49**:33, 1965.
3. Postlethwait, R.W., Willigan, D.A., and Ulin, A.W.: Human tissue reaction to sutures, Ann. Surg. **181**:144, 1975.

*EDITOR'S NOTE: Although the authors are to be commended both on their strong presentation for the single-layer wire technique and on their low anastomotic leakage rate, the reader is cautioned that similar results are obtainable by two-layer suturing or stapling techniques. Thus, this chapter is a statement *pro* this technique, not *con* others.

TABLE 17-1. Esophageal anastomosis using a single-layer wire technique

		Age	Leakage of esophageal anastomosis		
			No. of patients	Per-cent	Deaths
Esophagogastrostomy	189	26-82 (57.9)	7	3.7%	3
Esophagojejunostomy	317		3	0.9%	2
Esophagocolostomy	56		5	8.9%	1
TOTAL	562		15*	2.66%	6

*Most of the leakages (with esophagogastrostomy in every case, with esophagocolostomy in all but one case) occurred with anastomoses made in the neck.

4. Goligher, J.C.: Visceral and parietal suture in abdominal surgery, Am. J. Surg. **131**:130, 1976.
5. Matheson, N.A., and Irving, A.D.: Single layer anastomosis in the gastrointestinal tract, Surg. Gynecol. Obstet. **143**:619, 1976.
6. Maurya, S.D., Gupta, H.C., Tewari, A., Khan, S.S., and Sharma, B.D. Double layer versus single layer intestinal anastomosis: a clinical trial, Int. Surg. **69**:339, 1984.

CHAPTER 18 Critical postoperative care using the Swan-Ganz catheter

Ryoichi Motoki

The Swan-Ganz catheter, a flow-directed balloon-tipped catheter devised by Swan, Ganz et al.,[1] makes possible the bedside evaluation of hemodynamics in critically ill patients. Disorders of the circulatory system are often observed in patients whose esophageal cancer has been removed by surgery. Since they would develop severe complications causing multiple organ failure if they were treated improperly, careful postoperative management should be provided. For this purpose a clear understanding of the hemodynamics must be obtained by repeated right-side cardiac catheterization using the Swan-Ganz catheter. Adequate circulation must be maintained; if it fails, proper circulatory support must be begun.

TECHNIQUES

On the day before surgery the Swan-Ganz catheter is inserted percutaneously into the antecubital vein, floated into the pulmonary artery with the aid of a pressure monitor and oscilloscope, and advanced until the pulmonary wedge pressure is obtained. A preoperative hemodynamic measurement is carried out, and the catheter is left in place for more than 7 days.

Since the pulmonary wedge and systemic pressures are good estimates of the left-atrial and left-ventricular pressures, information about the pressures of the four cardiac chambers can be obtained. The cardiac output is also measured easily by the thermodilution technique with the aid of a thermistor and cardiac output computer. The vascular resistances can be calculated from the pressure differences and the cardiac output.

Twelve factors of hemodynamics, pressure, flows, and vascular resistance concerning systemic and pulmonary circulation are available. Mean pulmonary artery pressure (PAP), mean pulmonary wedge pressure (PWP) and mean right-atrial pressure (RAP) are measured with pressure transducers. Cardiac output (CO) is measured by the thermodilution technique with a cardiac output computer. The cardiac index (CI) is expressed as liters per minute per square meter of body surface. Mean systemic artery pressure (MAP), total peripheral resistance index (TPR), pulmonary arteriolar resistance index (PAR), left-ventricular stroke work index (LVSWI), right-ventricular stroke work index (RVSWI), left cardiac work index (LW), and right cardiac work index (RW) are calculated according to the following formulas:

$$MAP \text{ (mm Hg)} = \text{Diastolic artery pressure} + \text{Pulse pressure} \times \tfrac{1}{3}$$

$$TPR \text{ (dynes/sec/cm}^2) = (MAP - RAP) \times 79.92/CI$$

$$PAR \text{ (dynes/sec/cm}^2) = (PAP - PWP) \times 79.92/CI$$

$$LVSWI \text{ (g-m/beat/min)} = (MAP - PWP) \times CI \times 1000/\text{pulse rate} \times 0.0136$$

$$RVSWI \text{ (g-m/beat/min)} = (PAP - RAP) \times CI \times 1000/\text{pulse rate} \times 0.0136$$

$$LW \text{ (kg-m/beat/min)} = (MAP - PWP) \times CI \times 0.0136$$

$$RW \text{ (kg-m/beat/min)} = (PAP - RAP) \times CI \times 0.0136$$

Circulatory failure should be detected early and dysfunction should be corrected properly. Too much information may lead to misunderstanding or produce difficulty in understanding hemodynamics. We have devised a method of detecting disorders called a "hemodynamogram." The twelve hemodynamic factors measured or calculated are plotted on the radially arranged lines (Fig. 18-1). Normal values are located on the crossing points of the radial lines and the circle.

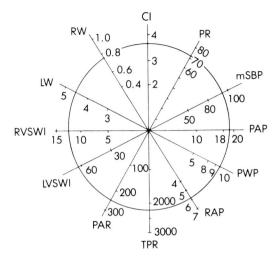

Fig. 18-1. Hemodynamogram. The twelve hemodynamic factors are plotted on the radially arranged lines. The crossings of the radial lines and the circle are each normal values. *PR,* Pulse rate; *mSBP,* mean systolic blood pressure.

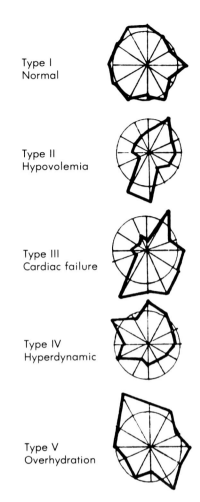

Hemodynamograms are classified according to CI and PWP into five groups, types I, II, III, IV, and V, which represent normal, hypovolemia, cardiac failure, hyperdynamic state, and hypervolemia, respectively (Fig. 18-2). The circulatory status of a patient can be understood easily from his hemodynamogram.

Another method of hemodynamic analysis is the myocardial function curve based on Starling's principle. Any movement to the upper left is thought to be improvement in myocardial function, and movement to the lower right, myocardial depression.

Fig. 18-2. Classification of hemodynamograms, with typical patterns: type I, normal hemodynamics (hemodynamogram almost identical with the circle); type II, hypovolemia (low CI and low PWP); type III, cardiac failure (low CI and high PWP); type IV, hyperdynamic state (high CI and low PWP); type V, overhydration or hypervolemia (high or normal CI and high PWP).

HEMODYNAMICS OBSERVED IN THE POSTOPERATIVE COURSE

Type I, with normal CI and PWP, is seen in a patient with normal hemodynamics. Since almost all factors in this type are within the normal range, the hemodynamogram is almost identical to the circle. The circulatory condition in type I is excellent and is the goal of therapy during the postoperative period.

Type II, with low CI and low PWP, is seen in a patient with hypovolemia. This type of abnormality is typically observed in patients with hemorrhagic shock. Besides low CI and low PWP, systemic pressure, cardiac work, and ventricular stroke work are lower than normal, and pulse rate and vascular resistance are higher. The type II hemodynamogram is often observed in the early

period after esophageal surgery. Tsuboi[2] studied the hemodynamics of patients who had undergone esophageal surgery. He found that the pulmonary arterial pressure and the pulmonary wedge pressure measured immediately after surgery were lower than those before surgery, though the lost blood had been replaced by transfusion. The sequestration of the effective extracellular fluid into the third space may play a major role in hypovolemia in the early postoperative period. When LVSWI is below 50 g-m/beat/min or CI is below 3.0 L/min., the disorder is critical and should be corrected by volume expansion as soon as possible. If intrathoracic and/or intraabdominal bleeding is strongly suspected, reoperation for hemostasis must be carried out.

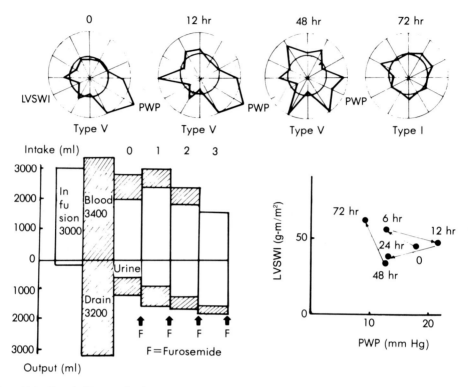

Fig. 18-3. Case 1. Hypervolemia resulting from overinfusion during surgery was detected by type V hemodynamogram; the condition was corrected by administration of furosemide. *Top,* Evolution of the hemodynamogram. *Lower left,* Fluid balance graphed. *Lower right,* LVSWI plotted against PWP.

Hemodynamograms resembling type II, with normal blood pressure, normal LVSWI (over 50 g-m/beat/min), and good peripheral circulation with high total peripheral resistance, is observed in some aged patients. Arteriosclerosis would account for the high vascular resistance. In such cases, no intensive volume expansion is necessary.

Type III, with low CI and high PWP, is seen in a patient with cardiac failure. This disorder is sometimes observed in the early period after esophageal surgery. Usually dobutamine hydrochloride (Dobutrex) is effective in correcting the abnormality. Changes in pulmonary function occur after esophageal surgery and are characterized by decreased lung volumes, decreased compliance, and transpulmonary shunting. Hypoxia caused by depressed lung function would lead to depression of cardiac function including cardiogenic shock with myocardial infarction or severe arrhythmia. Clinically, at the onset of any hypotensive episode in the postoperative period, cardiogenic shock should be ruled out by a hemodynamic study with the Swan-Ganz catheter before fluid administration is started, because lung edema will develop rapidly when a massive amount of fluid has been infused into patients with

cardiogenic hypotension.

Type IV, with high CI and low PWP, is seen in a patient with a hyperdynamic condition of the circulatory system. Generally, low blood pressure accompanying the type IV hemodynamogram is characteristically observed in warm shock status or the hyperdynamic state of septic shock. Patients with liver cirrhosis or an arteriovenous shunt are also implicated in this abnormality. Few patients who have undergone esophageal surgery show type IV hemodynamograms associated with sepsis or hepatic failure.

Type V, with high or normal CI and high PWP, is seen in a patient with hypervolemia. The cardiac performance is slightly increased by elevated cardiac preload. The causes of hypervolemia in postoperative patients seem to be overinfusion, renal failure, and/or redistribution of sequestered body fluid back into the circulating volume. The redistribution usually begins 32 to 48 hours after esophageal surgery and follows the elevation of PWP and PAP. Patients with these hemodynamics often develop pulmonary complications. There are many causes for postoperative pulmonary complications. The elevation of hydrostatic pressure across the pulmonary capillary wall is thought to play a role in accumulation of fluid in

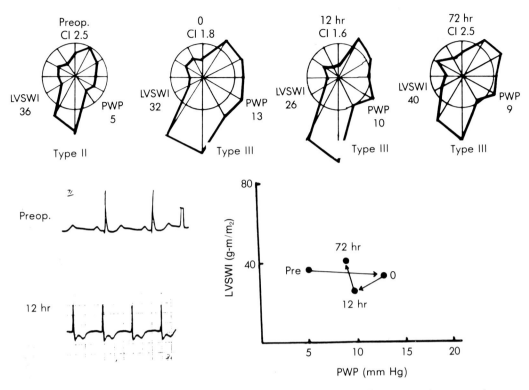

Fig. 18-4. Case 2. Type III hemodynamogram associated with hypotension suggested postoperative myocardial infarction. *Top,* Evolution of the hemodynamogram. *Lower left,* Changing electrocardiogram. *Lower right,* LVSWI plotted against PWP.

the interstitial and intraalveolar spaces. Therefore, the attempt to reduce PWP might be effective in preventing initiation or aggravation of pulmonary complications. Mean PWP should be kept below 10 mm Hg, if possible, with the infusion rate decreased and the urine output increased by administration of furosemide, mannitol, and/or dopamine.

CASE EXAMPLES

The following are examples of the application of information gained from Swan-Ganz catheterization.

Case 1: overhydration (Fig. 18-3)

A 70-year-old male patient had resection of the thoracic esophagus for cancer of the mid-esophagus. Because his blood pressure was unstable during the operation, he was thought to be hypovolemic. However, the hemodynamogram taken immediately after the operation showed type V, the overhydration type. His hemodynamics returned to normal after administration of diuretics.

Case 2: acute cardiac failure (Fig. 18-4)

A 64-year-old male patient with lower thoracic esophageal cancer had a history of angina. Resection of the thoracic esophagus was carried out although his cardiac function was not satisfactory. The postoperative hemodynamogram showed type III, the cardiac failure type, with ischemic change in the electrocardiogram. Cardiac function recovered with intensive cardiac support.

REFERENCES

1. Swan, H.J.C., Ganz, W., Forrester, J., et al.: Catheterization of the heart in man with use of a flow-directed balloon-tipped catheter, N. Engl. J. Med. **285:**447, 1970.
2. Tsuboi, M.: Studies on the postoperative pulmonary complications of the esophageal cancer, J. Jpn. Surg. Soc. **78:**223, 1977.

DISCUSSION—Chapters 14 to 18

Gordon Franklin Murray

It is not widely appreciated that Dr. Willy Meyer's description of successful esophageal resection at the annual meeting of the American Medical Association in 1913 was met with indifference.[1] Much of this apathy was due to ignorance of thoracic problems and their proposed solutions. In contrast, the preceding four chapters from the United Kingdom, France, Hungary, and Japan emphasize modern concern for the reduction of perioperative morbidity and mortality relating to esophageal resection and reconstruction. What has not changed since Dr. Meyer's presentation is the formidable challenge that complications of esophageal resection present to the thoracic surgeon. Patients often suffer from malnutrition or extreme debility, and many are of advanced age, with significant pulmonary and cardiovascular disease. These problems contribute to postoperative complications, which may be catastrophic. Furthermore, many patients are seen late in the course of their disease, which is complicated by advanced esophageal obstruction, malignant esophagorespiratory fistula, or perforation. Hope for survival is often not realistic, and symptomatic relief can be difficult to achieve (the mean survival is not infrequently 3 to 5 months and rarely exceeds one year).

Realizing that cure remains an elusive goal, the surgeon should give primary consideration to the attainment of effective palliation focused on early restoration of the patient's ability to swallow. Exactly how to achieve relief of the patient's dysphagia, however, makes for a very difficult and often confusing decision. When the options are examined, it becomes readily apparent that complications of specific morbidity are very much related to the surgeon's selection of available methods and techniques of resection and reconstruction. These factors include operative exposure, type of conduit, route of conduit, anastomotic techniques, and level of reconstruction. Recognition of those factors that portend an undesirable result in a particular patient should alert the surgeon to alter the operative approach.

PRETREATMENT EVALUATION

The extremely poor outlook for patients with carcinoma of the esophagus demands careful definition of the extent of disease prior to the selection of treatment. Pretreatment judgment concerning the operability of a lesion is of obvious importance. It is recognized that incomplete resection does not offer any other palliation than the abolition of dysphagia and control of aspiration; anorexia, continued weight loss, and cachexia inexorably lead to early death. An ill-advised radical resection in some patients may result in excessive operative mortality and morbidity and may deny a gratifying short-term improvement by radiation in a few individuals. Knowledge of carcinoma of the esophagus with extensive lymphatic metastasis clearly militates against the use of aggressive resectional therapy. The presence of extraesophageal mediastinal disease may be suggested by azygos venography, lymphangiography, abnormalities of the esophagogram, and computed tomography. Bronchoscopy is most important in all patients with lesions suspected of invading the trachea or main bronchi. We have demonstrated previously that mediastinoscopy is of value in accessing mediastinal extension of carcinoma of the esophagus in patients without endobronchial extension.[2] Lymphatic drainage of the esophagus, similar to mediastinal extension of bronchogenic carcinoma, involves lymph node stations accessible to the mediastinoscope. Fixed perinodal metastasis provides positive evidence of extension of disease beyond the esophagus. This finding has the same grave significance as extraesophageal extension identified by bronchoscopy. The ominous implication of such pathology was apparent for the patients in this series, who survived only 1 to 4 months. Also, nearly all our patients with distant celiac metastasis undergoing resection were found to have extension of cancer outside the esophagus in the mediastinum at thoracotomy. In our study, all patients with celiac nodal metastasis were dead within a year (mean survival, 6 months), and palliative surgical resection provided no improvement in length of survival. On the other hand, the favorable prognostic value of negative mediastinoscopy and celiotomy was also demonstrated in the study. The majority of such patients were alive and free of disease 2 years following operation. It is clear that such patients are prime candidates for resectional therapy.

Combined mediastinoscopy and celiotomy should be considered in all patients presumed to have operable carcinoma of the thoracic esophagus. Mediastinoscopy alone is of value in the assessment of carcinoma of the upper thoracic and midthoracic esophagus. Selection of surgical treatment based on assessment of lymphatic metastasis can avoid excessive morbidity and identify favorable candidates for aggressive excisional therapy. There is accumulating evidence that patients with evidence of extraesophageal mediastinal spread and positive celiac nodes are not candidates for surgical resection. These patients should be spared the rigors of radical therapy, since its benefits are so often outweighed by its complications.

OPERATIVE INTERVENTION

The operative challenge is made more formidable by associated malnutrition and pulmonary complications. Patients with severe obstruction present in a dehydrated, debilitated, anemic, and anergic state. Cardiopulmonary reserve is diminished, and resistance to infection is lowered because of impaired antibody production and decreased phagocytic activity of leukocytes. Although some of the complications are not preventable, adequate preoperative preparation and careful postoperative management can reduce attendant morbidity. Improved total parenteral nutrition and careful attention to the treatment of respiratory infection have enhanced markedly the safety of aggressive surgical intervention, with significant reductions in major wound, infectious, and cardiorespiratory complications. However, the primary purpose of this discussion will be to focus on complications directly related to surgical resection of the esophagus—that is, anastomotic leak, persistent obstruction, and gastroesophageal reflux.

Anastomotic leak following esophageal resection is a devastating complication and has been responsible for 30% to 50% of reported deaths. Important etiologic factors include undue tension, inadequate blood supply, unsatisfactory suture technique, and residual tumor. The stomach has become the preferred conduit because of its excellent blood supply and adequate length to bridge almost all defects. Esophagogastrectomy is a safe procedure, and the one anastomotic reconstruction with stomach (as opposed to three with interposed colon or jejunum) is extremely reliable. A very satisfactory operative technique is that first advocated by Ivor Lewis[3] in 1946, consisting of initial abdominal exploration and mobilization of the stomach followed immediately by a right thoracotomy, esophagectomy, and high esophagogastric anastomosis. This right-sided approach avoids the difficult anastomosis below the aortic arch presented by a left thoracotomy, and ensures tumor-free margins. Anastomotic technique has been further enhanced by end-to-side reconstruction of the fundus (avoiding the ischemic T anastomosis inherent in the gastric tube procedure) and the development of the automatic stapler. Current information strongly suggests that the stapler is an effective means of creating the esophagogastric anastomosis. The use of wire suture in one layer for esophagocolonic and esophagojejunal anastomosis is also appropriately emphasized in the present series of chapters.

The favorable implications of an anastomotic leak in the neck not withstanding, the requirement to achieve the additional distance may jeopardize a successful operation. The Lahey clinic group[4] recently reported an incidence of dehiscence of only 1.7% in patients who underwent transthoracic resection, compared with a disturbing 15.4% in comparable patients undergoing extrathoracic resection with a cervical anastomosis. The authors indicated maximal stretching of the stomach to reach the neck, with subsequent impairment of blood supply. This observation, if correct, has application to management decisions regarding lesions of the lower esophagus. In the latter circumstance, removal of left gastric lymph nodes and establishment of adequate proximal tumor margin are ensured by partial gastric resection. It would be certainly unwise to compromise these principles by insistence on a cervical reconstruction. For interposition procedures, careful management of the vascular pedicle to secure good arterial supply and venous drainage is critical in avoiding an anastomotic leak or even loss of the conduit. Provision of adequate space at the thoracic inlet is also essential, particularly if the conduit is advanced through the anterior mediastinum. Compression of the interposed segment may lead to impaired blood supply and gangrene of its cervical component.

Several mechanisms contribute to persistent or recurrent obstruction following esophageal resection. Stricture of the anastomosis is usually a delayed complication, occurring 3 to 6 months after reconstruction. Two related factors have been discussed: (1) inadequate blood supply at the suture line and (2) a small leak with focal infection producing excessive scarring. Reflux esophagitis is also a major cause of anastomotic stricture. Mechanical obstruction can result from excessive redundancy in patients with interposed segments, particularly colon. Compression at the thoracic outlet or constriction by a too small opening in the diaphragm may spoil an otherwise excellent result. In the abdomen, a vascular pedicle placed anterior to the stomach may result in pyloric obstruction or gastric impingement on the pedicle. Dysphagia related to tumor recurrence underscores the importance of a wide operative margin, usually achieved by a near-total esophageal resection. Notably, lesions of the lower esophagus may be associated with spread of tumor along the lesser curvature, fixation of celiac lymph nodes, and invasion of the posterior peritoneum. Subtotal resection of this abdominal disease leaves residual tumor, which imposes the risk of early recurrent obstruction of the stomach at the hiatus. In my opinion, such metastatic involvement precludes palliative resection in these patients.

However, resection of upper esophageal carcinoma is often achieved by leaving residual tumor on the trachea, bronchus, or vertebral body. When tumor does infiltrate the tissue of the aorta, it is usually possible to separate the malignancy by careful resection. But, can the traditional transthoracic experience be translated to the management of patients by esophagectomy without thoracotomy?[5] In fact, fixation of the tumor to a contiguous tracheobronchial or vascular structure may require thoracotomy in as many as 25% of patients in whom extrathoracic resection is attempted. Importantly, most of these patients will have a stage III lesion in the upper esophagus. The planned operative procedure is usually abandoned because of fixation of tumor to the aorta, trachea, or bronchi; but, in some instances, emergency thoracotomy is undertaken for a tracheal disruption or hemorrhage. It would appear that knowledge of carcinoma of the upper esophagus with mediastinal extension clearly militates against the election of the extrathoracic resectional technique.

Complications secondary to gastroesophageal reflux include erosive esophagitis, anastomotic stricture, and pulmonary aspiration with pneumonitis and lung abscess. Factors contributing to greater morbidity in the presence of reflux are inadequate pyloroplasty or pyloromyotomy, recurrent laryngeal nerve paralysis, and an indwelling nasogastric tube stenting the anastomosis. Reflux may be mitigated at the original operation by fundoplasty, particularly in the instance of primary esophagogastrectomy. Pyloroplasty is probably not necessary when the stomach is entirely brought into the chest. However, reflux with the left-sided approach is a more treacherous complication. The denervated intraabdominal stomach empties poorly, and pyloroplasty is mandatory. When an interposition procedure is elected, a long (8-cm) segment of intraabdominal colon or jejunum is advisable to discourage reflux. In the presence of gastroesophageal reflux, recurrent laryngeal nerve injury is a serious complication because of the secondary aspiration that often occurs. Although paralysis may result from mediastinal dissection, the complication is best averted by avoiding cervical retraction on the tracheoesophageal groove, particularly during exposure or anastomosis of the cervical esophagus. The injury is particularly morbid when a high cervical anastomosis is contemplated.

In summary, selective utilization of available procedures for the operative management of patients requiring esophageal resection seems optimal. Recognition of all the pathologic features of esophageal carcinoma that merit consideration of alternative methods should improve operative results and reduce morbidity.*

REFERENCES

1. Meyer, W: Extrathoracic and intrathoracic esophagoplasty in connection with resection of the thoracic portion of the esophagus for carcinoma, JAMA **62**:100, 1914.
2. Murray, G.F., Wilcox, B.R., and Starek, P.J.K.: The assessment of operability of esophageal carcinoma, Ann. Thorac. Surg. **23**:393, 1977.
3. Lewis, I.: The surgical treatment of carcinoma of the esophagus: with special reference to a new operation for growths of the middle third, Br. J. Surg. **34**:18, 1946.
4. Shahian, D.M., Neptune, W.B., Ellis, F.H., Jr., et al.: Transthoracic versus extrathoracic esophagectomy: mortality, morbidity, and long-term survival, Ann. Thorac. Surg. **41**:237, 1986.
5. Murray, G.F.: Esophagectomy without thoracotomy, Ann. Thorac. Surg. **41**:233, 1986.

*EDITOR'S NOTE: There is no substitute for the experienced esophageal surgeon with appropriately judgmental selection of the operative procedure to be employed and the technical skills to carry it out, or any variation indicated by unanticipated anatomic or pathologic findings.

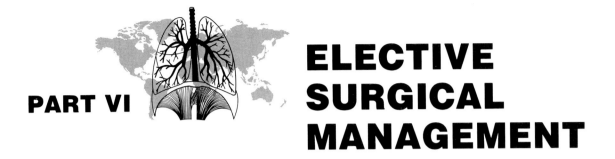

PART VI ELECTIVE SURGICAL MANAGEMENT

CHAPTER 19 Recognition and treatment of the early lesion

Guo Jun Huang

Carcinoma of the esophagus is more prevalent in China than in most other countries, its age-adjusted mortality being 31.66 per 100,000 in males and 15.93 per 100,000 in females. The incidence is much higher in certain parts of north central China, such as Linxian county of the Henan province, where the age-adjusted mortality reaches as high as 161 per 100,000 in males and 103 per 100,000 in females. In some parts of this county one person in four dies eventually of this malignancy.[1,2]

However, despite the high incidence of esophageal carcinoma in China, most patients coming to the hospitals are at late stages of their disease, and early cases are seen only infrequently in most medical centers. In my series of 1874 cases of esophageal carcinoma treated surgically from 1958 to 1982 at the Cancer Institute and Hospital of the Chinese Academy of Medical Sciences in Beijing, stage I carcinoma, that is, carcinoma in which the cancerous invasion is confined to only the mucosa or mucosa and submucosa without metastasis to lymph nodes or other organs, was seen in only 3% of the cases.[3] Similar situations occur in Japan, where Endo and associates[4] reported that early cases represented 3.3% of 846 resected cases of esophageal carcinoma over a period of 14 years, and Nabeya and Arai[5] collected only 177 cases from 1966 to 1979.

Absence of marked symptoms and lack of awareness of the disease on the part of patients as well as medical workers may account chiefly for the rarity in the discovery of early esophageal carcinoma. On the other hand, difficulties in identifying high-risk subjects and lack of a simple and efficient diagnostic tool may also account for the frequent nonrecognition of the disease at its early stage.

Methods to improve early detection of esophageal carcinoma have been the subject of intensive investigation. Double-contrast roentgenography by either barium and air[6-8] or barium followed by water[9] has been frequently used with good results in disclosing mucosal and muscular wall changes of early esophageal carcinoma. Modern fiberesophagoscopy used either alone or in conjunction with vital staining by toluidine blue[10,11] or Lugol's solution[4] also permits more detailed examination and more accurate biopsy of mucosal changes.

Abrasive cytology by means of a balloon catheter, so-called balloon cytology, has been widely used in China since 1961 in high-incidence areas of esophageal carcinoma as a means of mass screening for the detection of this disease, resulting in discovery of a large number of early cases, and for the detection and followup of esophageal dysplasia, which is also prevalent in these areas and known to develop into carcinoma in a high percentage of cases. Balloon cytology is thus of merit in identifying esophageal dysplasia in high-risk persons for whom periodic followup examinations can lead to the discovery of carcinoma at its very early stage. Balloon cytology is also used in medical centers now as a basic technique for the detection of early esophageal carcinoma that is equally as indispensable as other traditional methods.

It is the purpose of this communication to present briefly our experience in the recognition and treatment of early esophageal carcinoma, with special reference to the use of balloon cytology.

RECOGNITION
Awareness of early symptoms

Clinical studies of early esophageal carcinoma in high-incidence areas in China have shown that approximately 90% of patients have mild but definite symptoms related to swallowing. The most common are retrosternal discomfort or pain and a sense of friction, burning, or slow passage during swallowing of food. These symptoms usually come and go for months or even years, causing the patient no great concern until they become increasingly constant and severe. They appear only on deglutition and are more marked when the food is coarse or hastily eaten.

The symptoms of early esophageal carcinoma should be distinguished from those of chronic pharyngitis and esophagitis, which are also common in high-incidence areas of esophageal carcinoma. Patients with chronic pharyngitis or esophagitis usually complain of an obstructive or foreign-body sensation or of a boring, distending discomfort in the hypopharynx and the upper retrosternal region. These symptoms occur while the patient is not eating or when he merely performs the act of swallowing, but are absent on actual ingestion of food, in sharp contrast to the symptoms of early esophageal carcinoma, which appear only on swallowing food. Final differentiation, however, depends on cytologic and/or endoscopic examination.

It is apparent that public education to increase the level of awareness of both medical workers and the general population of the symptoms of early esophageal carcinoma is of importance in the early recognition of this malignancy.

Identification of high-risk subjects

Since the etiologic factors of carcinoma of the esophagus are not yet fully understood, it is difficult to clearly define high-risk persons for this malignancy. Certain preexisting diseases of the esophagus, such as long-standing caustic stricture, achalasia, peptic or fungal esophagitis, and Barrett's esophagus, are known to predispose to esophageal cancer. Esophageal diverticulosis, in my experience, is not a predisposing factor to cancerous development, although carcinoma may occur at the site of a diverticulum. Chronic nutritional deficiencies, consumption of certain moldy foods and pickled vegetables, and excessive exposure to tobacco and alcohol have all been documented to increase the risk of esophageal carcinoma.[12]

Severe dysplastic change of the esophageal epithelium, irrespective of its causes, however, is considered the major precancerous change of the esophagus. In high-incidence areas of esophageal carcinoma in China, there is a close correlation between the incidence of esophageal carcinoma and that of esophageal dysplasia. In a mass screening by balloon cytology of 17,388 subjects between 40 and 65 years of age carried out in Linxian county in 1984, normal cytology was found in 32.2%, mild dysplasia in 37.3%, marked

dysplasia in 26.4%, near-carcinoma in 1.9%, and carcinoma in 2.3%. Follow-up cytologic studies in this county in another series of over 500 subjects with severe dysplasia for 5 to 8 years revealed that about 40% displayed a regression to mild dysplasia or normal epithelium, about 20% showed persistence of severe dysplasia, another 20% fluctuated between severe and mild dysplasia, and the remaining 15% to 20% progressed to carcinoma. In a group of 11,011 individuals with normal epithelium, only 13 (0.12%) developed cancer during the same period.[13] Shu and associates,[14] in a follow-up study of 530 cases with marked dysplasia and another 530 cases with mild dysplasia, each group for 1 to 12 years, found 79 cases (14.9%) of carcinoma in the first group and only 5 (0.9%) in the second group. In their control study of 477 cases with normal cytology followed for 1 to 5 years, however, no carcinoma was found.

It may be seen from the foregoing that severe dysplasia of the esophageal epithelium is an unstable intermediate state that on one hand may regress to normal epithelium but on the other may progress into carcinoma in a high percentage of cases. Thus, persons with severe dysplasia of the esophagus are considered at high risk of developing esophageal carcinoma, and should be followed regularly at least once yearly by balloon cytology or fiberesophagoscopy.

Diagnosis of early esophageal carcinoma

The combined use of balloon cytology, roentgenography, and fiberesophagoscopy is very important in the diagnosis of early esophageal carcinoma. Balloon cytology is used in patients thought to have carcinoma of the esophagus, either with or without symptoms. When balloon cytology is positive for carcinoma of usual cell types and x-ray film shows definite filling defects of the esophagus, the diagnosis of esophageal carcinoma is established and treatment may be resorted to without delay. In early esophageal carcinoma, roentgenography may show no abnormality or only very slight wall stiffness or very fine mucosal abnormalities, such as thickening, irregularity, tortuosity, convergence or interruption of mucosal folds, fine superficial filling defects, or minute ulcerations.[7,8] In patients with symptoms in whom double-contrast barium swallow examination fails to show definite abnormality, balloon cytology is indicated and is usually followed by fiberesophagoscopy. The latter may be aided by intraluminal staining with toluidine blue or Lugol's solution in cases in which the lesion is faint or barely perceptible. Endoscopic findings of early esophageal carcinoma consist of congestion or superficial maceration of the mucosa, patches of mucosal thickening, minute plaque-like elevations, or granular appearance of the mucous membrane. Wang and associates[10] reported, in a group of 62 early esophageal carcinoma patients with positive cytology, a positive staining of the lesion by toluidine blue in 57, or 91.9%, of the cases, and biopsy of the stained mucosa was positive for carcinoma in 52, or 83.9%, of the cases. Both false-positive and false-negative results were seen, however, in a small number of cases.

A negative esophagoscopic and/or roentgenographic finding does not rule out early esophageal carcinoma unless repeated balloon cytology is also negative.

Xu and associates[15] collected 220 cases of esophageal carcinoma of all stages in which preoperative examinations by balloon cytology, roentgenography, fiberesophagoscopy, and endoscopic biopsy had all been done, and found a diagnostic accuracy of 87.3% by balloon cytology, which was comparable to that of roentgenography (90.5%), fiberesophagoscopy (94.5%), and endoscopic biopsy (92.3%). In the 24 patients of this series with stage I disease, however, the accuracy of balloon cytology was 95.8%, which was superior to that of roentgenography (62.5%), fiberesophagoscopy (83.3%), and endoscopic biopsy (87.5%). Huang[16] reported that in a group of 80 patients with stage I esophageal carcinoma first detected by balloon cytology, the positive diagnostic rate by roentgenography was only about 50%, and by fiberesophagoscopy, 75%.

It can be seen therefore that balloon cytology is a sensitive diagnostic method in the detection of early esophageal carcinoma, and is clinically as important as roentgenography and fiberesophagoscopy. It should be understood, however, that balloon cytology cannot indicate the location and extent of the lesion, which must be determined by careful roentgenography and fiberesophagoscopy.

TREATMENT

Carcinoma in situ or intramucosal carcinoma of the esophagus is clinically latent and may remain so for a long time. But eventually the growth will break through the basal layer of the epithelium and become a submucosal or early infiltrative carcinoma, which then develops with increasing rapidity. Clinically it is extremely difficult to tell when a carcinoma in situ becomes infiltrative, and to rule out infiltrative carcinoma when biopsy

shows carcinoma in situ. In a group of 23 untreated patients with early esophageal carcinoma diagnosed by cytologic examination, as reported by Pei and associates,[17] the average survival period was 43.6 months (range, 20 to 78 months) from the time of cytologic diagnosis.

It is our opinion that for early carcinoma of the esophagus, surgery remains the treatment of choice. This is especially true when one takes into consideration the fact that more than one third of early esophageal carcinoma is carcinoma in situ that is not only radiotherapy resistant but perhaps also chemotherapy resistant.

In our series of 253 patients with early (stage I) esophageal carcinoma treated surgically,[18] the 5-year survival was 89.9% and the 10-year survival 60.0%.

There was a resectability rate of 100% and a 30-day operative mortality of 2.4% (6 of 253). Pathology showed carcinoma in situ in 99 cases (39.1%) and early infiltrative (submucosal) carcinoma in 154 cases (60.9%).

In the majority of patients with early esophageal carcinoma the surgeons could not feel any abnormality of the esophagus during operation, and the location and extent of the lesion or lesions had to be determined by meticulous preoperative endoscopic examination, sometimes with the aid of intraluminal staining. In about one third of the cases, however, the lesion could be felt through the muscular coat of the esophagus as localized thickening of the mucosa with poorly defined margins. In doubtful cases, careful direct observation of the mucosa through an esophagotomy as advocated by Akiyama et al.,[19] plus intraluminal staining with either toluidine blue or Lugol's solution, is advisable to obtain a cancer-free margin of resection and to avoid incomplete eradication of multicentric cancerous lesions. As soon as the portion of the esophagus is resected, it should be examined immediately by the pathologist to verify the extent of the lesion and completeness of resection.

CONCLUSION

The fact that early esophageal carcinoma is seen only infrequently in medical centers may be attributable to (1) absence of marked symptoms, (2) lack of awareness of the disease on the part of patients as well as medical workers, (3) difficulty in identifying high-risk subjects, and (4) lack of a simple and efficient diagnostic tool. Abrasive cytology by means of a balloon catheter (balloon cytology) has been widely used in China in high-incidence areas of esophageal carcinoma as a means of mass screening for the detection of this disease, with the discovery of a large number of early cases, and for the detection and follow-up study of esophageal dysplasia, which is also prevalent in these areas and known to develop into carcinoma in a high percentage of cases. Balloon cytology is of merit in identifying esophageal dysplasia in high-risk persons for whom periodic follow-up examinations can lead to the discovery of carcinoma at its very early stage. Balloon cytology is now an indispensable method for the detection of early esophageal carcinoma, and has proved to be a simple, efficient, and useful diagnostic tool that is as important as barium roentgenography, fiberesophagoscopy, and endoscopic biopsy.

REFERENCES

1. Li, J.Y.: Epidemiology of esophageal cancer in China, Natl. Cancer Inst. Monogr. **62:**113, 1982.
2. Yan, C.S.: Research on esophageal cancer in China: a review, Cancer Res. **40:**2633, 1980.
3. Huang, G.J., Wang, L.J., Liu, J.S., et al.: Surgery of esophageal carcinoma, Semin. Surg. Oncol. **1:**74, 1985.
4. Endo, M., Yamada, A., Ide, H., et al.: Early cancer of the esophagus: diagnosis and clinical evaluation, Int. Adv. Surg. Oncol. **3:**49, 1980.
5. Nabeya, K., and Arai, Y.: Early carcinoma of the esophagus: definition and review of 177 cases collected in Japan, J. Jpn. Bronchoesophagol. Soc. **32:**393, 1981.
6. Suzuki, H., Kobayashi, S., Endo, M., and Nakayari, K.: Diagnosis of early esophageal cancer, Surgery **71:**99, 1972.
7. Wang, Z.Y.: Radiological appearances in early esophageal carcinoma, J. Soc. Med. **73:**849, 1980.
8. Shirakabe, H.: Early detection of carcinoma of the esophagus: the UICC Fukuoka Symposium on Fundamentals and Clinical Aspects of Digestive Tract Tumors, Fukuoka, Japan, 1984, Tsukushi Kaikan, p. 45.
9. Goldstein, H.M., and Dodd, G.D.: Double-contrast examination of the esophagus, Gastrointest. Radiol. **1:**3, 1976.
10. Wang, G.Q., Chang, F.B., Tian, Z.J., and Tang, J.: Clinical application of intraluminal toluidine blue staining in the diagnosis of early esophageal carcinoma, Chin. Med. J. **60:**93, 1980.
11. Huang, G.J., Shao, L.F., Zhang, D.W., et al.: Diagnosis and surgical treatment of early esophageal carcinoma, Chin. Med. J. **94:**229, 1981.
12. Li, M.X., and Cheng, S.J.: Etiology of carcinoma of the esophagus. In Huang, G.J., and Wu, Y.K., editors: Carcinoma of the esophagus and gastric cardia, Berlin, 1984, Springer-Verlag, pp. 25-51.
13. The Coordinating Group for the Research of Esophageal Carcinoma, Henan Province, and the Chinese Academy of Medical Sciences: Studies on relationship between epithelial dysplasia and carcinoma of the esophagus, Chin. Med. J. **1:**110, 1975.
14. Shu, Y.J., Yang, X.Q., and Jin, S.P.: Further investigation of the relationship between dysplasia and cancer of the esophagus, Chin. Med. J. **60:**39, 1980.
15. Xu, D.Y., Zhang, D.Y., Li, D., and Niu, W.H.: A comparison of diagnostic rates in 220 cases of esophageal carcinoma by balloon cytology, roentgenography, fiberesophagoscopy, and endoscopic biopsy, Cancer Res. Prev. Treat. **12:**162, 1985.
16. Huang, G.J.: Early detection and surgical treatment of esophageal carcinoma, Jpn. J. Surg. **11:**399, 1981.
17. Pei, Y.H., Zhang, Y.D., Hou, J., et al.: Natural evolution and follow-up study of early esophageal carcinoma in 23 cases, Cancer Res. Prev. Treat. **9:**75, 1982.
18. Shao, L.F., Huang, G.J., Zhang, D.W., et al.: Detection and surgical treatment of early esophageal carcinoma. In Proceedings of the Beijing Symposium on Cardiothoracic Surgery, Beijing, 1981, China Academic Publishing and John Wiley & Sons, Inc., pp. 168-171.
19. Akiyama, H., Kogure, T., and Itai, Y.: Role of esophagotomy in the surgical treatment of esophageal cancer, Int. Surg. **59:**478, 1974.

Recognition and treatment of the early lesion

DISCUSSION

Kenneth Charles McKeown

Environmental factors appear to play an important part in the incidence of carcinoma of the esophagus. Epidemiologic studies show that the condition is common in certain countries and in particular regions of the same country. Marked changes occur in the incidences over short distances and even between one district and another. The ethnic origin of patients is also important, as exemplified by the high incidence of carcinoma in the Bantu tribesmen in the Transkei district of South Africa (70 per 100,000) as compared with the much lower incidence in the white population. Regions of very high incidence are in the Linxian county in the Henan province in northern China, where 141 per 100,000 of the population dies of the disease and in northeast Iran, in the region south of the Caspian Sea, where the Gonbad district has a peak incidence of 174 cases per 100,000 of the population.[1]

Because the presenting symptom of dysphagia does not occur until the growth has encircled 75% of the lumen, most patients present at a late stage of the disease. In only 3 percent of cases is the disease confined to the mucosa or the submucosa (stage I) when the patient is submitted to surgical excision. This clinical fact calls for measures to obtain an earlier diagnosis, and these measures include the institution of screening programs, education of the population, and an awareness on the part of the medical attendant.

In countries of high incidence, *population* screening programs have been introduced, as in northern China. In Western countries the disease is much less common, and population screening programs are not appropriate, but it has been recognized that certain clinical conditions such as reflux esophagitis or achalasia often precede the onset of carcinoma,[2] and there is therefore a case to be made for screening *individuals* who because of previous esophageal disease are at high risk.[2]

In screening programs there are three options — routine double-contrast radiology, fiberoptic endoscopy, and esophageal cytology. Double-contrast radiology will demonstrate an established lesion in 62.5% of cases, though in cases of carcinoma occurring in association with achalasia, the lesion, often situated well above the narrowed segment, might well be overlooked in the distended and atonic esophagus. In cases of achalasia the presentation and detection of the disease are often late and the outlook is therefore bad.[3] Fiberoptic endoscopy, often assisted by intraluminal staining with toluidine blue or Lugol's iodine, can detect early malignancies in areas of esophageal dysplasia and has the advantage of making it possible for an immediate biopsy to be obtained. Esophageal cytology, by the use of either the brush or the balloon, provides a high degree of accuracy, in 95.8% of cases as outlined by Huang. The combination of balloon cytology and fiberoptic endoscopy provides a sound basis for early diagnosis and indeed for the detection of dysplasia and premalignant lesions. There is an interesting parallel between these procedures for the early detection of esophageal cancer and cervical cytology and colposcopy in the detection of cancerous or precancerous lesions in the cervix uteri.

At operation the small early lesion is much easier to cope with than the extensive lesion, often adherent to vital structures, which is the usual experience in countries where screening programs are not in existence. The mortality of 2.4% quoted by Huang is far lower than that recorded by experienced surgeons in the West, where, even in the most expert hands, the mortality may be between 10% and 20%.[4] In the less experienced hands of the occasional esophageal surgeon, the mortality is nearer 50%.

In studies of the survival times after operation in Western series, there is a marked tendency to early recurrence, and only 60% of patients survive the first year. If the patient survives the second year, the survival curve flattens out and prospects improve.[4] Review of reports mainly from Western series shows that the 5-year survival rate is about 12%.[5] The figures of a 5-year survival of 89.9% and a 10-year survival of 60.0% are quite exceptional and perhaps emphasize that the very early diagnosis is allowing radical and curative surgery to be performed.

REFERENCES

1. Gillis, C.R., and Hole, D.J.: International geographical and local difference in carcinoma of the oesophagus. In Silber, W.P.P., editors: Carcinoma of the oesophagus, Rotterdam, 1978, Balkema, pp. 60-82.

2. Hennessey, T.P.J.: Tumours of the oesophagus. In Hennessey, T.P.J., and Cuschieri, A., editors: Surgery of the oesophagus, London, 1986, Bailliere Tindall.

3. McKeown, K.C.: Clinical features of carcinoma of the oesophagus, J. R. Coll. Surg. Edinb. (In press.)

4. McKeown, K.C.: The surgical treatment of carcinoma of the oesophagus (a review of 478 cases), J. R. Coll. Surg. Edinb. **30:**1, 1985.

5. Earlam, R., and Cunha-Melo, J.R.: Oesophageal squamous cell carcinoma. I. A critical review of surgery, Br. J. Surg. **67:**381, 1980.

CHAPTER 20 Surgical management of adenocarcinoma at the gastroesophageal junction

Da Wei Zhang

From 1958 to 1985, a total of 973 patients with carcinoma of the gastric cardia were admitted to the Cancer Hospital of the Chinese Academy of Medical Sciences for surgical treatment. Of the series, 729 patients had their tumors resected, for an overall resectability rate of 74.9%. This clinical experience will serve as the basis for the discussion of this chapter.

Two points are to be clarified before I proceed to various facets of the surgical treatment of carcinoma of the gastric cardia. First is the extent of the cardiac region. Anatomically, the gastric cardia encompasses the area where tubular and branched tubular cardiac glands exist. The extension of these glands covers a range of 0.5 to 4 cm, usually about 2 cm from the gastroesophageal junction. Inferentially, we at the Chinese Academy of Medical Sciences designate carcinoma of the gastric cardia as adenocarcinoma arising at this area and/or involving the gastroesophageal junction. Any squamous carcinoma involving this junction is designated as esophageal carcinoma in order to avoid confusion.[1] Carcinoma of the gastric cardia, unlike that arising from other parts of the stomach, presents unique clinical manifestations, requires special surgical care, and bears a much poorer prognosis. Therefore it is justified to consider carcinoma of the gastric cardia as an independent entity.

SYMPTOMS, SIGNS AND DIFFERENTIAL DIAGNOSIS

Because of the funnel-shaped geometry of the gastric cardia, blockage of food passage by tumor growth at this region does not occur as early as in the esophageal lumen. Dysphagia, if present, appears later in the clinical course compared with carcinoma of the esophagus, and signifies an advanced stage.

Early symptoms include substernal discomfort, intermittent epigastric aching, some postprandial distention, and dyspepsia. These symptoms are rarely severe enough to alert the patient to seek medical advice.

Upper gastrointestinal hemorrhage, manifested as hematemesis or melena, occurs in about 5% of patients with carcinoma of the gastric cardia.[2] Not infrequently, massive bleeding with shock may be the initial symptom. There may be no complaint of dysphagia, and the attending physician may fail to make the correct diagnosis. More than half of these patients were operated upon by laparotomy under the diagnosis of a bleeding ulcer but were eventually found to have carcinoma of the gastric cardia. Therapeutic results among this small subgroup were poor, largely because of rather high operative morbidity and mortality.

In early carcinoma of the gastric cardia, only minimal changes may be seen roentgenologically. Among these are minute mucosal deformities, a tiny niche, and a nonprominent but fixed filling defect.[3] Fiberoptic endoscopy, along with brush cytology and biopsy, is a must in establishing a final diagnosis in these cases. Radiologic manifestations in more advanced cases can be easily recognized. Destruction of mucosa, soft-tissue mass, filling defect and niche, tortuous and asymmetric narrowing of the cardiac channel, infiltration of the distal esophagus, the fundus, or the lesser curvature, and moderate degree of dilatation of the distal esophagus are common findings presenting in variable combinations.[3]

In my institute 973 cases of carcinoma of the cardia were subjected to operative treatment from 1958 to 1985. During the same period 10 patients

TABLE 20-1. Collective data of results of surgical treatment of carcinoma of the gastric cardia in China

Authors	No. of cases explored	No. of cases resected	Resectability (%)	Mortality (%)
Zhang, Y.D., et al.[7] (1982)	1742	1251	71.8	2.4
Shao, L.F., et al.[8] (1982)	963	791	82.1	3.4
Author's series (1986)	973	729	74.9	1.5

were diagnosed as having carcinoma of the cardia preoperatively, yet were found to have no tumor on exploration. Achalasia, peptic esophagitis, benign stricture, and peptic ulcer of the gastric cardia were among the final diagnoses. Some authors have stressed the importance of the presence of mucosal destruction and soft-tissue mass in establishing a diagnosis of carcinoma of the cardia.[4,5] Whenever x-ray findings are inconclusive, positive balloon cytology and endoscopic biopsy results must be obtained before any operative intervention is attempted.

Rarely an invasive gastric carcinoma mimicking idiopathic achalasia radiologically, endoscopically, and manometrically may be seen.[6] The presence of anemia, positive stool guaiac test, and subtle changes in the fundus may help establish a correct diagnosis.

INDICATIONS FOR SURGICAL TREATMENT IN PATIENTS WITH CARCINOMA OF THE GASTRIC CARDIA

The acknowledged mode of treatment for carcinoma of the gastric cardia is surgery. Radiotherapy or chemotherapy share poor response rates. I suggest the following circumstances as indications for surgery. First, the diagnosis should be confirmed by positive roentgenologic, cytologic, and endoscopic findings. Remote metastases to lymph nodes, liver, adrenal glands, omentum, and peritoneum should be ruled out by ultrasonography, CT scanning, and/or peritoneoscopy. The ideal candidate should have a fair to good cardiopulmonary reserve and no serious ailment in other vital organs.

SURGICAL APPROACHES

Left posterolateral thoracotomy through the bed of the seventh rib or the seventh intercostal space has been the route of entry most frequently adopted in our institute. The abdomen would then be opened through a radially placed incision over the dome of the left hemidiaphragm. This approach provides excellent exposure of the gastroesophageal junction. The incision can be easily extended into a thoracoabdominal incision by dividing the left costal arch in case total gastrectomy or colonic or jejunal interposition is necessary.

In patients with poor cardiopulmonary reserve partial gastrectomy and inversion extraction esophagectomy without thoracotomy may be indicated. The greater curvature of the stomach is tailored into a slender tube long enough to reach the lower neck to anastomose with the cervical esophagus. However, there is a risk of not obtaining a tumor-free cut margin on the stomach side because of the intended preservation of enough stomach tissue along the greater curvature. Another approach that is an option for patients with low cardiopulmonary function is a combined sternum-splitting and abdominal incision, which allows a posterior mediastinal esophagogastrostomy without entering the pleural cavity. Its disadvantage is the limited exposure of the posterior esophageal bed. In this particular technique the use of stapled esophagogastrostomy or esophagojejunostomy is recommended.

SURGICAL RESULTS

Table 20-1 compares the surgical results recently reported in China with those of my series. The data show rather high resectability rates of 71.8% to 82.1% and reasonable resection mortality of 1.5% to 3.4%.

One point worthy to be mentioned is the frequent practice of proximal partial gastrectomy, sparing resection of the spleen or part of the pancreas, in these series.

The overall 5-year survival rates for the three groups listed in Table 20-1 were 15.4%, 24.5%, and 19.1%, respectively.

Among various factors influencing the postresection long-term results, lymph node metastasis, carcinomatous invasion to the gastric serosa, and the nature of resection are three determinants of proven significance. Table 20-2 shows the 5-year

TABLE 20-2. Collective data of 5-year survival rates as influenced by the three major determinants (percent)

Authors	Lymph node metastasis		Invasion to gastric serosa		Nature of resection	
	−	+	−	+	Radical	Palliative
Zhang, Y.D., et al.[7]	26.8	8.3	21.0	14.1	19.8	8.1
Shao, L.F., et al.[8]	35.0	17.9	—	—	33.3	14.4
Author's series	40.0	12.4	22.1	11.5	23.3	9.9
	($p < 0.0001$)		($p < 0.01$)		($p < 0.001$)	

survival rates related to these determinants in the same series listed in Table 20-1.

Obviously there is little that can be done by surgeons to reverse the first two determinants during operation. For decades there has been interest in early detection and early treatment of carcinoma of the gastric cardia. Yet the majority of patients present at advanced stages of the disease. In the present series, 75.1% of patients had lymph node metastases at operation. To improve the results of surgery, the only effort a surgeon can make is to attain completeness of tumor resection by dissecting all the involved lymph nodes and ensuring tumor-free edges of both esophageal and gastric margins.

PROXIMAL SUBTOTAL GASTRECTOMY OR EXTENDED RESECTION

Whether to perform proximal subtotal gastrectomy or extended resection is a problem of much debate in surgical treatment of carcinoma of the gastric cardia. Some surgeons claim en-bloc resections of the diseased stomach, spleen, tail of the pancreas, omentum, and regional lymph nodes improve survival.[9,10] Others compare long-term results after partial gastrectomy and total gastrectomy, finding no difference between these two groups. These surgeons propose that total gastrectomy is indicated only when cancer involves the body of the stomach.[11] Sugimachi et al.[12] reported that prophylactic splenectomy in total gastrectomy for stomach cancer has no beneficial effect on long-term survival in cases having metastatic lymph nodes in the hilum of the spleen. In cases without node metastasis, the survival rate was higher in the nonsplenectomy group. A higher incidence of postoperative infections and a shorter period of survival in patients who died of recurrence were also noted among the splenectomized patients. Some authors note that no difference had been found in oper-

TABLE 20-3. Mean survival in 230 cases of nonresectable cardiac cancer

Type of surgery	No. of patients	Mean survival (mo)
Exploration only	140	5.5
Esophagogastric bypass	85	6.4
Gastrostomy or jejunostomy	5	3.7

ative mortality between subtotal gastrectomy and extended resections. Likewise, there was no difference in the long-term survival rates between the two groups.[13]

In our institute either total gastrectomy or extended resection has been performed in only a limited number of patients, 14 cases and 23 cases, respectively. The mean survivals were 8.4 months and 19.7 months, respectively. Among total gastrectomy patients, only one lived longer than 12 months. In the group with extended resection, there were two postoperative deaths and two long-term survivors. One lived 6 years and the other 8 years after operation. For a lesion extending distally no farther than one third the length of the lesser curvature, proximal partial gastrectomy is the operation of choice. The preservation of a distal gastric pouch provides better digestive function and spares patients the late complications of total gastrectomy.[11]

PALLIATIVE TREATMENT FOR NONRESECTABLE CASES

Table 20-3 illustrates the mean survival for various palliative operations in patients whose tumors had been found nonresectable at operation and who had severe dysphagia. In all, there were 244 nonresectable cases in my series, with follow-up data in 230. Neither gastrostomy nor bypass operation increased the life span of these patients. However, esophagogastric bypass did alleviate dysphagia and make the patients happy to resume

TABLE 20-4. Resectability and 5-year survival rates of the group treated by combined regimen versus the control (surgery alone) group

Therapeutic modalities	Resectability %	5-year survival %
Irradiation + surgery (n = 145)	84.8	25.0 (19/76)
Surgery alone (n = 828)	73.2	18.2 (87/478)
	p = 0.27	p = 0.25

a nearly normal diet. Gastrostomy or jejunostomy should be reserved only for those who are severely dysphagic and in whom situations are unsuitable for bypass operations.

SURGICAL TREATMENT FOR RECURRENT DYSPHAGIA

Benign cicatricial stenosis and recurrence of carcinoma at the anastomotic site are the two possible causes for recurrent dysphagia. Endoscopy is performed first in an attempt to ascertain the etiology. For benign anastomotic stenosis, dilatation is attempted. If this fails and if the general condition of the patient allows a second thoracotomy, and there is no sign of remote metastasis, the patient may be reoperated upon. The narrowed anastomosis is exposed through an incision on the wall of the intrathoracic stomach pouch. The scar tissue is trimmed away and the anastomotic opening enlarged.

When local recurrence occurs without evidence of distant metastasis, resection of the anastomosis and reconstruction of the alimentary tract are attempted. In my series, three patients had been operated upon in this way, and all recovered with satisfactory function of swallowing. In these cases the intervals between the two thoracotomies were 9, 15, and 25 months. The recurrent tumors were all localized, with sizes ranging from 3 to 5 cm in diameter. Resection of the anastomosis and a new esophagogastrostomy were performed without real difficulty. One of the three patients died of tumor metastasis 2 years after the second thoracotomy. The other two were living and well at the sixth and twentieth months after the second operation.

COMBINED PREOPERATIVE RADIOTHERAPY AND SURGERY IN THE TREATMENT OF CARCINOMA OF THE GASTRIC CARDIA

The rationale for preoperative irradiation is threefold: to devitalize the cancer cells so as to reduce the risk of dissemination during surgical intervention; to sterilize the microscopic deposits of tumor cells inaccessible to surgery so as to reduce the chance of local recurrence; and to eliminate carcinomatous infiltrations into the adjacent structures, thus facilitating resection. Clinical trial has confirmed that in the treatment of squamous esophageal carcinoma a combined regimen improves resectability and long-term survival.[14]

Starting in the late 1970s, a similar regimen has been tested among patients with adenocarcinoma of the gastric cardia. Table 20-4 demonstrates the preliminary results.

We must confess that combined preoperative irradiation and surgery does not show any superiority in the treatment results for cancer of the gastric cardia in the present series, being quite different from the results reported by Wilson et al.[15]

CARCINOMA OF THE GASTRIC CARDIA AFTER DISTAL PARTIAL GASTRECTOMY

More and more case reports have appeared in the literature dealing with the occurrence of gastric cancer in the gastric stump after distal partial gastrectomy. An incidence of 2.2% in a series of 2273 cases has been reported.[16] The diagnostic criteria for a postgastrectomy stomach pouch carcinoma are (1) partial distal gastrectomy performed for noncancerous diseases and (2) time interval between the gastrectomy and the onset of the carcinoma no less than 5 years. Among the newly developed tumors 15.6% to 35.7% were located at the gastric cardia.[17-19] Some authors have confirmed a statistically increased incidence in gastric stump carcinoma 12 years or more after gastrectomy, but failed to confirm that gastric ulcer and Billroth II anastomosis may lead to a higher prevalence of stump carcinoma.[20] After resection of the distal stomach, the loss of acid production, regurgitation of alkaline jejunal content into the gastric stump, and the development of atrophic gastritis and intestinal metaplasia are all possible predisposing factors.[17,18,21] In the author's institute five patients conforming to the above-mentioned diagnostic criteria were treated surgically. Completion total gastrectomy was carried out in three cases, with subsequent end-to-side or Roux-en-Y esophagojejunostomy. In two patients we managed to preserve a cuff of normal stomach attached to the original gastroenterostomy by partially removing the proximal stomach. A medium-sized artery, named the posterior gastric artery by some authors,[19,22] was found nourishing this remaining portion of the stomach in these two cases.[19,22]

REFERENCES

1. Li, L., and Pan, G.L.: Pathology of carcinoma of the gastric cardia. In Huang, G.J., and Wu, Y.K., editors: Carcinoma of the esophagus and gastric cardia, 1984, pp. 118-119.
2. Sun, C.F., et al: Diagnosis and management of massive bleeding from cancer of the gastric cardia, Chin. J. Surg. **20**:165, 1982. (In Chinese.)
3. Wang, Z.Y., and Su, J.H.: Radiologic diagnosis. In Huang, G.J., and Wu, Y.K., editors: Carcinoma of the esophagus and gastric cardia, 1984, pp. 207-210.
4. Wang, G.Q., and Huang, G.J.: Analysis of 7 cases falsely diagnosed as carcinoma of cardia of the stomach, Cancer Res. Prev. Treat. **2**:54, 1975. (In Chinese.)
5. Du, S.Q., et al.: Cases misdiagnosed as esophageal or gastric cardiac cancer: an analysis of 37 cases, Chin. J. Oncol. **4**(1):48, 1982. (In Chinese.)
6. McCallum, R.W.: Esophageal achalasia secondary to gastric carcinoma, Am. J. Gastroenterol. **71**:24, 1979.
7. Zhang, Y.D., et al.: Surgical treatment of 4310 cases of carcinoma of the esophagus and gastric cardia, Chin. J. Oncol. **4**:1, 1982. (In Chinese.)
8. Shao, L.F., et al.: Results of surgery in 3155 cases of carcinoma of the esophagus and gastric cardia, Chin. J. Surg. **20**:19, 1982. (In Chinese.)
9. Skinner, D.B.: En bloc resection for neoplasms of the esophagus and cardia, J. Thorac. Cardiovasc. Surg. **85**:59, 1983.
10. Wada, T.: Appleby's operation for advanced carcinoma of the stomach, Jpn. J. Surg. **80**:1448, 1979.
11. Kaibara, N., et al.: Carcinoma of the upper portion of the stomach: proximal partial gastrectomy or total gastrectomy, Jpn. J. Cancer Clinic **30**(9):1052, 1984. (In Japanese.)
12. Sugimachi, K., et al.: Critical evaluation of prophylactic splenectomy in total gastrectomy for the stomach cancer, Jpn. J. Cancer Clinic **30**(9):1057, 1984. (In Japanese.)
13. Papachriston, D.N., et al.: Adenocarcinoma of the gastric cardia, Ann. Surg. **192**:58, 1980.
14. Huang, G.J., et al.: Combined preoperative irradiation and surgery in esophageal carcinoma, Chin. Med. J. **94**:73, 1981.
15. Wilson, S.E., et al.: Cancer of the distal esophagus and cardia: preoperative irradiation prolongs survival, Am. J. Surg. **150**:114, 1985.
16. National Cooperative Group for Carcinoma of the Stomach: Gastric stump carcinoma: etiological and diagnostic features in 51 cases, Chin. J. Oncol. **5**:305, 1983. (In Chinese.)
17. Takahashi, T., et al.: Studies on carcinoma of the remnant of stomach after distal gastrectomy, Jpn. J. Cancer Clinic **30**(14):1773, 1984. (In Japanese.)
18. Ohyama, T., et al.: Clinicopathological study on carcinoma of the gastric stump, Jpn. J. Cancer Clinic **30**(1):43, 1984. (In Japanese.)
19. Zhang, G.C., et al.: Proximal partial gastrectomy and esophagogastrostomy in postgastrectomy cardiac cancer patient, Chin. J. Surg. **19**(9):520, 1981. (In Chinese.)
20. Domellöf, L., and Janunger, K.G.: The risk of gastric carcinoma after partial gastrectomy, Am. J. Surg. **134**:581, 1977.
21. Feldman, F., et al.: Primary gastric stump cancer, Am. J. Roentgenol. **115**(2):257, 1972.
22. Suzuki, K., et al.: Incidence and surgical importance of the posterior gastric artery, Ann. Surg. **187**:134, 1978.

Surgical management of adenocarcinoma at the gastroesophageal junction

DISCUSSION

F. Henry Ellis, Jr.

The decreasing incidence of carcinoma of the stomach in the Western world has not included lesions that develop in the region of the gastroesophageal junction. As a result, patients with adenocarcinoma in this location constitute a sizable proportion of those who are candidates for resection. In my experience with esophagogastrectomy for cancer, more than one half of the operations have been for adenocarcinoma of the cardia.[1,2] I am in almost complete agreement with the views expressed by Zhang in his detailed and carefully analyzed review of a large group of patients with adenocarcinoma at the gastroesophageal junction who were treated at the Cancer Institute in Beijing. By way of comment, I will emphasize some of the important points in this chapter.

The high resectability rate and low hospital mortality reported by Zhang are commendable and surpass results obtained by most Western surgeons. He prefers a limited resection, with intrathoracic esophagogastrostomy when possible, avoiding more radical procedures involving a thoracoabdominal incision with splenectomy, partial pancreatectomy, and total gastrectomy unless these are required to remove macroscopic tumor. My associates and I have found that the more radical resective procedures only increase morbidity and mortality and have no favorable effect on longevity, and we too favor a limited resection through a left thoracotomy with intrathoracic esophagogastrostomy for most cancers involving the gastroesophageal junction. Some surgeons prefer the transhiatal approach without thoracotomy when resecting lesions in this location,[3] but I have limited the use of this technique mostly to early-stage lesions in the upper thoracic or cervical esophagus. Shahian and associates[4] found that morbidity and mortality were higher when this approach was used for lower thoracic esophageal lesions than when the transthoracic route was employed, although survivorship was not adversely affected.

Combined forms of therapy using preoperative irradiation or chemotherapy or both in addition to surgery in treating esophageal cancer are now under investigation in many centers.[5,6] However, the data reported from China do not support the use of preoperative irradiation for adenocarcinoma at the gastroesophageal junction. The advantages of this combined form of therapy favored by Wilson et al.[7] are not impressive, since the results at 2 years were no different statistically between patients receiving irradiation and surgery and those treated with surgery alone. Similarly, chemotherapy as adjunctive therapy for patients with carcinoma involving the gastroesophageal junction treated surgically was found by a group at the Memorial Sloan-Kettering Cancer Center to have no advantage over surgery alone.[8]

It has long been my view that any appreciable improvement in long-term survivorship for patients with carcinoma of the esophagus or cardia or both will require earlier diagnosis than is now possible. Although the results of protocols employing combined forms of therapy at a few major centers should be analyzed carefully, in my opinion they probably will demonstrate little impact on long-term survivorship, since more than one half of the patients most likely have metastatic disease at the time treatment is initiated. This view is supported by the fact that the stage of the lesion is the major determinant of long-term survival.[2] It is also consistent with Zhang's data because nodal involvement, which was present in 75% of his patients, had a major impact on 5-year survival. Survival after palliative management of technically nonresectable lesions was no different from that in untreated patients, although the quality of life in patients undergoing such procedures was better because of restoration of the swallowing mechanism.

It is of interest that plastic intubation of the obstructing carcinoma was not employed in Zhang's patients. Although such techniques are not without risk, they are particularly applicable to nonresectable lesions of the gastroesophageal junction and in my opinion warrant wider use by our Chinese colleagues.

Zhang has had relatively limited experience with reresection for anastomotic recurrences, and his optimistic view contrasts with my experience.[9] Of 18 patients with documented anastomotic recurrence after esophagogastrectomy at the Lahey Clinic, 12 had disseminated disease. Six patients without disseminated disease and one other whose original operation was done elsewhere underwent reexploration, but reresection was possible in only four of these patients. The average length of survival after reresection in the four patients was 12 months, somewhat less than that reported by Zhang, although admittedly the data on this point are sparse.

The Lahey Clinic experience with carcinoma of the esophagus and cardia is summarized later in this volume (Chapter 46). The overall operability rate between January, 1970, and January, 1986, was 80%. Of the 271 operations performed, 143 were done for adenocarcinoma of the cardia, of which 120 (83.9%) were resections. Only one of these patients died within 30 days after operation, for a hospital mortality of 0.9%. In contrast to other reports, we have found no statistically significant difference between survivorship of patients with squamous cancer of the esophagus and those with adenocarcinoma at the gastroesophageal junction. The 5-year actuarial survival of patients with carcinoma of the cardia was 15%, slightly less than that reported by Zhang, although probably not statistically so. Curative resections, however, were accompanied by a 5-year survival rate similar to that reported by Zhang, 18% as opposed to 0% for palliative resections.

REFERENCES

1. Ellis, F.H., Jr., Gibb, S.P., and Watkins, E., Jr.: Overview of the current management of carcinoma of the esophagus and cardia, Can. J. Surg. **28**:493, 1985.
2. Ellis, F.H., Jr., Gibb, S.P., and Watkins, E., Jr.: Esophagogastrectomy: a safe, widely applicable, and expeditious form of palliation for patients with carcinoma of the esophagus and cardia, Ann. Surg. **198**:531, 1983.
3. Goldfaden, D., Orringer, M.B., Appelman, H.D., and Kalish, R.: Adenocarcinoma of the distal esophagus and gastric cardia: comparison of results of transhiatal esophagectomy and thoracoabdominal esophagogastrectomy, J. Thorac. Cardiovasc. Surg. **91**:242, 1986.
4. Shahian, D.M., Neptune, W.B., Ellis, F.H., Jr., and Watkins, E., Jr.: Transthoracic versus extrathoracic esophagectomy: mortality, morbidity, and long-term survival, Ann. Thorac. Surg. **41**:237, 1986.
5. Steiger, Z., Franklin, R., Wilson, R.F., Leichman, L., Seydel, H., Loh, J.J.K., Vaishamapayan, G., Knechtges, T., Asfaw, I., Dindogru, A., Rosenberg, J.C., Buroker, T., Torres, A., Hoschner, D., Miller, P., Pietruk, T., and Vaitkevicius, V.: Eradication and palliation of squamous cell carcinoma of the esophagus with chemotherapy, radiotherapy, and surgical therapy, J. Thorac. Cardiovasc. Surg. **82**:713, 1981.
6. Bains, M.S., Kelsen, D.P., Beattie, E.J., Jr., and Martini, N.: Treatment of esophageal carcinoma by combined preoperative chemotherapy, Ann. Thorac. Surg. **34**:521, 1982.
7. Wilson, S.E., Hiatt, J.R., Stabile, B.E., and Williams, R.A.: Cancer of the distal esophagus and cardia: preoperative irradiation prolongs survival, Am. J. Surg. **150**:114, 1985.
8. Fein, R., Kelsen, D.P., Geller, N., Bains, M., McCormack, P., and Brennan, M.F.: Adenocarcinoma of the esophagus and gastroesophageal junction: prognostic factors and results of therapy, Cancer **56**:2512, 1985.
9. Ellis, F.H., Jr., and Gibb, S.P.: Anastomotic recurrence after esophagogastrectomy for cancer: is there a place for reresection? Probl. Gen. Surg. **2**:436, 1985.

Surgical management of adenocarcinoma at the gastroesophageal junction

DISCUSSION

Robert Giuli

My opinion on this subject is now established and is based on a series of consistent statistical observations.

OBSERVATION 1

The first, which was the subject of a publication in 1972,[1] presented the results of a statistical analysis in one hospital department of the treatment for 135 adenocarcinomas of the anatomic cardia. The procedures performed were divided into 82 *upper polar gastrectomies* and 53 *total gastrectomies*. In the latter group, there were 14 total gastrectomies done in principle for an anatomic lesion apparently limited to the cardia, and 39 total gastrectomies done of necessity, either because of the actual extension of the cancerous lesion (27 of 39) or for a macroscopic invasion of the satellite lymph node chains of the stomach (12 of 39).

Individual study of each resection specimen provides a few observations. The extension of the tumor to the stomach can occur irrespective of any nodal involvement, since the pathologic study of the 39 total gastrectomy specimens, done *of necessity,* led to the observation in six cases (15.3%) that there was no involvement *of the lymphatic chains that were examined.* In all other cases, there was a consistent invasion of the right gastric nodes and, in some cases, of the pyloric (three), splenic (seven), or hepatic (four) nodes. The actuarial survival of these patients was 10% at 5 years.

In comparison, study of the 14 other total gastrectomies led to the observation of uninvolvement of all nodes in three (21.4%) of the cases. For the other patients, the celiac nodes were neo-plastic. We observed in two instances invasion of the *splenic* and *pyloric* nodes in very limited tumors of the gastroesophageal junction.

Finally, we noted, in 82 patients having undergone an *upper polar* gastrectomy taking only the celiac nodes, a *total lymphatic uninvolvement,* apparently favorable for the prognosis, in 34 patients (41.4%).

It was surprising to find, in the comparative study of these two groups of patients, striking results: for 82 patients undergoing upper polar gastrectomy, despite apparently favorable lymphatic uninvolvement in 34 cases, the overall survival was only 17.4% at 3 years, falling to 0 at 4 years. On the other hand, the survival rate for systematic total gastrectomy, in the same period of time, was a stable of 40% at 5 years. According to classical methods of statistical testing, there was a *highly significant* difference between the two percentages of survival.

From that time on, when we had for the first time advocated total resection of the stomach, whenever the patient could tolerate it, we have continued to gather data confirming this opinion. A second evaluation, 3 years later, involved 162 upper polar gastrectomies, and despite negative celiac nodes in one third of the patients (54), revealed an actuarial survival of 0% at the fourth year.

OBSERVATION 2

Our second overall evaluation[2] was done within the framework of the Group OESO in 1979 (see Chapter 33). We collected, from 22 different European teams, 2400 cases of resected tumors of the esophagus, in which were included 530 tumors of the cardia. The 5-year survival rate of 530 patients undergoing operation[2] was 19% (24-14) or 26% (33-19).* Again, two types of operation (upper polar and total gastrectomy) were compared for long-term results. Their distribution according to tumor size indicated that almost three fourths of "small" tumors of the cardia were treated by partial resection, while, among 109 total gastrectomies, almost nine tenths were performed for "large" tumors—those with a diameter of at least 4 cm.

Despite this feature, the results obtained favored *total* excision, the overall survival of which *doubles* (36%; 50-22) that of upper polar gastrectomy (18%; 24-12). The upper limit of the interval of confidence for partial gastrectomies scarcely reached the lower limit of that for total gastrectomies.

Even if we did not take into account the spread that we had seen in the statistics of one single department,[1] with *nil* survival following upper polar excision at 4 years, the differences seen in the present OESO study would be statistically significant.

Following total excision, the number of fistulas (12%) was less than half of that following partial gastrectomy (24%). The long-term *recurrence rate* (6%) was one-third that noted after partial gastrectomy (17%).

The comparison of the two procedures in terms of lymphatic spread leads one to assert more strongly the justification for a total resection of the stomach. For patients who survived surgery, the 5-year survival after upper polar gastrectomy, in favorable cases with negative lymph nodes (70 patients), reached 36%. In comparison, total gastrectomy in patients with negative nodes produced a 5-year survival of 70%. This survival remained at 48% in cases even with lymphatic invasion (52 cases).

In the group of operations limited to the upper pole of the stomach—resections with *high esophageal anastomoses* (that is, above the aortic arch), there was a survival rate apparently higher than the rates mentioned previously (23%; 41-5). It was, again, half that of total gastrectomy in which a long segment of esophagus (more than 4 cm) had been resected (46%; 64-28).

---

*Intervals of confidence. The first percentage represents all patients undergoing operation and the second those surviving surgery.

OBSERVATION 3

We carried out an analysis of the circumstances of onset of recurrence or metastasis following esophageal resection. The possibility of tumor recurrence appeared to increase progressively from the upper third (41%) down to the lower third of the esophagus (49%), then to decrease significantly after resection of the cardia (39%). In the latter situation, the very high percentages of *esophageal* (73%), *mediastinal* (21%), or even *cervical* recurrences (7%) are especially striking. Such findings, corroborated by those made with regard to involvement of the level of esophageal transsection *more than 4 cm* from the tumor (19%), present justification for more extensive surgery for tumors of the cardia. To avoid late recurrences, the excision should be extended, not only to the whole of the stomach, but also to a *very high level in the thoracic esophagus*.

CONCLUSIONS

The different data from these statistical evaluations, and the personal impression that I have derived from past experience in the treatment of these tumors, justify, at this time, the most extended form of surgical resection.

My present policy is to propose total gastric resection and subtotal esophagectomy for these patients, with anastomosis of a colonic transplant in the neck, all in one stage. Present postoperative care permits safe operation via three incisions—abdominal, left thoracic, and cervical—without changing the position of the patient, but rather simply mobilizing the left arm, which is prepared using sterile technique and draped in the field at the beginning of the procedure.

In retrospect, the validity of the results obtained does not seem to legitimize undertaking, within the Group OESO, a prospective randomized trial on the surgical *technique* for tumors of the cardia. On the other hand, additional treatments, especially chemotherapy, will logically be our preoccupation.

REFERENCES

1. Giuli, R., Estenne, B., and Lortat-Jacob, J.L.: Bilan de 135 interventions pour cancer du cardia: valeur de la gastrectomie totale, Ann. Chir. **26**:15, 849, 1972.
2. Giuli, R., and Gignoux, M.: Treatment of carcinoma of the esophagus: retrospective study of 2400 patients, Ann. Surg. **192**:44, 1980.

CHAPTER 21 Squamous cell carcinoma of the esophagus

John Wong and King Fun Siu

Over half of all squamous cell carcinomas of the esophagus occur in the middle third, defined endoscopically to be situated between 24 and 32 cm from the incisor teeth or radiologically where the bulk of the tumor overlies the fifth to eighth thoracic vertebrae. The second commonest site is the lower third, and the least common is the upper third. In 1946 Ivor Lewis[1] and, 1 year later independently, Norman Tanner[2] described the abdominal and right-chest approach to resect esophageal cancers of the middle third; reconstruction was accomplished using the stomach, and the anastomosis was made high in the chest. This operation was first performed in Hong Kong in 1954 by G.B. Ong, who has since introduced new operations and rediscovered old ones to deal with esophageal cancers of diverse sites.[3-6]

PRINCIPLES OF TREATMENT

No single operation has the versatility to cope with cancers at all levels of the esophagus, and surgeons must possess a repertoire of procedures that could be employed for tumors at various locations and of different stages. While there may be personal preferences for a particular technique, this preference must be tempered with the reality of having to deal with tumors of the commonest site of the esophagus—that is, the middle third— as well as the advanced stage of disease seen in the majority of unselected patients.

That resection offers the best results in terms of palliation or cure is now widely acknowledged. However, to justify this surgical policy implies that an acceptably low mortality can be achieved even for advanced disease, since otherwise the benefits gained by those who survive the operation are negated by the many who succumb.

If resection is deemed unsuitable because of extensive locoregional or metastatic disease or poor general status, a bypass procedure is the next

choice because its palliative potential is superior to intubation, radiotherapy, or chemotherapy, individually or in combination.

Depending on how restrictive the selective criteria are for resection, the results of resection and consequently also of bypass vary. Thus when only fit patients with confined disease are chosen for resection, relatively few resections (with respect to the total population of afflicted patients) will be carried out and the results will predictably be good.[7] Since comparatively fit patients would then undergo a bypass operation, this group of patients would also do well. On the other hand, if resection were applied to patients with advanced disease, the overall results for resection would be poor and even worse for bypass.[8-10] Patients with very advanced disease are far less able to tolerate any form of treatment than their counterparts with earlier stages, but they are also the group with the worst symptoms and thus stand to gain most from a successful surgical outcome. In the face of this dilemma, the surgeon's mandate must be to palliate whenever possible even though the clinical burden is an unenviable one.

Surgical approaches for resection

The objectives of resection are to extirpate the primary tumor and its involved lymphatic drainage, to obtain adequate resection margins, both proximally and distally, and to remove any adjacent expendable soft tissue that has been infiltrated. Because of the risk of anastomotic recurrence following even apparently wide resection margins, the concept of "total esophagectomy" has been advanced, and as much as a 10-cm margin in both directions has been advocated.[11,12] In practice, however, the length of clear resection margins obtainable is determined by the location of the tumor, the sites of periesophageal lymphatic metastases, and the surgical approach employed. Although there is usually no major impediment to a long distal margin, the proximal margin is limited anatomically by the cricopharyngeus and, functionally, by swallowing difficulties if the whole esophagus is removed.

Most surgeons who subscribe to the total esophagectomy concept accept a subtotal resection (which includes the whole thoracic esophagus) and make the anastomosis at or above the level of the clavicle, whether this anastomosis is achieved in the thorax[13] or in the neck.[4,11] Only when the tumor is in the upper third of the esophagus would an anastomosis close to the cricopharyngeus be contemplated.[6]

For carcinoma of the upper third of the esophagus—that is, in the cervical and superior mediastinal segments—a transthoracic approach is not required. A cervical lesion can be resected through a cervical and abdominal approach; for a superior mediastinal segment lesion, an upper sternotomy and an abdominal approach would suffice.[6,14] In both these situations, the normal segment of the thoracic esophagus is mobilized by hand through the enlarged esophageal hiatus.

For carcinoma of the middle and lower thirds of the esophagus we prefer the two-phase abdominal and right-chest approach, in which the whole thoracic esophagus is removed (under vision), and make the anastomosis at the apex of the right pleural cavity.[13] Lesions in the abdominal esophagus can be dealt with either through the left chest, with or without a laparotomy, or by a transhiatal approach as for cervical lesions.[15]

Reconstruction

The three interdependent factors to be considered in reconstruction are (1) the organ of substitution, (2) the route of the placement of the substitute, and (3) the level of the anastomosis.

The stomach, when intact and free of disease, is the first choice for esophageal substitution. The advantages are that only one anastomosis is required and the intestinal tract is left intact. The disadvantages are that the stomach is a bulky organ and postoperative gastric stasis may occasionally develop whether or not a drainage procedure has been added. The second choice for substitution is the colon. The advantages are that it is easy to prepare and an adequate length is nearly always available. The disadvantages are that the vascular anatomy may be unsuitable for a specific part of the colon (in which case another segment could be chosen), three anastomoses are required, and bowel preparation may not be satisfactory.

The third choice is the jejunum. The advantages are that it is clean and for short segment replacements the vasculature is usually adequate. The disadvantages are that, for long loops, it is difficult to prepare, the marginal vascular arcades may be deficient, and there is a redundancy of the intestine in relation to the mesentery. In fat patients, it may be impossible to prepare a jejunal loop that reaches the neck. Because there are no compelling advantages, the jejunum remains the last option for replacement except when only the lower esophagus is removed.

If the subcutaneous or retrosternal route is selected, the anastomosis will inevitably be in the neck. When placed in the posterior mediastinum (orthotopic route) or close to it, the anastomosis could be in the chest or in the neck.

The original two-phase operation described by Lewis[1] and Tanner[2] (with an intrathoracic anastomosis) was extended by Ong and Kwong[4] and McKeown[11] to a three-phase operation in which a cervical phase for the anastomosis was added. The rationale was that a cervical anastomotic leakage is less hazardous than one in the chest and that a more complete esophagectomy can be carried out. The disadvantages are that a three-phase operation takes longer to perform, an additional length of substitute is required (even though the length of esophagus resected is not necessarily increased), and the cervical dissection is associated with a higher incidence of swallowing problems postoperatively.

Recent results of the two-phase operation would indicate that an equivalent length of the esophagus can be removed through the chest when the anastomosis is performed at the apex of the right pleural cavity (Fig. 21-1).[13,16] Furthermore, since the anastomotic leakage rate is very low using this approach, the two-phase operation would appear to possess the advantages of the three-phase operation and not incur any of its penalties.

Of the three available routes for the placement of the substitute, the orthotopic route is the shortest, followed by the retrosternal and the subcutaneous routes. There is an increase of approximately 2 cm from the orthotopic to the retrosternal route and then a further 2-cm increase to the subcutaneous routes—a difference of nearly 4 cm from the orthotopic to the subcutaneous route.[17] The advantage of using the orthotopic route is that dissection in another plane is not required and it is the shortest distance from the abdomen to the neck. However, the main disadvantage is that if residual disease remains in the mediastinum, the substitute can be invaded or compressed by subsequent growth of the tumor. The retrosternal route has the advantages that it is away from the tumor bed and that the avascular tunnel can be easily prepared. The two disadvantages are (1) that if there is a tear in the mediastinal

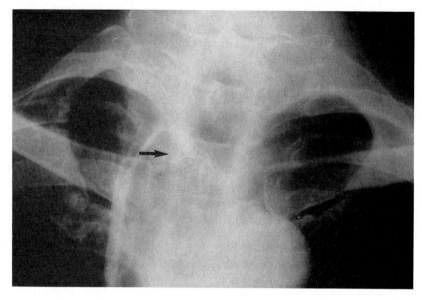

Fig. 21-1. Postoperative plain x-ray film of the neck showing the line of anastomotic staples *(arrow)* above the level of the clavicles.

pleura, the substitute may prolapse into the pleural cavity and pull on the anastomosis and, in the case of jejunum or colon, also undergo torsion and (2) that tumor recurrence in the thoracic inlet may compress the substitute in this confined space. The subcutaneous route offers the safest placement of the substitute, but it is also the longest and angulates over the xiphisternum and the clavicular heads. It is also cosmetically unattractive, but should an anastomotic leak occur or the loop become gangrenous, early detection is assured and management of these complications is somewhat easier.

Use of stomach

The abdominal and right-chest approach (Lewis-Tanner operation). To resect a tumor in the middle and lower thirds of the esophagus, this approach has broad appeal. It is by far our most frequently performed operation.

The abdomen is opened through an upper midline incision extending from the xiphisternum to just below and to the left of the umbilicus. A self-retaining "upper-hand" retractor facilitates the dissection around the esophageal hiatus. The stomach is examined for evidence of peptic ulcer disease, and the hiatal region is palpated for the presence of metastatic lymph nodes. If the stomach is suitable for substitution, mobilization is begun by separating the greater omentum from the gastroepiploic arcade. Detachment is commenced in the center and then extended to the right, as far as the front of the pancreas. Con-

genital adhesions from the transverse mesocolon to the posterior wall of the stomach and to the greater omentum are divided. Further mobilization is directed to the left side toward the splenic hilum. Particular care should be taken in dividing the upper short gastric vessels (which may be very short), to avoid damage to the spleen. From the upper posterior wall of the stomach, one or two veins issue directly from the stomach to the splenic vein, and these should be ligated. When the whole greater curve of the stomach has been freed, it is turned upward and the left gastric vessels are exposed and divided. If celiac lymph node metastases are present, they are dissected off the pancreas and left on the stomach to be resected later.

Kocher's maneuver is usually required. In addition to incising the peritoneum on the lateral side, the peritoneal attachment of the transverse mesocolon is separated from the front of the second part of the duodenum. Next, the lesser omentum is divided. This is commenced at the medial border of the portal structures, then along the hepatic and gastric arteries, and finally toward the cardia. The lesser curvature is thus released from tethering by the lesser omentum. The part of the lesser omentum between the undersurface of the liver and the esophagus is thick and often contains medium-sized vessels; these have to be ligated.

The stomach is now freed up to the hiatus, and the esophagus is separated from the muscular crura of the diaphragm on both sides and from the aorta posteriorly. The peritoneum in front of

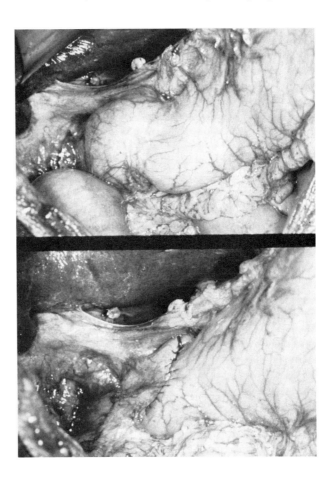

Fig. 21-2. Appearance of the pyloroduodenal area before *(above)* and after *(below)* a Heineke-Mikulicz pyloroplasty using two layers of continuous sutures.

the esophagus is divided, and the fibrous crus lying anteriorly is identified. Artery forceps are applied to this portion of the diaphragm, which is divided. The incision is extended for 4 to 5 cm and the pericardium exposed. Because this part of the diaphragm is traversed by phrenic vessels, the divided edges are transfixed.

By placement of long, narrow Deaver retractors into the enlarged hiatus, the distal esophagus can be dissected under vision up to the level of the inferior pulmonary veins. Bleeding points from the pleura or the aorta can be coagulated. If doubt exists with respect to the resectability of a middle-third tumor, a hand may be introduced into the right pleural cavity to evaluate the fixity of the tumor. Using only clinical assessment, barium swallow, endoscopy, and findings obtained at the abdominal phase of the operation, we have had only one occasion in over 150 thoracotomies on which we have not been able to proceed with a resection.

The site for the division of the gastroesophageal junction, the lower resection margin, is then examined. If celiac or left gastric lymph node metastases are present, the line of transection is 3 or 4 cm distal to the palpable edge of the lymph node. If the lymph nodes are not clinically involved, then a site nearer the gastroesophageal junction may be divided. Branches of the left gastric vessels crossing the line of transection are separately divided.

A Heineke-Mikulicz pyloroplasty is usually performed for this operation. In a patient whose stomach is judged to be short and in whom the subcutaneous or retrosternal route is selected, thus necessitating a cervical anastomosis, a pyloroplasty is omitted. In these circumstances the addition of a pyloroplasty may shorten the stomach and so place the upper anastomosis, as well as the pyloroplasty or pyloromyotomy, under tension. When a pyloroplasty is made, the pyloroduodenal junction is divided longitudinally for 2 cm on either side of the pylorus. Closure is by a continous suture using absorbable material, the first layer taking the redundant mucosa of the stomach and the mucosa and submucosa of the duodenum and, with the same suture, the returning second layer taking only the seromuscular layer on both sides (Fig. 21-2). The end of the knot is clipped with a metal clip to mark its po-

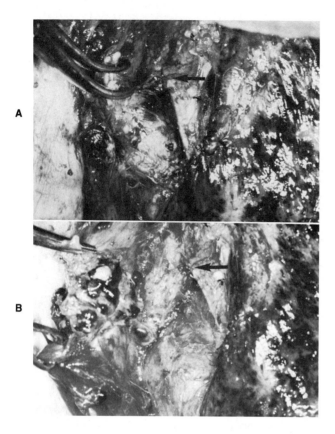

Fig. 21-3. A, The tumor and subcarinal metastatic lymph nodes being dissected from the trachea, carinal bifurcation *(arrow)*, main bronchi, and pericardium. B, After mobilization of the tumor and lymph nodes.

sition radiologically. The abdomen is then closed.

The patient is turned onto the left side, and a right fifth-space posterolateral thoracotomy is performed. The posterior end of the sixth rib is divided. It is useful to have one-lung anesthesia, but the operation can be carried out with both lungs inflated; in patients with poor cardiorespiratory reserve, one-lung anesthesia may be contraindicated. Since many of the patients have had tuberculosis or inflammatory pulmonary disease, adhesions are common and require careful dissection and hemostasis.

Mobilization of the thoracic esophagus is commenced by dividing the pleura over the junction of the azygos vein to the superior vena cava, and the azygos vein is divided between clamps. The caval end is transfixed. The pleura is divided proximally over the trachea, and the vagus nerve is identified and divided. The pleural incision is extended to the apex of the right chest along the lateral border of the trachea. The pleura over the right main bronchus is then incised, and pulmonary branches of the vagus are divided between clamps. Lymph nodes in the groove between the right main bronchus and the pericardium are freed and left attached to the esophagus. Vessels issuing from the pericardium to the lymph nodes are co-

agulated with diathermy. Division of the pleura distally exposes the right inferior pulmonary vein, and the esophagus is separated from the pericardium. The anterior esophagus is freed to its abdominal hiatus.

Next, the esophagus is separated from the posterior wall of the trachea, the carina, and the main bronchi; the left recurrent laryngeal nerve may be seen lateral and behind the trachea, and is preserved. Subcarinal lymph nodes are detached from the pericardium and the undersurface of the tracheal bifurcation (Fig. 21-3). Vessels in this region are ligated or coagulated by diathermy. By retraction of the esophagus posteriorly, the left inferior pulmonary vein is exposed and the lymph nodes in the groove between the left inferior pulmonary vein and the left main bronchus are likewise dissected free. The anterior aspect of the esophagus is now cleared in its entire length and remains attached only posteriorly and to the left pleura.

Attention is turned to the posterior aspect of the esophagus. Mobilization is begun by dividing the upper and lower tributaries of the azygos vein (the hemiazygos veins) as they arch across the esophagus to form the main trunk. Usually three or four branches are ligated. An incision is made

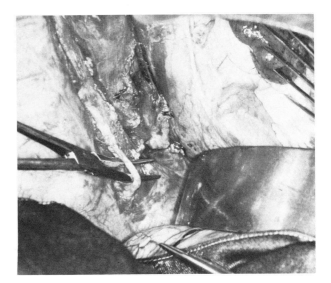

Fig. 21-4. The thoracic duct in front of the descending thoracic aorta above the esophageal hiatus is identified and freed, ready for division.

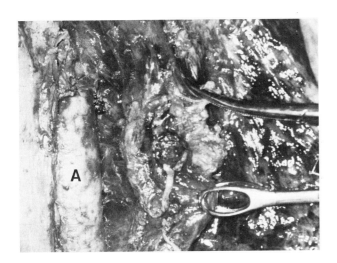

Fig. 21-5. Posterior mobilization of the esophagus is completed and the descending thoracic aorta *(A)* is exposed. Same patient as shown in Fig. 21-3.

in the pleura lying in front of the upper hemiazygos and extended upward to join the incision previously made from the front. By mobilization of the posterior aspect of the esophagus above the azygos vein, it is completely freed and circumscribed. Dissection is then continued downward along the anterior border of the lower hemiazygos. After division of the pleura, the connective tissue is reflected forward, exposing the thoracic aorta. The thoracic duct, lying on the front of the descending aorta, is identified and divided near the esophageal hiatus (Fig. 21-4). A clip is placed to mark the site of division of the duct. The pleura over the aorta just above the diaphgram is divided, and this joins the pleural division previously made on the anterior aspect. The thoracic duct and connective tissue are reflected off the

front of the aorta, toward the esophagus, until the left pleura is reached (Fig. 21-5). Usually there are no esophageal arteries of significance supplying the lower part of the thoracic esophagus, but near the upper end, just distal to the aortic arch, at least one large branch, and maybe five or six smaller ones, require ligation. The esophagus is now attached only to the left pleura, which is divided. The whole esophagus is free.

Difficulties in dissection of the esophagus arise when the tumor has infiltrated into adjacent structures. In particular, dissection of a tumor that has involved the trachea or bronchi must be done with special care, since injury of the tracheal wall is difficult to repair and such a mishap has a high chance of proving fatal. Should a hole be made, repair can be carried out by direct suture if the

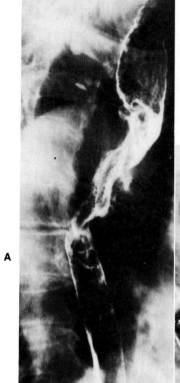

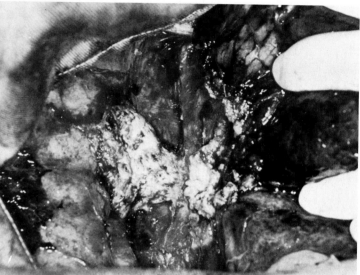

Fig. 21-6. A, Barium swallow showing marked angulation of the esophageal axis and proximity of the tumor to the vertebrae. **B,** The tumor had infiltrated extensively to the vertebrae, aorta, distal trachea, and bronchi. Resection was incomplete, and there was substantial residual tumor. The patient lived for 5 months.

defect is small, but if it is large a pedicled pericardial or intercostal flap will be required. The repaired site is subsequently buttressed by the substitute, which is usually the stomach. If the tumor has infiltrated the pericardium, excision of a cuff of pericardium presents no difficulty. Parts of the involved lung can also be resected, and the lung edge sutured. It is rare for the tumor to have infiltrated the aorta to the extent that the plane of cleavage is obliterated; if this is the case, some tumor may have to be left on the aortic wall. Occasionally tumor infiltration into the vertebrae will also render resection incomplete (Fig. 21-6). Enlarged lymph nodes anywhere in the mediastinum can be removed. This may include anterior and left paratracheal nodes (Fig. 21-7), apical pleural cavity nodes, and those along the left main bronchus and left pleura.

Once the whole esophagus has been freed, the stomach is brought into the chest and divided at the site previously determined. A large Satinsky clamp is placed on the distal gastric side and a crushing clamp on the proximal side before division with a diathermy knife. The esophagus at the apex of the pleural cavity is similarly clamped and divided after the nasogastric tube has been withdrawn to just above the site of transection. The mediastinum is therefore bared and final hemostasis obtained before the anastomosis is made (Fig. 21-8).

The Satinsky clamp on the proximal esophagus is released and six stay-sutures are placed equidistantly around the circumference of the esophagus. The esophageal lumen is irrigated with saline in order to wash away any debris (Fig. 21-9).

If the anastomosis is to be made by stapler, the gastric opening is used to introduce the instrument (Fig. 21-10). The method of stapling in this situation has previously been described,[13] but suffice for it to be mentioned here that we use the largest stapler that can be accommodated in the esophagus, since there is an inverse relationship between the size of the stapler and the occurrence and severity of postoperative anastomotic stricture.

When a hand anastomosis is employed, the gastric opening is closed in the same manner as for the pyloroplasty. A separate gastrotomy is made on the posterior wall just below the apex

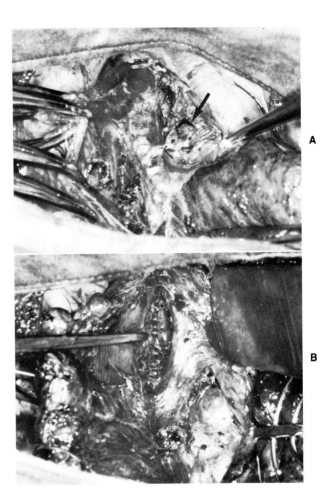

Fig. 21-7. Extensive metastases to **(A)** anterior tracheal lymph nodes (lying behind superior vena cava and indicated by forceps and arrow) and **(B)** left paratracheal lymph nodes (indicated by forceps).

of the stomach, and the anastomosis is completed with a single layer of continous suture, using a synthetic absorbable monofilament material (Fig. 21-11). As a rule, the stapler technique is preferred for an anastomosis at the apex of the right pleural cavity because it is simpler, it achieves more accurate tissue apposition, and there is less spillage of gastric contents into the mediastinum. On completion of the operation, the stomach traverses the whole length of the right thorax (Fig. 21-12). The chest is closed with drainage.

Resection of the upper third of the esophagus. A carcinoma in the cervical segment can be resected through a cervical incision, and a tumor in the superior mediastinal segment can be resected through an upper split-sternum incision[6,14]; in both cases the normal distal thoracic esophagus is mobilized from the abdomen by hand.

The cervical exposure is obtained through a transverse supraclavicular incision. After mobilization of the carotid sheath and the thyroid gland, the esophagus is visualized. The left recurrent laryngeal nerve is identified and protected throughout the operation (Fig. 21-13). Even when the nerve appears adherent to tumor or involved lymph nodes, it is important to preserve the nerve, since damage to or sacrifice of the nerve will not only cause vocal cord palsy but also will predispose to aspiration pneumonia and death. If the tumor is lying in the superior mediastinal segment and cannot be mobilized via the cervical exposure alone, the upper sternum is split to the second intercostal space (Fig. 21-14).

After mobilization of the tumor and adjoining lymph nodes from the nearby structures and particularly from the back of the trachea, the rest of the esophagus is freed via the abdomen—the most distal part under vision and the intervening portion around the tracheal bifurcation by finger dissection. During this phase of the mobilization it is essential to stay close to the esophageal wall to avoid damage to the azygos vein and the thoracic portion of the left recurrent laryngeal nerve. When mobilization is complete, the whole esophagus with the attached stomach (freed by upper midline laparotomy as with the Lewis-Tanner op-

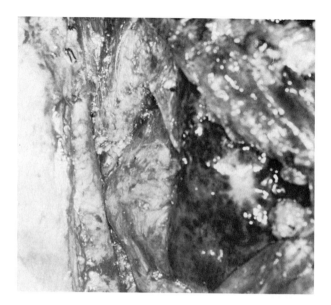

Fig. 21-8. The posterior mediastinum after being cleared of tumor and metastases; the trachea, bronchi, pericardium, and aorta are shown. Same patient as shown in Figs. 21-3 and 21-5.

Fig. 21-9. The upper esophagus is transected at the apex of the right chest and the esophageal lumen opened with six stay-sutures placed in its circumference. The nasogastric tube is visible in the esophageal lumen.

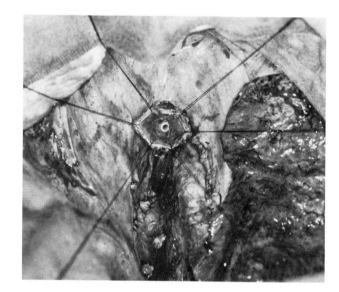

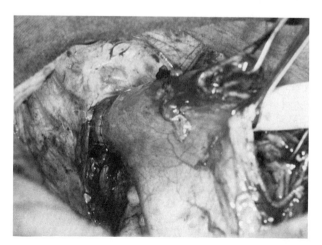

Fig. 21-10. The stapler has been introduced through the gastric opening after transection of the gastroesophageal junction, the anvil (in the esophagus) approximated with the stapler, and the stapler fired.

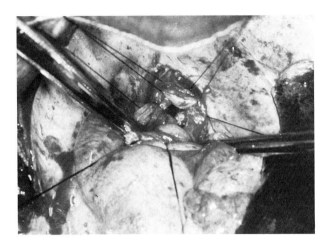

Fig. 21-11. A hand anastomosis being made between the stomach and the esophagus at the apex of the right chest with a single layer of continuous suture.

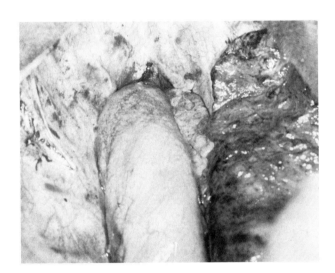

Fig. 21-12. Completed reconstruction for a middle-third tumor. The stomach lies in the right pleural cavity, and the fundus is at the apex of the chest.

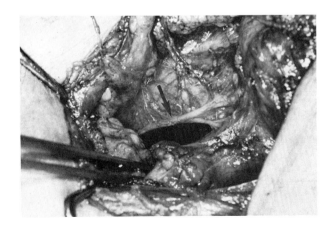

Fig. 21-13. A cervical tumor (indicated by forceps) is separated from the trachea. The left recurrent laryngeal nerve *(arrow)* is identified and protected throughout the operation.

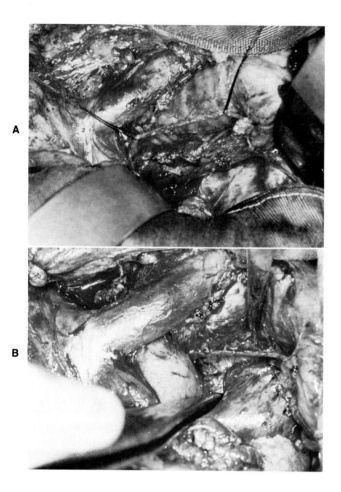

Fig. 21-14. The upper sternum has been divided to expose and resect a tumor of the superior mediastinal segment. The left recurrent laryngeal nerve (freed and held by sutures) is safeguarded during mobilization of the tumor **(A)**, and its integrity confirmed at the completion of reconstruction with stomach **(B)**.

eration) is brought up to the neck and the gastroesophageal junction divided. This sequence is always possible if a sternotomy has been added; but when only a cervical incision is made, it is usually necessary to divide the gastroesophageal junction during the abdominal phase, since it may be difficult or impossible to accomplish this in the neck. The proximal esophagus is freed to just below the cricopharyngeus and divided. Anastomosis at this site is usually performed by hand because this is simpler and more expeditious. If there is a sufficient length of esophageal stump, a stapler may be used. The need to preserve the left recurrent laryngeal nerve is again emphasized.

Other forms of gastric substitution. Apart from the whole-stomach preparation for esophagoplasty already described, other variations include the reverse gastric tube of Heimlich[18] and Gavriliu, and the isoperistaltic gastric tubes described by Yamagishi et al.[19] and Postlethwait,[20] both of which are prepared from the greater curvature, the former based on the left gastroepiploic vessels and the latter the right. Tubulari-

zation of stomach has also been described by Akiyama et al.,[21] the only departure from the whole-stomach preparation being that the proximal lesser curvature is resected to release the tethering by the left gastric arcade and to obtain more complete clearance of the lymph nodes at the cardia.

Little, if any, advantage seems to accrue from the use of the greater curvature gastric tubes as first-choice techniques for substitution, because their preparation adds to the complexity of the operation without offering additional tumor clearance or functional benefits. In addition, one or more long suture lines are required, a potential source of morbidity. On the other hand, the gastric tube proposed by Akiyama et al.[21] has theoretical merit, although we have not found resection of the lesser curvature necessary to allow the stomach to reach the pharynx for anastomosis.[5,22] Furthermore, tumor recurrence from having left clinically normal lymph nodes in the region of the cardia has been rare, and patients with overt lymph node involvement at this site from a middle-third tumor are usually incurable and often die from disseminated malignancy within a few months.

Pyloroplasty or no drainage. The fact that esophageal cancer surgeons with large experience differ in their practice as to whether to perform a pyloroplasty or pyloromyotomy when the whole stomach is used for reconstruction indicates that the difference, if any, of adding one drainage procedure or the other is only marginal. On the other hand, trials on the need for pyloroplasty in this situation have been meager.[23,24] To date, 100 patients have been entered into our prospective controlled trial, and follow-up has passed 2 years. Preliminary results showed that the only significant difference was a prolonged gastric emptying time (at 6 months after operation) in the group of patients who did not receive a pyloroplasty, and, also in this group, a small number of patients suffered from gastric stasis with symptoms of distention after meals and some degree of regurgitation. However, these symptoms were not severe, and the two patients who had this complication declined further operation. The very small number of patients who did not have a pyloroplasty and subsequently developed outlet problems were insufficient to show a significant difference, in statistical terms, from those who were drained, but this complication is a real one and conceded by most surgeons who do not perform pyloroplasty. On the other hand, patients with pyloroplasty in our series have suffered no ill effects from the procedure; the question then arises as to whether all patients should have a pyloroplasty in order to benefit the very few who might require this. Because we have been unable to identify prospectively those few patients who need pyloroplasty, it would be our current recommendation that unless the patient has a short stomach and an anastomosis in the neck is necessary, a pyloroplasty should be added when the whole stomach is used for reconstruction.

Use of colon

If the vasculature of the colon is suitable and the bowel is well prepared, use of the colon represents the simplest method of reconstruction, if the stomach is not available, or for bypass. The right colon, left colon, and transverse colon are equally satisfactory; it is desirable to have the substitute placed in an isoperistaltic manner (Fig. 21-15). The right colon and the transverse colon are based on the middle colic vessels, and the left colon is based on the ascending branch of the left colic vessels.[25-28] The left colon has the advantage of being less bulky than the right.

When the anastomosis is made in the neck, correct orientation of colon presents no difficulty,

since the upper abdomen and the neck are exposed simultaneously. When colon replacement is performed in the right chest in a two-phase operation, it is essential to ensure that the colon is not twisted. This complication can be avoided by suturing the proximal colon to the distal esophagus in their correct alignment before the patient is turned for the right thoracotomy. In this way an axial anastomosis can be made without fear of rotation of the colonic loop.

The length of the colon is always adequate to replace the whole esophagus, and usually excess colon has to be resected to eliminate redundancy. Since the anastomotic arcade runs very close to the colonic wall, there is no discrepancy between mesenteric and colon lengths as occurs when a long jejunal loop is used.

Because of the ease of preparation and good functional result, for some surgeons colon is the first choice for esophageal substitution when a subtotal esophagectomy has been performed. However, three anastomoses are required for this method of replacement. If the stomach is left intact, the colonic loop is placed in the retrogastric position and the colon may then be anastomosed to the front or back of the stomach. Otherwise, if no stomach remains, the colon may be anastomosed end-to-end to the duodenum.

Use of jejunum

The use of jejunum for esophagoplasty is the third and last option, because it is tedious to prepare a long jejunal loop and the blood supply may be inadequate (in 25% of patients) to develop a loop that reaches the neck.[15,29] Furthermore, in obese patients it may be impossible to prepare such a long loop; even if it were possible, there may be discrepancy between the length of the mesentery and that of the intestine.

To avoid fruitless dissection of the mesentery only to find the vasculature inadequate, the upper four jejunal vessels are first identified and bulldog clamps placed across them to test the adequacy of the anastomotic arcades. This and subsequent steps in vascular dissection are greatly assisted by the use of a fiberoptic light to rapidly visualize the main vessels and arcades so that the avascular planes may be opened readily for the clamps to be applied (Fig. 21-16). Once the vasculature has been found to be adequate, the peritoneum of the mesentery is reflected to the anastomotic arcade, and the connective tissue, which includes fat, lymphatic vessels, lymph nodes, and nerves, is removed from the main jejunal vessels. The arteries and veins are divided and ligated separately and mobilized from each other.

The proximal end of the jejunal loop is usually

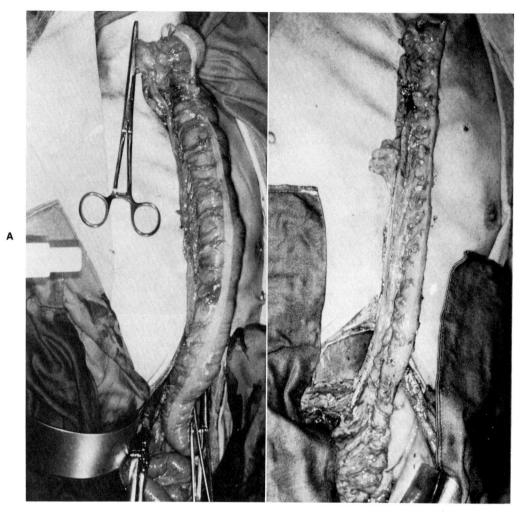

Fig. 21-15. The right colon, based on the middle colic vessels, has been mobilized and readily reaches the neck (**A**). The left colon, based on the ascending branch of the left colic vessels, also is quite adequate for total esophageal replacement (**B**); it is less bulky than the right colon.

10 to 15 cm from the duodenojejunal junction, and following division of four jejunal vessels the loop should reach the neck. For shorter lengths of esophageal replacement, division of two or three jejunal vessels should suffice.

When a long loop has been prepared, even in thin patients there is nearly always an excess of intestinal coils in relation to the mesentery (Fig. 21-17, *A*). This discrepancy is undesirable because adhesions that form between the redundant coils may cause obstruction. This may also produce a sense of fullness and distention after meals. When the loop is placed in the subcutaneous route, it appears unsightly. Therefore it is advantageous, though not essential, to resect part of the middle of this excess intestine and reanastomose the two ends (Fig. 21-17, *B*). A straight jejunal loop can thus be formed.[15] If a gastrec-

tomy has been performed, a Roux-en-Y configuration of the long jejunal loop is functionally satisfactory.

If a segmental interposition loop is required, a second segment of the jejunum is resected so that the distal end can be returned to the infracolic compartment for anastomosis to the proximal jejunum. The pedicled interposition loop is then placed in the retrocolic and retrogastric position and the distal end of the jejunal loop anastomosed to the front of the stomach. If the stomach has been resected, the distal end of an interposition loop can be anastomosed to the duodenal stump. When the upper end of the loop is to be anastomosed to the cervical esophagus, the loop can be placed in the retrosternal or subcutaneous position; when the anastomosis is in the right chest, as for the colon, correct alignment of the jejunum must be ensured.

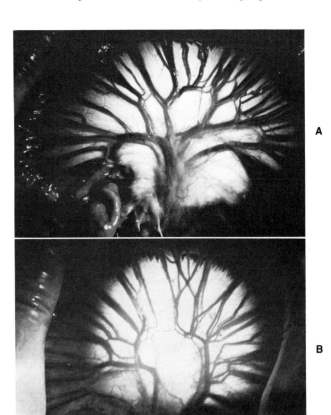

Fig. 21-16. Transillumination of the small bowel mesentery to identify the location of jejunal vessels and their anastomotic arcades (**A**). An incomplete arcade, which renders the preparation of a long jejunal loop futile (**B**).

As a rule, after a Polya gastrectomy the jejunum is unsuitable to prepare a long loop to reach the neck. If a shorter length of loop is required, then even after a Polya anastomosis the upper jejunum could still be used as a substitute.

A free jejunal graft with microvascular anastomosis has very little place in substitution for the esophagus in the neck or in the thorax after resection for carcinoma. Two teams of surgeons are required for a three-phase operation, and the net result is the preservation of a segment of the thoracic esophagus, which is a dubious advantage and, to some, a risk. Since the conventional methods of substitution are simpler and proven to be satisfactory, perhaps only in a patient who has had previous gastrectomy and colectomy and whose jejunal vasculature does not support a pedicled loop would a free jejunal graft represent the final option for reconstruction using the gastrointestinal tract. The complications of free jejunal graft operations are not inconsiderable.[30]

Anastomosis

A variety of hand anastomotic techniques have been described, and proponents of a particular method claim the superiority of their technique by citing the low incidence of anastomotic failures. The methods differ in the number of layers of suture, the material used, whether the sutures are placed in an interrupted or a continuous manner, and whether additional protection is afforded, such as by invagination or omental graft. However, these variations are finite. Currently most experienced surgeons employ a single layer of interrupted sutures for anastomosis, and a leakage rate of not more than 5% should now be achieved after resection. As often stated, provided that the blood supply between the esophagus and the substitute is adequate and there is no tension at the anastomosis, the precise technique is probably of less critical importance. Our current method of hand anastomosis is a single layer of continuous suture using an absorbable monofilament synthetic material (Fig. 21-18).

That a stapled esophagogastric anastomosis is associated with a very low leakage rate would indicate that mucosa-to-mucosa apposition is not essential, and, furthermore, the presence of necrotic tissue within the staples (which is an inevitable accompaniment of the stapler tech-

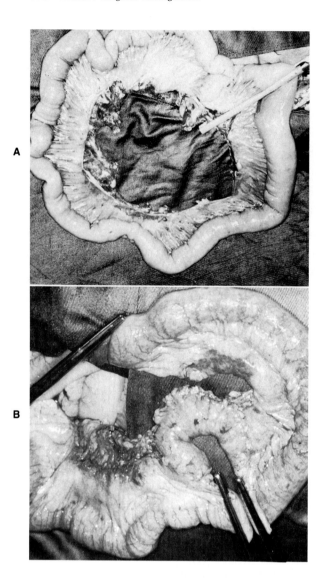

A

B

Fig. 21-17. A, A long jejunal loop is being prepared. Four main jejunal vessels have been divided, and the blood supply is satisfactory. There is excessive intestinal length in relation to the mesentery. **B,** Redundancy of the intestine is resected in the middle of the loop to straighten it.

nique) does not predispose to anastomotic leakage.[31] However, a stapled anastomosis is associated with a high incidence of postoperative strictures, and this is in part related to the size of the stapler used. In our series of patients, the risk of developing anastomotic stricture using the EEA stapler is about 20% regardless of the size used, and about 10% for the ILS. With two larger ILS staplers, namely 29 mm and 33 mm, the risk of stricture is negligible and is less than with our hand technique. The smallest ILS stapler (25 mm) produces the highest stricture rate of the whole range of sizes of staplers—in excess of 25%. The largest size stapler that fits into the esophageal lumen is selected, in order to minimize the risk of postoperative stricture. Strictures, when they occur, can be easily managed by bougienage in an average of two sessions and usually under local anesthesia. Recurrence of the stricture after adequate bougienage is uncommon.

Because of the low incidence of anastomotic failures, the ease with which a stricture can be dealt with, and the precision it offers in making an esophagogastrostomy at the apex of the right chest, our practice has been to use the stapler for anastomosis in the two-phase operation whenever this is possible.

RESULTS

In the 3 years between 1982 and 1985, of 311 unselected patients with carcinoma of the esophagus admitted to Queen Mary Hospital in the Department of Surgery, University of Hong Kong, 250 agreed to any form of treatment recom-

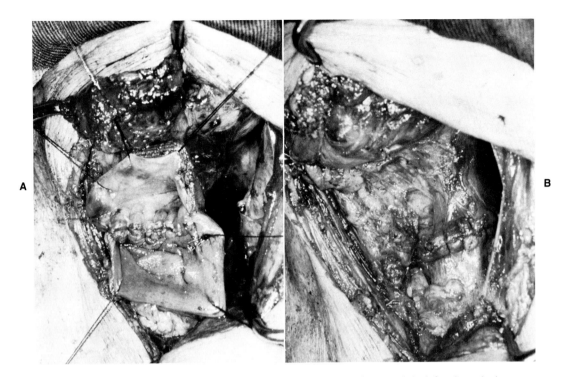

Fig. 21-18. A hand anastomosis between the cervical esophagus *(above)* and the left colon substitute *(below)*, both of which correspond closely in size. A continuous suture on the posterior wall is made (**A**). The external appearance after completion of the anastomosis is shown in (**B**).

mended. Of these patients, 230 were operated upon; 189 underwent resection and 34 had bypass operations. Only seven patients were explored (through the abdomen) and found not suitable for a definitive procedure. Resection was deemed curative if all macroscopic tumor was removed from the mediastinum and no extrathoracic disease was present. Resection was palliative if residual tumor was evident, gross metastatic lymph nodes were present in the mediastinum or had reached the extremes of the mediastinum, extrathoracic lymph nodes were involved, or liver metastases were found. There were 93 patients in the curative group and 95 in the palliative group. One patient had a staged resection but died before reconstruction could be carried out. Bypass operation was performed on 34 patients who had extensive local disease as evidenced by bronchoscopic finding of infiltration into the tracheobronchial tree, who were unfit for a thoracotomy, or who had disseminated disease.

With this treatment policy, the 30-day mortality for resection was 6%, the 3-month mortality was 13%, and the 3-year actuarial survival was 30%. When divided into curative and palliative resection groups, the actuarial survival at 3 years was 50% and 10%, respectively.

For bypass operations, the 30-day mortality was 35% and the 3-month mortality was 52%. No patient survived beyond 14 months.

Leakage from the anastomosis and other sites was 6% for the resection group and 23% for the bypass group. The hand anastomosis for the resection group fared as well in terms of leakage as the stapled anastomosis (3% versus 4%, respectively), but the incidence of postoperative anastomotic strictures was high for the stapler group (15%) in comparison with the hand anastomosis group (9%). For patients who survived the operation, a normal meal could be taken by the vast majority, the proportion increasing with time.

CONCLUSION

Resection for carcinoma of the esophagus could be accomplished in three quarters of unselected patients, in half of whom the resection was deemed curative and resulted in a 50% chance of living 3 years. Those with advanced disease had a much lower chance of long-term survival, but all patients who underwent resection obtained good palliation. Resection even in patients with advanced disease can now be achieved with acceptably low mortality and complication rates.

In contrast, patients undergoing a bypass operation, which is reserved only for those with far advanced disease and previously not considered surgical candidates, face a much greater operative risk. However, in these patients even intubation carries a high risk, and a lesser degree of palliation is afforded.

From our data, it would appear that about 15% of unselected patients with carcinoma of the esophagus have some prospect of a long survival; the remainder can only expect palliation lasting a few months. Palliation by operation is nonetheless worthwhile, since it converts death from total dysphagia into death from malignant cachexia.

REFERENCES

1. Lewis, I.: The surgical treatment of carcinoma of the oesophagus with special reference to a new operation for growths of the middle third, Br. J. Surg. **34**:18, 1946.
2. Tanner, N.C.: The present position of carcinoma of the oesophagus, Postgrad. Med. J. **23**:109, 1947.
3. Ong, G.B.: The Kirschner operation: a forgotten procedure, Br. J. Surg. **60**:221, 1973.
4. Ong, G.B., and Kwong, K.H.: The Lewis-Tanner operation for cancer of the oesophagus, J. R. Coll. Surg. Edinb. **14**:3, 1969.
5. Ong, G.B., and Lee, T.C.: Pharyngogastric anastomosis after oesophago-pharyngectomy for carcinoma of the hypopharynx and cervical oesophagus, Br. J. Surg. **48**:193, 1960.
6. Ong, G.B., Lam, K.H., Lam, P.H.M., and Wong, J.: Resection for carcinoma of the superior mediastinal segment of the esophagus, World J. Surg. **2**:497, 1978.
7. Huang, G.J., Shao, L.F., Zhang, D.W., Li, Z.C., Wang, G.Q., Liu, S.X., and Chang, F.B.: Diagnosis and surgical treatment of early esophageal carcinoma, Chin. Med. J. **94**:229, 1981.
8. Ong, G.B., Lam, K.H., Wong, J., and Lim, T.K.: Factors influencing morbidity and mortality in esophageal carcinoma, J. Thorac. Cardiovasc. Surg. **76**:745, 1978.
9. Wong, J.: Management of carcinoma of oesophagus: art or science? J. R. Coll. Surg. Edinb. **26**:138, 1981.
10. Wong, J., Lam, K.H., Wei, W.I., and Ong, G.B.: Results of the Kirschner operation, World J. Surg. **5**:547, 1981.
11. McKeown, K.C.: Total three-stage oesophagectomy for cancer of the oesophagus, Br. J. Surg. **63**:259, 1976.
12. Skinner, D.B.: En bloc resection for neoplasms of the esophagus and cardia, J. Thorac. Cardiovasc. Surg. **85**:59, 1983.
13. Wong, J.: Stapled esophagogastric anastomosis in the apex of the right chest after subtotal esophagectomy for carcinoma, Surg. Gynecol. Obstet., 1986. (In press.)
14. Orringer, M.B.: Partial median sternotomy: anterior approach to the upper thoracic esophagus, J. Thorac. Cardiovasc. Surg. **87**:124, 1984.
15. Wong, J., and Ong, G.B.: Esophagogastrectomy for carcinoma of the abdominal esophagus and gastric cardia. In Nyhus, L.M., and Baker, R.J., editors: Mastery of surgery, Boston, 1984, Little, Brown & Co., pp. 582-590.
16. Siu, K.F., Cheung, H.C., and Wong, J.: Shrinkage of the esophagus after resection for carcinoma, Ann. Surg. **203**:173, 1986.
17. Ngan, S.Y.K., and Wong, J.: Lengths of different routes for esophageal replacement, J. Thorac. Cardiovasc. Surg., **91**:790, 1986.
18. Heimlich, H.J.: The use of a gastric tube to replace the esophagus as performed by Dr. Dan Gavriliu of Bucharest, Rumania, Surgery **42**:693, 1957.
19. Yamagishi, M., Ikeda, N., and Yonemoto, T.: An isoperistaltic gastric tube: new method of esophageal replacement, Arch. Surg. **100**:689, 1970.
20. Postlethwait, R.W.: Surgery of the esophagus, New York, 1979, Appleton-Century-Crofts, p. 464.
21. Akiyama, H., Hiyama, M., and Hashimoto, C.: Resection and reconstruction for carcinoma of the thoracic oesophagus, Br. J. Surg. **63**:206, 1976.
22. Lam, K.H., Wong, J., Lim, S.T.K., and Ong, G.B.: Pharyngogastric anastomosis following pharyngolaryngoesophagectomy: analysis of 157 cases, World J. Surg. **5**:509, 1981.
23. Hsu, H.K., Huang, M.H., Chien, K.Y., Liu, R.S., and Yeh, S.H.: Functional evaluation of using stomach as an esophageal substitute, J. Surg. Assoc. ROC **17**:186, 1984.
24. Mannell, A., Hinder, R.A., and San-Garde, B.A.: The thoracic stomach: a study of gastric emptying, bile reflux and mucosal change, Br. J. Surg. **71**:438, 1984.
25. Belsey, R.: Reconstruction of the esophagus with left colon, J. Thorac. Cardiovasc. Surg. **49**:33, 1965.
26. Postlethwait, R.W.: Colonic interposition for esophageal substitution, Surg. Gynecol. Obstet. **156**:377, 1983.
27. Scanlon, E.F., and Staley, C.J.: The use of the ascending and right half of the transverse colon in esophagoplasty, Surg. Gynecol. Obstet. **109**:99, 1958.
28. Wilkins, E.W.: Long-segment colon substitution for the esophagus, Ann. Surg. **192**:722, 1980.
29. Ong, G.B., Lam, K.H., Wong, J., and Lim, T.K.: Jejunal esophagoplasty for carcinoma of the esophagus, Jpn. J. Surg. **10**:15, 1980.
30. Stell, P.M., Missotten, F., Singh, S.D., Ramadan, M.F., and Morton, R.P.: Mortality after surgery for hypopharyngeal cancer, Br. J. Surg. **70**:713, 1983.
31. Steichen, F.M., and Ravitch, M.M.: Mechanical sutures in esophageal surgery, Ann. Surg. **191**:373, 1980.

22 The current role of partial esophagectomy in the surgical treatment of middle- and lower-third esophageal carcinoma

Louis Couraud, Abdullah Hafez-Alqudah, Philippe Clerc, and Serge Meriot

The application to squamous esophageal carcinoma of the concept of systemic disease that affects the whole upper aerodigestive tract synchronously or successively leads surgeons to consider systematic and extended resection of the entire esophagus instead of limiting themselves to the classical partial resection, which generally extends only 5 to 8 cm above the upper margin of the tumor. Complete resection undoubtedly carries greater risk than partial resection, but should restricted and elective indications deprive elderly patients of optimal therapy? On the other hand, an improved prognosis has not clearly been demonstrated as compared with the benefits of partial esophagectomy. We feel there remain numerous indications for partial esophagectomy. We accept the unquestionably justified indications for total esophagectomy but will focus discussion on the current indications for partial esophagectomy to demonstrate its wide applicability. Our findings are based on our experience with 390 partial esophagectomies performed for carcinoma between 1970 and 1984.

MATERIAL AND METHODS

Of the 390 patients with partial resection of the lower esophagus, 355 were men (91%) and 35 were women (9%). All patients were clinically and anatomically symptomatic. The histologic types were as follows:

Squamous cell carcinoma (more or less differentiated): 235 cases (60%)
Adenocarcinoma: 144 cases (37%)
Undifferentiated or others: 12 cases (3%)

Groupings were based on lymph node involvement, operative technique, and long-term results. Complementary therapy and gastric cancers that had spread to the cardia were excluded as factors for grouping purposes. The tumor was situated in the lower third of the esophagus in 262 cases (67%) and in the middle third in 128 cases (33%).

Sometimes the patient was elderly; 86 patients were over 70 years of age. A large number (26%) had an associated serious illness: respiratory disorders (26 cases), cardiovascular problems (31 cases), previous cancer (12 cases), and alteration of hepatic functions (many alcoholics).

Each patient underwent an esophageal resection with mediastinal lymph node excision more than 5 cm from the upper margin of the tumor, including resection of the lesser curvature of the stomach, followed by reanastomosis at the top of an isoperistaltic gastric tube created from the length of the greater curvature[1] (Fig. 22-1). For old and debilitated patients, the operation was, whenever possible, carried out through a single approach. Left thoracotomy with subaortic anastomosis was done in 246 cases (228 thoracotomies, 18 thoracoabdominal incisions), and left thoracotomy with anastomosis above the aortic arch was performed in 21 cases. In 123 cases, the operation was carried out through an abdominal incision followed by a right thoracotomy. Except for patients who underwent only palliative resection—that is, those in whom a neoplastic segment remained (21%) and all of whom died within 18 months despite complementary radiotherapy and chemotherapy—patients had isolated surgical resection without supplementary oncologic treatment.

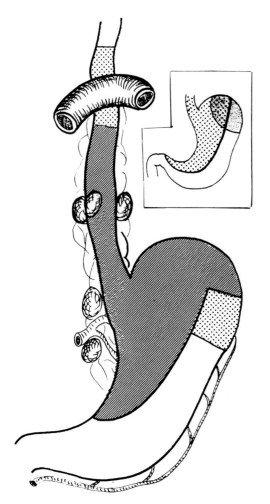

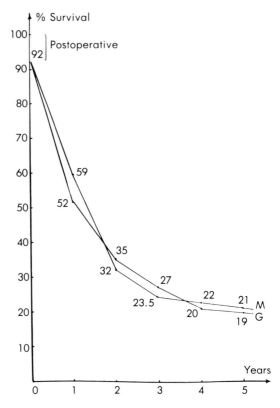

Fig. 22-2. Survival curves of 318 partial esophagectomies (1970 to 1984), with follow-up from 1 to 14 years. Squamous cell carcinoma (M), 21%; adenocarcinoma (G), 19%; average, 20.75%.

Fig. 22-1. Schematic operative drawing showing our different aims in the partial esophagectomy: esophagectomy, mediastinectomy, isoperistaltic gastric tube, hand-made end-to-end anastomosis. *Inset,* Lymphatic drainage of the cardia and lesser curvature of the stomach. (Modified from Pissas, A., Doyon, J.F., Sarrazin, R., and Bouchet, Y.: J. Chir. **116**:583, 1979.)

RESULTS

The overall operative mortality during the first 2 months was 7.6% (30 of 390). However, the low mortality for patients under 70 years of age (18 of 304 patients, 6%), must be compared with the higher rate among those over 70 (18 of 86 patients, 14%). The postoperative period of hospitalization varied between 15 and 20 days. Complications were as follows:

1. Morbidity (15%) involved mainly cardiovascular and respiratory problems of various degrees of severity. Sometimes hepatic insufficiency was present.

2. Anastomotic fistulas were rare (9 cases, 2%) but always severe, causing 5 deaths.

Survival rates were as follows in 318 patients with a follow-up of 1 to 14 years: 57% after 1 year, 34% after 2 years, 26% after 3 years, 22% after 4 years, and 20.75% after 5 years (Fig. 22-2). After 5 years the survival rate rose to 27% if patients with only palliative interventions were excluded. The survival rate for patients with adenocarcinomas, 19% after 5 years, differed only slightly from the rate for patients with squamous cell carcinoma (21%).

Among patients who underwent an apparently satisfactory resection the cause of death is known for only 133. In these death resulted from metastases to other organs (55%), locoregional involvement (33%), and other diseases (12%). We were unable to determine precisely the number of deaths caused by recurrence of esophageal carcinoma, but fewer than 20% of the patients showed dysphagia caused either by external compression referable to mediastinal recurrence or by neoplastic recurrence from the esophagus.

DISCUSSION
Relationship of partial resection and recurrence

Assuming that esophageal cancer is often multicentric and requires the most extensive surgery possible, it can be seen that resections do not necessarily lead to recurrence. Numerous postmortem or clinical studies have proved the multicentric character of neoplastic degeneration at every level of the upper aerodigestive tract. With the aid of vital staining (toluidine blue), Pradoura et al.[2] revealed 98 "synchronous" cancers out of 652 (15%) cancers of the upper aerodigestive tract. Even if the cancer appears unicentric, a multicentric development, although not as prevalent, can occur, as it did in 11 of 108 cases (10%) studied by Reboud et al.[3] Undoubtedly, the rate of multicentricity is very high in some circumstances among old and debilitated people, in those with immunodeficiency, and in patients whose tumors have reached an advanced stage, taking into account findings located below the tumor.

The reported frequency of synchronous cancers seems overestimated, at least in cases in which there is a strong indication for surgery. Specifically, the level of esophageal recurrence seems below that forecast. On the other hand, a systematic study of 50 cases using vital staining (toluidine blue) during endoscopy and again over the operative specimen[4] revealed only two positive findings with regard to endoscopic site (+9 cm for an adenocarcinoma, +10 cm for a squamous cell carcinoma) and an apparently extramucosal finding at +8 cm in an operative specimen (6%).

Spread to the esophageal wall is less likely to result in unsuccessful surgery than is periesophageal mediastinal lymph node spread. Akiyama et al.[5] give percentages of 9.8% for the esophageal wall and 29.4% for the upper mediastinum, according to the location of the main tumor.

Overall, if the pharyngolarynx is left in place, resection is considered "imperfect." Total esophagectomy is only slightly less imperfect than partial esophagectomy. Each individual case must be evaluated as to comparative risks and benefits.

Morbidity and mortality comparisons

From the viewpoint of morbidity and mortality, partial esophagectomy remains a comparatively less serious operation than total esophagectomy.

Bronchoalveolar complications are infrequent in patients with partial resections wherein the anastomosis is located at the subaortic or the thoracic inlet (5.6% in our experience); in this procedure the upper part of the esophagus is retained. Such complications occur much more frequently at the upper esophageal sphincter. In these cases, dyskinetic problems associated with swallowing and regurgitation of acids create more respiratory complications and require intensive care.

Looking at mortality in comparative periods provides evidence of a constant increase in mortality resulting from subtotal versus total esophagectomy.[6-12] Reportedly the rate for total esophagectomy ranges from 10% to 30%, while that for partial esophagectomy[9,13] has been 5% to 8% for the last 10 years. The only evidence to the contrary is that of Akiyama et al.,[5] who reported a 1.4% mortality, but it remains to be seen whether the rate will be this low under the statistical screening and treatment conditions of Western nations.

These statistics are impressive despite significantly restrictive contraindications for total esophagectomy as follows:

Age over 70 years
Obesity or major, rapid deterioration of overall condition
Recent ischemic myocardiopathy
FEV_1 and FEV_1/VC decreased below 50% of their theoretical values[14]

In addition, the development of hepatic insufficiency rules out total esophagectomy. The age limit for candidates for partial esophagectomies can surpass 80 years if good general health prevails. Furthermore, a respiratory function test that reveals 30% or 35% of the FEV_1 and FEV_1/VC theoretical values does not constitute an absolute contraindication if a single left thoracotomy approach is to be used.

In situations that do not meet the outlined indications, the available options include doing nothing or carrying out (1) a resection without thoracotomy but including lymph node excision, as proposed by Orringer,[15] or (2) a partial esophagectomy, preferably through a single operative approach. We prefer by far the latter solution whenever possible.

Cure rates

Unquestionably, partial esophagectomy may be a curative operation. We have found that 20.75% of our patients live longer than 5 years (27% if only satisfactory complete anatomic resections of gross tumor are included). These figures can be improved by total esophagectomies only if they achieve better removal of the esophageal wall and a more extended periesophageal lymph node excision. However, measuring the rate of improvement of survival is difficult. With the exception of the series of Akiyama et al.,[5] which reports a

TABLE 22-1. The different kinds of esophagectomies performed in our unit between January 1, 1983, and December 31, 1985

Procedure		No. of patients
Total esophagectomies	(3 operative approaches)	17
Subtotal esophagectomies—anastomosis at the upper pole of right hemithorax	(2 operative approaches)	34
Partial esophagectomies	(1 operative approach—left)	62

5-year survival rate of 34.6% (15.3% in 23 cases with periesophageal lymph node involvement and 53.8% in 23 cases without involvement of the lymph nodes), among 52 cases with 5-year follow-up the prognosis after extensive operations does not improve greatly; in general, the 5-year survival varies from 20% to 30%. Factors that explain the difficulty in comparing these approaches include:

1. The anatomic differences among clinical cases
2. The more or less restrictive aspects of surgical indications
3. The usual imprecision of TNM classification

CONCLUSIONS

Total esophagectomy remains the best possible resectional operation for cancers of the esophagus. Therefore one must attempt the highest possible esophagectomy with the highest possible extension of mediastinal lymph node excision. But partial esophagectomy must not be considered as only a palliative procedure; it is also a potentially curative operation.

In *poor-risk* patients, the indications for esophagectomy must be considered as part of a thorough endoscopic evaluation, including search for small neoplastic sites with the aid of vital staining with toluidine blue. The following findings hold:

1. If a second highly placed neoplastic site is found, total esophagectomy is to be considered very hazardous. There is still recourse to palliative measures (chemoradiotherapy, transesophageal intubation).
2. In the absence of a second highly placed neoplastic site, the surgical indication depends on evaluation of each technique's risk. Although total esophagectomy may be theoretically preferable, in our opinion partial resection should be chosen if there are unreasonable increases in operative risk.

We have seen various indications for esophagectomy in our unit since 1983. The most important factors to weigh are the degree of precariousness of the state of the patient, the widest operative indications, and our predisposition to performing partial esophagectomy (see Table 22-1). Finally, improvements in postoperative care have minimized the contraindications for the procedure in elderly patients. Therefore we feel that partial esophagectomy has a place of paramount importance despite encouraging results with total esophagectomy.

REFERENCES

1. Boerema, I.: Oesophagus resection with restoration of continuity by a gastric tube, Arch. Chir. Neerland. **4**:120, 1952.
2. Pradoura, J.P., Colonna d'Istria, J., Jausseran, M., Gaillard, M., Giudicelli, R., Fuentes, P., and Reboud, E.: L'oesophage du cancereux ORL, Sem. Hop. Paris. **60**:839, 1984.
3. Reboud, E., Pradoura, J.P., Fuentes, P., and Giudicelli, R.: Multicentric esophageal carcinoma: yield of total endoscopy and vital staining. In DeMeester, T.R., and Skinner, D.B., editors: Esophageal disorders: pathophysiology and therapy, New York, 1985, Raven Press, pp. 347-353.
4. Couraud, L., Hafez, A., Velly, J.F., Levy, F., and Pierchon, M.-S.: Contribution à l'étude des cancers oesophagiens multifocaux par imprégnation au bleu de toluidine: implications thérapeutiques, Ann. Chir. **39**:211, 1985.
5. Akiyama, H., Tsurumaru, M., Kawamura, T., and Ono, Y.: Principles of surgical treatment for carcinoma of the esophagus: analysis of lymph node involvement, Ann. Surg. **194**:438, 1981.
6. Giuli, R., and Gignoux, M.: Treatment of carcinoma of the esophagus, Ann. Surg. **192**:44, 1980.
7. Maillet, P., Baulieux, J., Boulez, J., and Benhaim, R.: Carcinoma of the thoracic esophagus: results of one-stage surgery (271 cases), Am. J. Surg. **143**:629, 1982.
8. Postlethwait, R.W.: Carcinoma of the thoracic esophagus, Surg. Clin. North Am. **63**:933, 1983.
9. Morand, G., Lion, R., Wihlm, J.M., and Witz, J.P.: Les résultats des exérèses sub-totales de l'oesophage. In Cancers de l'oesophage, Paris, 1984, Editions Maloine, pp. 128-130.

10. Skinner, D.B.: En bloc resection for neoplasms of the esophagus and cardia, J. Thorac. Cardiovasc. Surg. **85**:59, 1983.

11. Fuentes, P., Giudicelli, R., Riera, P., and Reboud, E.: Les procédés de remplacement de l'oesophage, In Cancers de l'oesophage, Paris, 1984, Editions Maloine, pp. 154-158.

12. Griffith, J.L., and Davis, J.T.: A twenty year experience with surgical management of carcinoma of the esophagus and gastric cardia, J. Thorac. Cardiovasc. Surg. **79**:447, 1980.

13. Couraud, L., and Meriot, S.: Le traitement des cancers du tiers inférieur et du tiers moyen de l'oesophage par résection et gastroplastie tubulée isopéristaltique, Chirurgie **108**:703, 1982.

14. Elman, A., Boudinet, A., Flammand, Y., Metrot-Magny, C., and Levy, D.: Les contre-indications fonctionnelles respiratoires à la chirurgie oesophagienne. In Cancers de l'oesophage, Paris, 1984, Editions Maloine, pp. 17-20.

15. Orringer, M.B.: Palliative procedures for esophageal cancer, Surg. Clin. North Am. **63**:941, 1983.

16. Pissas, A., Doyon, J.F., Sarrazin, R., and Bouchet, Y.: Le drainage lymphatique de l'estomac, J. Chir. **116**:583, 1979.

CHAPTER 23 Use of tubular isoperistaltic gastroplasty after total or partial esophagectomy

Louis Couraud, Abdullah Hafez-Alqudah, Philippe Clerc, and Serge Meriot in collaboration with Francisco París and Manuel Tomas-Ridocci

During the 1960s, when Sweet's operation was the basic technique for esophageal replacement using the stomach, we adopted an operative model, put forward by Boerema[1] in 1952, of esophageal replacement by an isoperistaltic gastric tube created from the whole length of the greater curvature. This choice was based on several objectives:

To avoid bringing into the thorax a substitute that was too wide or distended, but rather a tube whose caliber was similar to that of the esophagus

To achieve neoplastic lymph node removal, frequent in the paracardial region

To achieve a mobile and vascularized substitute at less risk than with colonic interposition needed after total gastrectomy

At the present time more than 500 partial or total replacements of the esophagus have been performed using this technique. We believe this experience has confirmed the qualities of the tubular isoperistaltic gastroplasty—long length of the tube, good arterial supply, benefits in tumor ablation as confirmed by recent studies, and adaptability for long-term use. This technique has been adopted by many highly experienced authors since 1970.[2-6]

OPERATIVE PROCEDURE

The operation consists of the following steps (Fig. 23-1).

1. Ligation and division of the left gastric artery and lymph node dissection of the celiac axis

2. Division of the gastrocolic ligament and mobilization of the stomach, carefully conserving the arterial supply (right gastroepiploic vessel) to the greater curvature (eventually performing the Kocher maneuver and duodenopancreatic mobilization)

3. Ligation and division of the arterial supply of the lesser curvature on its horizontal section underneath the branches of the left gastric artery

4. Resection of the fundus, vertical section of the lesser curvature, and half of the anterior and posterior walls of the stomach. The remaining gastric tube, 3.5 to 5 cm wide, can be used upward to a point 3 to 4 cm above the last vascular arcade. If the vascular arcade is unsuitable, a slightly wider tube must be maintained. The tubular gastroplasty can be made cleanly either over a curved hemostatic clamp or, preferably, by using a GIA stapler. We have always used a second inverting suture.

5. End-to-end gastroesophageal anastomosis in the thorax or into the neck

VASCULAR ANATOMY AND LYMPHATIC DRAINAGE

The isoperistaltic gastric tube of the greater curvature is better supplied arterially than the entire stomach, and makes a longer substitute. Whereas the mobilization of the entire stomach entails a zone of decreased blood supply at the fundus, specifically the point of gastroesophageal anastomosis, the gastric tube, which is well sup-

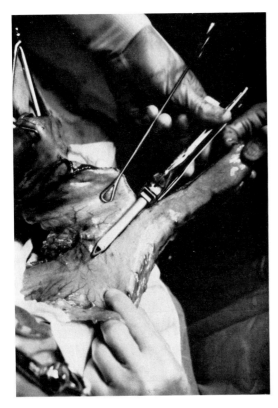

Fig. 23-1. Operative procedure for tubular gastroplasty after total or partial esophagectomy.

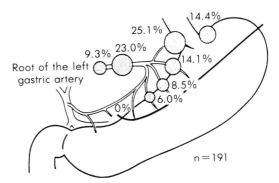

Fig. 23-2. Rate of positive lymph nodes in the superior gastric region (per number of cases). (From Akiyama, H., Tsurumaru, M., Kawamura, T., and Ono, Y.: Ann. Surg. **194**: 438, Oct. 1981.)

plied by its vascular arcade, does not suffer ischemia. Moreover, the lesser curvature impedes the ascent of the stomach. Also, the curvilinear resection on the gastric walls allows a better expansion of the greater curvature, and therefore permits creation of a tube that rises as high as, if not higher than, the entire stomach.

The tube's quality and vitality can be seen in our results in 390 interventions: (1) no tubular necrosis; (2) a low rate of gastroesophageal fistulas (9 cases, 2%).

The lesser curvature at the point of emergence of the left gastric artery's branches is a zone of lymphatic confluence of esophageal and gastric origin, which is important to excise.

The frequency of lymph node involvement of the left gastric artery's region has been measured by Akiyama et al.[2]:

    61.5% in cancers of the lower third of the esophagus

    32.8% in cancers of the middle third of the esophagus

    31.8% in cancers of the upper third of the esophagus

This lymph node involvement can extend along the vertical part of the lesser curvature to the fourth arterial branch. Therefore, for safety the resection must pass at the same level as, or below, the fifth branch of the left gastric artery (Fig. 23-2).

The areas and the direction of lymphatic drainage of the stomach have been studied by Pissas et al.[7] The lymphatic glands of the stomach are extensively linked to those of the esophagus. The field of lymphatic drainage of the cardia, the lesser curvature, and the juxtaposed half of the anterior and posterior gastric walls is directed toward the glands of the left gastric artery and celiac axis.

A valvular system prevents the circulation of the lymph toward the greater curvature. But major blockage by neoplastic lymph node involvement of the lesser curvature may cause an inversion of the current toward the greater curvature.

Therefore, surgical resection of the lesser curvature represents ablation of an area of lymphatic propagation of the esophageal carcinoma. The greater curvature, a site protected from lymph node involvement, can be used to create the tube, if neoplastic recurrence has not occurred there.

As a result, the tubular gastroplasty is an operation better adapted to treat esophageal cancers than conservation of the entire stomach. But it rapidly becomes inadequate when cancers spread to the cardia. In these cases it is preferable to carry out total gastrectomy.

POSTOPERATIVE STUDIES

Radiologically the substitute tube is completely satisfactory. It is slightly wider than the normal esophagus, but this ensures that it is sufficiently wide to avoid stenosis. The barium swallow shows emptying at normal speed, without stasis.

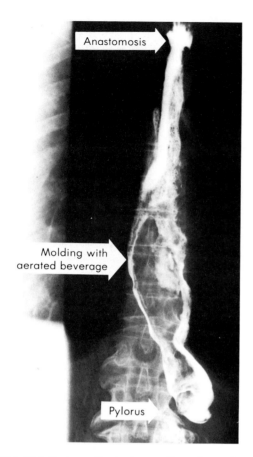

Anastomosis

Molding with
aerated beverage

Pylorus

Fig. 23-3. Postoperative barium swallow after replacement of the esophagus by isoperistaltic gastric tube.

Contrary to the case with ascent of the whole stomach, the tube is not subjected to gaseous distention and unless technical errors occur, it is not the site of thoracic alimentary stasis (Fig. 23-3). Therefore, it does not cause bronchopulmonary shifting, blocking of the bronchoalveolar drainage, or recurrent bronchopneumopathies, which often result from intrathoracic gastric distention.

Manometric studies have been performed to evaluate motor activity of both types of gastroplasty—isoperistaltic gastric tube (five patients) and total stomach (five patients). The motor behavior of both esophageal substitutes has been assessed following dry swallows and other stimuli—intraluminal injection of 30 ml of water or 0.1N hydrochloric acid and pill swallowing, as described previously.[8] Following dry swallows there was no response either with the gastric tube or with total gastroplasty, and neither esophageal substitute responded to stimuli (Fig. 23-4).

Our data indicate no active contribution from gastric tube or total stomach to the transmission of food in the digestive tract. Vagus division prob-

ably explains absence of motility in both cases. Nevertheless no alimentary stasis occurs either. In our opinion the presence of a normal proximal segment of the esophagus will act as a motor pump and help the transit of the alimentary bolus through the substitute, especially when the tube has the same inner diameter as the normal esophagus.

DISCUSSION

The isoperistaltic gastric tube appears to present anatomic, carcinoma ablation, and functional advantages when compared with total gastroplasty. However, replacement of all or part of the esophagus by a gastric tube is not perfect or totally safe.

Study of the mid-term and late complications and sequelae in a series of 318 tubular gastroplasties for cancer, in which 180 patients lived for more than a year, revealed the following phenomena (see Table 23-1):

Absence of compressive problems

Delayed occurrence of transdiaphragmatic hernias (eight cases, 4.5%)

Frequent postprandial and postoperative diarrhea, almost all disappearing after 3 months

Extremely frequent small-stomach syndrome, which becomes rare after 3 months and disappears after 1 year

Delayed appearance of pylorospasm (6% of secondary pyloroplasties needed after 1 year despite 8% [26 of 318] initial pyloroplasties)

Frequent severe reflux esophagitis; 28% in the first months, dropping to 5% after 1 year; the 5% was badly tolerated

Appearance of stenoses in the anastomotic site or in the adjacent esophagus; 9% required esophageal dilatation between 3 months and 1 year, but only 4% after 1 year

Overall, esophageal replacement remains a mutilating operation with undeniable sequelae. The isoperistaltic gastric tube does not completely avoid these inconveniences. Long-term follow-up of the functional results of esophageal replacement substitutes for benign stenosis (isoperistaltic gastric tubes, antiperistaltic tubes, colonic interposition) shows that, after the difficulties of the first year when most complications occur, the tubular isoperistaltic gastroplasty yielded stable results, with no tendency toward deterioration. Patients with esophageal cancer who have survived 5 years confirm this good long-term result.

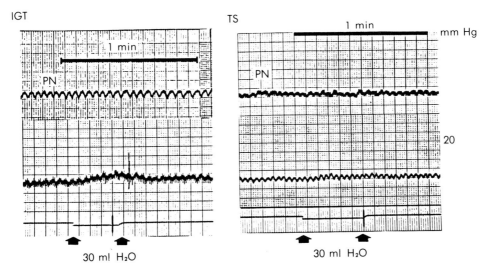

Fig. 23-4. Absence of motor response after intraluminal injection of 30 ml of distilled water. *IGT,* Isoperistaltic gastric tube; TS, total stomach; *PN*, pneumogram.

TABLE 23-1. Postoperative complications and sequelae (percent)

Complications or sequelae	Immediate (before 3 mo)	Secondary (from 3 to 12 mo)	Late (after 1 yr)
Cardiorespiratory	0	0	0
Diaphragmatic hernias	0	1	2.5
Diarrhea	Approx. 50	5	1
Small-stomach syndrome	Approx. 100	30	1
Pylorospasm			6 (requiring secondary pyloroplasty)
Reflux esophagitis	28		5
Anastomotic stenosis and dilatations	0	9	4

REFERENCES

1. Boerema, I. Oesophagus resection with restoration of continuity by a gastric tube. Arch. Chir. Nederland. **4**:120, 1952.
2. Akiyama, H., Tsurumaru, M., Kawamura, T., and Ono, Y.: Principles of surgical treatment for carcinoma of the esophagus: analysis of lymph node involvement, Ann. Surg. **194**:438, 1981.
3. Maillet, P., Baulieux, J., Boulez, J., and Benhaim, R.; Carcinoma of the thoracic esophagus: results of one-stage surgery (271 cases), Am. J. Surg. **143**:629, 1982.
4. Couraud, L., and Meriot, S.: Le traitement des cancers du tiers inférieur et du tiers moyen de l'oesophage par résection et gastroplastie tubulée isopéristaltique, Chirurgie **108**:703, 1982.
5. Stephen, S.J., and Uragoda, C.G. Some technical modifications in esophageal resection for carcinoma, Thorax **27**:228, 1972.
6. Gignoux M., Segol, P., Olivier, J.M., and Brieard, H.: L'oesophago-gastro-plastie cervicale dans le traitement du cancer de l'oesophage thoracique, Lyon Chir. **74**:262, 1978.
7. Pissas, A., Doyon, J.F., Sarrazin, R., and Bouchet, Y.: Le drainage lympatique de l'estomac, J. Chir. **116**: 583, 1979.
8. Moreno-Osset, E., Tomas-Ridocci, M., París, F., Mora, F., Garcia-Zarza, A., Molina, R., and Pastor-Benages, A.: Motor activity of esophageal substitute, Ann. Thorac. Surg. (In press.)

DISCUSSION—Chapters 21 to 23

Earle W. Wilkins, Jr.

The principal issues in this discussion relate to (1) the elective surgical management of squamous carcinoma of the esophagus and (2) the role of partial esophagectomy in its management. The fact that Couraud and his colleagues include 41% nonsquamous tumors in their discussion (Chapter 22) in no way alters the impact of this particular commentary. The goal will be to discuss what is generally, worldwide, accepted as the standard or the norm in the surgical management of esophageal carcinoma.

RESECTION FOR SQUAMOUS CARCINOMA

Technical considerations in surgery for carcinoma involving the esophagus at any level can be reduced to certain finite considerations: surgical access to the esophagus, the viscus to be utilized for its replacement, the route or anatomic positioning of the substitute, and the level and technique of anastomosis.

Access. The options are numerous, primarily depending on the level of the tumor. They include left thoracoabdominal, left transthoracic, combined right thoracic and abdominal or right thoracoabdominal, combined abdominal and cervical, and transcervical with or without median sternotomy. The access chosen, in general, is determined by the level of tumor and the appropriate length of proximal margin. Experienced esophageal surgeons tend to have their own preferred approaches.

Viscus. Here the options are limited to three: stomach, colon, and jejunum. The stomach may be used as a transpositioned organ, being brought up isoperistaltically to the desired level, or as a reversed greater curvature tube, with the remainder being left in the abdominal location. The colon utilized depends on its arterial supply. In general, the left hemicolon is more suitable. It is placed in isoperistaltic direction. The jejunum may be used as a long loop or Roux limb deriving arterial supply from its abdominal mesentery or

as a free graft with microvascular anastomoses. (Gastric antrum and sigmoid colon have been similarly utilized for free grafts.)

Route. The preferred sites for placement of the substituting viscus are the posterior mediastinum (orthotopic position) and the anterior mediastinum (retrosternal position). However, the viscus may be brought up through either pleural space or even anterior to the sternum in the subcutaneous location.

Anastomosis. The surgeon must decide whether he or she prefers the anastomosis to lie within the thorax or in the neck. And the surgeon must decide whether it should be done by the manual placement of sutures or with the mechanical stapling device.

• • •

Wong is absolutely correct when he states that "surgeons must possess a repertoire of procedures that could be employed for tumors at various locations and of different stages." Management of the patient with carcinoma of the esophagus is not for the inexperienced or casual surgeon. Seventeen options have been listed for consideration, and even the experienced surgeon is advised to think through the possibilities in planning strategy and technique for a given patient.

Wong's report on the elective management of squamous cell carcinoma of the esophagus is an extraordinarily thorough and well-organized presentation of the subject. In addition to the options of techniques already mentioned, two points deserve emphasis and commentary.

1. General thoracic surgeons universally agree "that resection offers the best results in terms of palliation or cure." This is especially true in the stage I tumors picked up early in the evolution of symptoms or by screening techniques before the development of symptoms, usually in patients studied in areas of high geographic risk.[1] Unfortunately, in the usual North American experience patients are seldom encountered with stage I carcinomas. In those patients with stage II or III tumors, there has been remarkably little increase in survival of patients undergoing resection for

squamous carcinoma in the past 30 years. At the Massachusetts General Hospital, for instance, Sweet[2] reported in 1952 his 5-year patient survival statistics, "21% for patients with negative nodes and 7.5% for those with positive nodes." In 1983 Katlic and Grillo[3] at the same hospital reported 12% overall survival for stage II or III patients (actually 24% for stage II carcinomas and 6% for stage III). The latter study included an era of utilization of preoperative radiation therapy in selected cases.

There is a convincing need for adjuvant therapy in addition to extirpational surgery. A glimmer of hope has now appeared with the combined utilization of chemotherapy and radiation along with surgery.[4] At this time some form of protocol for combined therapy is advisable for *all* patients with squamous carcinoma of the esophagus. The Massachusetts General Hospital preference is for two cycles of cisplatin and 5-fluorouracil preoperatively with radiation postoperatively for patients with positive nodes or evidence of mediastinal invasion, then followed by six additional cycles of chemotherapy. More recently this postoperative chemotherapy has been limited to those patients who have shown response to preoperative treatment.[5]

2. In a malignant tumor of the potentially lethal nature of esophageal carcinoma, it is of the utmost importance that the therapy applied have nonlethal implications. Surgeons argue that one must "fight fire with fire." On the other hand, where only 12% of patients survive 5 years (Massachusetts General Hospital), one cannot afford to have a high hospital mortality following surgery. In their cumulative 1980 report, Earlam and Cunha-Melo[6] report 29% hospital deaths and 4% 5-year survivals. Their commentary that resection of esophageal squamous carcinoma has "the highest hospital mortality of any routinely performed surgical procedure to date" is devastating. A guiding principle in surgery should be that, when hospital mortality exceeds 5-year survival, the indications for and technique of a given surgical procedure should be seriously questioned and thoroughly reviewed.

The principal causes of operative mortality are (1) overzealous selection of patients for resections (particularly relating to age, pulmonary function, and extent of tumor), (2) anastomotic leakage, and (3) postoperative respiratory complications. Whatever the technical options chosen for resection, particular attention must be paid to the technique of anastomosis. Preservation of blood supply, avoidance of tension, avoidance of excessive trauma to the edges to be approximated, and use of interrupted sutures are more important than the material used. I do prefer a two-layer manually performed anastomosis to Wong's one-layer. His stated "leakage rate of not more than 5%" is commendable, but the goal should be 1% or less. Some have achieved this. I have no experience with stapled esophageal anastomoses, but Donnelly et al.[7] report no direct anastomotic leaks in 100 consecutive stapled anastomoses. The incidence of late stricture in stapled anastomoses as reported by Wong certainly requires careful monitoring.

ROLE OF PARTIAL ESOPHAGECTOMY

Definitions must first be established. *Total* technically means removal of the entire esophagus, including the cricopharyngeus. With very rare exceptions, surgeons do not use this operation. What esophageal surgeons in practice call "total esophagectomy" is usually resection of the abdominothoracic esophagus to within 2 cm of the cricopharyngeus sphincter with placement of the anastomosis in the neck. The purpose of this technique is twofold: (1) to minimize intramural recurrence of carcinoma and (2) to render management of an anastomotic leak, should it occur, technically easier and prognostically less ominous. Although substantive reasons, these are not categorically imperative. *Subtotal,* or near-total, esophagectomy is a more appropriate and exact term for this procedure. *Partial* esophagectomy, then, by definition, becomes anything less than subtotal, with the anastomosis performed within the thorax at an appropriate margin level above the carcinoma. Couraud is correct that "the gravity of complete resection is undoubtedly higher than that of partial resection." Preservation of the cricopharyngeus is essential to maintenance of normal swallowing mechanics and prevention of aspiration with its often fatal consequence. In addition, it is important to maintain normal innervation of the larynx, which is essential to avoidance of aspiration. Unless involved by gross tumor, the recurrent laryngeal nerves should be spared.

Partial esophagectomy remains the standard procedure for both squamous cell carcinoma and adenocarcinoma. One does indeed need to exercise caution about the extent of carcinoma submucosally above the tumor, more particularly in adenocarcinoma. Frozen-section pathologic analysis of the proximal resection margin is advisable.

This is an era when efforts are moving in opposing directions from the standard procedure of partial esophagectomy: (1) avoidance of thoracotomy with transhiatal esophagectomy (in my opinion, certainly a less "radical" procedure) and (2) extended procedures with en bloc "mediastinectomy"[8] and/or subtotal esophagectomy with cervical anastomoses. There seems to be no clearcut preferred procedure at least in terms of altered long-term survivals. The morbidity of the various techniques bear close monitoring as experience accumulates and time passes. Unless and until distinct advantages appear from such operations, the general thoracic surgeon may be well advised to continue use of the generally accepted standard, the partial esophagectomy. For the thoroughly trained esophageal surgeon, there is no substitute for individualization of indications and surgical techniques.

TUBULAR ISOPERISTALTIC GASTROPLASTY

In our experience it has rarely been necessary to use tubular isoperistaltic gastroplasty, although its rationale seems quite à propos when extensive lesser curvature resection is required because of left gastric nodal metastases. Our experience with it as a technical exercise dates back to the work of Sweet in extensive proximal gastrectomy for stricture.[9] Its potential hazard lies at the critical anastomotic point where the gastric tube suture line intersects the circumferential esophagogastric line. Leakage at this juncture is a risk.

A final point of Couraud's conclusion merits comment. If one does less than a total esophagectomy, or even subtotal esophagectomy, careful preoperative investigation of what would remain of the esophagus is an essential. This should include normal radiographic procedures plus computed tomography, thorough endoscopic visualization, and, as he suggests, careful screening with toluidine blue vital staining. To this one

should add intraoperative reevaluation. In experience at Massachusetts General Hospital, although multiple upper airway and alimentary tract carcinomas are common, multiple esophageal primary carcinomas have been unusual.

In conclusion, one should not arbitrarily discard the properly planned and executed partial esophagectomy.

REFERENCES

1. Shao, L., Li, Z., Liu, S., and Wong, M.: Surgical treatment of 210 cases of early carcinoma of the esophagus and gastric cardia, Zhonghua Waike Zazhi **19**(5):259, 1981.
2. Sweet, R.H.: The results of radical surgical extirpation in the treatment of carcinoma of the esophagus and cardia: with five-year survival statistics, Surg. Gynecol. Obstet. **94**:46, 1952.
3. Katlic, M.R., and Grillo, H.C.: Carcinoma of the esophagus: a current perspective. In Choi, N.C., and Grillo, H.C., editors: Thoracic oncology, New York, 1983, Raven Press, pp. 279-301.
4. Steiger, Z., Franklin, R., Wilson, R.F., et al.: Eradication and palliation of squamous cell carcinoma of the esophagus with chemotherapy, radiotherapy and surgical therapy, J. Thorac. Cardiovasc. Surg. **82**:713, 1981.
5. Carey, R.W., Hilgenberg, A.D., Wilkins, E.W., Jr., et al.: Preoperative chemotherapy followed by surgery with possible postoperative radiotherapy in squamous cell carcinoma of the esophagus: evaluation of chemotherapy component, J. Clin. Oncol. **4**:697, 1986.
6. Earlam, R., and Cunha-Melo, J.R.: Oesophageal squamous cell carcinoma: 1. A critical review of surgery, Br. J. Surg. **67**:381, 1980.
7. Donnelly, R.G., Sastry, M.R., and Wright, C.D.: Esophagogastrectomy using end-to-end anastomotic stapler: results of the first 100 patients, Thorax **40**:958, 1985.
8. Skinner, D.B.: En bloc resection for neoplasms of the esophagus and cardia, J. Thorac. Cardiovasc. Surg. **85**:59, 1983.
9. Sweet, R.H., Robbins, L.L., Gephart, F.T., and Wilkins, E.W., Jr.: The surgical treatment of peptic ulceration and stricture of the lower esophagus, Ann. Surg. **139**:258, 1954.

CHAPTER 24 En bloc resection for esophageal carcinoma

David B. Skinner

En bloc resection of esophageal cancer is indicated for patients in whom cure of localized or regional disease may be possible. It is a more extensive operation than a standard esophagectomy of the type which has been practiced routinely for the past 50 years.

RATIONALE

The development and application of an en bloc resection for esophageal cancer are based upon the classical theories of carcinogenesis and mechanisms of neoplastic spread. Most theories of neoplasia accept a single locus of cellular change as the origin of a cancer. Following a period of localized multiplication and spread within the tissue of origin, the neoplasm acquires the ability to penetrate adjacent dissimilar tissue. At some point, spread to remote sites by either lymphatic or hematogenous routes occurs. Lymphatic spread is typically in the adjacent region initially, whereas hematogenous spread is generally systemic. The time relationship between onset of lymphatic and onset of hematogenous spread of cancers remains unknown.

The role of surgery in the cure of cancer is limited to cases in which the disease is localized in the site of origin and adjacent tissues, and occasionally in patients with early lymphatic spread in the region. All other uses of surgery to treat any type of cancer are palliative and designed to eliminate or reduce symptoms and complications caused by the tumor mass. For most organs, curative surgery applies the principle of an en bloc resection of tissues surrounding the site of origin of the neoplasm in an effort to obtain complete local and regional control of those cancers that have not disseminated. In many organs, for truly localized cancers surgery alone achieves 5-year survival rates of 60% or more.

Until recently, surgery for esophageal cancer was widely regarded as palliative, and long-term cures were considered to be accidental. The reasons for this pessimistic attitude about surgical treatment of esophageal cancer are several. When esophageal cancer becomes symptomatic by causing dysphagia, the disease is already at an advanced stage. Because of the ability of esophageal smooth muscle to distend without sensation of increased pressure, almost circumferential invasion of the esophageal wall by a cancer is required before the presenting symptom of dysphagia occurs.[1] Since the diametric capacity of the esophagus is several centimeters, there are no small early esophageal cancers causing the symptom of dysphagia. As a result, many cases are systemic or regionally advanced at the time of presentation and there are no hopes for surgical cure in such cases. In fact, the 5-year survival rate for treatment of symptomatic esophageal cancer has been so low (5% range) in many series that some have proposed that esophageal cancer is different from other types of cancer and must be a systemic disease from its onset.

A second reason for the lack of enthusiasm for attempted curative resection of esophageal cancer is the location of the esophagus. Its proximity to vital organs, the small amount of surrounding tissue that can be removed, and difficulties in exposure have made the application of en bloc resection principles seem impossible to many.

Third, inaccessibility of the esophagus for detailed study has made preoperative staging, and selection of patients for possible cure, rather difficult. There has been no consistent agreement on a pathologic staging system that has been widely adopted, predictive of prognosis, and usable for patient selection.

Recent information has led to a reexamination of these three reasons why en bloc resection has not been applied more consistently in the treatment of esophageal cancer. Numerous investigators now demonstrate that esophageal cancer can be diagnosed with a high degree of sensitivity and specificity by esophageal cytology.[2,3] High-

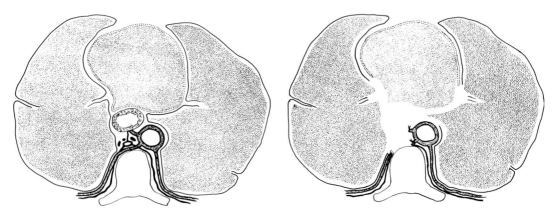

Fig. 24-1. Diagram showing the structures immediately adjacent to the esophagus in the posterior mediastinum and outlining the extent of the radical resection to include removal of adjacent pericardium, pleura bilaterally, arterial and venous supply to the esophagus, lymphatic drainage through the thoracic duct, and the azygos vein system in the posterior mediastinum. When complete, the dissection leaves only the myocardium, lungs, aorta, and vertebral bodies remaining in the posterior mediastinum.

risk groups of patients for development of esophageal neoplasia are known, and the application of cytologic screening can lead to early diagnosis of presymptomatic esophageal cancer in a number of instances.[4,5] When such patients with asymptomatic tumors less than 2 cm in size, and without penetration through the esophageal wall, without lymph node metastases, and without systemic metastases are treated by surgical resection, high cure rates (85% at 5 years) are reported.[6] This indicates that esophageal carcinoma behaves in a manner similar to carcinomas in other organs for which local extensive resections offer good prospects for surgical cure. Clearly, esophageal carcinoma is not a systemic disease from its onset.

Review of the embryology of esophageal development and the anatomic relationships of the esophagus to other structures demonstrates that an en bloc resection of the esophagus within an envelope of surrounding healthy tissue is achievable. This was first pointed out by Logan for carcinomas of the cardia,[7] and subsequently extended for carcinomas at all levels within the esophagus.[8] As with any digestive tract cancer, the tumor-bearing esophagus should be removed with its "serosa" and mesentery included in the resection. Embryologically, there is a mesoesophagus suspending the esophagus dorsally from the aortic arch distally, and determining the direction of lymphatic drainage and vascular supply. Removal of this dorsal mesoesophagus can be achieved by dissecting on the wall of the aorta and vertebral bodies, and including the azygos vein and thoracic duct within the dissection along with the dorsal lymphatic and fatty tissues adjacent to the esophagus. As with any muscle, the

esophageal longitudinal muscle must have sites of origin and insertion. Anatomic studies demonstrate that the subpleural and subpericardial fibrous tissue serves as a site of muscle attachment for the esophagus, and in effect provides a serosal-like function in this regard. It is quite feasible anatomically to remove the adjacent pericardium and pleura where they abut on the esophagus as part of the en bloc resection of the total organ. Such an analysis of the embryology and anatomy of the esophagus indicates that en bloc resection principles can be applied to removal of this organ when cure may be achievable. For complete removal of the tumor-bearing esophagus and cure of patients with early spread into tissues adjacent to the mucosa, such an en bloc resection is logical and recommended (Fig. 24-1).

Cephalad to the aortic arch, the lymphatic spread of the esophagus is more circumferential and extends into the cervical lymph node chains. These too can be removed along with the esophagus to provide a more complete regional control for carcinoma of the upper one third.

The availability of a substantial number of esophagectomy specimens and knowledge of prognosis permit multivariant analysis of factors influencing prognosis for esophageal cancer. Such information can serve as the basis for a refined staging system for the pathologic classification of esophageal cancer. This in turn provides the basis for preoperative clinical staging. Such a multivariant analysis shows that only the degree of esophageal muscular wall penetration, and the presence and number of lymph node metastases influence prognosis as independent variables.[9] Size of the primary tumor, the degree of cellular

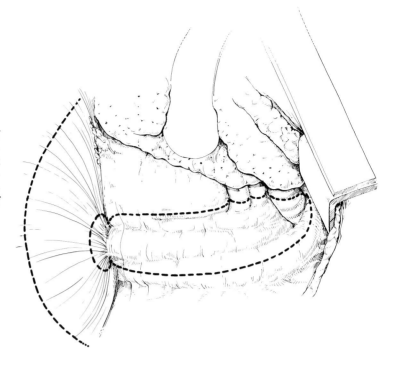

Fig. 24-2. Outline of the extent of radical dissection in the mediastinum performed through a left thoracotomy to include pericardium, pleura, and a cuff of diaphragm on the lateral aspect of the esophagus.

differentiation, the level of location within the esophagus, and the cell type (adenocarcinoma versus squamous carcinoma) do not influence prognosis independently of the depth of wall penetration and lymph node metastases.

The availability of computed tomography (CT) scans of the chest and abdomen, radionuclide scans, and the upcoming availability of magnetic resonance imaging permit new methods for visualizing esophageal and mediastinal tissues before surgery, and offer the promise that reasonably accurate clinical staging can be achieved based upon evidence of probable wall penetration and enlarged lymph nodes. This in turn offers the promise that choices can be made as to whether therapy for esophageal cancer offers any hope of cure, or whether only palliation should be the objective.[10]

With this information, it appears that the role for en bloc esophagectomy can be defined. This operation should be undertaken in patients in whom preoperative staging indicates that the disease may be localized to the esophagus itself or with only early spread through the wall, or to immediately adjacent lymph nodes. The anatomic principles for en bloc resection, surgical techniques, and knowledge of potential complications and risk are well worked out. The surgeon and the physician treating patients with esophageal cancer have choices to make on the basis of whether the disease is potentially curable.

SURGICAL TECHNIQUE

The concept of en bloc resection is not one of a more extensive removal of remote lymph nodes, but rather a removal of the tumor-bearing esophagus with an envelope of all available surrounding tissue in an effort to provide thorough local and regional control of the cancer and its early spread. If there are remote lymph node metastases more than 10 cm from the primary tumor, or if there is evidence of systemic disease, the patient is incurable by surgery, and an en bloc resection is not indicated.

The first step in the operation is the assessment of possible spread of disease. This is done by thorough preoperative review of available scans and staging procedures. At operation, organs available for inspection such as liver and lungs are evaluated for possible metastatic disease missed by preoperative studies. The limits of the en bloc resection are identified, usually 10 cm proximal and distal to the palpable tumor. Lymph nodes are excised for frozen-section examination at these limits of the planned resection. Positive lymph nodes or cancer tissue at such a remote site indicates no hope for curative resection, and a more limited resection for palliation is considered. The distance of 10 cm from the proximal tumor is chosen on the basis of pathology studies documenting submucosal and intramural spread of esophageal primary cancers up to this distance

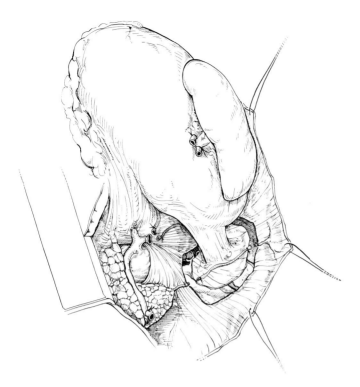

Fig. 24-3. Following division of the splenic vessels and removal of the mediastinum from the colon and mesocolon, the stomach and spleen are retracted anteriorly to provide exposure to the celiac axis and hiatus. The left gastric artery is ligated at its origin, and the left inferior phrenic artery is divided as it comes from under the adrenal gland. A cuff of diaphragm is resected surrounding the tumor mass. Through the enlarged hiatus, the thoracic duct and azygos vein are divided near the aortic hiatus.

in potentially curable cases, but not beyond.[11]

The plan for achieving 10-cm margins dictates the surgical approach. For carcinomas whose proximal extent is 10 cm or more below the aortic arch pulsation on esophagoscopy, operation is performed through a left thoracotomy (Fig. 24-2). This provides optimal exposure for meticulous dissection around the primary tumor mass when it is near the esophageal hiatus, and provides good access to the upper abdomen for removal of the proximal stomach and adjacent left gastric lymph nodes and perigastric tissue near the hiatus. Thoracotomy is performed in the sixth interspace. The diaphragm is detached around its periphery to expose the upper abdomen. Lymph nodes are biopsied from the mediastinum 10 cm cephalad to the palpable tumor, and at the celiac axis. The tumor mass itself is palpated to be sure that it is not fixed to adjacent structures. If these initial findings are favorable, en bloc resection is begun.

Because of its proximity to the tumor and because lymph node drainage along the short gastric vessels represents regional and not remote spread, the spleen is mobilized and included in the resection. After division of the splenic vessels, the dissection is carried along the splenic artery to the celiac axis. The left gastric artery is ligated and divided. All tissues in the retroperitoneum cephalad to the pancreas are swept up into the esophageal hiatus (Fig. 24-3). A margin of diaphragm muscles around the hiatus is excised with

the specimen, using cautery for hemostasis. This removal of a rim of diaphragm with the esophagus opens the hiatus widely. Through the aperture, it is straightforward to identify the thoracic duct and origins of the azygos vein on the vertebral bodies. These are ligated and divided to start the mediastinal dissection. Points for transection on the stomach are identified 10 cm distal to the tumor mass on both the greater and the lesser curvature. The omentum is dissected from the colon and included in the gastric part of the resection. Adenocarcinoma arising within the tubular esophagus is regarded as a primary esophageal cancer rather than a primary gastric carcinoma. For such adenocarcinomas, we do not routinely practice total gastrectomy. However, if the cancer is clearly of gastric origin, current data suggest that a total gastrectomy is advisable.

After completion of the abdominal dissection, the diaphragm is replaced in its original site by retractors, and the chest dissection begins. An incision is made in the pleura overlying the aorta. Periaortic tissues are swept toward the esophagus. The bronchoesophageal vessels are ligated and divided. Medially the dissection is continued on the aortic wall until the vertebral bodies are reached. The right intercostal artery and left intercostal veins are ligated together as they pass from the aorta medially. This permits access under the azygos vein on the surface of the vertebral bodies. The hemiazygos vein is ligated as it courses under the aorta, as is the accessory hemi-

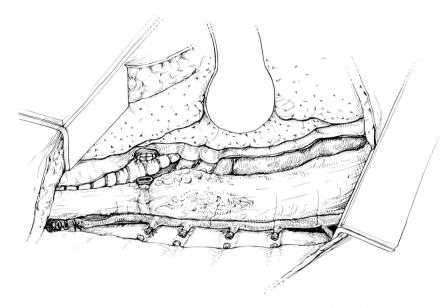

Fig. 24-4. Extent of the en bloc resection of the posterior mediastinum through a right thoracotomy for middle-third carcinoma. The azygos vein is divided flush with the vena cava, and the branches to the azygos are divided as they pass onto the vertebral bodies. The pericardium is incised anteriorly to the pulmonary ligament and onto the pulmonary veins. The subcarinal lymph nodes are removed with the specimen.

azygos vein. As the vertebral body is cleared, the dissection progresses toward the right chest. The extensions of the right intercostal arteries and veins are again divided as they pass off into the right thorax, completing the posterior dissection.

Superiorly, the dissection is carried through the pleura to the wall of the esophagus at the pre-selected 10-cm mark above the tumor. The vagus nerves are divided at this level. The pericardium is entered on the back of the pulmonary veins and atrium. The pleuropericardial reflection on the left side is incised from the pulmonary hilum down to the diaphragm. By pulling on the edge of the incised pericardium, the surgeon can identify from within the pericardium the reflection of the pericardium off the right pulmonary veins without difficulty. An incision in this pericardium leads to entry into the right pleural cavity, and the right pleuropericardial reflection is incised from within the pericardium. When this is done, the only remaining attachment of the mediastinal structures encasing the esophagus is the right pulmonary ligament, which is easily divided. Now the esophagus is completely mobilized within a sheath of hopefully healthy surrounding tissues. The only place at which the esophagus is actually seen is at the upper margin of the dissection, 10 cm proximal to the tumor.

If the primary tumor is an adenocarcinoma, and all glandular epithelium is included within the esophagus at the site of transection below the aortic arch, an anastomosis of the colon or stomach may be made to the esophagus at this point. If the primary carcinoma is squamous cell, dissection is carried on the wall of the esophagus up to the neck, and a subtotal esophagectomy is done in every case because of the approximately 10% likelihood of multifocal squamous cell carcinoma.

The organ used for esophageal reconstruction depends principally on the surgeon's choice. In highly favorable cases in which the patient's condition is quite stable after the resection, we prefer the use of an isoperistaltic colon segment because this avoids the risk of postoperative reflux esophagitis, which follows esophagogastrostomy in approximately 30% of patients. This is unfortunately proving true even in cases in which the esophagogastric anastomosis is made in the neck. However, the colon is unsuitable for use as an interposition in some patients because of previous or concurrent colonic disease, and the preparation of the colon for interposition adds extra time and trauma to an already lengthy and extensive operation.

For carcinomas of the middle third of the esophagus closer than 10 cm to the aortic arch, the operation is done through a right thoracotomy (Fig. 24-4). A similar dissection is carried out, with the exception that the abdominal portion of the resection is not necessary in cases in which the primary tumor is more than 10 cm above the hiatus. Once again the dissection begins on the vertebral body by incising the right pleura and dissecting underneath the intercostal vessels, azygos vein, and thoracic duct until the medial wall of the aorta is reached. The right intercostal vessels are ligated at this point, and the bronchoesophageal arteries are ligated flush with the aorta. This dissection is carried distally for 10 cm and proximally for as much distance as available until the base of the neck is reached.

Anteriorly the azygos vein is divided flush with the vena cava and oversewn. The tracheoesophageal groove is dissected, with care being taken to preserve the recurrent laryngeal nerves. Subcarinal lymph nodes are dissected with the specimen, and the pericardium is entered at its reflection off the top of the atrium. The right pleuropericardial groove is incised to open the pericardium widely where it is adjacent to the tumor. By dissection within the pericardium, the left pleuropericardial groove is entered. This mobilizes the entire esophagus with the exception of the left pulmonary ligament, which is divided.

A place for transection of the esophagus is identified 10 cm proximal to the tumor or at the highest point available, and the esophagus is removed. The organ chosen for replacement is mobilized and passed up through the posterior mediastinum. Normally this is done through a separate incision and by a second team working in the abdomen while the en bloc resection is being done transthoracically. The thoracic and abdominal incisions are closed, and the final anastomosis is done in the neck.

For carcinomas arising above the aortic arch, the preferred exposure is a transverse cervical incision with a partial sternotomy to provide full exposure of the esophagus and trachea down to the level of the aortic arch. Bilateral modified radical neck dissections are carried out to remove all fibrofatty and lymphatic tissues from the carotid sheath and bring them into the resection plane adjacent to the esophagus. The jugular vein, vagus nerve, and carotid arteries are preserved but skeletonized with the removal of their surrounding tissues. The recurrent nerves are readily identified as they join the tracheoesophageal groove at the level of the aortic arch and the right subclavian artery. The nerves are preserved and tissues posterior to the nerve are dissected free onto the wall of the esophagus. Exposure obtained through this approach is excellent.

Below the aortic arch the esophagus is removed by dissection on its muscular wall, which can be done without a full sternotomy or thoracotomy by dissecting upward through the hiatus and downward from the partial sternotomy incision. The organ chosen for replacement is advanced through the posterior mediastinum and anasto-

mosed to the esophagus as high as possible. If the tumor involves the cricopharyngeus, laryngectomy is necessary and the anastomosis is done to the hypopharynx. If free margins can be obtained and the larynx still preserved, the anastomosis may be done at the cricopharyngeal sphincter muscle.

POSTOPERATIVE MANAGEMENT, MORBIDITY, AND MORTALITY

For patients with an extensive mediastinal dissection around the lung roots and including removal of the thoracic duct, a large amount of fluid replacement is required in the first 24 to 48 hours after surgery. This is presumably due to fluid sequestration at the site of the lymphatic beds. After 48 to 72 hours such fluid is mobilized apparently through expanding lymphatic collaterals.

Because of this large fluid load, many patients have decreased pulmonary compliance and require respirator support for approximately 72 hours after surgery. When the diuretic phase is well established, efforts begin to wean the patient from the respirator. Other than this requirement for additional respirator support, management of patients undergoing en bloc esophagectomy is similar to that for patients undergoing the traditional routine esophagectomy.

In addition to technical considerations, the principal complications, as expected, are cardiac and pulmonary. When postoperative complications of all types are considered, approximately one half of patients have a complication—a morbidity rate similar to that from a standard esophagectomy.

Among 11 en bloc esophagectomy cases recently reviewed, the 30-day hospital mortality was 1, or 10%. An additional two patients died after the first month in and out of the hospital from causes that could be related to the surgical procedure. This mortality rate in the range of 10% is quite comparable to that reported in a number of series for standard esophagectomy, and is nearly identical to the mortality rate for standard esophagectomy performed in our clinic during the same time interval in 36 patients.

RESULTS

Survival following en bloc esophagectomy is influenced by operative mortality, which is a randomly scattered event unrelated to cancer staging, by a possible impact of preoperative or postoperative adjuvant chemotherapy or radiation, and by the stage of the tumor based upon the two factors of degree of wall penetration and lymph node status. In our series, preoperative radiation or chemotherapy had a negative impact on patient survival that was statistically significant.[10] When those cases classified as 30-day hospital mortality or receiving preoperative adjuvant therapy are excluded, the impact of staging on survival is even more dramatic. Following en bloc esophagectomy, 2-year and 5-year survival respectively in patients without full-thickness wall penetration and lymph node spread was 78% and 55%. When there were one to four positive lymph nodes but no full-thickness spread, 2-year survival was 64%, and 5-year survival was 30%. When there was full wall penetration but no positive lymph nodes, survival was 56% and 15% respectively. However, when both full wall penetration and positive lymph nodes were present, 2-year survival was only 12% and 5-year survival 2%.

En bloc esophagectomy seems particularly valuable in patients with early spread in the local region, because a dissection limited to the wall of the esophagus is unlikely to produce long-term survivors among patients with full-thickness wall penetration or regional lymph node metastases. Because of the importance of these staging factors to prognosis, it is not possible to compare the results of different kinds of esophageal resection among different clinics unless the staging is clearly specified. In our clinic, patients treated by en bloc resection for a variety of reasons have had better survival curves than those of comparable stage treated by standard esophagectomy. However, there is no pretention that this is a randomized trial. Such a randomized trial is unlikely to resolve the issue, because the more extensive resection produces more tissue for pathology analysis and is thereby likely to lead to more precise staging, which influences the results.

A second factor speaking in favor of the more extensive resection when disease is potentially curable is the observation that local mediastinal or anastomotic recurrences as the primary site of recurrence occur in only 5% of surviving patients. Hence, the argument for en bloc esophagectomy is based both on excellent local and regional control of the disease and on apparent improved survival in patients whose cancers are beginning the process of local and regional penetration.

SUMMARY

En bloc esophagectomy is a surgical technique for obtaining more thorough removal of the tissue surrounding the primary tumor of the esophagus. It is not conceived as an extended lymph node dissection, which would be of dubious value outside the immediate region of the tumor. Although a somewhat lengthier operation, en bloc esophagectomy can be performed with morbidity and mortality comparable to those of standard esophagectomy in our own series and in other series reported. The operation appears to have a sound anatomic and embryologic rationale. Results achieved appear beneficial for patients with early local and regional spread of the disease, and the operation is effective in preventing mediastinal and anastomotic recurrences. En bloc esophagectomy is advocated for patients who may have potentially curable esophageal cancer at all levels within the esophagus and regardless of cell type.

REFERENCES

1. Sweet, R.H.: The results of radical surgical extirpation in treatment of carcinoma of the esophagus and cardia with five-year survival statistics, Surg. Gynecol. Obstet. **94:**46, 1952.
2. Dowlatshahi, K., Skinner, D.B., DeMeester, T.R., Zachary, L., Bibbo, M., and Wied, G.L.: Evaluation of brush cytology as an independent technique for detection of esophageal carcinoma, J. Thorac. Cardiovasc. Surg. **89:**848, 1985.
3. Gephart, T., and Graham, R.M.: The cellular detection of carcinoma of the esophagus, Surg. Gynecol. Obstet. **108:**75, 1959.
4. Dowlatshahi, K., Mobarhan, S., and Daneshbod, A.: Clinical studies of carcinoma of the esophagus in north Iran, Digestion 16(3):237, 1977.
5. Livstone, E.M., and Skinner, M.D.: Tumors of the esophagus. In Berk, J.E., editor: Bockus gastroenterology, vol. 2, Philadelphia, 1985, W.B. Saunders Co., pp. 819-821.
6. Huang, K.C., et al.: Diagnosis and surgical treatment of early esophageal carcinoma. In Stipa, S., Belsey, R.H.R., and Moraldi, A., editors: Medical and surgical problems of the esophagus, vol. 43, New York, 1981, Academic Press, pp. 269-299.
7. Logan, A.: The surgical treatment of carcinoma of the esophagus and cardia, J. Thorac. Cardiovasc. Surg. **46:**150, 1963.
8. Skinner, D.B.: En bloc resection for neoplasms of the esophagus and cardia, J. Thor. Cardiovasc. Surg. **85:**59, 1983.
9. Skinner, D.B., Dowlatshahi, K.D., and DeMeester, T.R.: Potentially curable cancer of the esophagus, Cancer **50:**2571, 1982.
10. Skinner, D.B., Little, A.G., Ferguson, M.K., Soriano, A., and Staszak, V.M.: Selection of operation for esophageal cancer based on staging, Ann. Surg. (In press.)
11. Miller, C.: Carcinoma of the thoracic oesophagus and cardia: a review of 405 cases, Br. J. Surg. **49:**507, 1962.

25 Transhiatal esophagectomy without thoracotomy for esophageal carcinoma

Mark B. Orringer

BACKGROUND AND HISTORY

In almost every reported major series of esophageal resections for carcinoma, *pulmonary complications* following a combined thoracoabdominal procedure and *sepsis* from disruption of an intrathoracic esophageal anastomosis are the leading causes of postoperative complications and death. Although some recently reported exceptional series indicate a hospital mortality for esophageal resection of less than 5%[1-3] in most reports, mortality ranges from 15% to 40%[4-6] and averages 33%.[7] Transhiatal "blunt" esophagectomy without thoracotomy and esophageal reconstruction with a cervical esophagogastric anastomosis offer several advantages over the standard transthoracic approach. The operation not only minimizes the physiologic insult to the patient by avoiding a thoracotomy but also places the anastomosis in the neck, where the consequences of disruption are seldom serious.

Transhiatal esophagectomy dates back to the days before successful endotracheal anesthesia was available. Denk reported the first blunt transmediastinal esophagectomy without thoracotomy using a vein stripper to avulse the esophagus from the posterior mediastinum of cadavers.[8] The British surgeon Gray-Turner reported the first successful transhiatal esophagectomy for carcinoma, and he reestablished continuity of the alimentary tract with an antethoracic skin tube at a later stage.[9] As endotracheal anesthesia became feasible, however, direct transthoracic esophagectomy became the standard operation, and transhiatal esophagectomy without thoracotomy was virtually forgotten. For the most part, transhiatal esophagectomy has been used most commonly in patients undergoing resection of pharyngeal or cervical carcinomas, where after laryngopharyngectomy and removal of an essentially normal thoracic esophagus, the stomach has been used to restore alimentary tract continuity.[10-12] Until relatively recently, there were few reports of the use of transhiatal resection for the diseased intrathoracic esophagus.[13,14] My personal experience with nearly 300 patients undergoing transhiatal esophageal resection both for benign and for malignant disease,[15-18] as well as the reported experience of others with this technique,[19-22] has provided justification for my belief that a thoracotomy is seldom required in order to resect the esophagus either for benign or for malignant disease.

INDICATIONS AND CONTRAINDICATIONS

I approach virtually every patient who is felt to be a candidate for esophageal resection for carcinoma as though a transhiatal resection will be possible. Bronchoscopic evidence of tracheobronchial *invasion* by the tumor is an absolute contraindication to this technique. Patients with *biopsy-proven* distant metastatic disease (e.g., hepatic nodule or supraclavicular lymph node) are not considered candidates for esophagectomy, because of their markedly limited life expectancy. Within reason, a tissue diagnosis of metastatic disease is demanded before a patient is designated unsuitable for esophageal resection. In our experience, CT scan criteria for resectability of esophageal carcinoma have not proven reliable, and I emphasize that *contiguity* of the esophageal tumor with the aortic or prevertebral fascia is *not* synonymous with *invasion*. Among our last 152

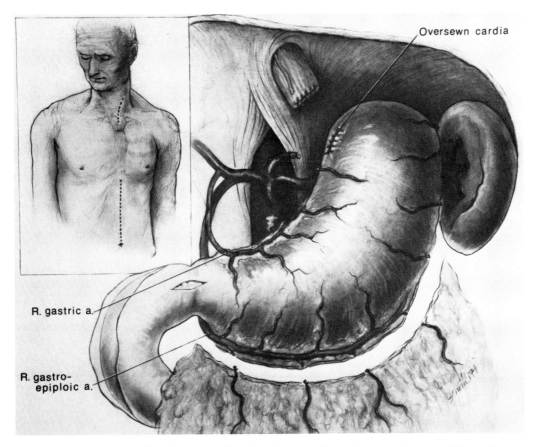

Fig. 25-1. Gastric mobilization for esophageal replacement bases the stomach on the right gastric and right gastroepiploic vascular arcades after division of the left gastric and left gastroepiploic vessels. A pyloromyotomy and Kocher maneuver are routine. (From Orringer, M.B., and Sloan, H.: J. Thorac. Cardiovasc. Surg. **70:**836, 1975.)

consecutive patients with carcinoma of the intrathoracic esophagus, transhiatal resection has been possible in all but five regardless of the findings of the CT scan. The single most important contraindication to transhiatal esophagectomy is the assessment by the surgeon palpating the tumor through the diaphragmatic hiatus that there is fixation to adjacent tissues, which makes proceeding with a blunt resection dangerous. The surgeon *must* be prepared to open the thorax and perform a standard esophageal resection, and should not view his or her inability or unwillingness to persist with a difficult transhiatal resection as an indication of defeat.

TECHNIQUE

The patient is positioned supine, with the neck extended by a small folded sheet placed beneath the scapulae. The head is turned to the right, and the occiput is stabilized on a head ring. The op-

erative field extends from the mandible to the pubis and laterally to both midaxillary lines. A radial artery catheter for continuous intraoperative monitoring is secured in place, and the arms are padded and placed at the patient's side so that the surgeon and assistants have access to the neck, chest, and abdomen. Exposure in the abdomen is greatly enhanced by use of a self-retaining table-mounted upper abdominal retractor.

The abdominal procedure

Through an upper midline incision, the stomach is inspected for any evidence of tumor invasion (e.g., involvement by celiac axis lymph node metastases or infiltration of the gastric wall) that might preclude use of the stomach as an esophageal substitute. Gastric mobilization begins along the greater curvature of the stomach, where the course of the right gastroepiploic artery is carefully identified (Fig. 25-1). The greater omentum is mobilized away from the high greater curvature of the stomach by dividing and ligating

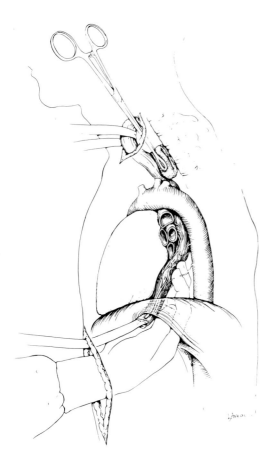

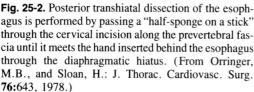

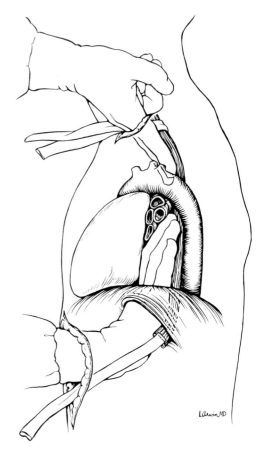

Fig. 25-2. Posterior transhiatal dissection of the esophagus is performed by passing a "half-sponge on a stick" through the cervical incision along the prevertebral fascia until it meets the hand inserted behind the esophagus through the diaphragmatic hiatus. (From Orringer, M.B., and Sloan, H.: J. Thorac. Cardiovasc. Surg. **76:**643, 1978.)

Fig. 25-3. Anterior transhiatal dissection of the esophagus is a mirror-image of the posterior dissection, this time performed with the volar aspects of the fingers against the anterior esophagus and avoiding injury to the carina. (From Orringer, M.B.: Transhiatal blunt esophagectomy without thoracotomy. In Cohn, L.H., editor: Modern technics in surgery: cardiothoracic surgery, New York, 1983, Futura Publishing Co.)

the short gastric and left gastroepiploic vessels far enough away from the stomach to avoid ischemic necrosis. Care is taken to avoid injury to the spleen. The greater omentum is then similarly freed from the low greater curvature of the stomach, with care being taken to preserve the right gastroepiploic artery. Mobilization of the greater omentum is carried out to the level of the pyloroduodenal area.

The avascular gastrohepatic omentum along the lesser curvature of the stomach is incised, the right gastric artery is identified and preserved, and gastric mobilization along the high lesser curvature is continued by dividing the terminal branches of the left gastric artery near the stomach. If lymph nodes involved by metastatic tumor can be dissected away from the celiac axis vessels, they are removed with the tumor. But rather than risk major hemorrhage, when celiac axis nodal metastases are extensive, the left gastric

artery is divided as close to the stomach as possible. A pyloromyotomy is performed routinely to prevent delayed gastric emptying, which may follow the vagotomy that accompanies the esophagectomy. A generous Kocher maneuver is carried out to maximize the upward reach of the mobilized stomach. A 14 French rubber jejunostomy tube, secured in place with a Witzel maneuver, is inserted routinely in all of our patients undergoing esophageal resection.

The gastroesophageal junction is then encircled with a rubber drain and retracted downward as gentle blunt mobilization of the lower 5 to 10 cm of the esophagus from the mediastinum is carried out through the diaphragmatic hiatus. The hiatus is gently dilated, one finger at a time, until the hand can be inserted into the posterior mediastinum. Intraarterial blood pressure is monitored during this and subsequent portions of the transhiatal dissection to prevent prolonged hypotension, which may result from displacement of the heart by the hand inserted into the posterior mediastinum. The tumor-containing portion of the intrathoracic esophagus is grasped and "rocked" from side to side to document that the esophagus is in fact mobile and amenable to transhiatal resection.

The cervical procedure

Through an oblique incision that parallels the anterior border of the left sternocleidomastoid muscle, the sternocleidomastoid muscle and carotid sheath are retracted laterally and the trachea and thyroid gland medially as the prevertebral fascia is approached. It may be necessary to ligate the middle thyroid vein and/or inferior thyroid artery. The cervical esophagus is identified immediately anterior to the prevertebral fascia. During the entire cervical dissection, the recurrent laryngeal nerve in the tracheoesophageal groove is protected from retractors to avoid nerve injury, which may result in cricopharyngeal motor dysfunction and disastrous complications from aspiration. The cervical esophagus is separated from the trachea and encircled with a rubber drain. This drain is then retracted superiorly with one hand, as the volar aspects of the fingers, closely applied to the esophagus, are used to sweep away the loose fibroareolar esophageal attachments within the superior mediastinum.

The transhiatal dissection

With upward traction on the rubber drain encircling the cervical esophagus, and one hand through the diaphragmatic hiatus posterior to the esophagus, a "half-sponge on a stick" is gently inserted downward through the cervical incision along the prevertebral fascia, sweeping the esophagus anteriorly, until the sponge stick from above meets the hand from below (Fig. 25-2). Posterior mobilization of the esophagus is now complete. A 28 French Argyle Saratoga sump catheter inserted through the cervical incision and downward into the mediastinum permits evacuation of blood and facilitates inspection of the mediastinum through the diaphragmatic hiatus in a relatively dry field. The anterior esophageal dissection is performed as a mirror image of the posterior dissection, this time keeping the volar aspects of the fingers against the anterior aspect of the esophagus (Fig. 25-3). As the carina is approached, pressure should be exerted posteriorly against the esophagus, sweeping it away from the membranous trachea and the pericardium. If the tumor is fixed to the tracheobronchial tree or aorta in this region, persistent dissection

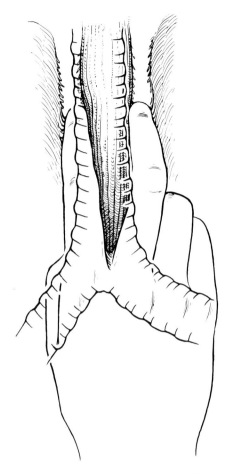

Fig. 25-4. Lateral transhiatal dissection of the esophagus is performed by the hand inserted upward from the diaphragmatic hiatus into the superior mediastinum until the circumferentially mobilized upper esophagus is palpated. (From Orringer, M.B.: Transhiatal blunt esophagectomy without thoracotomy. In Cohn, L.H., editor: Modern technics in surgery: cardiothoracic surgery, New York, 1983, Futura Publishing Co.)

may result in injury to the membranous trachea or to the aorta. When a "half-sponge on a stick" inserted through the cervical incision, anterior to the esophagus, meets the surgeon's hand inserted from below along the anterior esophagus, the anterior esophageal mobilization has been completed.

After circumferential mobilization of the upper 5 to 8 cm of the esophagus through the cervical incision and the lower 8 to 10 cm of the intrathoracic esophagus through the abdominal incision, the right hand is then inserted through the diaphragmatic hiatus anterior to the esophagus and is advanced upward behind the trachea until the index and middle fingers can palpate the circumferentially mobilized upper esophagus and lateral attachments, which are still intact (Fig. 25-4). The esophagus is "trapped" against the

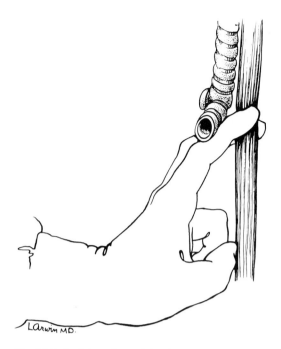

L.Arwin M.D.

Fig. 25-5. Avulsion of remaining lateral esophageal attachments by downward raking motion of hand. The esophagus is trapped against the prevertebral fascia by the index and middle fingers. (From Orringer, M.B.: Transhiatal blunt esophagectomy without thoracotomy. In Cohn, L.H., editor: Modern technics in surgery: cardiothoracic surgery, New York, 1983, Futura Publishing Co.)

prevertebral fascia by the index and middle fingers as a downward raking motion of the hand avulses any small remaining periesophageal attachments (Fig. 25-5). When the entire thoracic esophagus is mobile, several centimeters of esophagus are drawn upward into the cervical incision, and the GIA surgical stapler is used to divide the esophagus in the neck. A rubber drain is sutured to the divided distal esophagus with a heavy no. 1 silk suture. Traction on the stomach then draws the intrathoracic esophagus into the abdomen, pulling its attached rubber drain through the mediastinum. The cervical and abdominal ends of the rubber drain traversing the mediastinum are then secured with hemostats, and the esophagogastric esophagus is divided with several applications of the GIA surgical stapler. The divided cardia is oversewn with a running 4-0 polypropylene Lembert stitch. In most normal patients, if the mobilized stomach is placed on the anterior thorax, it will be seen that the gastric fundus will reach 2 to 4 cm above the level of the clavicles, particularly if the fibroareolar tissue along the distal branches of the left gastric artery is cleaned away from the lesser curvature of the stomach (Fig.

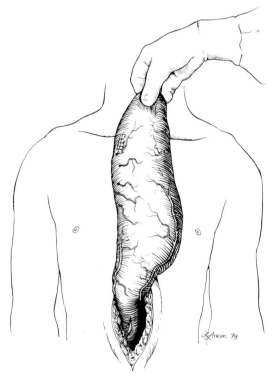

Arwin 79

Fig. 25-6. Cephalad reach of the mobilized stomach placed on the anterior chest wall usually extends 2 to 4 cm above the level of the clavicles. The high greater curvature of the gastric fundus, *not* the divided cardia, reaches most superiorly to the neck. (From Orringer, M.B.: Esophageal replacement using stomach substernally and after blunt esophagectomy. In Nyhus, L.M., and Baker, R.J., editors: Mastery of surgery, Boston, 1984, Little, Brown & Co.)

25-6). If the stomach reaches to the clavicles on the anterior thorax, it will clearly reach to the neck through the posterior mediastinum, which is the shortest distance between the abdominal cavity and the cervical esophagus. Before positioning of the stomach into the posterior mediastinum, both pleurae are inspected through the diaphragmatic hiatus both manually and by direct vision, and if entry into either chest has occurred during the esophagectomy, a chest tube is inserted and connected to underwater seal. After identification of the portion of the gastric fundus that will reach most superiorly to the neck, this point on the stomach is sutured to a transmediastinal rubber drain with several fine silk sutures (Fig. 25-7). Gentle traction on the cervical end of the transmediastinal drain draws the gastric fundus through the diaphragmatic hiatus and into the posterior mediastinum. With a combination of traction on the mediastinal rubber drain and guidance by the hand inserted through the diaphragmatic hiatus from below, the stomach is manipulated into the posterior mediastinum until the fundus is visible at the cervical end of the incision. The gastric fundus is then suspended in the neck by suture to the prevertebral fascia with two interrupted 3-0 polypropylene sutures.

Before the cervical esophagogastric anastomosis is begun, the abdominal portion of the operation is completed to prevent contamination by exposure to intraoral bacteria, which may occur once the cervical esophagus is opened. The jejunostomy tube is brought out through a separate left-upper-quadrant stab wound, and the jejunum is tacked to the anterior abdominal wall with several fine sutures. The mediastinum is not drained through the abdomen. The abdominal incision is closed and isolated from the field as the cervical anastomosis is constructed (Figs. 25-8 and 25-9). The cervical esophagogastrostomy is performed with a single layer of interrupted 4-0 polyglycolic acid suture, and a nasogastric tube is inserted into the intrathoracic stomach for postoperative gastric decompression. The neck wound is irrigated and closed loosely over a ¼-inch rubber drain.

Transhiatal esophagectomy and proximal partial gastrectomy for carcinoma of the gastroesophageal junction

This technique is also applicable for patients with tumors involving the gastroesophageal junction. In most of these patients, the stomach can be divided with a 4- to 6-cm gross margin from the tumor, still preserving the entire greater curvature length, including that point which will reach most superiorly to the neck, and saving a major portion of the upper stomach, which is usually discarded in the performance of a hemigastrectomy for these tumors (Fig. 25-10). When this technique is used for tumors of the gastroesophageal junction, it is important that the surgeon not divide the cervical end of the esophagus until he or she is satisfied that there is an adequate gastric margin distal to the tumor so that gastric division preserving the entire greater curvature is possible. If, in error, the surgeon mobilizes the entire thoracic esophagus and then divides the cervical end only to find that the tumor is so extensive that a proximal hemigastrectomy is required to resect it, he or she will be faced with insufficient gastric length to reach to the divided cervical esophagus—a disastrous situation.

With localized gastroesophageal junction tumors, after the mobilized thoracic esophagus and stomach have been placed upon the anterior abdominal wall, the stomach is divided with a GIA

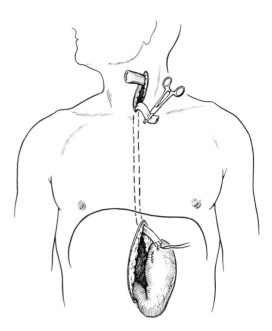

Fig. 25-7. Suturing to the transmediastinal rubber drain that point on the high greater curvature of the stomach which reaches most cephalad to the neck. (From Orringer, M.B.: Esophageal replacement using stomach substernally and after blunt esophagectomy. In Nyhus, L.M., and Baker, R.J., editors: Mastery of surgery, Boston, 1984, Little, Brown & Co.)

stapler applied well away from palpable tumor (Fig. 25-11). A greater-curvature gastric tube is thereby created. The gastric staple suture line is oversewn with a running 4-0 polypropylene inverting Lembert stitch. The stomach is then positioned in the posterior mediastinum as described previously, and the anastomosis is performed on the anterior gastric wall, away from the gastric staple suture line (Fig. 25-12).

RESULTS

I have performed a transhiatal esophagectomy without thoracotomy in 147 patients with carcinoma of the intrathoracic esophagus. One hundred and fourteen (78%) were men, and 33 (22%) women. The patients ranged in age from 38 to 92 years and averaged 61 years of age. Twenty-two percent of these patients were 70 years of age or older. Eighty-six percent had experienced weight loss, which averaged 21 pounds. Of the 147 tumors, 8 occurred in the upper esophagus, 62 in the midesophagus, and 77 in the distal esophagus. Stomach was used to reconstruct the esophagus in 142 (97%) of these patients, colon being required in five patients who had undergone prior gastric resections. I am convinced that the

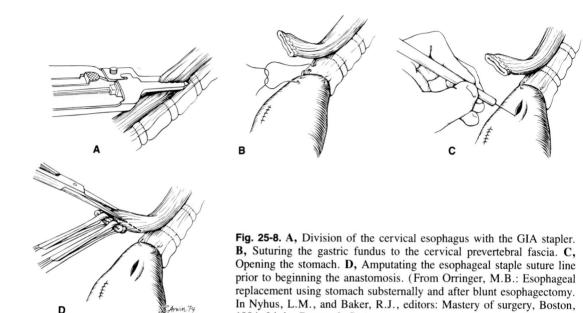

Fig. 25-8. **A,** Division of the cervical esophagus with the GIA stapler. **B,** Suturing the gastric fundus to the cervical prevertebral fascia. **C,** Opening the stomach. **D,** Amputating the esophageal staple suture line prior to beginning the anastomosis. (From Orringer, M.B.: Esophageal replacement using stomach substernally and after blunt esophagectomy. In Nyhus, L.M., and Baker, R.J., editors: Mastery of surgery, Boston, 1984, Little, Brown & Co.)

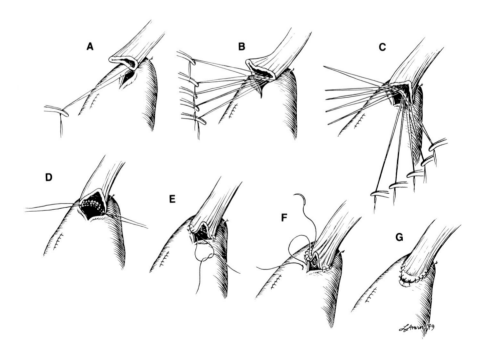

Fig. 25-9. Construction of the cervical esophagogastric anastomosis. **A** to **D,** Completion of the two posterior quadrants with knots tied on the inside of the lumen. **E** to **G,** Completion of the anterior two quadrants of the anastomosis. (From Orringer, M.B.: Esophageal replacement using stomach substernally and after blunt esophagectomy. In Nyhus, L.M., and Baker, R.J., editors: Mastery of surgery, Boston, 1984, Little, Brown & Co.)

normal stomach will *always* reach to the neck for a cervical esophagogastric anastomosis.

Measured intraoperative blood loss has ranged from 125 to 3600 ml and has averaged 890 ml. One or two chest tubes have been inserted intraoperatively because of entry into one or both pleural cavities during the esophagectomy in 96 (65%) of these patients. Three patients sustained posterior membranous tracheal tears intraoperatively, and these were repaired without incident. Postoperative complications have included recurrent laryngeal nerve paresis in 35 (24%); chylothorax in three (2%), and anastomotic leak in nine (6%). Since adoption of a policy of strictly avoiding placement of any retractors against the tracheoesophageal groove during the cervical portion of the operation, recurrent laryngeal nerve injury has occurred only four times in our last consecutive 65 patients undergoing transhiatal esophagectomy. There have been no intraoperative deaths or reexplorations for postoperative bleeding. Nine hospital deaths (mortality of 6%) occurred— from aspiration pneumonia (2), retroperitoneal or mediastinal abscess (2), pulmonary embolism (1), respiratory insufficiency (1), cardiac arrhythmia (1), mesenteric vascular accident (1), and hepatic failure (1). Seventy-nine percent of the patients surviving operation have been discharged from the hospital within 14 days of operation, and another 9% within 21 days. Thus 88% of patients surviving transhiatal esophagectomy for carcinoma have been discharged from the hospital with comfortable swallowing within 3 weeks of operation.

The actuarial survival following transhiatal esophagectomy for intrathoracic esophageal carcinoma is shown in Table 25-1. The 5-year survival for middle-third tumors has been 12% and that for lower-third tumors 30%. The mean survival time for middle-third tumors has been 19 months, and that for lower-third tumors 39 months. The effect of tumor stage and location upon 12- and 24-month survival following transhiatal esophagectomy is shown in Table 25-2. These data are not dissimilar from the recently reported survival statistics following radical transthoracic esophagectomy,[23] further justifying our belief that it is the biologic nature of the tumor and its stage at the time of operation, rather than the extent of resection, that determine survival in these patients.

SUMMARY

Transhiatal esophagectomy without thoracotomy and esophageal replacement with a cervical esophagogastric anastomosis provide safe and efficient palliation, and occasionally cure, for the patient with carcinoma of the intrathoracic esophagus. This procedure, by avoiding a thoracotomy, reduces the physiologic insult of esophageal resection in these debilitated patients, and the elimination of an intrathoracic esophagogastric anastomosis avoids the hazards of sepsis from an anastomotic leak. In addition, this approach provides the maximum surgical margin that is possible, thereby minimizing the incidence of suture line tumor recurrence. Clinically significant gastroesophageal reflux rarely occurs with a cervical esophagogastric anastomosis, in contrast to its frequent occurrence when the anastomosis is performed within the chest. Our hospital mortality of 6% and the fact that 88% of our patients surviving operation have left the hospital within 3 weeks of surgery justify our continued use of this operation.

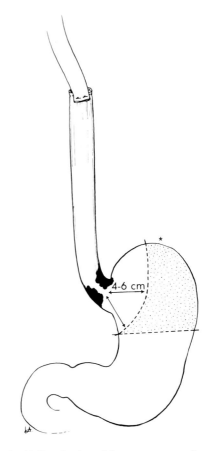

Fig. 25-10. Proximal partial gastrectomy performed for localized gastroesophageal junction tumors provides a 4- to 6-cm gross margin beyond the tumor while preserving the entire greater curvature, including the point *(asterisk)* that reaches most cephalad. A standard hemigastrectomy for such a tumor wastes valuable stomach *(stippled area)* that can be used for esophageal replacement. (From Orringer, M.B., and Sloan, H.: J. Thorac. Cardiovasc. Surg. **76:**643, 1978.)

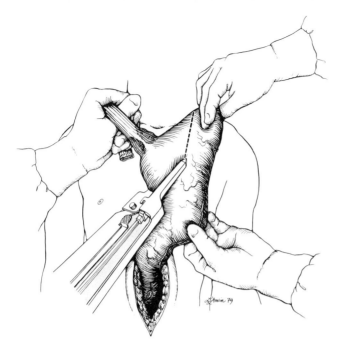

Fig. 25-11. Performance of a partial proximal gastrectomy after a transhiatal esophagectomy for a tumor of the gastroesophageal junction. A gastric "tube" is created as the entire greater curvature is preserved for the subsequent esophageal replacement. (From Orringer, M.B.: Esophageal replacement using stomach substernally and after blunt esophagectomy. In Nyhus, L.M., and Baker, R.J., editors: Mastery of surgery, Boston, 1984, Little, Brown & Co.)

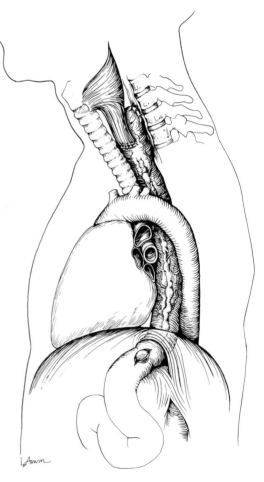

Fig. 25-12. Final position of the mobilized intrathoracic stomach in the original esophageal bed in the posterior mediastinum. The gastric fundus is suspended in the neck from the prevertebral fascia, an end-to-side cervical esophagogastric anastomosis has been performed, and the pylorus comes to rest several centimeters below the diaphragmatic hiatus. (From Orringer, M.B., and Sloan, H.: J. Thorac. Cardiovasc. Surg. **76:**643, 1978.)

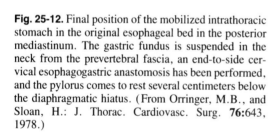

TABLE 25-1. Actuarial survival following transhiatal esophagectomy for carcinoma

Site*	Number	Percent survival after operation						Mean survival time (mo)
		6 mo	12 mo	24 mo	36 mo	48 mo	60 mo	
Upper third	8	75	60	0	0	0	0	11
Middle third	55	73	42	20	15	12	12	19
Lower third	75	82	64	48	34	30	30	39

*Differences among these groups are statistically significant (p = .01).

TABLE 25-2. Effect of tumor stage and location upon 12- and 24-month survival following transhiatal esophagectomy for carcinoma

TNM tumor stage*	Middle-third carcinomas				Distal-third carcinomas			
	Number	Mean percent survival		Mean survival time (mo)	Number	Mean percent survival		Mean survival time (mo)
		12 mo	24 mo			12 mo	24 mo	
0-I	8	83	62	41	3	100	100	—
II	5	40	40	19	8	100	69	72
III	35	39	13	14	61	61	40	32
IV	7	43	0	9	3	0	0	4

*Differences among these groups are statistically significant (p = .001).

REFERENCES

1. Akiyama, H., Tsurumaru, M., Kawamura, T., et al.: Principles of surgical treatment for carcinoma of the esophagus: analysis of lymph node involvement, Ann. Surg. **194**:438, 1981.

2. Ellis, F.H., Jr., and Gibb, S.P.: Esophagogastrectomy for carcinoma: current hospital mortality and morbidity rates, Ann. Surg. **190**:699, 1979.

3. Piccone, V.A., LeVeen, H.H., Ahmed, N., et al.: Reappraisal of esophagogastrectomy for esophageal malignancy, Am. J. Surg. **137**:32, 1979.

4. Ellis, F.H., Jr.: Carcinoma of esophagus, Cancer **33**:264, 1983.

5. Giuli, R., and Gignoux, M.: Treatment of carcinoma of the esophagus: retrospective study of 2400 patients, Ann. Surg. **192**:44, 1980.

6. Postlethwait, R.W.: Complications and deaths after operations for esophageal carcinoma, J. Thorac. Cardiovasc. Surg. **85**:827, 1983.

7. Earlam, R., and Cunha-Melo, J.R.: Oesophageal squamous cell carcinoma. I. A critical review of surgery, Br. J. Surg. **67**:381, 1980.

8. Denk, W.: Zur Radikaloperation des Osophagus, Karzentralbl. Chirurg. **40**:1065, 1913.

9. Gray-Turner, G.: Excision of thoracic esophagus for carcinomas with construction of extrathoracic gullet, Lancet **2**:1315, 1933.

10. Akiyama, H., Sato, Y., and Takahashi, F.: Immediate pharyngogastrostomy following total esophagectomy by blunt dissection, Jpn. J. Surg. **1**:225, 1971.

11. LeQuesne, L.P., and Ranger, D.: Pharyngolaryngectomy with immediate pharyngogastric anastomosis, Br. J. Surg. **53**:105, 1966.

12. Ong, G.B., and Lee, T.C.: Pharyngogastric anastomosis after oesophagopharyngectomy for carcinoma of the hypopharynx and cervical esophagus, Br. J. Surg. **48**:193, 1960.

13. Kirk, R.M.: Palliative resection of oesophageal carcinoma without formal thoracotomy, Br. J. Surg. **61**:689, 1974.

14. Thomas, A.N., and Dedo, H.H.: Pharyngogastrostomy for treatment of severe caustic stricture of the pharynx and esophagus, J. Thorac. Cardiovasc. Surg. **73**:817, 1977.

15. Orringer, M.B.: Transhiatal esophagectomy without thoracotomy for carcinoma of the thoracic esophagus, Ann. Surg. **200**:282, 1984.

16. Orringer, M.B.: Transhiatal esophagectomy for benign disease, J. Thorac. Cardiovasc. Surg. **90**:649, 1985.

17. Orringer, M.B., and Orringer, J.S.: Esophagectomy without thoracotomy: a dangerous operation? J. Thorac. Cardiovasc. Surg. **85**:72, 1983.

18. Orringer, M.B.: Technical aids in performing transhiatal esophagectomy without thoracotomy, Ann. Thorac. Surg. **38**:128, 1984.

19. Bains, M.S., and Spiro, R.H.: Pharyngolaryngectomy, total extrathoracic esophagectomy and gastric transposition, Surg. Gynecol. Obstet. **149**:693, 1979.

20. Cordiano, C., Fracastoro, G., Mosciaro, O., et al.: Esophagectomy and esophageal replacement by gastric pull-through procedure, Int. Surg. **64**:17, 1979.

21. Szentpetery, S., Wolfgang, T., and Lower, R.R.: Pull-through esophagectomy without thoracotomy for esophageal carcinoma, Ann. Thorac. Surg. **27**:399, 1979.

22. Tryzelar, J.F., Neptune, W.B., and Ellis, F.H., Jr.: Esophagectomy without thoracotomy for carcinoma of the esophagus, Am. J. Surg. **143**:486, 1982.

23. Skinner, D.B.: En bloc resection for neoplasms of the esophagus and cardia, J. Thorac. Cardiovasc. Surg. **85**:59, 1983.

DISCUSSION—Chapters 24 and 25

Alberto Peracchia

The treatment of esophageal cancer has aroused great interest from the beginning of this century. In 1913, at the American Medical Association meeting, Willy Mayer[1,2] discussed the best approaches for surgical treatment, without much interest from the audience. This led him and other surgeons to constitute the American Association for Thoracic Surgery with the purpose of discussing the specific problems related to esophageal cancer.[3] In 1937, Fisher[4] published a thorough analysis of the different techniques used for the treatment of esophageal cancer. He reviewed the indications for extrapleural, transpleural, and extrathoracic routes of access.

The debate concerning surgical approach to cancer of the thoracic esophagus, extent of resection, and role of adjuvant therapy is not solved yet. No agreement has been reached other than to consider the long-term results of treatment unsatisfactory.

The Skinner and Orringer reports clearly express this controversy. They support two interesting techniques, which reflect two opposite philosophical attitudes in the management of esophageal cancer.

Some general observations can be made from our experience with 2082 patients with esophageal cancer between 1967 and 1985. There were 1755 cases of squamous cell carcinoma of the esophagus, and 327 cases of adenocarcinoma of the gastric cardia.

The rationale for this classification is based on different biologic and clinic behavior of the two types of neoplasm. Adenocarcinoma of the gastric cardia differs from squamous esophageal carcinoma not only histologically but, above all, for its pattern of natural history, age of incidence, spread, and a peculiar response to chemotherapy and radiotherapy.[5-7] As a consequence, a different surgical approach is advocated for adenocarcinoma of the cardia—total gastrectomy and extensive esophageal resection.[6]

Finally, it is important to underscore that staging of gastric cancer differs from that of esophageal carcinoma. Moreover, evaluation of the mo-dalities and sites of recurrence and of survival rates makes it difficult to consider together epidermoid carcinoma of the esophagus and adenocarcinoma of the cardia.

ORRINGER'S REPORT

Esophagectomy without thoracotomy was originally proposed and performed for intrathoracic esophageal carcinoma.[8] The technique has been recently popularized by Orringer with the same indication.

Orringer's choice in the treatment of intrathoracic esophageal carcinoma is based on technical considerations: the high incidence of bronchopulmonary complications after thoracotomy and the catastrophic effects of an anastomotic dehiscence in the mediastinum.

The incidence of postoperative respiratory complications that are not due only to the particular biologic conditions of the patients operated upon for esophageal carcinoma can be significantly decreased if anesthesia is carried out by experts in esophageal surgery. Reduced postoperative mechanical ventilation and continued peridural analgesia have limited bronchopulmonary complications to 10.5% in our series of 506 patients operated upon between 1980 and 1985.

No significant difference in the incidence of respiratory complications was found between patients who underwent total esophagectomy by thoracotomy (8.5%) and those who did not have thoracotomy (13%). Similar results were observed by Shahian et al.[9]

Lack of experience did not account for the higher rate of complications after esophagectomy without thoracotomy, since this technique was applied until December, 1986, to a total of 166 patients, 67 of whom had intrathoracic carcinoma.

The incidence of leak was 4.3% in our series of 298 cases of stapled intrathoracic esophagogastric anastomosis, and the mortality for leak was 0.6% (2 cases, or 15% of those with anastomotic leak). This is in agreement with the experience of Fekete et al.[10] Anastomotic stenosis was found in 8% of this group of patients, requiring an average of 4.8 dilatations. Orringer reports a 50% incidence of anastomotic stenosis in the neck, some of which (14%) required repeated dilatations. Since he states that surgery for esophageal carcinoma is aimed at curing dysphagia, it is doubtful how one can consider the quality of life improved, given this high incidence of anastomotic stricture.

The 24% incidence of recurrent laryngeal nerve paresis, considered by Orringer as a "devastating complication,"[11] suggests that, when it is possible to gain a proximal distance of at least 10 cm from the macroscopic margin of the tumor, a high intrathoracic anastomosis is preferable to a cervical anastomosis.

We agree with Orringer in that esophagectomy without thoracotomy is, from a technical standpoint, a safe operation in both benign and malignant disease. However, based on oncologic criteria, this technique should not be applied to every patient with esophageal cancer. The main issue is that it is not possible to perform a radical mediastinal lymphadenectomy without opening the chest. This also generates staging problems and difficulty in comparison of results.

Orringer believes that esophageal cancer is a systemic disease from its onset and, therefore, that surgery has only a palliative role. In contrast, Huang et al.[5,7] have shown an 85% 5-year survival rate in patients with tumors less than 2 cm in diameter without full penetration of the esophageal wall and without lymph node metastasis. This emphasizes the importance of an early diagnosis but also demonstrates that surgery still can be curative in selected cases.

Esophagectomy without thoracotomy is routinely performed for hypopharyngeal and cervical esophageal carcinoma. We prefer to open the diaphragm according to Pinotti,[13] in order to obtain adequate exposure of the lower mediastinum. An illuminating retractor is used to improve the view of the operative field. Small tumors located at the thoracic inlet or at the cardia can be resected without thoracotomy.

SKINNER'S REPORT

The rationale for Skinner's surgical therapy is the removal of the primary tumor along with cellular tissue and regional lymph nodes, so that radiotherapy and chemotherapy can eventually complete the eradication of the neoplastic tissue. DeMeester[12] has applied this principle to lung carcinoma with nodal metastases. We believe that the same holds true for esophageal carcinoma.

In our experience, the ratio between esophagectomy with thoracotomy and without thoracotomy is 10:1. We prefer thoracotomy for intrathoracic carcinoma when there are no contraindications, such as severe respiratory failure, poor general condition, and/or advanced age.

Our surgical approach consists of a median laparotomy and right thoracotomy through the fifth intercostal space when the tumor is localized at the level of the carina or below. The esophagogastric anastomosis is performed at the apex of the chest, at least 10 cm above the upper margin of the tumor. When the tumor is localized above the carina, right thoracotomy is performed first, followed by laparotomy and cervicotomy for accomplishment of the anastomosis. The resection is extended to the supramesocolic lymph nodes and to the mediastinal structures, including lymph nodes, thoracic duct, and areolar tissue. The azygos vein and the pericardium are not removed as described by Skinner.

We share Skinner's approach to the treatment of esophageal carcinoma, with the exception that we do not consider together epidermoid carcinoma of the esophagus and adenocarcinoma of the gastric cardia. We think that resection should be extended to the whole stomach, greater omentum, and spleen in stage I or II adenocarcinoma of the cardia.

Oncologic criteria, as correctly stressed by Skinner, should represent the guidelines for the surgeon. We are also convinced that resection aimed to cure should be extensive, primarily when the disease is localized.

Postoperative intensive care differs in our experience from that advocated by Skinner. We prefer early extubation of the patient, at the end of operation after esophagectomy without thoracotomy, and after 2 or 3 hours if thoracotomy is performed. This has decreased the incidence of respiratory complications to 10% in the patients who have had resections.

CONCLUSIONS

Postoperative mortality (within 30 days) reported by Orringer (8%) and Skinner (10%) is acceptable, and is similar to that in our experience. In our 506 patients with epidermoid carcinoma of the esophagus, postoperative mortality was 5.9%. In 59 patients who underwent esophagectomy without thoracotomy, postoperative mortality was 3.8%, even though most of the patients were over 70 and in poor general condition.

Comparison of survival rates in Orringer's and Skinner's reports is somewhat difficult, because of the differing approaches to staging and data presentation. The excellent 3-year and 5-year survival rates (78% and 55%, respectively) reported by Skinner after en bloc resection, in patients without wall infiltration and without nodal metastasis, are remarkable.

Esophagectomy without thoracotomy is, in our opinion, an excellent technique, with low morbidity but with oncologic limitations. It represents the ideal approach in patients with cervical esophageal or cardia tumors. However, on the basis of our experience, we believe that thoracotomy does not significantly increase morbidity and mortality, and that an intrathoracic anastomosis is no less safe than an anastomosis in the neck.

The "en bloc" resection proposed by Skinner is the technique of choice in patients with limited intramediastinal tumors, in whom a radical resection could result in cure. However, even if there is local-regional spread of the disease, an adequate debulking provides the basis for more effective adjuvant therapy.

Finally, new staging methods are needed for a better understanding of the prognostic factors and for a better comparison of the long-term results of therapy.

REFERENCES

1. American Medical Association: Minutes of 64th Annual Session, Minneapolis, Minn., June 1913.

2. Meyer, W.: Extrathoracic and intrathoracic esophagoplasty in connection with resection of the thoracic portion of the esophagus for carcinoma, JAMA **63:**62, 1914.

3. Murray, G.F.: Esophagectomy without thoracotomy, Ann. Thorac. Surg. **41:**233, 1986.

4. Fisher, A.W.: Erfolgreiche Entferming eines Krebses der Speiserohore im mittleren Brustteil nach dem abdominocollaren Durchzugsverflaren, Uerh. Dtsch. Ges. Chir., 1937, p. 498.

5. Huang, G.T.: Surgery of esophageal carcinoma, Sem. Surg. Oncol. **1:**74, 1985.

6. Holscher, A.H., and Siewert, J.R.: Surgical treatment of the adenocarcinoma of the gastroesophageal junction: results of a European questionnarie (GEEMO), Dig. Surg. **2:**1, 1985.

7. Huang, K.C., et al.: Diagnosis and surgical treatment of early esophageal carcinoma. In Stipa, S., Belsey, R.H.R., and Moraldi, A., editors: Medical and surgical problems of the esophagus, New York, 1981, Academic Press, pp. 296-299.

8. Denk, W.: Zur radicaloperation des esophagus karzinoms, Zentralbl. Chir. **40:**1065, 1913.

9. Shahian, D.M., Neptune, W.B., Ellis, F.H., and Watkins, E.: Transthoracic versus extrathoracic esophagectomy: mortality, morbidity and long-term survival, Ann. Thorac. Surg. **41:**237, 1986.

10. Fekete, F., Breil, P., Ronsse, H., Tossen, J.C., and Langonnet, F.: EEA stapler and omental graft in esophagogastrectomy, Ann. Surg. **193:**825, 1981.

11. Orringer, M.B.: Transhiatal esophagectomy without thoracotomy for carcinoma of thoracic esophagus, Ann. Surg. **200:**282, 1983.

12. DeMeester, T.R.: The staging issue: unification of criteria. In Delarue, N.C., and Echapasse, H., editors: Lung cancer. International trends in general thoracic surgery, vol. 1. Philadelphia, 1985, W.B. Saunders Co., pp. 37, 41.

13. Pinotti, H.W.: Via de acceso transdiafragmatico al esofago toracico y al mediastino anterior, Salvat Editores, 1984.

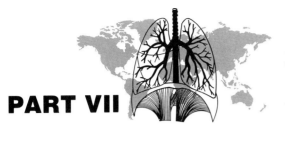

PART VII

SOME SPECIAL ELECTIVE SURGICAL TECHNIQUES

26 **Synchronous combined abdominothoracocervical esophagectomy: the team approach**

Eric M. Nanson

In 1946 Ivor Lewis[1] described his operation of esophagectomy for carcinoma of the esophagus. He used a right lateral thoracotomy and performed an esophagogastric anastomosis in the right upper chest. First, an abdominal incision was required to mobilize the stomach. This incision was then closed and the patient was repositioned and redraped for the lateral thoracotomy and the thoracic part of the procedure, which involved the mobilization of the esophagus, the enlargement of the esophageal hiatus, and the drawing up of the stomach into the chest. The esophagogastric anastomosis was then performed after resection of the esophagus with its growth.

The disadvantage of this operation was that it involved a two-stage procedure. The patient had to be repositioned and redraped, which potentially added to the shock of the operation, prolonged the procedure, and was a problem for the anesthetic and operating teams. In 1950 Milnes Walker and Nanson, working at Bristol Royal Infirmary, evolved the synchronous combined approach, based on the same principle as that commonly used for excision of the rectum. It has been further refined in an extensive experience.[2]

THE PRINCIPLES OF THE OPERATION

The principles of the operation can be stated in the following manner.

Principle 1

Carcinoma of the esophagus, if suitable for excision, should be treated by total esophagectomy. Carcinoma of the esophagus has a potential for extensive submucosal spread, as well as submucosal lymphatic embolization with satellite growths developing distant from the primary site. Therefore, wide excision plus resection of adjacent lymph nodes is indicated to achieve any possibility of cure.

Principle 2

The stomach provides the best substitute for the excised esophagus. The stomach fundus can be readily brought up into the neck for anastomosis. (Fig. 26-1). The vascularity is secure, hinged on the right gastric and right gastroepiploic vessels. The stomach acts as an excellent conduit without risk of distention, provided it is totally within the area of negative intrathoracic pressure. Only one anastomosis is required.

Principle 3

The higher the esophagogastric anastomosis, the less problem there is with gastric reflux. The higher the anastomosis, the more tubular the stomach becomes. Provided the pyloric sphincter is rendered incompetent by either a plasty or myotomy procedure, there are no sphincters between the cricopharyngeus muscle and the duodenum. The upper esophagus appears to be more resistant to acid gastric reflux than the lower esophagus. The stomach is totally vagotomized by the esophagectomy, and therefore its acidity is low.

Principle 4

The esophagogastric anastomosis should be of the "ink-well" variety. This technique discourages reflux.

Principle 5

The pylorus must be sited at the esophageal hiatus. (See Fig. 26-1.) This ensures that the whole stomach lies totally in a negative pressure area, and therefore abdominal pressure will not act upon it to favor reflux.

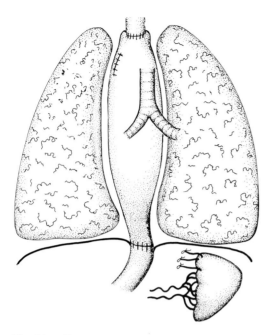

Fig. 26-1. Esophagogastric anastomosis done in the neck to fundus of stomach. Note pylorus at hiatus, and tubular shape of stomach.

Principle 6

Two teams facilitate the operation. The abdominal team can explore the abdomen and assess operability from the point of view of subdiaphragmatic metastatic spread. The abdominal team can mobilize the stomach and enlarge the esophageal hiatus and assess esophageal operability by passing a hand up into the posterior mediastinum to assess the fixation and extent of the lesion. The abdominal team, working in conjunction with the thoracic team, can help mobilize a difficult lower-third growth.

The patient only has to be positioned and draped once, thereby diminishing possible shock and reducing the risk of inadvertent contamination of the wounds. The incisions can be closed seriatim. Once the abdominal team is finished and the stomach passed up into the chest, the abdominal wound can be closed. Once the thoracic esophagus has been mobilized and removed, the stomach fundus can be passed up into the neck and the thoracic incision closed. Then the esophagogastric anastomosis can be done through the cervical incision. From the points of view of anesthesia and operative trauma, this is a very quiescent and benign period for the patient, so that the vital anastomosis can be done meticulously and deliberately, with as much time being taken as is necessary to ensure that it is leak-proof. The two-team approach shortens the time of the operation to about 2 hours.

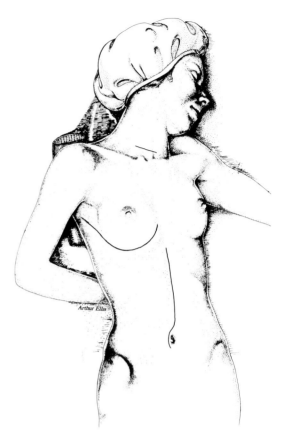

Fig. 26-2. Positioning of the patient and locations of the three incisions.

Principle 7

The chest must be opened through an extensive anterior thoracotomy. This enables the abdomen to be flat on the operating table for the abdominal team. The thoracolumbar spine can be twisted some 30 degrees elevating the right anterior chest. This enables the thoracic team to enter the chest by either the third or the fourth anterior intercostal space, depending on the level of the tumor. Rib spreaders allow the chest to open like an oyster. The upper thoracic cage hinges upward easily. Once the root of the right lung has been mobilized and the pulmonary ligament divided, the whole right lung can be rotated forward through the incision and usually rest on the front of the sternum, so that the anesthetist can continue to ventilate it throughout the operation. This obviates the necessity for compression and collapse of the right lung.

Principle 8

The neck incision facilitates the crucial esophagogastric anastomosis. It is more easily done on the right side through a short supraclavicular incision. The thoracic team, on the right side, is appropriately placed to do the cervical procedure as well. By a combined approach from the neck and the right thoracic apex, the cervical esophagus can be mobilized to the cricoid cartilage and the gastric fundus can be passed into the cervical incision, so that the esophagogastric anastomosis is conveniently performed at the level of the skin surface.

SOME POINTS ON TECHNIQUE THAT FACILITATE THE OPERATION

1. *Each* team consists of surgeon, his or her assistant, and an instrument nurse. The surgeons are usually side by side on the right side of the operating table unless the abdominal surgeon is left handed, in which case he or she may stand on the opposite side. The assistants normally stand on the left side of the operating table.
2. The patient is positioned with the pelvis flat on the table, but the right chest is raised about 30 degrees on a sandbag.
3. The right arm is positioned as in Fig. 26-2, with the hand tucked under the right loin and the elbow over the edge of the table. This allows ready access into the axilla.
4. In the female, the chest incision is inframammary and the breast is turned up to expose the pectoralis major muscle, which is divided transversely in either the third or the fourth intercostal space. If the esophageal lesion is in the lower third, the fourth space is used.
5. The intercostal incision extends from the sternum to the head of the rib. The internal mammary vessels are secured and divided. This enables the upper flap of the chest to open as a trap door. If more exposure is required, an appropriate costal cartilage may be divided.
6. The root of the lung is mobilized by dividing the azygos major vein as it arches forward and by dividing the vagal branches to the lung. The pulmonary ligament is divided. This opens the entire posterior mediastinum and exposes the full length of the thoracic esophagus.
7. The lung is then rotated forward out of the wound onto the front of the sternum, where it is covered with a moist saline pack and allowed to ventilate freely during the thoracic procedure. The surgeon thus works behind and below the right lung (Fig. 26-3).

8. The abdominal team normally begins first and explores the abdomen for evidence of metastatic spread. If this is absent, the surgeon then mobilizes the abdominal esophagus. He or she enlarges the esophageal hiatus, if necessary, by dividing one or the other crus. The surgeon can then pass a hand up into the posterior mediastinum and assess to a large degree the resectability of the esophageal lesion. If this is favorable, the thoracic team begins, and the two work simultaneously.
9. The abdominal team mobilizes the stomach, separating the great omentum. It is very careful to maintain the integrity of the right gastric and right gastroepiploic vessels and their arcades. The veins are just as important as the arteries.
10. The abdominal team mobilizes the duodenum and the head of the pancreas by a Kocher maneuver so that the pylorus will reach the level of the esophageal hiatus. It performs either a pyloroplasty or a pyloromyotomy, to render the pyloric sphincter incompetent and permit free gastric drainage.
11. When the thoracic team has mobilized the esophagus, the stomach is drawn up into the chest, guided by the abdominal team from below to ensure that there is no twisting and that the pylorus lies at the hiatus.
12. The thoracic team then divides the lower esophagus at the cardia and closes the stomach in a routine manner. Then it moves to the neck and opens that area by retracting the sternocleidomastoid muscle laterally and the midline structures medially, exposing the cervical esophagus medial to the carotid sheath. Care is taken to preserve the right recurrent laryngeal nerve. The mobilization of the cervical esophagus is facilitated by passing one or two fingers from the chest in the posterior mediastinum into the prevertebral area of the lower cervical region. The esophagus is then divided about 2 cm below the cricopharyngeus muscle and the entire distal esophagus is removed.
13. The fundus of the stomach is guided into the neck and held there temporarily. It is suspended from the apex of the chest cavity by interrupted sutures, to remove tension from the subsequent suture line. The chest is closed in a routine manner with underwater tube drainage.
14. Finally, the esophageal anastomosis is done to the fundus of the stomach in an inkwell manner (Fig. 26-4). If the surgeon prefers to use a circular stapling device, this is done

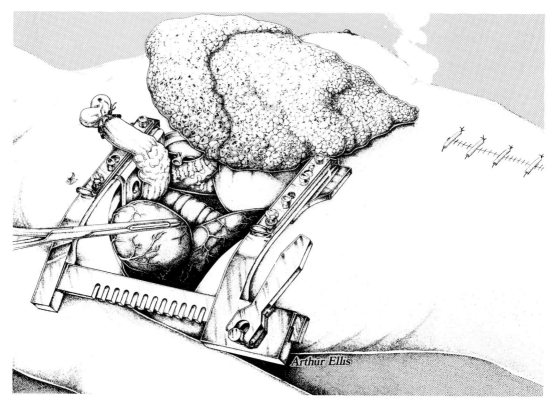

Fig. 26-3. Extent of exposure obtained through a right anterior thoracotomy. The lung has been mobilized onto the front of the sternum. The clamp is across the cardia of the mobilized stomach.

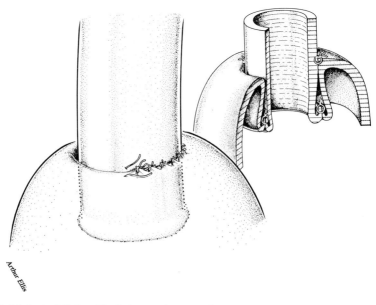

Fig. 26-4. Method of "inkwelling" the esophagogastric anastomosis to protect the suture line and control reflux.

before the chest is closed. The anastomosis is accomplished over a nasogastric tube that is positioned in the upper two thirds of the intrathoracic stomach.

SUMMARY

The virtues of this technique are as follows:
1. The operating time is shortened.
2. No repositioning is needed.
3. The right lung can be ventilated throughout the operation.
4. The two teams help each other in the region of the esophageal hiatus.
5. The cervical esophagogastric anastomosis can be done at skin level carefully and deliberately after the abdomen and chest have been closed.
6. A near-total esophagectomy is achieved.

ACKNOWLEDGEMENTS

I wish to thank Mr. Norman C. Tanner, who in 1948 introduced me to the surgery of the esophagus while he was working as registrar at St. James Hospital in Balham. I also wish to pay tribute to Professor R. Milnes Walker, who was Professor of Surgery at the University of Bristol while he was a senior lecturer on the professorial unit. Professor Milnes Walker encouraged and helped in the development of this operation.

I also wish to acknowledge the help and skillful artistry of Professor J.B. Carman, Department of Anatomy, University of Auckland, who with his departmental artist Mr. Arthur Ellis was responsible for drawing of the diagrams.

REFERENCES

1. Lewis, I.: The surgical treatment of carcinoma of the oesophagus with special reference to a new operation for growths of the middle third, Br. J. Surg. **34:**18, 1946.
2. Nanson, E.M.: Aust. N.Z. J. Surg. **45:**340, 1975.

Synchronous combined abdominothoracocervical esophagectomy: the team approach

DISCUSSION

Frederick Griffith Pearson

This technique of esophagectomy, which was developed by Nanson and Milnes Walker as long ago as 1950, was little publicized in subsequent years, and is not widely known or appreciated today. Nanson described the technique and presented his experience at a Canadian Royal College meeting in 1965, since which time I have continued to use this approach for selected cases requiring a total thoracic esophagectomy and reconstruction with a cervical anastomosis. Indeed, it is my operation of choice in most patients with operable, squamous cell carcinoma of the thoracic esophagus at all levels, including the lower third. The functional results obtained with a cervical esophagogastrostomy appear to be predictably good, the morbidity from an anastomotic leak in the neck is usually inconsequential, and the risk of tumor recurrence at the anastomosis is minimized.

TECHNIQUE

The technique is clearly and concisely described in Nanson's report, with emphasis on all of the important details. To take best advantage of this technique, it is essential to use two complete teams: two surgeons, two instrument nurses, two cauteries, and so on. With experience, and the use of this two-team approach, most operations are readily accomplished within 3 hours or less. Certain technical points warrant emphasis.

1. The right anterolateral thoracotomy through the third or fourth intercostal space must be carried anteriorly to the sternal margin, and posteriorly as far back into the axilla as possible. If

this is done, adequate exposure is predictably obtained. I find it preferable to collapse the right lung rather than elevate the ventilated lung out of the right hemithorax, as described by Nanson. Lung collapse is achieved through the use of a double-lumen orotracheal tube, or a bronchial blocker. Once the inferior pulmonary ligament has been divided, the collapsed right lung can be retracted anteriorly to provide exposure of the esophagus in its middle third (lower trachea and subcarinal compartment). The lung may be retracted inferiorly for exposure at and above the level of the azygos vein. Surprisingly, the most awkward access through this incision is in the lower third of the esophagus, where the esophagus lies behind the right side of the heart. Most of this latter dissection is more easily achieved by dissection from below, through the dilated hiatus.

2. Mobilization of the stomach is straightforward and is clearly described in Nanson's report. Significant additional length is obtained by extensive Kocherization of the duodenum, following which the pylorus should lie at the level of the esophageal hiatus. If the stomach is undamaged by previous surgery, there is no problem with gastric length, allowing a tension-free cervical reconstruction. I do not add a pyloroplasty in patients with a normal pylorus and duodenum, and no prior history of peptic ulcer disease. The incidence of prolonged, delayed gastric emptying has been minimal, and there has been no greater incidence of this complication in patients without a pyloroplasty. Duodenogastric reflux with "bile gastritis" is a known complication following pyloroplasty and is occasionally trou-

blesome even in the "upright stomach." If the stomach is stabilized in the posterior mediastinum by closing the right mediastinal pleura, a further cause of delayed gastric emptying is prevented. If the mediastinal pleura is not closed, the body of the stomach may be markedly displaced into the right chest, resulting in a gastric reservoir lying over the hemidiaphragm with acute angulation of the lumen at the diaphragmatic hiatus.

3. Recurrent nerve palsy is a known complication of this technique of thoracic esophagectomy. I believe the injury usually occurs from the cervical dissection and can be prevented by deliberately avoiding compression or traction on the nerve during this stage of the procedure. Metal retractors applied in the region of the tracheoesophageal groove should not be used to displace the airway medially.

4. The cervical esophagogastrostomy is done in end-to-side fashion, anastomosing the end of the cervical esophagus to that part of the greater curvature of the stomach which can be elevated to the highest level in the neck. Two layers of absorbable, interrupted suture are used (4-0 Vicryl). The posterior aspect of the stomach is secured to the prevertebral fascia with two or three interrupted sutures in order to prevent tension at the anastomosis when the patient is upright.

ADVANTAGES

Nanson's approach affords good exposure for total thoracic esophagectomy, including a radical resection with lymphadenectomy when indicated. The subcarinal and retrotracheal esophagus is readily mobilized under direct vision through the anterolateral thoracotomy. The lower third of the esophagus is usually more easily mobilized from below through the dilated hiatus.

Excellent functional results are usually obtained with the upright stomach, maintained in its posterior mediastinal position, and anastomosed in the neck. In the absence of other pathology, gastroesophageal reflux is never a significant problem with this reconstruction. The only precaution advised is elevation of the head of the bed on 6-inch blocks, and avoidance of large meals immediately before retiring.

If two experienced teams are used, there is no alternative approach that results in such relatively short operating time.

Using this approach, one has the option of doing the esophagectomy without thoracotomy in selected cases of cancer involving the distal third of the esophagus. This decision can be made from the findings at laparotomy and the transhiatal dissection of the distal esophagus.

CHAPTER 27 Transabdominal esophagogastrectomy for the poor-risk patient

Manjit S. Bains

My standard approach for resection of a distal thoracic esophageal carcinoma is through a laparotomy and a separate right thoracotomy with an esophageal anastomosis placed within the chest. On occasion, an extrathoracic esophagectomy may be done through transhiatal and cervical exposures. However, both are extensive procedures and the associated physiologic insult is accompanied by substantial morbidity and mortality.

Over the past 6 years, for low-lying lesions, I have been able to perform an esophagogastrectomy through a transabdominal approach only, using the EEA stapler to accomplish an end-to-end anastomosis. This method has been applied only to a small number of patients in whom the transhiatal dissection of palpable tumor was possible. The singular advantage of this technique is the conversion of a prolonged procedure to a more expeditious one, possibly minimizing the morbidity by not entering the chest cavity or exploring the neck. This technique has been employed in 20 patients and has *not* yielded a morbidity or survival advantage over the standard technique. One early patient died from peritonitis resulting from an anastomotic leak. There have not been any major complications in the last 10 patients in whom this surgical approach was utilized.

TECHNIQUE OF TRANSABDOMINAL RESECTION

A laparotomy is done through a midline incision extending from the xiphoid process to 2 cm below the umbilicus. The liver and celiac nodes are carefully evaluated for metastases. The triangular ligament of the left lobe of the liver is divided and the peritoneum incised around the esophageal hiatus. For low-lying tumors of the esophagus, one can readily assess the resectability by exploration through the esophageal hiatus. Invasion of the pericardium or the aorta may preclude even a palliative resection. However, tumor involvement of the diaphragm is excised with a rim of normal muscle. The distal esophagus is mobilized through a dilated hiatus to include the periesophageal tissues present between the pericardium anteriorly, the adventitia of the aorta posteriorly, and the pleural reflections laterally. I believe that the exposure of the lower esophagus to the inferior pulmonary veins from the transhiatal approach is superior to the exposure obtained by the transthoracic approach. In a patient with a wide costal arch, and with the use of a self-retaining Goligher retractor (Fig. 27-1), one can dissect the esophagus with its surrounding periesophageal tissue almost to the subcarinal region. We do *not* feel that a satisfactory peribronchial or subcarinal node dissection can be done through this approach.

A decision is made at this point as to whether to do further esophageal resection and reconstruction through a right thoracotomy approach or to continue the extrathoracic dissection of the esophagus with anastomosis in the neck. Completion of the resection through this exposure is made if extensive local disease or limited metastatic disease in the liver is present and the approach is technically feasible. There is an advantage in avoiding a thoracotomy in frail, elderly, or very obese individuals to minimize pulmonary problems, provided the abdominal exposure enables completion of the anastomosis above the palpable esophageal tumor with the EEA stapler.

The stomach is mobilized along the greater curvature, dividing the gastrocolic ligament and preserving the right gastroepiploic and right gastric vessels but dividing the left gastric, left gastroepiploic, and short gastric vessels. A Kocher maneuver is *not* routinely performed. The celiac nodes are dissected and included with the spec-

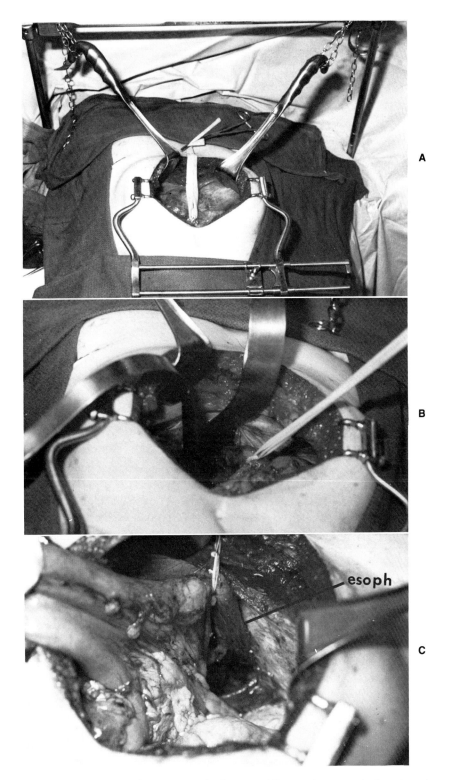

Fig. 27-1. A, A self-retaining Goligher retractor in place, providing good exposure in the epigastrium. The Penrose drain is around the esophagus. **B,** A close-up view of the exposure provided with the self-retaining retractor. The Harrington retractor at top is positioned in the esophageal hiatus, retracting the esophageal hiatus and pericardium anteriorly. It, too, can be supported on the Goligher for a consistently reliable exposure. **C,** The mobilized esophagus in the esophageal hiatus.

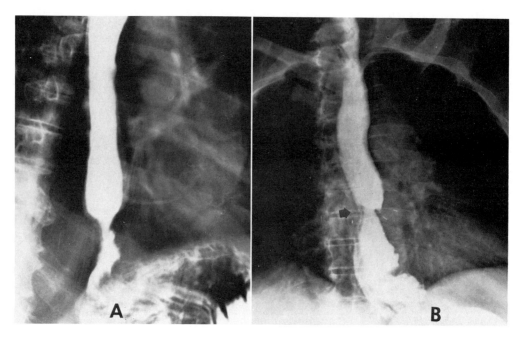

Fig. 27-2. A, Esophagram showing a large tumor at the gastroesophageal junction. **B,** Esophagram after resection, with the anastomosis marked by the arrow above the level of the inferior pulmonary vein.

imen. Through the lesser sac, the peritoneum is incised along the superior border of the pancreas, and all node-bearing tissue overlying the esophageal crurae and the abdominal aorta is swept up with the mobilized stomach. A pyloric drainage procedure is routinely performed. My preference is to do a hemipyloromyomectomy, excising the anterior half of the pyloric muscular ring, leaving the intact mucosa to pout through the seromuscular defect.[1] From 5 to 7 cm of normal esophagus above the tumor and 7 to 10 cm of stomach inferiorly are resected; the margins are routinely assessed for clearance with frozen-section pathology studies. The stomach is transected by applying first a TA-90 stapler, usually with 4.8-mm staples, across the stomach from the left side of the fundus toward the lesser curvature. The stapler is not placed all the way across the stomach. The 5 to 7 cm of stomach toward the midportion of lesser curvature is divided with the electrocautery and the open portion subsequently used for introduction of the EEA stapler. Two traction sutures are placed, at the 2-o'clock and 10-o'clock positions, and the esophagus is transected 5 cm above the proximal palpable tumor border. The resected specimen is submitted to pathology for frozen-section analysis of resection margins. A purse-string suture using 2-0 or 3-0 Prolene is placed about the esophageal margin in an over-and-over fashion. The appropriate-size EEA stapler is then selected. Two satisfactory doughnuts

of tissue must be obtained from the stapler with adequate exposure. The anastomosis is usually above the level of the inferior pulmonary veins (see Figs. 27-2 and 27-3).

If there is concern about an intact anastomosis or if the margin tests positive for tumor cells, a revision of the anastomosis is made through a separate right thoracotomy incision or a cervical incision may be made for completion of extrathoracic dissection and supraclavicular anastomosis. The gastrotomy along the lesser curvature is closed and the TA staple line reinforced with interrupted 3-0 silk sutures for seromuscular approximation over the staples. One pleural cavity is intentionally entered and drained. This is important for drainage of the mediastinum into the pleura rather than into the peritoneum in case of anastomotic leak. The stomach is loosely anchored to the diaphragm at the hiatus. The peritoneal cavity is not drained. The stomach is routinely decompressed with a Salem sump nasogastric tube.

RESULTS

Four of the 20 patients treated by transhiatal resection were completely obstructed and had limited liver metastases, one patient had a sigmoid lesion suspected of being carcinoma, and two patients were extremely obese. All other pa-

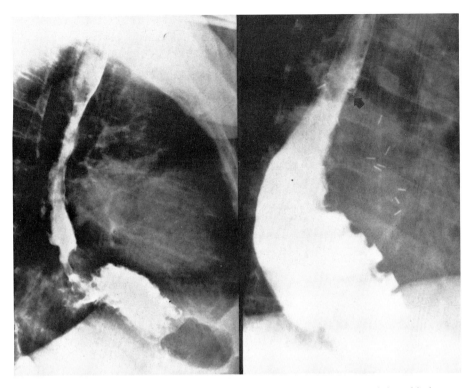

Fig. 27-3. Esophagram showing large tumor at the gastroesophageal junction *(left),* with the anastomosis indicated by the arrow *(right)* almost at the level of the left main bronchus.

tients had locally advanced disease. One patient died of peritonitis secondary to an anastomotic leak, and a second patient died of a cerebrovascular accident while recovering from postoperative pneumonia. Of the remaining 18 patients, one required a thoracotomy for closure of a disrupted TA staple line along the lesser curvature of the stomach, with a subsequent uneventful course. There are 12 patients now alive (range, 4 to 67 months), with two at 65 and 67 months.

COMMENTS

In cancer of the esophagus, distant metastases, including metastases to the liver, are contraindications to resection. However, patients (except those with tracheoesophageal fistula) suspected of having direct extraesophageal extension or periesophageal or celiac node metastases without distant metastasis are surgically explored with the intent of resection of all tumor if possible. I prefer to approach distal esophageal tumors through a midline laparotomy and a separate right posterolateral thoracotomy incision. If the resection is clearly palliative or if the general condition of the patient is not optimal, an extrathoracic resection

through a transhiatal and cervical exposure is considered. Even though most resections for esophageal carcinoma are palliative, there is a definite advantage in resecting all known tumor. The transabdominal approach can achieve this palliative resection in many patients with tumors in the lower third of the esophagus. I also prefer to perform the esophagogastrostomy anastomosis using the EEA stapler whenever possible. With this, anastomotic leaks are less frequently observed than with manual anastomosis. Because I am comfortable with the transhiatal dissection and the use of the EEA stapler, I recommend this abdominal approach for patients in whom exposure is satisfactory and adequate length of esophagus proximal to the tumor can be excised. This has been possible in nearly 10% of esophagectomies I have performed.

In none of the patients was this approach predetermined. The decision was made at the time of surgery in all instances. In five patients this approach was abandoned because of unsatisfactory anastomosis, and the procedure was completed in a conventional fashion through a thoracotomy approach. The procedure remains limited to distal esophageal tumors in medically high-risk patients.

CONCLUSION

Esophageal resection for carcinoma, whenever possible, provides satisfactory palliation, if not cure. The resection may be performed through the conventional Ivor Lewis[2] approach or trans-hiatally as popularized by Dr. Orringer.[3] In a select group of patients with low-lying lesions, a satisfactory resection can be performed transabdominally through the esophageal hiatus using an EEA stapler for the anastomosis, without thoracotomy or cervical incision.

REFERENCES

1. Bains, M.S., and Spiro, R.H.: Pharyngolaryngectomy, total extrathoracic esophagectomy and gastric transposition, Surg. Gynecol. Obstet. **149**:693, 1979.
2. Lewis, I.: The surgical treatment of carcinoma of the oesophagus, with special reference to a new operation for growths of the middle third, Br. J. Surg. **34**:18, 1946.
3. Orringer, M.B.: Transhiatal esophagectomy without thoracotomy for carcinoma of the thoracic esophagus, Ann. Surg. **200**:282, 1984.

Transabdominal esophagogastrectomy for the poor-risk patient

DISCUSSION

Frederick Griffith Pearson

Bains reports experience with 20 patients operated on during the past 6 years, who had a carcinoma of the distal esophagus managed by a low, intrathoracic esophagogastrostomy using a laparotomy and transhiatal approach without thoracotomy. The decision to use this method of reconstruction following resection was made at the time of exploration in a group of poor-risk patients. This method of reconstruction was selected as a possibly less morbid procedure than either esophagectomy without thoracotomy and a cervical reconstruction, or a thoracoabdominal approach.

The author notes that this technique had morbidity and mortality comparable to those of the alternative methods of reconstruction. One death occurred as a result of peritonitis secondary to a leak at the anastomosis, and another from complications of postoperative pneumonia; a third patient required reoperation because of disruption of the staple line along the lesser curvature of the stomach. Furthermore, in five additional patients, the intrathoracic anastomosis was considered unsatisfactory, and the anastomosis was redone through a thoracotomy.

OPERATIVE TECHNIQUE

The operative technique is clearly described and is straightforward. The stomach is mobilized in the usual fashion. The EEA stapler is passed through a part of the lesser curvature incision that is left open until the esophagogastric anastomosis has been done. I concur with the observation that good exposure of the distal third of the intrathoracic esophagus is possible through a transhiatal approach, and allows a precise dissection up to the level of the inferior subcarinal compartment. The subcarinal glands themselves are not well visualized or easily accessible using this technique. A hemipyloromyomectomy is the preferred method for gastric drainage and is added routinely.

COMMENT

Bains has certainly demonstrated that a resection and intrathoracic reconstruction can be done through a laparotomy alone. I am doubtful, however, that this approach will actually reduce morbidity and mortality in a high-risk group of patients. I think it is unlikely that resecting the remaining intrathoracic esophagus using the combined transhiatal and cervical exposure (without thoracotomy) will add significantly to the risk. There is no comparison between the morbidity of an anastomotic leak in the neck and that of an intrathoracic leak. I agree with the author's indications for esophagectomy without thoracotomy in patients with selected tumors in the distal esophagus, but would choose abdominocervical exposure without thoracotomy for such patients.

CHAPTER **28** Median sternotomy in radical surgery for esophageal carcinoma involving cervical and upper thoracic segments

Juan J. Boretti

Radical surgical treatment of malignant lesions of the upper esophagus through conventional standard anterolateral and posterolateral thoracic incisions has been recognized as difficult to perform, because of several factors:

1. The highly situated lesion in the narrow superior bony thorax is relatively inaccessible by conventional thoracotomy. This has led to the employment of combined transpleural, abdominal, and cervical incisions, either concurrently or sequentially, in order to accomplish an adequate esophageal mobilization followed by gastric replacement or colon interposition.[7]

2. Each of these steps provides only a limited exposure of the organ, the lesion, and the surrounding structures. Consequently, appraisal of local conditions and the stage of the disease is difficult through these separate incisions. This constitutes a drawback when hasty changes from preoperative planning have to be made in the operating room.

3. In consecutive approaches there may be controversy regarding the proper order of the steps of the surgical procedure.

4. The anterolateral thoracic approach offers a limited surgical field for mobilization of the esophagus under direct vision. Dissection by this route often is cumbersome, even with the ipsilateral lung selectively deflated.

5. The posterolateral thoracotomy has none of these shortcomings but carries the nuisance of closing the thoracic incision, repositioning the patient, and redraping the operative field.

6. These latter two procedures may not permit a thorough contralateral lymph node dissection.

With these factors in mind, a nonconventional anterior approach with sternum-splitting has been recently attempted in selected cases to resect both benign and malignant lesions. Early results of this brief experience seem encouraging from both surgical and oncologic perspectives.

BACKGROUND PERSPECTIVE

Since 1981, esophagectomy without thoracotomy has been frequently employed by our group for treatment of esophageal carcinoma and other nonmalignant lesions. With this technique, subtotal or total esophagectomies with cervical anastomosis can be performed in one stage and the procedure carried out with the patient in the supine position. The stomach has been generally used as the esophageal substitute, except in one case in which the colon was employed.[2]

Although often considered an unwise oncologic procedure, experience gained with these independent cervical and abdominal incisions has shown that blunt dissection in most circumstances allows a satisfactory resection of lesions located at upper or lower ends of the esophagus. In these cases the esophageal wall in the middle third is usually free of neoplastic infiltration and a blunt mobilization can be carried out through the hiatus of the diaphragm.[3] However, this approach is not so appropriate for tumors lying across the thoracic inlet in the lower cervical and upper thoracic esophagus, in middle-third lesions, and when adjacent mediastinal structures are involved.

At one time, a one-stage combined procedure through separate cervical, thoracic, and abdominal incisions with a two-team approach was used (Harrison and Pickett's technique).[4] Direct access through a right anterolateral thoracotomy allowed sharp dissection of the middle esophagus but frequently did not meet the requirements for a thorough en bloc excision of compromised contiguous upper mediastinal fat and lymph nodes. Such traditional combined cancer operations were often associated with a significant morbidity, and cure of cancer patients was seldom achieved.

Experience with surgical management of tracheal, vascular, and mediastinal lesions through a sternum-splitting approach led us to consider this route as expeditious and safe for handling malignant and nonmalignant esophageal lesions. With median sternotomy it is possible not only to excise the upper and middle intrathoracic esophagus but also to dissect the anterior, bilateral, and subcarinal tracheal node groups under direct vision. When this approach is used to treat esophageal tumors, extension of the incision into the neck proves helpful for radical neck dissection and for ease of performing the proximal anastomosis. Once the cervical esophagus and upper and middle thoracic esophagus are freed, the sternotomy is extended caudad with an abdominal midline incision, in order to mobilize the stomach or colon to be used as an esophageal substitute.

In terms of preoperative risk assessment, this approach has hazards and contraindications similar to those of other conventional thoracic procedures.

Having employed this technique in several cases, I found that it had been previously described in Waddell and Scannell's[5] and Orringer's[6] reports, in which the use of total or partial median sternotomy, respectively, was advocated. I fully agree with these authors and understand that my work is the reaffirmation of the technique published by Waddell and Scannell,[5] to whom full credit should be given.

OPERATIVE TECHNIQUE

The patient is placed in the supine position, with the neck slightly extended and the head turned to the left. General anesthesia with tracheal intubation is used. The endotracheal tube employed should allow lateral movements of the trachea during dissection. Caution should be taken that unnoticed airway obstruction by kinking does not occur during these maneuvers. Spiraled wire-embedded endotracheal tubes are recommended to avoid this intraoperative accident. A central venous catheter is positioned in the superior vena cava through a vein of the *right* arm. This is important because the left innominate vein will be divided to gain adequate exposure of the mediastinum. A radial artery line and electrocardio-

graphic monitoring are routinely used.

The abdomen, anterior chest, and neck are prepared and draped. The incision is made along the right sternocleidomastoid muscle to the suprasternal notch and is continued downward with the median sternotomy incision. Sternum splitting by means of an electric or pneumatic saw is then accomplished (Fig. 28-1). Pleural opening can ordinarily be avoided by asking the anesthetist to deflate the lungs at this stage. However, opening of the pleura does not have further consequences, providing chest tubes are placed before final closure. A sternal retractor provides generous exposure of the operative field. If necessary, a self-retaining Adson retractor positioned in the neck provides additional maneuverability for dissection (Fig. 28-2).

Once thymic and mediastinal fat is dissected away, the cervical and thoracic great vessels are exposed in the anterior mediastinum. The left innominate vein is divided between vascular clamps (Fig. 28-3) to enable restoration of its continuity by an end-to-end anastomosis at completion of the procedure. This is an important technical point to gain access to the aortic arch and its branches. These are carefully freed and surrounded with tapes. The course of the left recurrent laryngeal nerve behind the aortic arch is identified to prevent inadvertent injury. By gentle spreading of the vascular clamps on the ends of the innominate vein and lifting of the aorta forward and to the left, comfortable exposure of the treachea and both paratracheal lymph node areas is gained. The trachea is then cautiously dissected free and encircled with tapes, with care being taken to avoid injury to the recurrent laryngeal nerves in the tracheoesophageal groove.

Alternate shifting of tracheal sling tapes to the right and to the left permits sharp mobilization of the anterior surface of the esophagus under direct vision from the subcarinal level to the thoracic inlet (see Fig. 28-3), thus avoiding injury to the posterior membranous trachea. Dissection of the cervical esophagus is carried out, with the sternocleidomastoid muscle and the carotid sheath being retracted laterally. The trachea and the thyroid gland are retracted medially, and the right laryngeal nerve is identified in the tracheoesophageal groove. The esophagus is freed posteriorly from the prevertebral fascia. The vagus and the recurrent laryngeal nerves should, whenever possible, be carefully preserved in order to prevent postoperative vocal cord dysfunction, impaired swallowing, and tracheobronchial aspiration. The omohyoid, sternothyroid, and sternohyoid muscles may be transected at this stage for additional exposure. Use of rigid retractors must be gentle to avoid recurrent laryngeal nerve trauma.

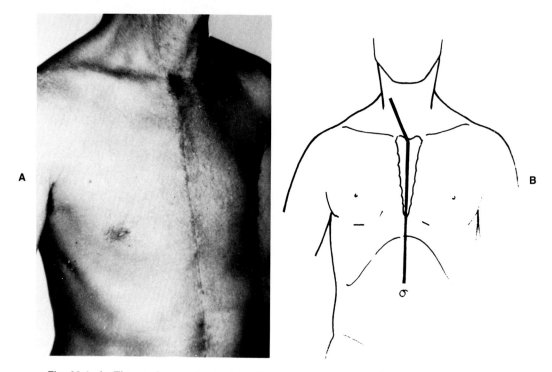

Fig. 28-1. A, The continuous skin incision for anterior approach is shown in this postoperative view. **B,** Diagram of the incision.

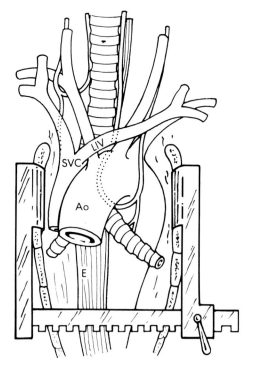

Fig. 28-2. Diagram of the extensive operative field obtained after placing the sternal retractor. *SVC,* Superior vena cava; *LIV,* left innominate vein; *E,* esophagus; *Ao,* aorta.

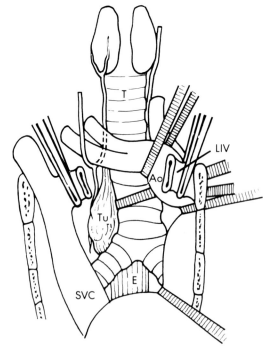

Fig. 28-3. Division of the left innominate vein gives additional exposure. Vascular clamps enable reanastomosis at the end of the procedure. Note sling tapes around aorta, cervical trunks, and trachea, which facilitate esophageal exposure. Gentle lifting of the aorta forward and to the left provides ready access to the upper midesophagus. The trachea can be exposed to the carina and both main bronchi. *SVC,* Superior vena cava; *Tu,* tumor; *LIV,* left innominate vein; *E,* esophagus; *T,* trachea; *Ao,* aorta.

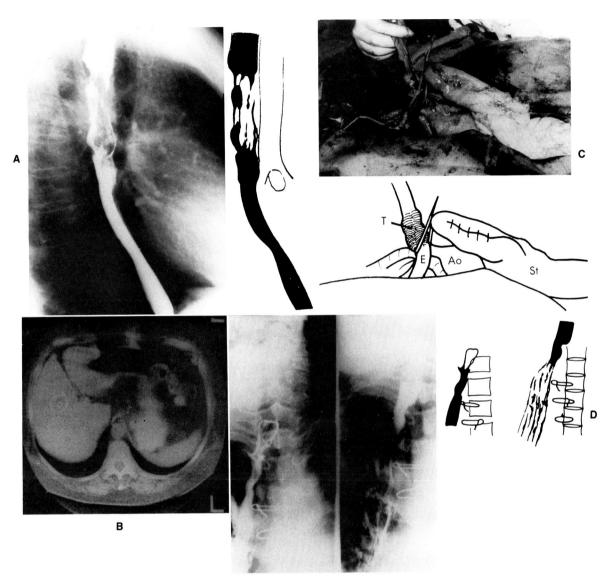

Fig. 28-4. Patient 5, Table 28-1. **A,** Preoperative esophagogram showing an upper-third filling defect behind the tracheal aerogram. Biopsy revealed a squamous cell carcinoma. **B,** CT scan demonstrates an intrahepatic nodule in same patient. After its removal through the abdominal incision, histologic examination revealed a benign hamartoma. **C,** Pictorial view of the operative field in the anterior approach. The esophagus has been freed to the neck incision and the tumor isolated. Note oversewn gastric fundus brought high without tension. It is positioned in the posterior mediastinum, before the proximal anastomosis is begun. *Ao,* Aorta; *T,* tumor; *St,* stomach; *E,* esophagus. **D,** Postoperative esophagogram.

Completion of esophageal freeing from the neck down to both main bronchi through this anterior route is done under direct visual control. By gentle pulling of the aortic arch to the left and the trachea to the right, exposure of the left paratracheal area is obtained and a meticulous dissection of the fat pad bearing lymph nodes is done in a cephalad direction to the left side of the neck. Again, care is exercised at this point to avert undesirable left recurrent laryngeal nerve injury. Removal of the right paratracheal lymph nodes

en bloc with the ipsilateral cervical groups is accomplished as well. Sharp excision of subcarinal nodes is somewhat more difficult, but it may also be carried out along with the tracheobronchial groups over both main bronchi.

During the surgical procedure, two different situations may be encountered:

1. A *resectable* esophageal lesion, in which a radical curative excision may be done (see Table 28-1 and Figs. 28-4 to 28-6)
2. A *nonresectable* malignant tumor involving

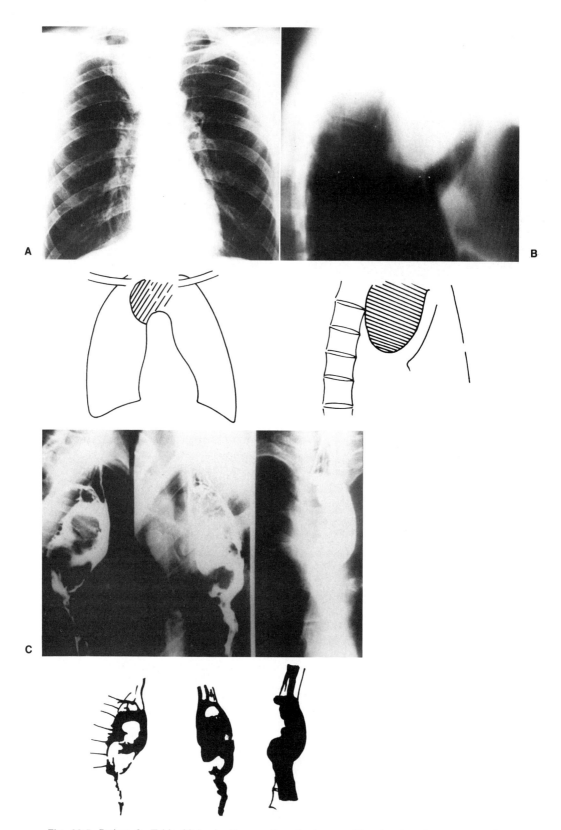

Fig. 28-5. Patient 2, Table 28-1. **A,** Preoperative chest x-ray film showing the presence of a mediastinal mass in the superior mediastinum. **B,** Lateral film in the same case shows the tumor in the posterior mediastial compartment. Note contact of the tumor with the tracheal wall. Bronchoscopic examination showed only a moderate forward displacement of the trachea without involvement. **C,** Preoperative esophagogram showing a bulky filling defect in the upper intrathoracic esophagus. This image was attributed to an intramural esophageal tumor that was clinically suspected of being a leiomyosarcoma.

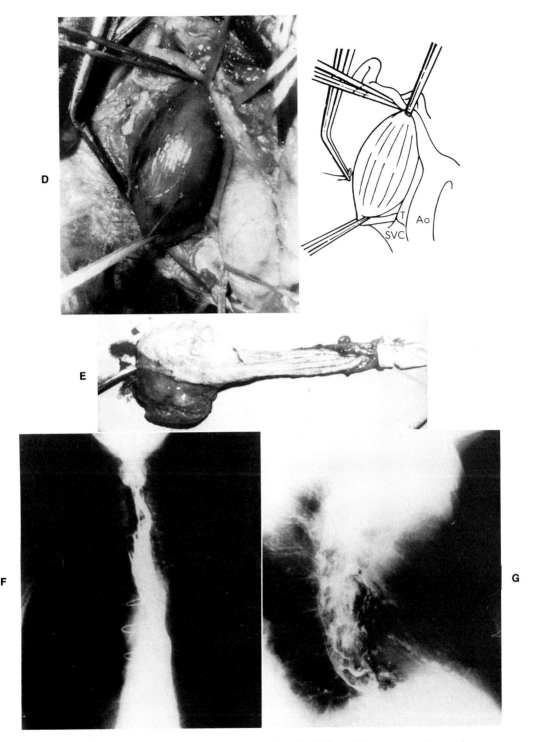

Fig. 28-5, cont'd. D, View of the same case at operation. By lifting of sling tapes on the esophagus, the tumor is conveniently exposed. *SVC,* Superior vena cava; *T,* trachea; *Ao,* aorta. **E,** Surgical specimen. Subtotal esophagectomy with intramural tumor in the upper end. Histologic examination revealed a benign leiomyoma with necrosis. **F,** Esophagogram on the ninth postoperative day showing the cervical esophagogastric anastomosis. **G,** Same case, lateral view. Note the stomach in the posterior mediastinum and signs of mild tracheobronchial aspiration of contrast medium. Regurgitation subsided a few weeks later.

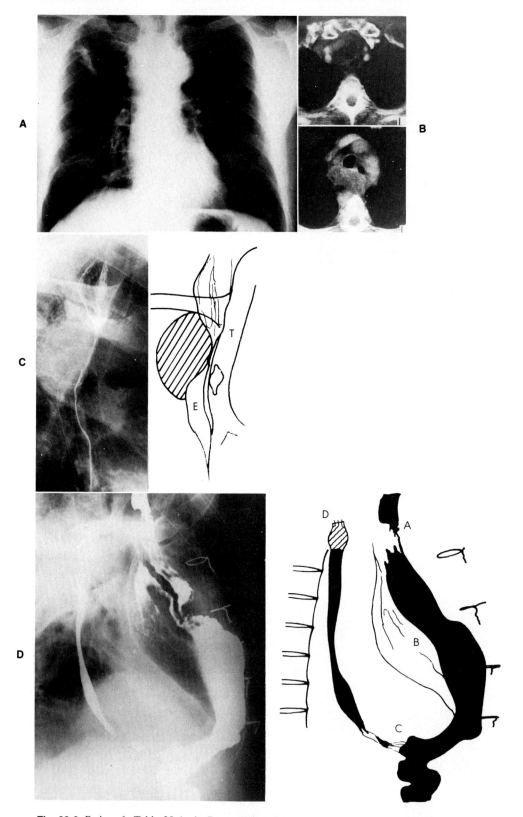

Fig. 28-6. Patient 6, Table 28-1. **A,** Preoperative chest x-ray film showing a mass in the superior mediastinum and an infiltrate in the right upper lobe. **B,** CT scan shows a large tumor in the posterior mediastinum with esophageal involvement. **C,** Preoperative esophagogram showing marked upper-third stenosis causing severe dysphagia. Endoscopy revealed a firm nondilatable stricture at 25 cm from the incisors. *E,* Esophagus; *T,* trachea. **D,** Barium swallow on the tenth postoperative day shows palliative bypass procedure carried out through anterior approach. *A,* Proximal esophagogastric anastomosis in the neck. *B,* The stomach positioned in the anterior mediastinum. *C,* Distal end of in situ esophageal body with end-to-side anastomosis to gastric antrum. Gastroesophageal reflux of contrast medium refilling the body of the esophagus. *D,* Oversewn upper end of the body of the esophagus in the cervical area.

vital adjacent mediastinal structures, in which a palliative bypass technique is feasible (see Fig. 28-6 and Table 28-1)

In both situations the procedure is carried out through the midline abdominal incision. In the former, esophageal intrathoracic dissection is completed through a medial phrenic incision. The stomach is mobilized, preserving the right gastric and right gastroepiploic arteries and the gastroepiploic arcade. The duodenum may be mobilized, if necessary, to obtain the required length of the gastric conduit for esophageal substitution. A pyloroplasty is routinely made in order to ensure good gastric emptying. The gastroesophageal junction is transected and oversewn in two layers. The stomach is brought cephalad to the neck through the posterior mediastinum. Care is taken to avoid undue tension at the cervical anastomosis. The highest portion of the gastric fundus is selected, and a two-layer esophagogastric anastomosis (end-to-side) with nonabsorbable interrupted sutures is accomplished (see Fig. 28-4, *C* and *D*.) For a bulky fundus, resection of the sternoclavicular joint may be considered in order to widen the thoracic inlet and avoid compression at this site. Suspension of the gastric fundus from the prevertebral fascia with anchoring nonabsorbable interrupted sutures prevents tension on the anastomotic suture line.

Adequate protection of bone edges is taken during digestive tract anastomoses to minimize the risk of sternal wound infection and possible subsequent dehiscence.

When the tumor is nonresectable (see Fig. 28-6), the proximal esophagus is transected and its thoracic end above the tumor is oversewn with nonabsorbable interrupted sutures. With the esophageal body being left in its mediastinal bed, the cardia is divided transabdominally, the stomach mobilized, and a pyloroplasty performed as previously described. This is followed by an end-to-side anastomosis of the distal end of the esophageal body to the antrum of the stomach. The stomach is elevated out of the abdomen and delivered to the neck along the anterior mediastinum. The esophagogastric anastomosis is performed in an identical fashion to that in resected cases.

A feeding jejunostomy for nutritional support is usually carried out in both resected and nonresected cases. A nasogastric tube is positioned across the anastomosis for gastric decompression, to avoid reflux and possible aspiration in the immediate postoperative period.

An end-to-end anastomosis of the divided ends of the left innominate vein is performed before closing the sternum. If either pleural cavity has been entered, chest tubes are placed. A separate closed-tube drainage system near the cervical anastomosis is routinely employed.

POSTOPERATIVE COURSE

Postoperative incisional pain from sternotomy is ordinarily more tolerable than in lateral thoracotomies. Because impairment of ventilation is lessened, pleuropulmonary complications are minimal and postoperative courses uneventful.

Some distressing complications have occurred, including transient vocal cord dysfunction, impaired swallowing, and tracheobronchial aspiration with inadvertent trauma either to the vagus or recurrent laryngeal nerve. If anastomotic leaks supervene, they are usually transient and heal spontaneously with conservative management. This is in sharp contrast to the catastrophic consequences of intrathoracic anastomotic leakage, which results in extended hospital stays and high mortality.

These last two complications lend credence to the utility and safety of adjuncts such as the decompressing nasogastric tube and the feeding jejunostomy. Both should be maintained until anastomotic leaks are ruled out by contrast radiographic swallow and the patient is able to resume an oral diet.

When a radical cervicomediastinal lymphadenectomy is performed, pleural effusion or even chylothorax is likely to appear. However, these complications usually subside in a few days with management by thoracentesis.

CLINICAL CASES

During 1985, six esophageal surgical procedures were performed using a completely anterior approach with contiguous cervicotomy, median sternotomy, and midline abdominal incisions (see Fig. 28-1). Four patients had esophageal carcinomas. Three of them were located in the upper thoracic esophagus (see Table 28-1). The fourth was a middle-third carcinoma in which surgical resection was not satisfactory because dissection under direct visual control was not feasible. The patient, who had associated malnutrition and chronic bronchopulmonary suppurative disease, died on the ninth postoperative day with anastomotic leakage and sepsis. Although a middle-third esophageal carcinoma case is not a strict indication for the anterior approach, the fatal outcome may be more attributable to the patient's prior general condition and malnutrition than to the approach per se.

One patient had a nonresectable malignant me-

TABLE 28-1. Summary data on patients and procedures

Patient	Age	Sex	Pathology	Site of lesion
1	65	M	Esophageal carcinoma	Upper third
2	41	M	Esophageal leiomyoma with necrotic changes	Upper third
3	60	M	Esophageal carcinoma	Upper third
4	58	M	Esophageal carcinoma	Middle third
5	57	F	Esophageal carcinoma	Upper third
6	54	M	Mediastinal carcinoma with esophageal involvement	Upper third

*This patient had ligation of left innominate vein instead of anastomosis.

diastinal mass with esophageal involvement. A bypass palliative procedure was done in this particular case (see Fig. 28-6).

Finally, one patient had a very large esophageal intramural tumor, initially suspected of being a leiomyosarcoma, and is a good example of the advantages of the anterior approach (see Fig. 28-5). In spite of the final histologic examination report disclosing a benign necrotic leiomyoma, it has been included here in order to illustrate some technical details of the procedure. Had it been a malignant tumor, the esophageal resection would have been easily performed through the anterior route with the technique described. In addition, the operative findings in this particular case suggest the use of this approach for enucleation of esophageal benign leiomyomas in selected cases. Surgical management of large, high leiomyomas by means of conventional techniques may be awkward through a lateral thoracotomy.

CONCLUSIONS

The anterior thoracic approach makes possible a ready and direct exposure of the esophagus from the neck to the tracheal bifurcation. This is accomplished by means of a continuous incision that includes a cervicotomy, a median sternotomy, and a midline abdominal incision. This approach has the following advantages:

1. Reduced incisional pain and discomfort from this approach result in a benign postoperative course with minimal or no respiratory complications.
2. Freeing of the esophagus from the trachea and surrounding tissues and organs may be achieved by means of sharp dissection under direct visual control, thus minimizing the risk of undesirable injury to any of these anatomic structures.
3. Removal of cervicomediastinal fat pads and lymph node groups may be meticulously accomplished under direct vision on both sides of the sagittal plane.
4. Blunt dissection of the lower third of the esophagus and gastric or colonic mobilization for esophageal substitution through the median abdominal incision present no difficulty.
5. This technically straightforward procedure may be carried out in the supine position, thus avoiding tedious intraoperative positional changes and field redraping.

In our opinion, lower cervical and upper thoracic esophageal lesions may be deemed as precise indications for the elective anterior approach. This opinion is by no means intended to deny the value of conventional thoracotomies, which have their own precise indications. The anterior surgical approach is a known technique, suitable for selected cases of esophageal carcinoma, with the aim of improving the meager therapeutic results in this disease.

ACKNOWLEDGEMENT

I wish to acknowledge the assistance of Dr. J.L. Sgrosso in surgery and in the preparation of the manuscript for this chapter.

REFERENCES

1. Sanderson, D.R., and Bernatz, P.E.: Malignant tumors of the esophagus and cardia of the stomach. In Payne, W.S., and Olsen, A.M., editors: The esophagus, Philadelphia, 1974, Lea & Febiger.
2. Boretti, J.J., Piazza, M., Della Bianca, J.A., Di Giorno, H., Novelli, J., and Rodriguiz Otero, J.: Esofagectomía sin toractomía, Rev. Argent Cirugía **43:**41, 1982.

Operation	Complications	Immediate results
Resection	Left cervical and upper arm venous thrombosis*	Good
Resection	Vocal cord dysfunction; transient	Good
Resection en bloc with cervicomediastinal lymph nodes	Pleural effusion	Good
Blunt resection	Esophageal leak	Death
	Sepsis	
Resection en bloc with cervicomediastinal lymph nodes	Gastric distention within thorax	Good
Palliative bypass	Acute respiratory failure	Good

3. Orringer, MB., and Orringer, J.S.: Transhiatal esophagectomy without thoracotomy: a dangerous operation? J. Thorac. Cardiovasc. Surg. **85:**72, 1983.
4. Harrision, A.W., and Pickett, W.H.: One-stage multiple approach operation for cancer of upper and mid-thoracic esophagus, Surgery **28:**771, 1950.
5. Waddell, W.R., and Scannell, J.G.: Anterior approach to carcinoma of the superior mediastinal and cervical segments of the esophagus, J. Thorac. Surg. **33:**663, 1957.
6. Orringer, M.B.: Partial median sternotomy: anterior approach to the upper thoracic esophagus, J. Thorac. Cardiovasc. Surg. **87:**124, 1984.

Median sternotomy in radical surgery for esophageal carcinoma involving cervical and upper thoracic segments

DISCUSSION

Frederick Griffith Pearson

Boretti describes an operative approach for exposure and resection of esophageal cancer situated in the upper third of the posterior mediastinum behind the mediastinal trachea. Although a high, right thoracotomy provides good exposure of the esophagus and related structures at levels below the lower half of the trachea, esophageal resection becomes progressively more difficult when the tumor lies in the narrowest part of the bony thorax immediately below the thoracic inlet. Boretti proposes the addition of median sternotomy for resection of tumors in the lower cervical and upper mediastinal esophagus. Boretti contends that the addition of sternotomy provides exposure that facilitates resection of the primary cancer itself along with the pretracheal, paratracheal, and subcarinal nodes and mediastinal fatty contents. He notes that this anterior approach was first described by Waddell and Scannell of Boston as long ago as 1957. The author reports experience with six patients in whom this approach was used during 1985.

OPERATIVE TECHNIQUE

The technique used in these cases is described in detail and is clearly defined with accompanying diagrams and photographs. The usual incision begins in the neck along the anterior border of one or other sternocleidomastoid muscle and is continued as a full median sternotomy into the upper abdomen. Exposure allows an easy cervical anastomosis, a neck dissection if indicated, controlled resection of the upper thoracic esophagus, and preparation of the stomach or colon for subse-

quent replacement. A single-stage operation is done, and no repositioning of the patient is required.

Exposure of the mediastinal trachea and the adjacent esophagus is obtained following division of the left innominate vein and displacement of the aortic arch anteriorly and to the left. This approach provides good exposure throughout most of the tracheal length, but may not afford optimal access at the level of the carina, main bronchi, and subcarinal compartment. Better exposure at the subcarinal level can be obtained using a transpericardial approach with vertical division of the anterior pericardium to expose the intrapericardial segments of the ascending aorta and superior vena cava. The posterior pericardium can then be divided vertically between these vessels down to the level of the superior border of the right main pulmonary artery. With division of the posterior pericardium in this way, the distal trachea and subcarinal compartment is readily accessible. We commonly employ this approach for resection of tumors involving the distal trachea or carina and find that it provides predictably good access.

If the mediastinal trachea is then encircled with a sling, it can be readily displaced to either side, thus affording direct access to the underlying esophagus and the paratracheal and paraesophageal areas on both sides. At the subcarinal level, a sling encircling either main bronchus facilitates exposure. With the use of this anterior approach, both recurrent laryngeal nerves can be identified and preserved throughout the full length of their courses in the esophagotracheal groove.

Mobilization of the stomach through the incision is straightforward. The importance of a complete Kocherization of this duodenum is appropriately emphasized.

ADVANTAGES

We have used this exposure in only four patients. Even with this limited experience, however, I would support Boretti's contention that this anterior approach is superior to any alternative operative exposure for difficult resections at and below the level of the thoracic inlet. I believe it has a clear application in selected cases. When a radical resection is indicated, this is the only approach that gives clear exposure of the pretracheal and paratracheal compartments, allowing a precise resection of the surrounding tissues and glands with the least potential for injury to the recurrent laryngeal nerves. I believe this approach will be more widely adopted as surgeons in other centers gain experience with this operation.

CHAPTER 29 Elective surgical techniques for cervical and postcricoid lesions

Kam-Hing Lam and William Ignace Wei

For anatomic reasons, squamous carcinoma arising from the cervical and postcricoid regions of the esophagus and hypopharynx gives rise to special problems in surgical management. The cervical portion of the esophagus, which is 5 to 6 cm in length, lies immediately below the hypopharynx and the larynx. A tumor located in the cervical esophagus would be so close to the larynx and hypopharynx that in surgical treatment, en bloc resection of all three structures is often necessary. The defect extending from the base of the tongue to the cardia is best bridged by bringing the stomach up to the neck for direct anastomosis to the pharynx.

The postcricoid area, 2 to 3 cm in height, is the lowermost and narrowest portion of the hypopharynx. A tumor at that site necessitates a circumferential pharyngectomy and laryngectomy. The amount of esophagus to be resected is controversial but, in view of the possibility of submucosal spread of carcinoma,[1,2] should not be less than 3 cm beyond the gross tumor margin. Therefore, if the cancer is limited to the hypopharynx alone, an adequate distal resection margin can be obtained while a short end of the cervical esophagus is preserved for anastomosis by a local or regional reconstructive method. However, in most instances, the tumor has some degree of extension into the esophagus, so that after adequate excision a safe and easy cervical anastomosis is not possible. It is therefore preferable to resect the whole esophagus and reconstruct with the stomach.

PREOPERATIVE ASSESSMENT

The usual investigative procedures are carried out. Special attention is paid to the radiologic extent of the disease shown on barium swallow, particularly its inferior aspect. This information, as pointed out earlier, will determine whether a limited resection of the hypopharymx will suffice or not. The same information is often not obtainable from endoscopy because the tumor obstructs passage of the instrument.

The upper extent of the tumor should be noted. If a cancer reaches the level of the tonsils, resection will have to include the palatoglossal fold and part of the soft palate. Stretching the stomach to such a high level makes the anastomosis unsafe because of possible tension. Other methods of reconstruction, such as myocutaneous flaps, are required.

Study of the whole length of the esophagus should not be omitted. A second tumor may be present in 10% to 15% of patients. In these, thoracotomy and esophagectomy under direct vision are indicated because blood supply to the tumor-bearing thoracic esophagus will be too proliferate to be dissected blindly.

Bronchoscopy is routinely performed to detect tracheal invasion so that appropriate resection can be included if required.

Assessment of cardiac and respiratory function is important. Although thoracotomy is not performed when the thoracic esophagus is dissected via the neck and the abdomen, the operation involves entering the mediastinum with possible contamination of the pleural cavities. In particular, the heart will be compressed during blind dissection of the lower thoracic esophagus through the hiatus. Venous return will be markedly impaired and cardiac output reduced by a situation not unlike cardiac tamponade. Momentary myocardial ischemia and arrhythmia may take place, and the heart should be able to withstand this condition.

OPERATIVE TECHNIQUES
Pharyngolaryngoesophagectomy and pharyngogastric anastomosis
Resection of laryngopharynx

This operation was first described by Ong and Lee in 1960,[3] when thoracotomy was included. LeQuesne and Ranger[4] subsequently described the procedure without thoracotomy.

Under oroendotracheal ventilation the patient is placed in the supine position. The neck is hyperextended with raised support behind the shoulders. The surgical area prepared stretches from the mandibular border to the symphysis pubis. A transverse incision at the level of the thyroid notch is made and skin flaps are raised to the hyoid bone above and to the suprasternal notch below.

Beginning along the anterior borders of the sternocleidomastoid muscles, the surgeon dissects free the laryngopharyngeal complex. The interval between the pharyngeal constrictor muscles and the carotid sheath is entered until the prevertebral fascia is reached. On the side of the lesion the thyroid lobe is included in the specimen to be resected, while the lobe on the contralateral side is preserved unless infiltrated by tumor. The internal laryngeal neurovascular bundle is divided, and the posterior pharyngeal wall separated from the prevertebral fascia.

The site of proximal resection is defined by dissection along the upper border of the hyoid bone. Care is taken to avoid damage to the lingual arteries along the upper border of the greater cornu of the hyoid bone. Muscles of the tongue attached to the hyoid are incised until the mucosa of the valleculae is reached.

Attention is now turned to the trachea, which is separated from the cervical esophagus. Preparation is then made for transection of the trachea and fashioning of a terminal tracheostomy. The site for the trachea is marked on the inferior neck skin flap, immediately above the sternal notch. Four small skin flaps made with a cruciate incision will avoid future tracheocutaneous stenosis.[5] After 5 minutes of oxygenation, the trachea is divided. With the patient maintained on Venturi jet ventilation, the terminal tracheostome is created by suturing the small skin flaps into corresponding slits in the trachea.

The next step includes transection of the pharynx and dissection of the esophagus. The hyoid bone is held with strong forceps and pulled forward. The pharynx is entered at the valleculae and divided well above the tumor, with the mucosal surface under direct vision (Fig. 29-1). The pharyngolaryngeal specimen is then wrapped in a large pack to avoid contamination. With the

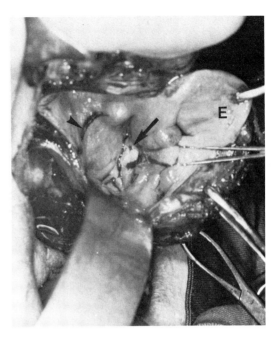

Fig. 29-1. Pharynx entered above hyoid bone. Tissue forceps holding epiglottis. Tumor in sight *(arrow)*. Posterior pharyngeal wall about to be divided along marking *(arrowhead)*.

pack held in one hand, the esophagus is put on stretch and the plane between it and the trachea is dissected downward into the mediastinum. With retraction to give good exposure, the upper part of the thoracic esophagus is freed under direct vision (Fig. 29-2). Lower down, dissection is carried out bluntly using wet gauze swabs. The carina can be reached from the neck. The remaining thoracic esophagus is dissected from below.

Preparation of the stomach and mediastinal dissection

Attention is now turned to the abdomen. Through an upper midline incision the stomach is prepared in the usual manner described in Chapter 25. It is important to free the duodenum extensively, until the entire inferior vena cava is exposed, so that the stomach can be stretched high into the upper neck. If necessary, the gastric arcade along the lesser curve can be divided to give extra length to the stomach. The abdominal esophagus is freed and the hiatus is defined. The crura of the diaphragm are divided to allow dissection of the lower thoracic esophagus. This is initially done under direct vision. For the remaining middle stretch of the thoracic esophagus,

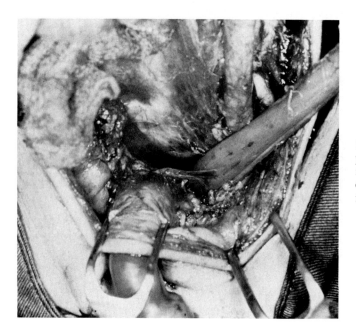

Fig. 29-2. Esophagus put on stretch by pulling on the pharyngolaryngeal specimen. Separation between trachea and esophagus continues into the mediastinum.

blind dissection with the right hand inserted into the mediastinum is required. It is important that the hand does not stray away from the esophageal wall. The posterior attachments are easily freed while the anterior attachment to the carina may require dissection with the finger hooked around it and stripping from above. Completion of dissection is verified by transmitting pulling action from abdomen to neck and vice versa.

On completion of dissection the gastroesophageal junction is divided and the cardia closed. The distal end of the abdominal esophagus is transfixed and attached to two pieces of long gauze swabs (Fig. 29-3). As the pharyngolaryngoesophagectomy specimen is removed via the neck, the gauze swabs are guided into the posterior mediastinum. They serve as tamponade for minor bleeding there. Pyloromyotomy is then performed. The fundus of the stomach is anchored to the ends of the gauze swabs, which are then withdrawn via the neck wound. By this action, together with gentle delivery with the other hand, the stomach is guided into the posterior mediastinum to appear at the root of the neck.

Pharyngogastric anastomosis

Pharyngogastric anastomosis is performed with two layers of interrupted sutures, inner catgut and outer silk. The posterior outer layer is put in first (Fig. 29-4), and continued until it is felt that tension will be increased if more of the stomach is sutured to the posterior pharyngeal wall. Then the fundus is opened through a T-shaped incision and the inner layer of sutures inserted. With this

completed, the anterior wall of the stomach is pulled up to the base of the tongue, which may descend somewhat to meet the gastric wall. The anterior outer layer is completed (Fig. 29-5). No anchoring sutures are necessary. The neck incision is closed after insertion of drains. The abdomen is closed without drainage. Two chest drains are routinely inserted.

Technical difficulties

Dissection in the neck is usually straightforward. If the trachea is infiltrated to a significant extent, resection of part of it will be necessary, and manubrium resection to allow a terminal tracheostomy at a lower level will be required.

At the time of mediastinal dissection, bleeding may be encountered. Retraction of the enlarged hiatus allows location and control of the bleeder. On rare occasions immediate thoracotomy may be necessary for identifying and ligating the bleeding vessel, particularly if it is the azygos vein. Blind and blunt separation of the trachea from the esophagus should be undertaken with care, so that the soft membranous posterior wall of the trachea is not torn. If a small vent is produced, it will subsequently be sealed off by the stomach. A large tear will require repair through a thoracotomy.

In the abdomen, the most vulnerable structure is the right gastroepiploic vein, on which the venous drainage of the entire stomach depends heavily. The fact that it drains to the superior mesenteric vein, along with the middle colic vein, puts it at risk of tension when the stomach is

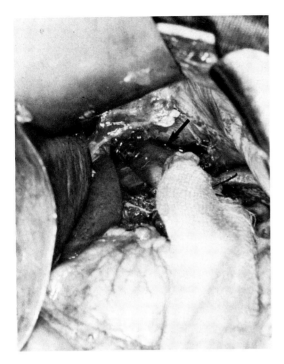

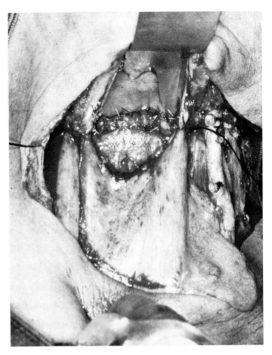

Fig. 29-3. Esophagus has been freed and gastroesophageal junction divided. Two pieces of long gauze swabs are attached to the distal end of the esophagus *(arrow)*, to be pulled into the posterior mediastinum as the esophagus is removed in the neck.

Fig. 29-4. Pharyngogastric anastomosis. Posterior rows of sutures in place.

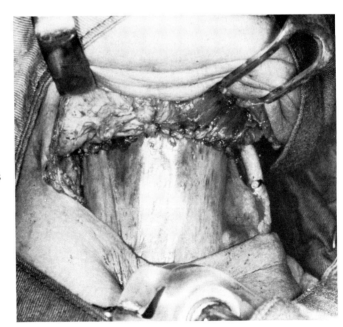

Fig. 29-5. Pharyngogastric anastomosis completed.

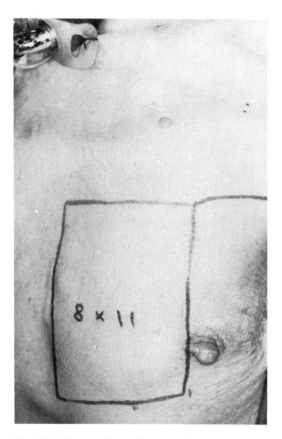

Fig. 29-6. Rectangular outline on skin overlying pectoralis major muscle.

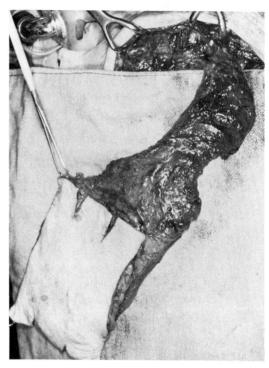

Fig. 29-7. Skin island, with underlying pectoralis major muscle, showing three slits on skin edge.

pulled up to the neck. The danger is enhanced if the transverse colon is retracted inferiorly at the same time. If drainage via this avenue is compromised from control of bleeding at that point, the right gastric vein will be the only remaining and barely adequate portal, if it has not been divided previously.

When the stomach is delivered through the posterior mediastinum, it is essential that the fundus lead the way. If a point closer to the cardia is taken as the apex of the gastric preparation, the greater curve will be redundant and may fold on itself to lie on the right side and give rise to obstruction.

Postoperative care

A nasogastric tube is not necessary, since ileus is minimal and gastric retention unusual. Feeding by mouth can be commenced in 48 hours, beginning with fluids. It is stepped up to a full diet on day 7 to 10. In case of anastomotic leakage, feeding is stopped and parenteral nutrition instituted.

The neck drains are retained for 2 to 3 days.

The chest drains are maintained until a yield of less than 100 ml of fluid per tube is obtained each day.

Humidified oxygen is given via a mask. Blockage of the trachea is prevented by frequent clearing of dried sputum and blood clots. Because coughing is ineffective, assistance in keeping the trachea clear is necessary.

Pharyngolaryngectomy with cervical esophagectomy and tubed pectoralis major myocutaneous flap reconstruction
Resection

Resection follows the same procedure as described earlier. After transection of the pharynx above the hyoid bone, the tumor is examined to determine whether the resection margins are adequate with cervical esophageal resection alone. A finger is inserted into the pharyngoesophageal lumen to palpate the lower border of the tumor while transection of the esophagus is carried at least 3 cm distal to that level. The specimen is removed and reconstruction performed.

Tubed pectoralis major flap reconstruction

The distance between the transected pharynx and esophagus is measured. The donor skin island

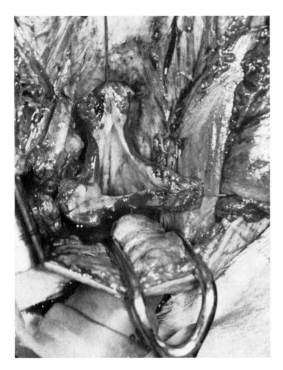

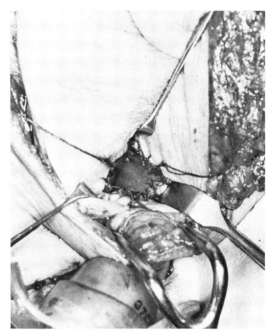

Fig. 29-9. Lower anastomosis completed.

Fig. 29-8. Three vertical slits, 2 cm in length each, are made on the esophageal end, for interdigitating into slits on the skin edge.

is marked out on the chest wall overlying the pectoralis major muscle (Fig. 29-6). A rectangular outline with a length equal to the height of the defect and a width of 7 to 8 cm is made. The pectoralis myocutaneous flap is raised, with the blood supply being based on the pectoral branch of the acromiothoracic vessels.[6] The prepared flap is brought up to the neck and rolled into a tube for anastomosis to the oropharynx and the esophagus.

Straightforward end-to-end anastomosis has a high chance of stricture formation. To reduce this, two slits are made on the anastomosing edge of the skin island (Fig. 29-7), which, together with the vertical suture line, make three slits. Three corresponding slits are made on the esophageal stump (Fig. 29-8). The esophageal projections thus produced are inserted into the slits in the skin island to produce an interdigitating anastomotic suture line (Fig. 29-9). Even with suture line contracture, the anastomosis does not become stenosed. Usually, the proximal anastomosis between the oropharynx and the skin tube, being much wider, does not require such an additional step, or may need only shallow slits on the skin edge alone.

A nasogastric tube is inserted before completion of the vertical suture line of the skin flap (Fig. 29-10). Subsequent management is straight-

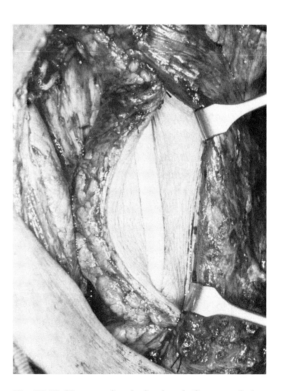

Fig. 29-10. Nasogastric tube in place before completion of vertical suture line of tubed pectoralis major myocutaneous flap.

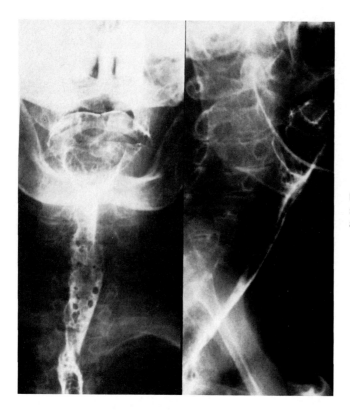

Fig. 29-11. Postoperative barium swallow showing intact mucocutaneous anastomosis and patent passage.

forward. Oral feeding is commenced on day 7 when integrity of the suture line has been demonstrated radiologically (Fig. 29-11).

RESULTS

After pharyngolaryngoesophagectomy and pharyngogastric anastomosis (gastric pull-up operation) the reported hospital mortality varies widely, between 0% and 31%.[1,7-10] Our previous report,[10] describing an experience of 157 such operations performed to 1979 for a variety of pathologic lesions, gave a hospital mortality of 31%. All deaths in hospital irrespective of length of stay were included.

With modification of the operative technique, the risk of this procedure has been reduced (see Table 29-1). The present hospital mortality is between 5% and 6%, and the postoperative complication rate 30%. Leakage of the pharyngogastric anastomosis occurs in about 10% of patients, neck wound infection in 5%, and chest infection in 15%.

Long-term postoperative functioning was studied in 136 patients who had survived more than 6 months.[11] It was found that their alimentary function was good and that 83% could take solid food. Regurgitation was present in 23% of patients, and gastric pathology in the form of chronic ulcers and/or gastritis occurred in five of the 136 patients.

The tubed pectoralis major myocutaneous flap was used for reconstruction of circumferential defects of the pharynx in eight patients. In two patients the anastomoses had been performed in a conventional end-to-end circular manner. In one of these two, the distal suture line leaked but subsequently healed with conservative management. This anastomosis became stenotic and required revision. The other six patients had the anastomoses performed in the interdigitating manner and were free from strictures, in spite of the fact that one had transient leakage. All these patients were able to take food normally. This is in contrast to the experience of Schuller[12] and Stell,[13] who reported postoperative swallowing difficulties in 17% and 70% of their patients, respectively. The difference is probably the result of the additional step we take in making an interdigitating anastomosis.

REFERENCES

1. Harrison, D.F.N.: Pathology of hypopharyngeal cancer in relation to surgical management, J. Laryngol. Otol. **84:**349, 1970.
2. Davidge-Pitts, K.J., and Mannel, A.: Pharyngolaryngectomy with extrathoracic esophagectomy, Head Neck Surg. **6:**571, 1983.

TABLE 29-1. Mortality and morbidity after pharyngolaryngoesophagectomy and pharyngogastric anastomosis

	No.	Mortality (%)	Anastomotic leak (%)	Wound sepsis (%)	Neck hemorrhage (%)	Chest infection (%)	Overall morbidity (%)
To 1979*	157	31	23	27	20	27	
1980-1981	38	18	18	34	16	29	53
1982-1983	31	6.5	6.5	6.5	3.2	13	29
1984-1985	22	4.5	9	4.5	4.5	18	32

*Data from Lam, K.H., Wong, J., Lim, S.T.K., and Ong, G.B.: World J. Surg. **5**:509, 1981.

3. Ong, G.B., and Lee, T.C.: Pharyngogastric anastomosis after oesophagopharyngectomy for carcinoma of the hypopharynx and cervical oesophagus, Br. J. Surg. **48**:193, 1960.

4. LeQuesne, L.P., and Ranger, D.: Pharyngolaryngectomy, with immediate pharyngogastric anastomosis, Br. J. Surg. **53**:105, 1966.

5. Lam, K.H., Wei, W.I., Wong, J., and Ong, G.B.: Tracheostome construction during laryngectomy: a method to prevent stenosis, Laryngoscope **93**:212, 1983.

6. Ariyan, S.: The pectoralis major myocutaneous flap, Plast. Reconstr. Surg. **63**:73, 1979.

7. Akiyama, H., Hiyama, M., and Miyazono, H.: Total esophageal reconstruction after extraction of the esophagus, Ann. Surg. **182**:547, 1975.

8. Pradhan, S.A., and Rajpal, R.M.: Gastric pull-up for cancers of the hypopharynx and cervical esophagus: our experience, J. Surg. Oncol. **26**:149, 1984.

9. Spiro, R.H., Shah, J.P., Strong, E.W., Gerold, F.P., and Bains, M.S.: Gastric transposition in head and neck surgery, Am. J. Surg. **146**:483, 1983.

10. Lam, K.H., Wong, J., Lim, S.T.K., and Ong, G.B.: Pharyngogastric anastomosis following pharyngolaryngoesophagectomy: analysis of 157 cases, World J. Surg. **5**:509, 1981.

11. Wei, W.I., Lam, K.H., Choi, S., and Wong, J.: Late problems after pharyngolaryngoesophagectomy and pharyngogastric anastomosis for cancer of the larynx and hypopharynx, Am. J. Surg. **148**:509, 1984.

12. Schuller, D.E.: Pectoralis myocutaneous flap in head and neck cancer reconstruction, Arch. Otolaryngol. **109**:185, 1983.

13. Stell, P.M.: Replacement of the pharynx after pharyngolaryngectomy, Ann. R. Coll. Surg. Engl. **66**:388, 1984.

Elective surgical techniques for cervical and postcricoid lesions

DISCUSSION

Frederick Griffith Pearson

Pharyngolaryngectomy may be indicated in patients with primary carcinoma of the hypopharynx, postcricoid area, or upper cervical esophagus. The authors report an extensive experience with a one-stage operation that involves total esophagectomy without a thoracotomy and a reconstruction with pharyngogastrostomy. Details of preoperative evaluation, operative technique, and postoperative management are presented. This operation was first described by Professor G.B. Ong from this same center in Hong Kong in 1960. Only during the past decade, however, has this approach become widely adopted by other centers.

LeQuesne and Ranger in England were using this same operation when I visited them in 1960, and we began using this method of reconstruction following pharyngolaryngectomy at Toronto General Hospital shortly thereafter. The indications for pharyngolaryngectomy have been the same, and for the past 20 years this has been our procedure of choice for such reconstructions. We have now operated on 70 patients and report results that are similar to those reported by Lam and Wei—an operative mortality of 5%, and generally excellent functional results. Reconstructions using colon, a myocutaneous flap, or an interposed segment of jejunum with microvascular anastomosis are used for those few patients in whom the stomach is not suitable (usually by virtue of previous gastric surgery).

OPERATIVE TECHNIQUE

Bronchoscopy and esophagoscopy are essential parts of the preoperative evaluation. There is an important incidence of synchronous second primary tumors in the esophagus, which warrants a methodical examination of the entire organ. Thin-slice CT scans define the gross extent of the tumor

more precisely than endoscopy, and these findings may modify the operation selected. For instance, tumors involving the tonsillar fossa require an upper resection margin, which cannot be safely reconstructed with the mobilized stomach.

Certain details of the operation itself warrant emphasis:

1. The operation should always be done with two surgical teams including the scrub nurses and instrument setup. In our own hospital, most of these patients are referred to the otolaryngologists, who undertake the resection. The laparotomy with gastric mobilization and reconstruction have been done by the thoracic surgeons.

2. Sufficient gastric length for a high pharyngogastric anastomosis is almost always possible, but requires extensive Kocherization of the duodenum. When necessary, additional length can be obtained by gentle but steady and sustained traction on the gastric fundus. Still greater length is obtained by extending the resection of the lesser curvature side of the stomach.

3. A tunnel of adequate diameter in the posterior mediastinum is essential and is most accurately assessed by manual examination of the mediastinal tunnel with one hand passed up through the diaphragmatic hiatus and the other down from the cervical incision. The authors describe their technique of introducing two gauze swabs into the posterior mediastinum, which act as packs for control of bleeding following the thoracic esophagectomy. The stomach is then stitched to the abdominal end of the swabs, which are then pulled out from above and thus deliver the apex of the gastric fundus into the neck. In recent years we have used an alternative technique, which is minimally traumatic and delivers the full available length of stomach into the neck without torsion. A long plastic sheath (an arthroscopy bag) is pulled over the stomach from fundus to pylorus. The uppermost part of the greater cur-

vature of the stomach may be secured to the apex of the plastic sheath, which is then drawn up through the posterior mediastinum into the neck. As the redundant folds of the sheath are pulled up into the neck, they exert a milking action on the mobilized stomach, bringing it into the neck without undue traction and avoiding any friction on the surface of the stomach itself.

4. The pharyngogastric anastomosis is easily done in two layers. This is a very broad anastomosis and is never complicated by stenosis unless there is a major dehiscence.

5. Care should be taken to preserve as much of the residual tracheal blood supply as possible. The full length of the membranous trachea is inevitably exposed by the thoracic esophagectomy. It is particularly important to preserve as much as possible of the posterolateral tracheal attachments, which carry the majority of the tracheal blood supply, which is segmental in nature.

6. Preservation of at least one lobe of the thyroid gland along with the associated parathyroid glands on the same side simplifies postoperative management and is nearly always possible to achieve.

7. The plastic surgery technique for tracheocutaneous anastomosis is an innovation with which we have had no experience, although stenosis at the tracheocutaneous junction has been an uncommon problem in our experience. The technique described further reduces the possibility.

ADVANTAGES

I believe this is the optimal operation and reconstruction following pharyngolaryngectomy for cancers of the upper respiratory tract. It is a one-stage operation with a single anastomosis, which is done expeditiously by two surgical teams. The intrathoracic esophagus in these cases is normal and can be easily and safely removed without thoracotomy. Alternative methods of reconstruction using a myocutaneous flap or free jejunal transplant do not provide better functional results. Anastomotic stenosis is a common problem with myocutaneous reconstruction. Jejunal interposition with a free transplant and microvascular anastomosis is technically more difficult, and even in the most experienced hands the technical failure rate is still somewhat higher than with pharyngogastrostomy.

CHAPTER 30

Esophageal reconstruction: free jejunal transfer or circulatory augmentation of pedicled intestinal interpositions using microvascular surgery

W. Spencer Payne and Jack Fisher

The feasibility of free intestinal transfer to the neck was demonstrated by Carrel and Guthrie about 80 years ago.[1] With the exception of sporadic, but seminal, clinical and laboratory reports in the 1950s and 1960s,[2-12] microvascular technology did not reach general clinical application until the early 1970s. As microvascular technology began to find application in many areas of surgery, patency rates for small-vessel anastomoses began to exceed 90% to 95%, and success rates with free intestinal transfer for reconstruction of the hypopharynx and cervical esophagus dramatically improved.[9,13-17]

This report concerns the Mayo Clinic experience with microvascular techniques in 38 patients undergoing esophageal reconstruction during the 4-year period from 1981 to 1985. The ages of the patients ranged from 7 to 69 years (mean, 40 years). Microvascular techniques were used for the following clinical circumstances: (1) free jejunal transfer for reconstruction of the pharynx and cervical esophagus in association with radical resections for cancer (laryngopharyngectomy), 23 patients; (2) elective free jejunal transfer for reconstruction of traumatic pharyngeal and cervical esophageal strictures (larynx preserved), 4 patients; (3) salvage of failed substernal colonic interposition with free jejunal transfer for reconstruction of hypopharynx and upper thoracic and cervical esophagus (larynx preserved), 5 patients; and (4) microvascular circulatory augmentation of the orad end of pedicled colonic interpositions (complex laryngopharyngeal, tracheoesophageal

defects), 6 patients. Of the 15 patients in groups 2 through 4, 12 had an intact larynx before microvascular reconstruction.

TECHNIQUE FOR RECONSTRUCTION AFTER LARYNGOPHARYNGECTOMY

Free jejunal transfer for reconstruction of the pharynx and cervical esophagus after an ablative surgical procedure for cancer has become an established technique (see Fig. 30-1). It has several advantages over previous reconstructive techniques.[18] It allows for a single-stage reconstruction at the time of the ablative procedure and is particularly useful for patients who have experienced failure of previous reconstruction. It is applicable to patients who have had previous irradiation or who are candidates for postreconstruction irradiation. The revascularized segment of bowel actually enhances local tissue healing and will support split-thickness skin grafts applied directly to it. Mobilization of the jejunal segment for transfer is considerably simpler than mobilization for colon, stomach, or regional myocutaneous or cutaneous flaps. Finally, with highly predictable local healing, the duration of hospitalizations and rehabilitations is greatly improved. Unfortunately, many patients treated with this procedure have limited survival because of their underlying malignancy, which is unaffected by the method of reconstruction. Whether the level of palliation of free jejunal transfer will con-

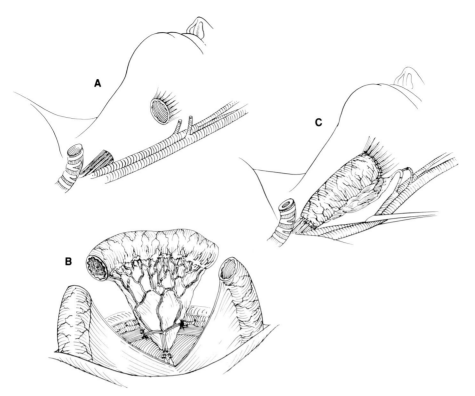

Fig. 30-1. Free jejunal transfer at time of laryngopharyngectomy. **A,** Circumferential defect of pharynx and cervical esophagus. **B,** Jejunal segment isolated with vascular pedicle. **C,** Jejuno-pharyngeal, jejunoesophageal anastomosis and arterial and venous microvascular anastomoses completed. (From DeSanto, L.W., Pearson, B.W., and Fisher, J. In English, G.M., editor: Otolaryngology, Philadelphia, 1983, Harper & Row, Publishers, Inc.)

tinue to justify its use over other techniques is yet to be determined.[18]

Technique of jejunal procurement

While the neck procedure is being done, a second surgical team performs laparotomy and identifies a suitable segment of jejunum approximately 40 cm distal to the ligament of Treitz (see Fig. 30-1, *B*). This point is selected on the basis of both a suitable caliber of bowel and an adequate length of mesenteric vessels for subsequent anastomosis. The isolated segment of jejunum to be used for repair is allowed to perfuse on a single vascular pedicle of mesenteric artery and vein until the time of transfer, to minimize the warm ischemic period. Bowel continuity can be immediately restored by end-to-end jejunostomy, and the mesenteric defect is closed after the isolated jejunum is transferred.

Technique of jejunal transfer and microvascular anastomosis

After the defect in the pharyngeal or esophageal continuity is well defined and the sites for prox-

imal and distal bowel anastomosis are well exposed, suitable recipient vessels in the neck are prepared. If the transfer is low in the neck, the preferred arterial recipient vessel is the transverse cervical artery. In the midneck region, the external carotid artery or one of its branches is used (see Fig. 30-1, *C*) or, in some cases, an end-to-side microvascular anastomosis is made to the common carotid artery. In the upper neck area, an artery of the external carotid system is used. An end-to-side venous anastomosis between the mesenteric vein and the internal jugular vein is preferred.

After the sites for the proposed bowel and vascular anastomoses are prepared, the jejunal segment is transferred to the neck by dividing the mesenteric vascular pedicle in the abdomen. Care must be taken to maintain an isoperistaltic orientation of the jejunal segment to be transferred. The proximal bowel anastomosis in the neck is performed first because often it not only is the more difficult to effect but also tends to stabilize the jejunum and permit orientation of the vascular pedicle for subsequent microvascular anastomosis without tension or angulation. The bowel anastomosis in the neck is performed with a single circumferential layer of multiple interrupted 3-0 polyglactin 910 (Vicryl) sutures. Warm ischemia is well tolerated by the jejunum for up to 2 to 3 hours, more than ample time to effect microvascular anastomosis and reperfusion. The vascular anastomoses are all performed by standard microvascular technique with 8-0 to 10-0 nylon monofilament sutures, depending on the vessel size. Systemic anticoagulation, hypothermia, and vascular flushing are not used. After completion of the vascular anastomoses, occluding microvascular clamps are released and the jejunal segment is allowed to be perfused. The distal jejunal anastomosis is then effected in the same manner as the proximal one (see Fig. 30-1, *C*). The use of the operative microscope has significantly improved the success rates of microvascular anastomosis.

TECHNIQUE FOR PHARYNGOESOPHAGEAL RECONSTRUCTION WITH INTACT LARYNX (12 PATIENTS)

Although the technique of free jejunal transfer is greatly facilitated by the absence of the larynx and pharynx, such is not the case when a functioning larynx is to be preserved. The larynx can usually be preserved when free jejunal transfer is used for the repair of benign traumatic cervical esophageal or pharyngeal stenoses or for longer, more distal reconstructions in which microvascular anastomosis is performed in the neck.

Our basic method is to approach the pharynx and cervical esophagus through an oblique left cervical incision parallel to the anterior border of the sternocleidomastoid muscle. With retraction of the carotid sheath laterally, the retropharyngeal-prevertebral space is entered just cephalad to the omohyoid muscle. The larynx is rotated medially, and the site of stenosis is identified by passing a rubber bougie down the esophagus via the mouth. With the site of the stricture identified, the cervical esophagus or pharynx is incised, and the stricture is removed circumferentially. If the site of resection is low in the neck or if the site of distal jejunal anastomosis is in the upper part of the chest, exposure is enhanced by division of the strap muscles (omohyoid, sternohyoid, and sternothyroid) and interruption of ipsilateral thyroid vessels. To gain access for still lower intrathoracic anastomoses, the sternocleidomastoid muscle can be disconnected from its sternoclavicular origin, the manubrium divided in the mid-

line, and its ipsilateral half removed en bloc with the medial two thirds of the clavicle and anterior end of the first rib. The latter exposure technique permits easy access to the upper end of a partially sloughed substernal colon[14]; also, the upper end of the native esophagus can be dependably exposed for anastomosis to the T-4 level. Experience suggests that median sternotomy is not a desirable incision for exposure of the substernal colon remnant. The technique for free jejunal transfer is as previously described.

PREOPERATIVE EVALUATION FOR COMPLETE RECONSTRUCTIONS

Examples of some of our more complex applications of free jejunal transfer and microvascular augmentation of pedicled colonic interposition are shown in Figs. 30-2 to 30-6. Thorough preoperative evaluation of patients presenting with complex reconstruction problems is essential. Although we have gained great confidence in the reliability of microvascular techniques for preserving or augmenting the blood supply of interposed bowel, we also believe that it is important to define potential alternative methods of reconstruction preoperatively. Such planning is especially important in patients who have undergone multiple operations, in whom preconceived strategies may prove to be unfeasible at the time of exploration. Thus, we thoroughly evaluate the entire gastrointestinal tract before operation, using contrast radiographic and endoscopic techniques to explore all sinuses, fistulas, and stomas and also normal enteric orifices. Occasionally, we have used selective angiography if the integrity of critical visceral vessels is in question because of previous operation or disease. Additionally, mechanical and antibiotic preparation of the large bowel is often desirable before operation even though it is not required for jejunal transfer.

The basic precept to be maintained is that the patient is to have successful reconstruction—the specific method to be used is of little consequence to the patient as long as it is effective. In this context, free jejunal transfer and microvascular circulatory augmentation become important, but not exclusive, methods of reconstruction.

A major consideration is the maintenance of airway and speech. Twelve of our patients had part or all of the larynx intact, and problems with aspiration and airway, access during operation, and wound closure were taken into consideration preoperatively.

Preoperative evaluation also includes oculoplethysmography with sequential bilateral carotid artery occlusion to determine the adequacy of cross-circulation when use of the common carotid artery as the recipient vessel is a potential. Impaired cross-circulation is a contraindication to use of the common carotid artery. Intraoperative electroencephalographic monitoring is used when the common carotid artery is to be occluded for microvascular anastomosis, even though good collateral circulation has been demonstrated preoperatively.

RESULTS

In three patients in whom preoperative oculoplethysmography showed inadequate collateral circulation, the transverse cervical vessels were used instead of the common carotid artery. In 10 patients, the common carotid artery was used, and intraoperative electroencephalographic monitoring was performed during cross-clamping of the carotid artery. The external carotid artery or its branches were the most commonly used recipient arteries. The internal jugular was the recipient vein in more than 90% of the cases. Of the 12 patients with an intact larynx, one had his larynx removed before reconstruction. Of the 11 remaining patients, one with a severe caustic injury had to have a laryngectomy at the time of microvascular reconstruction, one with an intact larynx after reconstruction required a permanent tracheostomy because of recurrent aspiration, and one had the laryngeal remnant anastomosed to the jejunal segment and speech was maintained. In the eight remaining patients, the larynx was undisturbed. Of this group of 12 patients, 11 have been maintained on an oral diet alone and one has required jejunostomy feedings. Two patients in group 1 (reconstruction associated with an esophagolaryngectomy for cancer) had thromboses of the microvascular anastomoses and complete loss of the entire free jejunal segments, which necessitated alternate reconstructions. Both had previously received irradiation and had extensive postirradiation changes in the neck area.

CONCLUSIONS

Microvascular techniques were used in 23 patients after ablative surgical procedures for cancer and in 15 patients who were classified as esophageal cripples. Free jejunal transfer was useful in cases of failed colonic interpositions, bridging defects up to 25 cm in length. Colonic interpositions with microvascular augmentation in the

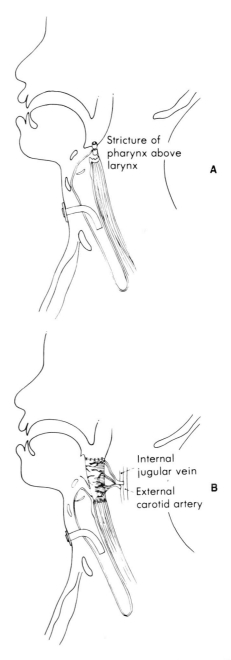

Fig. 30-2. An 18-year-old man who sustained mandibular fracture and neck injury in a vehicle accident required tracheotomy and repair of fracture. Subsequently, he developed inability to swallow or phonate and became dependent on tracheostomy for airway and gastrostomy for feeding. **A,** Examination revealed almost complete stenosis of pharynx at level of epiglottis. At cervical exploration, retrograde passage of bougie up esophagus via gastrostomy established site of stricture. Stricture and a portion of pharynx, supraglottic larynx, and epiglottis were excised. **B,** Defect was repaired with free jejunal transfer. (From McCaffrey, T.V., and Fisher, J.: Ann. Otol. Rhinol. Laryngol. **93**:512, 1984.)

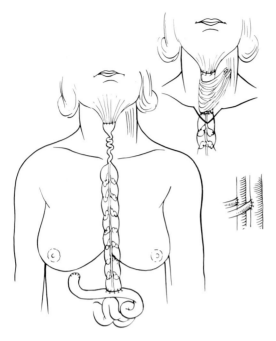

Fig. 30-3. A 68-year-old woman with previous total esophagogastrectomy reconstructed with colon sustained ischemic necrosis of cephalad end of colon. Esophageal continuity was reconstructed with free jejunal transfer using common carotid and internal jugular as recipient vessels.

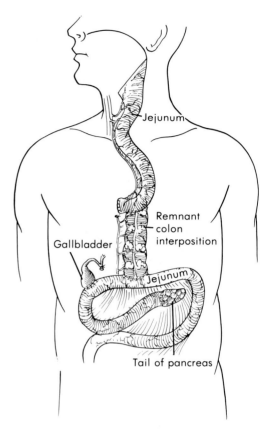

Fig. 30-4. A 55-year-old man with self-inflicted severe lye burn required emergency esophagectomy, gastrectomy, and pancreaticoduodenectomy. Six months later, substernal colonic interposition was carried out with ischemic sloughing of upper half. Pharyngocolonic defect was reconstructed with free transfer of 25-cm segment of jejunum.

neck can be used when the entire hypopharynx and esophagus require reconstruction. In this group of patients with benign and malignant disease, a microvascular operation successfully restored esophageal continuity, and all but one patient had restoration of a normally functioning swallowing mechanism. One patient with an intact larynx, although able to swallow, had laryngeal incompetence that required permanent tracheostomy to prevent aspiration. Close collaboration of experienced microvascular, laryngeal, and esophageal surgeons provides optimal technical support for both the planning and the technical performance of some of the more complicated reconstructions.

REFERENCES

1. Carrel, A. and Guthrie. Cited by Carrel, A.: The surgery of blood vessels, etc., Johns Hopkins Hosp. Bull. **18:**18, 1907.
2. Seidenberg, B., Rosenak, S.S., Hurwitt, E.S. and Som, M.L.: Immediate reconstruction of the cervical esophagus by a revascularized isolated jejunal segment, Ann. Surg. **149:**162, 1959.
3. Roberts, R.E. and Douglass, F.M.: Replacement of the cervical esophagus and hypopharynx by a revascularized free jejunal autograft: report of a case successfully treated, N. Engl. J. Med. **264:**342, 1961.
4. Hiebert, C.A. and Cummings, G.O., Jr.: Successful replacement of the cervical esophagus by transplantation and revascularization of a free graft of gastric antrum, Ann. Surg. **154:**103, 1961.
5. Jurkiewicz, M.J.: Vascularized intestinal graft for reconstruction of the cervical esophagus and pharynx, Plast. Reconstr. Surg. **36:**509, 1965.
6. Nakayama, K., Yamamoto, K., Tamiya, T., et al.: Experience with free autografts of the bowel with a new venous anastomosis apparatus, Surgery **55:**796, 1964.
7. Peters, C.R., McKee, D.M. and Berry, B.E.: Pharyngoesophageal reconstruction with revascularized jejunal transplants, Am. J. Surg. **121:**675, 1971.
8. Hopkins, D.M. and Bernatz, P.E.: Experimental replacement of the cervical esophagus, Arch. Surg. **87:**265, 1963.
9. McKee, D.M. and Peters, C.R.: Reconstruction of the hypopharynx and cervical esophagus with microvascular jejunal transplant, Clin. Plast. Surg. **5:**305, April 1978.

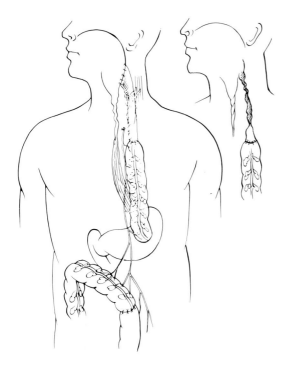

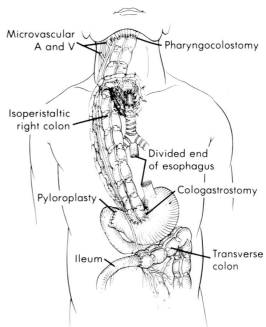

Fig. 30-5. A 44-year-old man with accidental ingestion of nitric acid sustained severe strictures at cricopharyngeus and throughout cervical esophagus. Subsequent colonic interposition sloughed cervical and pharyngeal portions. Attempts at tubed, deltopectoral flap reconstruction also necrosed. Free jejunal transfer successfully restored pharyngocolonic defect.

Fig. 30-6. A 43-year-old man sustained severe radiation injury to neck during treatment of a lymphoma; larynx, pharynx, cervical esophagus, and overlying skin were sloughed. In addition, there was a long, continuous, fistulous communication between thoracic esophagus and full length of membranous trachea. Esophagus was reconstructed by means of a subcutaneously placed isoperistaltic right colonic interposition between base of tongue and stomach. To prevent gastric reflux aspiration through huge tracheoesophageal fistula, the esophagogastric junction was interrupted. Because pedicled colon was to be anastomosed to heavily irradiated pharyngeal tissues, ileocecal artery and vein were anastomosed to common carotid and internal jugular vessels to augment perfusion of middle colonic vessels. Additionally, this permitted application of split-thickness skin graft to cover cervical portion of colon. The introitus of the tracheoesophageal stoma was lined with pedicled omentum and skin graft to effect complete reepithelialization of stoma. *A* and *V,* Arterial and venous microvascular anastomoses.

10. Androsov, P.E., et al. Cited by Chang, T.-S., Hwang, O.-L., and Wang, W.: Reconstruction of esophageal defects with microsurgically revascularized jejunal segments: a report of 13 cases, J. Microsurg. **2:**83, 1980.
11. Longmire, W.P., Jr.: A modification of the Roux technique for antethoracic esophageal reconstruction: anastomosis of the mesenteric and internal mammary blood vessels, Surgery **22:**94, 1947.
12. Jurkiewicz, M.J.: Reconstructive surgery of the cervical esophagus, J. Thorac. Cardiovasc. Surg. **88:**893, 1984.
13. Katsaros, J. and Tan, E.: Free bowel transfer for pharyngo-oesophageal reconstruction: an experimental and clinical study, Br. J. Plast. Surg. **35:**268, 1982.
14. Fisher, J., Payne, W.S. and Irons, G.B., Jr.: Salvage of a failed colon interposition in the esophagus with a free jejunal graft, Mayo Clin. Proc. **59:**197, 1984.
15. Hester, T.R., Jr., McConnel, F.M.S., Nahai, F., Jurkiewicz, M.J. and Brown, R.G.: Reconstruction of cervical esophagus, hypopharynx and oral cavity using free jejunal transfer, Am. J. Surg. **140:**487, 1980.
16. Gluckman, J.L., McDonough, J., and Donegan, J.O.: The role of the free jejunal graft in reconstruction of the pharynx and cervical esophagus, Head Neck Surg. **4:**360, 1982.

17. Chang, T.-S., Hwang, O.-L. and Wang, W.: Reconstruction of esophageal defects with microsurgically revascularized jejunal segments: a report of 13 cases, J. Microsurg. **2:**83, 1980.
18. DeSanto, L.W., Pearson, B.W., and Fisher, J.: Reconstruction of the pharynx and cervical esophagus. In English, G.M., editor: Otolaryngology, Philadelphia, 1983, Harper & Row, Publishers, Inc., pp. 1-15.

CHAPTER 31 Adenocarcinoma of the columnar epithelial–lined lower esophagus of Barrett

W. Spencer Payne, Molly K. McAfee, Victor F. Trastek, K. Krishnan Unni, and Alan John Cameron

At the Mayo Clinic, approximately 50% of esophageal cancers occur in the general region of the gastroesophageal junction, and 90% of these are adenocarcinomas. Almost all of the remaining cancers of the esophagus are squamous cell in type.[1]

There is justified confusion regarding the origins of adenocarcinomas that affect the esophagus. The rarity of adenocarcinoma, except about the gastroesophageal junction, has led many to assume that most cardial cancers are really nothing more than ordinary gastric cancers that happen to arise near the esophagus. Those rare and exceptional adenocarcinomas of the esophagus that develop remote from the cardia have been suggested to originate from the glandular epithelium of the deep and superficial secretory glands that are normally distributed throughout the length of the esophagus[2,3] or from commonly occurring congenital patches of ectopic columnar epithelium seen especially frequently in the upper thoracic or low cervical esophagus[4,5] (Fig. 31-1).

Of special interest has been the observation of adenocarcinoma arising from the columnar epithelial–lined lower esophagus (CELLE) of Barrett[6-14] (Fig. 31-2). Although it is common and, perhaps, justifiable to speak of histogenesis of cancers from similar types of tissues, the actual cause of esophageal malignancy, whether adenocarcinoma, squamous cell carcinoma, or other, is unknown, and our concepts of tumor cell origin may have to undergo some modification when carcinogenesis is more clearly defined. Already there are hints that cardial adenocarcinomas, although histologically similar to other gastric cancers, have not decreased in prevalence as have most gastric cancers arising elsewhere in the stomach.[15,16] Such observations suggest that adenocarcinomas in and about the gastroesophageal junction might have an origin quite different from ordinary gastric cancer or even the squamous cell cancer of the esophagus. Indeed, some have suggested that many, if not all, of the cardial adenocarcinomas might well have arisen from Barrett's epithelium, and that all traces of the benign CELLE might well have been destroyed by the neoplasm by the time the cancer is diagnosed.[14,17,18] Retrospective studies attempting to correlate diaphragmatic hernia and gastroesophageal reflux symptoms with the subsequent development of adenocarcinoma of the cardia have failed to define a clear correlation between antecedent reflux and subsequent cancer, despite the high correlation between reflux and Barrett's esophagus.[19-22] On the other hand, at least 25% of patients with Barrett's esophagus and cancer vehemently deny antecedent symptoms of reflux or even dyspepsia.[23,24]

Approximately 10% of individuals who underwent endoscopic investigation for gastroesophageal reflux had Barrett's esophagus.[10,13,25] The prevalence of Barrett's esophagus is especially high in scleroderma patients, in whom both incompetence and loss of clearing mechanism are so dominant.[26] Most institutions report that approximately 15% (range, 2% to 46%) of the cases of Barrett's esophagus diagnosed had an associated adenocarcinoma at the time of that diagnosis.[7,10,13,25] The location of such a neoplasm is either at the cephalically displaced squamocolumnar junction or within the columnar epithelial–lined segment of lower esophagus. Although such

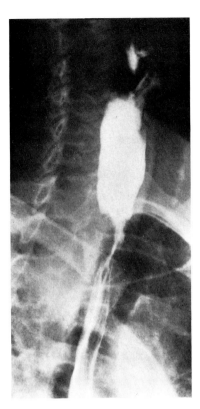

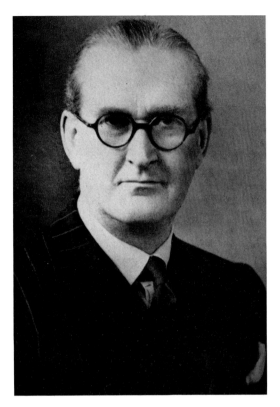

Fig. 31-1. Cancer arising from heterotopic rest of glandular epithelium in upper esophagus. Esophagogram of 46-year-old man with an 8-month history of high dysphagia. Multiple biopsies showed benign glandular mucosa at 20 cm from incisor teeth. Cytologic examination was positive for adenocarcinoma. Subsequent total esophagectomy with pharyngogastrostomy revealed a patch of benign ectopic glandular epithelium with contiguous invasive adenocarcinoma, stage III. The esophagus above and below was lined with normal squamous epithelium.

Fig. 31-2. Norman Rupert Barrett (1903-1979) was the first to draw attention to the phenomenon of columnar epithelial–lined lower esophagus, which bears his name and is still a clinical enigma. (From Payne, W.S.: Cardiopul. Med. **18**:8, fall/winter 1979.)

prevalence studies suggest an enormous risk of a patient with Barrett's esophagus developing cancer, incidence studies to date, although suggesting a significant increase in risk of malignancy in patients with Barrett's esophagus, do not approach the extravagant figures suggested by prevalence studies.[27,28]

For example, of 104 Mayo Clinic patients studied retrospectively who met specific diagnostic criteria for benign Barrett's esophagus,[27] only two patients had developed adenocarcinoma of the esophagus after followup of 3 to 15 years or more (mean followup, 8.5 years). The yearly incidence of esophageal carcinoma in initially benign Barrett's esophagus was 227 per 100,000, or approximately 30 times the expected rate. Ex-

pressed in other terms, this constituted one case of subsequent cancer in initially benign Barrett's esophagus per 441 patient-years of followup. In a similar study, Spechler et al.[28] found two adenocarcinomas in 105 male patients followed for a mean of 3.3 years—an incidence of 1 case per 175 patient-years. Obviously, longer followup or an even greater number of patients is required, but to date, age- and sex-adjusted survival rates for patients with benign Barrett's esophagus appear to be identical to those of the general population (see Fig. 31-3).

EXPERIENCE WITH BARRETT'S ESOPHAGUS WITH SIMULTANEOUS CANCER DIAGNOSIS

At the Mayo Clinic between 1970 and 1985, 62 patients underwent resection for invasive adenocarcinoma of the esophagus associated with

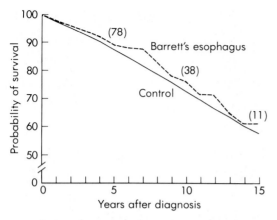

Fig. 31-3. Comparison of age- and sex-adjusted survival rates of 104 patients with Barrett's esophagus and a control population. Numbers in parentheses indicate subjects still at risk. (From Cameron, A.J., Ott, B.J., and Payne, W.S.: N. Engl. J. Med. **313:**857, 1985. Reprinted by permission of the New England Journal of Medicine.)

Barrett's esophagus (see Table 31-1). Those patients ranged in age from 36 years to 84 years (median, 60 years); 59 of the 62 were men. During this same period, one additional patient with just atypia and three additional patients with carcinoma in situ also underwent resection, but were excluded from the above 62 patients and the following staging-survival analysis.[29] Twelve (19%) had stage I disease ($T_1N_0M_0$), and only one of these died of recurrent disease, with a mean followup of 41 months. Thirteen (21%) of the 62 patients presented with stage II disease ($T_2N_0M_0$); six succumbed to disease and seven (54%) are alive without evidence of disease. Thirty-seven patients presented with stage III disease (T_1-$T_3N_1M_0$). In this stage III group, there were four operative deaths; at followup, four of the remaining 33 patients were living, but two of these had known recurrences (10.5% survival). Operative mortality was confined to the stage III disease group. All four patients with atypia or in situ cancer are living and well, with followup of 1 to 5 years after resection.

Of interest, and noted by others,[30] was the finding that the esophageal cancer was a second primary in six of the 62 patients; lung, colon, and vocal cord were the sites of the previous malignancies. Only half of the patients (30 of 62) had a past history suggestive of gastroesophageal reflux, and four of these had had previous operative antireflux procedures. Half had a history of alcohol or tobacco use, or both; 16 admitted to heavy alcohol abuse, and 35 of the 62 had 10 pack-years smoking histories. This was significantly less than that reported by Skinner et al.[24]

On pathologic examination, 35 of 62 resected specimens showed epithelial atypia (dysplasia) or carcinoma in situ in otherwise benign columnar epithelium adjacent to the invasive cancer. There did not appear to be any consistent predominant type of residual benign Barrett's columnar epithelium associated with neoplasm. Eight of the 62 resected specimens demonstrated multicentric malignancies within Barrett's epithelium (Fig. 31-4). A solitary focus of malignancy was more often the rule, and this was frequently at the squamocolumnar epithelial junction (Fig. 31-5).

Of special interest was the observation that five patients underwent resection of the esophagus during this period entirely on the basis of biopsy of the CELLE, which showed only marked atypia (dysplasia) in four patients and carcinoma in situ in one patient. In all five, this was the only histologic finding of concern, although endoscopy and roentgenography suggested nonspecific ulceration or nodularities in what appeared grossly to be benign Barrett's esophagus. In one patient, however, the esophageal roentgenogram was suggestive of malignancy. In three of these five, an obvious invasive cancer was defined in the surgical specimen. The other two surgical specimens showed only atypia (dysplasia) in one and carcinoma in situ in the other. Others have commented on the occurrence of the epithelial atypia and its association with cancer in Barrett's esophagus.[8,11,14,24,31-33] Our experience has led us to use this as an indication for resection, even in the absence of gross or microscopic evidence of invasive malignancy. One patient with biopsy-proven Barrett's esophagus developed invasive adenocarcinoma 20 years later. On retrospective review of the initial biopsy results, marked atypia (dysplasia) was apparent. These observations raise the question of whether there is urgency for resection in patients with demonstrated atypia in columnar epithelium. Nonetheless, we consider atypia (dysplasia) to be an ominous sign and would urge resection when it is encountered.

CONCLUSIONS

It is difficult to determine whether all patients with benign Barrett's esophagus with positive acid-reflux tests, irrespective of symptoms or complications, should have an antireflux procedure to prevent subsequent malignancy. Skinner[34] has suggested this approach and, indeed, that an effective antireflux procedure might prevent subsequent malignancy. It is our feeling that there is little evidence at hand to suggest reversal of atypia or regression of Barrett's epithelium by antireflux

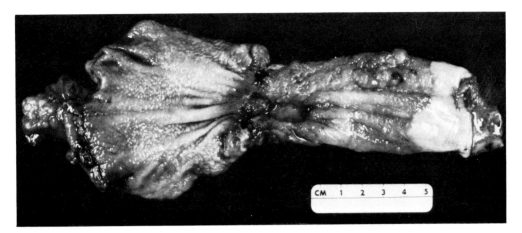

Fig. 31-4. Thoracic esophagus and lesser curvature of stomach show multicentric (2) foci of invasive carcinoma in Barrett's esophagus in 59-year-old man with an anatomic sliding esophageal hiatal hernia, without past history of gastroesophageal reflux symptoms or alcohol or tobacco abuse. He developed progressive dysphagia to solids. Subsequent roentgenography and endoscopy defined columnar epithelial–lined lower esophagus with squamocolumnar junction just above aortic arch and more distal invasive cancer near gastroesophageal junction. It was not until specimen was opened that the second, higher invasive cancer was appreciated.

TABLE 31-1. Location of squamocolumnar junction in Barrett's esophagus and site of adenocarcinoma arising in the columnar epithelium (62 patients)

Level of involved esophagus	Highest level of Barrett's esophagus	Highest location of carcinoma*
Upper third (to 24 cm)	2	1
Middle third (24 to 32 cm)	32	13
Lower third (32 cm to gastroesophageal junction)	28	48

*Eight of the 62 resected specimens demonstrated multicentric malignancies, and these were often diffuse and confluent.

procedures.[10,31,35] In view of the demonstrated inadequacies of biopsy because of sampling error and inadequacies of endoscopic evaluation, we have come to feel that it is the columnar epithelium that is at risk, and the first signs of epithelial atypia (dysplasia) should direct the surgeon to resection; antireflux procedures should be confined to those patients with benign Barrett's esophagus who manifest symptoms or complications. Considering our current knowledge of the incidence of subsequent cancer, it is doubtful that the value of prophylactic antireflux procedures can be demonstrated short of empiric operation on many hundreds of patients and probably many, many years of observation.

Furthermore, the risk of cancer developing in benign Barrett's epithelium in the absence of atypia (dysplasia) or carcinoma in situ is so low

that the risk of prophylactic resection does not seem justified at this time.

The problem of appropriate followup for patients with apparently benign Barrett's esophagus is unanswered. Obviously, such patients are at increased risk of developing subsequent adenocarcinoma, but the anticipated detection rate of one case per 441 patient-years of followup is low enough to frustrate patient compliance with annual or semiannual endoscopic examination. Brush or balloon cytology for early detection may prove to be a more acceptable alternative for the patient, but its ability to detect occult cancer in Barrett's esophagus or epithelial atypia (dysplasia) has not been fully exploited or defined in this particular setting. To date, we have not been able to detect occult malignancy in Barrett's esophagus by cytologic examination alone, although ob-

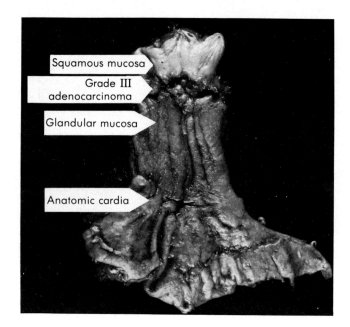

Squamous mucosa

Grade III
adenocarcinoma

Glandular mucosa

Anatomic cardia

Fig. 31-5. Adenocarcinoma developing at the site of a 5-cm cephalad displaced squamocolumnar junction. (From Hawe, A., Payne, W.S., Weiland, L.H., and Fontana, R.S.: Thorax **28:**511, 1973.)

vious biopsied malignancies have been accompanied by positive cytologic results. Of our 66 patients with invasive carcinoma, carcinoma in situ, or atypia, cytologic study was done just prior to resection in 42 patients. Of these, 27 (64%) findings were diagnostic of adenocarcinoma, five (12%) showed marked atypia, and 10 (24%) were false negatives.

For the present, at least, we recommend biennial endoscopy with appropriate biopsy and brush cytology, recognizing the limitations and empiricism of such recommendations.

REFERENCES

1. Payne, W.S., and Ellis, F.H., Jr.: Esophagus and diaphragmatic hernias. In Schwartz, S.I., Shires, G.T., Spencer, F.C., and Storer, E.H., editors: Principles of Surgery, ed. 4, New York, 1984, McGraw-Hill Book Co., pp. 1063-1112.
2. Lortat-Jacob, J.-L., Maillard, J.N., Richard, C.A., Fekete, F., Huguier, M., and Conte-Marti, J.: Primary esophageal adenocarcinoma: report of 16 cases, Surgery **64:**535, 1968.
3. Raphael, H.A., Ellis, F.H., Jr., and Dockerty, M.B.: Primary adenocarcinoma of the esophagus: 18-year review and review of the literature, Ann. Surg. **164:**785, 1966.
4. Heimark, J.J.: The occurrence and clinical significance of heterotopic gastric mucosa in the esophagus, thesis, Mayo Graduate School of Medicine, Rochester, Minn., 1955.
5. Rector, L.E., and Connerley, M.L.: Aberrant mucosa in the esophagus in infants and in children, Arch. Pathol. **31:**285, 1941.
6. Adler, R.H.: The lower esophagus lined by columnar epithelium: its association with hiatal hernia, ulcer, stricture, and tumor, J. Thorac. Cardiovasc. Surg. **45:**13, 1963.
7. Berardi, R.S., and Devaiah, K.A.: Barrett's esophagus, Surg. Gynecol. Obstet. **156:**521, 1983.
8. Haggitt, R.C., Tryzelaar, J., Ellis, F.H., and Colcher, H.: Adenocarcinoma complicating columnar epithelium–lined (Barrett's) esophagus, Am. J. Clin. Pathol. **70:**1, 1978.
9. Hawe, A., Payne, W.S., Weiland, L.H., and Fontana, R.S.: Adenocarcinoma in the columnar epithelial lined lower oesophagus, Thorax **28:**511, 1973.
10. Naef, A.P., Savary, M., and Ozzello, L.: Columnar-lined lower esophagus: an acquired lesion with malignant predisposition: report on 140 cases of Barrett's esophagus with 12 adenocarcinomas, J. Thorac. Cardiovasc. Surg. **70:**826, 1975.
11. Poleynard, G.D., Marty, A.T., Birnbaum, W.B., Nelson, L.E., and O'Reilly, R.R.: Adenocarcinoma in the columnar-lined (Barrett) esophagus: case report and review of the literature, Arch. Surg. **112:**997, 1977.
12. Sanfey, H., Hamilton, S.R., Smith, R.R.L., and Cameron, J.L.: Carcinoma arising in Barrett's esophagus, Surg. Gynecol. Obstet. **161:**570, 1985.
13. Saubier, E.C., Gouillat, C., Samaniego, C., Guillaud, M., and Moulinier, B.: Adenocarcinoma in columnar-lined Barrett's esophagus: analysis of 13 esophagectomies, Am. J. Surg. **150:**365, 1985.
14. Smith, J.L., Jr.: Pathology of adenocarcinoma of the esophagus and gastroesophageal region, and "Barrett's esophagus" as a predisposing condition, In Stroehlein, J.R., and Romsdahl, M.M., editors: Gastrointestinal cancer, New York, 1981, Raven Press, pp. 125-135.
15. Kalish, R.J., Clancy, P.E., Orringer, M.B., and Appelman, H.D.: Clinical, epidemiologic, and morphologic comparison between adenocarcinomas arising in Barrett's esophageal mucosa and in the gastric cardia, Gastroenterology **86:**461, 1984.

16. Sons, H.U., and Borchard, F.: Cancer of the distal esophagus and cardia: incidence, tumorous infiltration, and metastatic spread, Ann. Surg. **203:**188, 1986.

17. Webb, J.N., and Busuttil, A.: Adenocarcinoma of the oesophagus and of the oesophagogastric junction, Br. J. Surg. **65:**475, 1978.

18. Rogers, E., Iseri, O., Bustin, M., Goldkind, L., and Goldkind, S.F.: Adenocarcinoma of the esophago-gastric junction: a distinct entity (abstract), Gastroenterology **80:**1264, 1981.

19. Skinner, D.B.: Pathophysiology of gastroesophageal reflux, Ann. Surg. **202:**546, 1985.

20. Norton, G.A., Postlethwait, R.W., and Thompson, W.M.: Esophageal carcinoma: a survey of populations at risk, South. Med. J. **73:**25, 1980.

21. Allison, P.R., and Johnstone, A.S.: The oesophagus lined with gastric mucous membrane, Thorax **8:**87, 1953.

22. Michel, J.O., Olsen, A.M., and Dockerty, M.B.: The association of diaphragmatic hiatal hernia and gastroesophageal carcinoma, Surg. Gynecol. Obstet. **124:**583, 1967.

23. Smith, R.L., Boitnott, J.K., Hamilton, S.R., and Rogers, E.L.: The spectrum of carcinoma arising in Barrett's esophagus: a clinicopathologic study of 26 patients, Am. J. Surg. Pathol. **8:**563, 1984.

24. Skinner, D.B., Walther, B.C., Riddell, R.H., Schmidt, H., Iascone, C., and DeMeester, T.R.: Barrett's esophagus: comparison of benign and malignant cases, Ann. Surg. **198:**554, 1983.

25. Sarr, M.G., Hamilton, S.R., Marrone, G.C., and Cameron, J.L.: Barrett's esophagus: its prevalence and association with adenocarcinoma in patients with symptoms of gastroesophageal reflux, Am. J. Surg. **149:**187, 1985.

26. Cameron, A.J., and Payne, W.S.: Barrett's esophagus occurring as a complication of scleroderma, Mayo Clin. Proc. **53:**612, 1978.

27. Cameron, A.J., Ott, B.J., and Payne, W.S.: The incidence of adenocarcinoma in columnar-lined (Barrett's) esophagus, N. Engl. J. Med. **313:**857, 1985.

28. Spechler, S.J., Robbins, A.H., Rubins, H.B., et al.: Adenocarcinoma and Barrett's esophagus: an overrated risk? Gastroenterology **87:**927, 1984.

29. American Joint Committee on Cancer: Manual for staging of cancer, ed. 2, edited by O.H. Beahrs and M.H. Myers, Philadelphia, 1983, J.B. Lippincott Co., pp. 61-64.

30. Keen, S.J., Dodd, G.D., Jr., and Smith J.L., Jr.: Adenocarcinoma arising in Barrett esophagus: pathologic and radiologic features, Mt. Sinai J. Med. (N.Y.) **51:**442, 1984.

31. Harle, I.A., Finley, R.J., Belsheim, M., et al.: Management of adenocarcinoma in a columnar-lined esophagus, Ann. Thorac. Surg. **40:**330, 1985.

32. Levine, M.S., Caroline, D., Thompson, J.J., Kressel, H.Y., Laufer, I., and Herlinger, H.: Adenocarcinoma of the esophagus: relationship to Barrett mucosa, Radiology **150:**305, 1984.

33. Smith, R.R.L., Hamilton, S.R., Boitnott, J.K., and Rogers, E.L.: Spectrum of carcinoma arising in Barrett esophagus: a clinicopathologic study of twenty-five patients (abstract), Lab. Invest. **46:**78A, 1982.

34. Skinner, D.B.: The columnar-lined esophagus and adenocarcinoma (editorial), Ann. Thorac. Surg. **40:**321, 1985.

35. Burgess, J.N., Payne, W.S., Andersen, H.A., Weiland, L.H., and Carlson, H.C.: Barrett esophagus: the columnar-epithelial-lined lower esophagus, Mayo Clin. Proc. **46:**728, 1971.

CHAPTER **32** **Combined radical resection of adjacent organs involved by esophageal carcinoma**

Hideyuki Kawahara and Hiromasa Fujita

Carcinomas of the esophagus that secondarily invade the mediastinal structures are not uncommon.[1,2] Most of these carcinomas are incurable by surgical treatment because of existing distant metastasis. In some patients, however, despite extensive local spread the disease is confined to the chest with no distant metastasis at the time of surgery.[3] In such instances cure might be expected by effective surgical resections. Despite improved surgical techniques these carcinomas pose therapeutic problems for the surgeon. In particular, extension of the tumor into adjacent vital organs in the thorax has precluded the utilization of conventional surgical procedures.

In this section, some surgical techniques for resection of the thoracic aorta and the mediastinal trachea that have been invaded by the esophageal neoplasm are described.[4,5]

INDICATIONS FOR COMBINED RADICAL RESECTION

Our candidates for combined radical resection of adjacent vital organs are limited as follows: those with no distant metastases by extensive preoperative evaluation, those with no extensive lymphatic involvement, those with no severe skip lesions, and those with no medical contraindications.

RESECTION OF THE AORTA
Assessment of aortic involvement

Aortic invasion by the extension of the esophageal neoplasm should be accurately assessed pre-

operatively. In addition to standard esophagography and esophagoscopy, computed tomography (CT) has been introduced recently as a noninvasive method for assessing direct invasion into mediastinal structures. More recently, CT has been supplemented by pneumomediastinography (PMG) in an effort to increase the accuracy and to eliminate the false-positive rate.[6]

However, involvement of the aorta sometimes cannot be assessed by such preoperative evaluation. We believe, in these instances, that intraoperative utilization of the echogram (Fig. 32-1) may be beneficial in assessing aortic invasion.

Special problems in aortic resection

When direct invasion of the tumor into the aortic wall is predicted by preoperative evaluation, and combined resection of the aorta is almost a certainty, special attention is necessary prior to and during surgery.

Prevention of ischemic damage secondary to aortic cross-clamping. In operations on the descending thoracic aorta necessitating cross-clamping, it is generally accepted, though there is still some controversy, that some form of circulatory bypass of the clamped aorta is necessary to protect the spinal cord and other distal organs from ischemic damage.[7] Among various protective methods, we find that temporary extra-anatomic bypass or permanent aortoaortic bypass is best utilized in surgery of esophageal carcinoma, because it eliminates the complexities of extracorporeal circulation and eliminates the need for generalized heparinization, which may cause troublesome bleeding.

Extent of resection of the aorta. The extent of resection of the aortic wall with sufficient margins

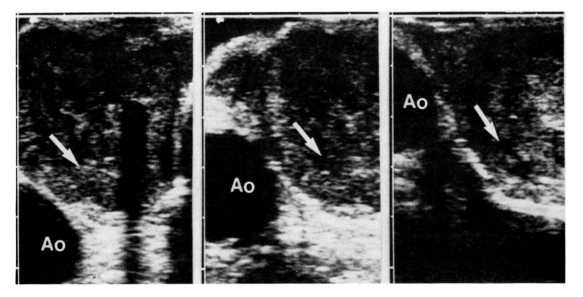

Fig. 32-1. Intraoperative ultrasonography showing the aorta, *Ao,* and a carcinoma of the esophagus *(arrow).* The "tumor slide" is displayed on the echogram in the case of no direct invasion, as is demonstrated here. (With permission of J. Machi, Operative ultrasonography, 1986.)

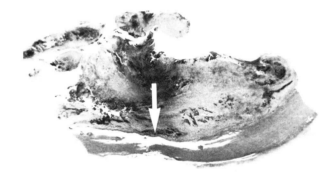

Fig. 32-2. Microscopic finding of the resected specimen from a 65-year-old man showing the semicircumferentially resected aorta and a carcinoma of the esophagus. This carcinoma, which infiltrated into the media of the aorta *(arrow),* was completely removed by this resection.

to ensure complete resection of the tumor is not well established. Our investigations on the resected specimen and postmortem study suggest that at least a 0.5-cm margin on each side of the aortic involvement should be achieved for complete removal of the tumor (see Fig. 32-2).

Operative approach. It is generally accepted in Japan that resection of the thoracic esophagus should be performed through a right thoracic approach, since mediastinal lymph node dissection can be accomplished without interference by the aortic arch.[8] However, surgery of the descending aorta is best approached from the left side. Which side to enter in performing combined esophagoaortic resection is therefore controversial. The decision may depend on the site of tumor location, the extent of resection, and reconstructive procedures necessary (see Table 32-1).

Operative technique

Segmental resection with permanent aortoaortic bypass. Segmental resection of the aorta is indicated in patients with extensive tumor involvement—one third or more of the circumference of the aorta—and perhaps in patients with direct invasion into the distal arch. In the latter instance, semicircumferential resection with patch repair seems technically difficult, since almost all direct invasion into the distal aortic arch is posterior.

CASE 1. A 70-year-old man with a carcinoma of the middle third of the esophagus underwent a two-stage procedure including subtotal esophagectomy, circumferential resection of the descending aorta, and retrosternal esophagogastrostomy.

At the first operation, the left chest was en-

TABLE 32-1. Resection of the thoracic aorta in the treatment of esophageal carcinoma invading the aorta

Patient	Method of aortic resection	Approach for aortic resection	Method of spinal protection
70-year-old man	Segmental resection	Bilateral thoracotomy	Aortoaortic permanent bypass
65-year-old man	Semicircumferential resection	Right thoracotomy	Axillofemoral bypass
66-year-old woman	Wedge resection	Right thoracotomy	None
74-year-old man	Semicircumferential resection	Left thoracotomy	Subclavian-aortic bypass

tered. The circumventing graft was placed in such a way as to bypass the tumor-bearing segment of the aorta, leaving the tumor untouched (Fig. 32-3, *A* and *B*). The aorta proximal and distal to the lesion was then transected between clamps, and each divided end of the aorta was sutured in two rows (Fig. 32-3, *C* and D). The chest was closed in routine manner, and the abdomen was entered with the patient in a supine position. The mobilized stomach was passed to the neck through a retrosternal tunnel and anastomosed to the transected cervical esophagus. The proximal and distal cut ends of the excluded esophagus were sutured with proximal decompressive drainage.

The second stage was performed 2 months later. During this operation, the right chest was entered and combined aortoesophagectomy was performed, with mediastinal lymph node dissection.

The advantages of this technique include the following: (1) The lumen of the alimentary tract is never exposed during the left thoracotomy, thus minimizing bacterial infection to the fabric aortic graft, and (2) the aortoaortic bypass is permanent, utilized during and after surgery. The disadvantage is that the magnitude of the operation is extended by the metachronous bilateral thoracotomy.

Semicircumferential resection with patch aortoplasty. This operation is indicated in patients in whom the aorta is involved in one third or less of its circumference.

The advantages of this method include the avoidance of extensive dissection and mobilization of the aorta and the sparing of almost all intercostal arteries, thus preventing possible postoperative neurologic complications. Either side of approach may be utilized in this procedure, but we recommend the left.

When semicircumferential resection of the aorta under cross-clamping is planned preoperatively, some form of arterial shunt should be placed prior to surgery. We recommend the axillofemoral bypass because it is accomplished with minimal technical difficulty, it has negligible physiologic effect on the patient, and it does not interfere with the operative field. Some attention should be paid to details in performing the axillofemoral bypass. An externally stented fabric graft should be selected and the graft should be coursed just lateral to the midclavicular line; both of these measures protect the graft from external compression during thoracotomy (see Fig. 32-4).

CASE 2. A 65-year-old man with a carcinoma of the upper third of the esophagus underwent subtotal esophagectomy, semicircumferential resection of the aorta with patch application, and lateral resection of the membranous trachea in a three-stage procedure.

In the first operation he underwent a left axillofemoral arterial bypass using an 8-mm PTFE graft.

In the second operation, a right thoracotomy was used (see Fig. 32-5). The normal esophagus was dissected free from its bed at both ends. The esophagus was then removed, leaving neoplastic tissue on the aorta, thus permitting aortic clamping distal to the left subclavian artery and again just distal to the lesion. The involved segment of the aorta was then resected semicircumferentially. The window defect was repaired with application of a woven Dacron patch (see Fig. 32-6). During this procedure, back bleeding from intercostal arteries was controlled by inserting fine occluding balloon catheters from the aortic lumen. The fabric graft was covered with a pedicled pleural flap.

For the third stage, esophageal reconstruction with subcutaneous esophagogastric anastomosis was performed 4 months later.

Subclavian-aortic bypass is another means of a temporary arterial shunting during surgery (see Fig. 32-7). The advantage of this procedure is that this shunting may be utilized only when it is necessary after exploration confirms aortic

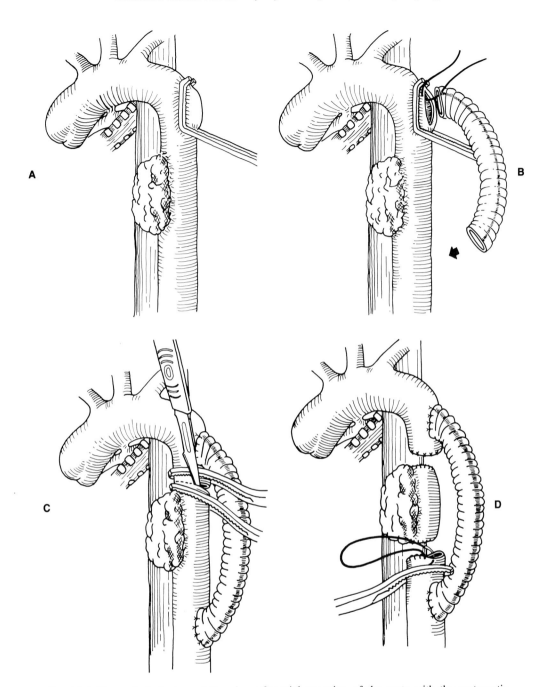

Fig. 32-3. The technical steps of the circumferential resection of the aorta with the aortoaortic permanent bypass. **A,** The tumor firmly adherent to the aorta. The partially occluding vascular clamp was applied to the proximal aorta. **B,** A linear longitudinal incision made and the preclotted woven Dacron graft, 20 mm in diameter, anastomosed using continuous sutures of 4-0 monofilament nylon sutures. **C,** The aorta cross-clamped and transected between the clamps. **D,** Each divided end sutured with continuous 4-0 monofilament nylon sutures.

invasion. However, a prolonged operation is inevitable during insertion and removal of the graft.

Wedge resection with lateral aortorrhaphy. This resection may be performed by side-clamping of the aorta. Because of its technical simplicity and elimination of the bypass procedure, the magnitude of the operation is no more than that of standard esophagectomy. The disadvantage of this method is that the extent of aortic resection is considerably limited both in circumference and in length. Direct invasion into the

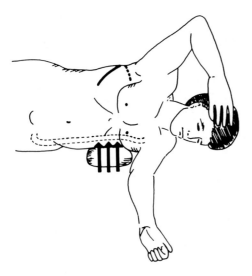

Fig. 32-4. Axillofemoral artery bypass in combined aortoesophageal resection. Placement lateral to midclavicular line avoids compression during posterolateral thoracotomy.

aorta by the esophageal neoplasm is usually more extensive than that which can be resected by simple side-clamping. The number of cases in which this technique is used, therefore, is small.

Complications

Various complications may occur during and after the combined aortoesophageal resection. The major complications directly related to this procedure are spinal cord ischemia and infection involving the fabric graft. The first of these may be eliminated by a carefully planned procedure minimizing the period of aortic clamping and by the effective utilization of temporary arterial shunting. Infection is related to intraoperative bacterial contamination, which may be minimized by careful surgical technique.

RESECTION OF THE TRACHEA

The tracheobronchial tree is frequently involved by carcinoma of the esophagus because

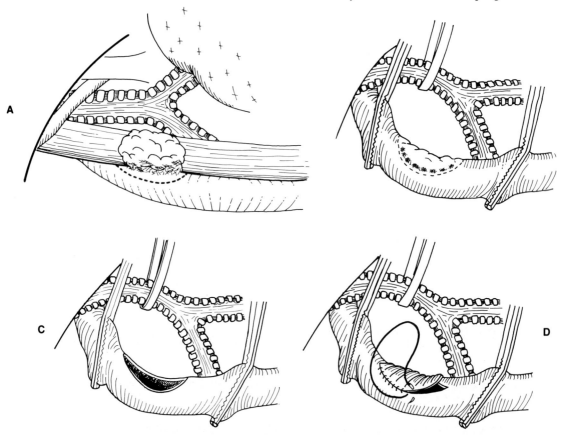

Fig. 32-5. The technical steps of semicircumferential resection of the aorta with patch application. **A,** Limited extension of tumor to wall of aorta. **B,** The esophagus has been removed, leaving tumor in aorta. **C,** Defect in aorta following semicircumferential resection. **D,** Suturing graft with woven Dacron patch.

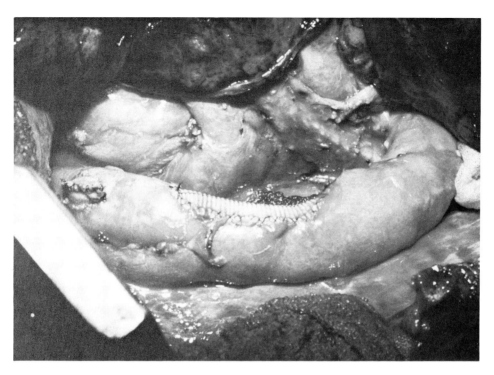

Fig. 32-6. Photograph of a 74-year-old man showing patch application following the semicircumferential resection of the aorta.

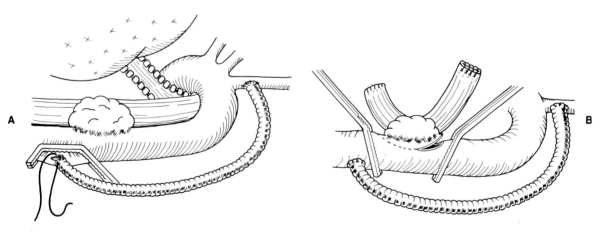

Fig. 32-7. The operative technique for semicircumferential resection of the aorta using subclavian-aortic bypass. **A,** After completion of the proximal anastomosis, a woven Dacron graft, 12 mm in diameter is anastomosed to the distal aorta by side-clamping. **B,** The involved segment of the aorta is then semicircumferentially resected during aortic cross-clamping.

of the proximity of the tracheal and esophageal walls. Most of these patients are not amenable to curative surgery. However, in a few selected patients, combined tracheoesophageal resection is justified in expectation of not only improving long-term survival but also providing better palliation. We find that there are considerable differences between resection of the trachea sec-

ondarily involved by carcinoma of the esophagus and that for a primary tumor of the trachea.

Preoperative evaluation of tracheal involvement

The location and extent of tracheal involvement should be precisely evaluated by bronchoscopy and computed tomography.

TABLE 32-2. Resection of the mediastinal trachea in the treatment of esophageal carcinoma invading the trachea

Site of tracheal invasion	Method of tracheal resection	Approach
Midmediastinal	Circumferential: 10 tracheal rings	Right thoracotomy, resection of manubrium
Upper mediastinal	Partial resection: 0.5 × 0.7 cm	Right thoracotomy
Tracheal carina	Lateral Y-shaped resection	Right thoracotomy
Cervicothoracic	Lateral resection: 1.5 × 3.2 cm, 8 tracheal rings	Right thoracotomy, partial midline sternotomy

Special problems in combined tracheoesophageal resection

The major problem in combined tracheoesophageal resection is the necessity for extensive resection of the tumor-bearing trachea and extensive dissection around the trachea during mediastinal lymphadenectomy. A second problem is the paradoxical movement of the membranous trachea during gasping or coughing after removal of the esophagus.

Such problems all too often lead to postoperative complications, including pneumonia and leakage of the tracheal anastomosis with resulting mediastinitis.

Approach

The surgical approach to the involved trachea is determined by the site of the segment to be resected (see Table 32-2). A right thoracotomy provides sufficient exposure of the mediastinal trachea, bifurcation, and right main bronchus. A partial midline sternotomy, usually from the sternal notch to the level of the second or third interspace, is indicated for lesions at the level of the thoracic inlet. In such an instance, dissection of the thoracic esophagus with mediastinal lymphadenectomy is performed by a concomitant right thoracotomy. The left approach may be indicated for patients in whom the left main bronchus is involved and mediastinal lymphadenectomy seems unnecessary.

Utilization of the pedicle flap of latissimus dorsi muscle

We have been utilizing the technique of intrathoracic application of a pedicle flap of the latissimus dorsi muscle in order to eliminate the aforementioned problems in a combined tracheoesophageal resection. The latissimus dorsi is used not only to reinforce the end-to-end tracheal anastomosis but also to close a window defect following lateral resection of the trachea. The latissimus dorsi is utilized because its dominant nutrient vessel is identifiable, its arc of rotation permits reaching intrathoracic locations, its functional loss is minimal, and it is very reliable.

Prior to opening of the chest, the muscle flap is fashioned through a standard thoracotomy incision with vertical extension, if necessary, without injuring the thoracodorsal vascular pedicle (see Fig. 32-8). The muscle flap is made as large as possible, usually 8 to 10 cm in width and 25 to 30 cm in length, so that intraoperative adjustments can be made.

Techniques

Circumferential resection with end-to-end anastomosis. Circumferential resection of the trachea is indicated for patients in whom one third or more of the circumference is involved by the extension of the esophageal tumor. However, the limits of resection of the trachea that permit direct reapproximation with a high degree of reliability are not completely established in combined tracheoesophagectomy. When performing this procedure, we recommend the use of the technique of intrathoracic application of a pedicle flap of the latissimus dorsi to support the anastomosis.

CASE 3. A 44-year-old man with dysphagia and subtotal obstruction of the midportion of the trachea underwent subtotal esophagectomy with retrosternal esophagogastrostomy and segmental resection of the mediastinal trachea comprising 10 tracheal rings, with end-to-end reapproximation.

The right chest was entered. The esophagus was densely adherent to the middle third of the mediastinal trachea, so that it was impossible to dissect between them (Fig. 32-9, *A*). The patient was rotated into the supine position and underwent resection of the sternal manubrium. The segment of trachea was circumferentially resected en bloc with the tumor-bearing esophagus, followed by an end-to-end anastomosis. Tracheal mobilization included a suprahyoid release and division of the right pulmonary ligament, which was essential to permit end-to-end anastomosis (Fig. 32-9, *B*). A pedicle flap of the latissimus dorsi was

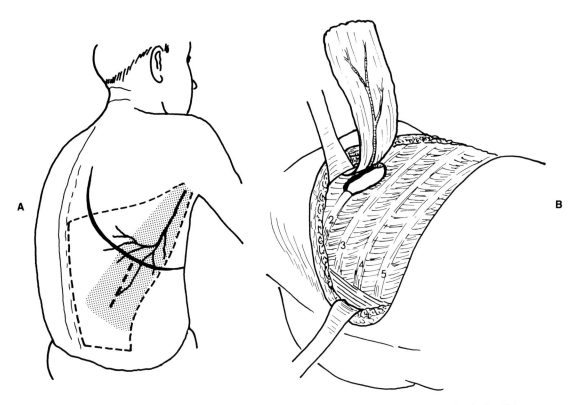

Fig. 32-8. Operative technique for fashioning the pedicle flap of the latissimus dorsi. **A,** Skin incision and the pedicle muscle flap. **B,** A 5-cm segment of the second rib resected, providing chest wall entrance for the pedicle flap.

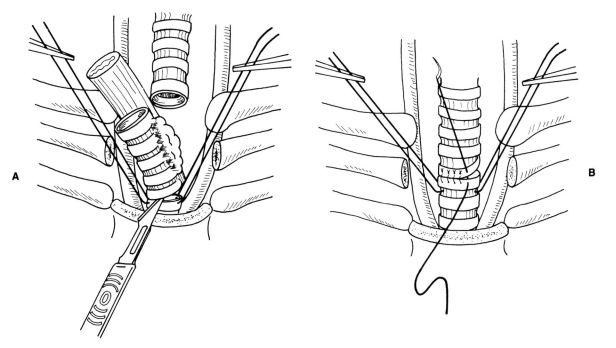

Fig. 32-9. Operative technique for combined tracheoesophageal resection. The esophageal carcinoma infiltrates the middle mediastinal trachea. Resection of the sternal manubrium provides sufficient exposure of the involved trachea. **A,** Traction sutures placed in the distal trachea and the circumferential resection being performed. **B,** After placement of sutures on the membranous trachea, sutures on the lateral and anterior wall are placed and tied one by one, knots on the outside.

transposed into the thorax and wrapped around the suture line (Fig. 32-8, *B*). Neck flexion was maintained for 10 days postoperatively.

Lateral resection with insertion of a pedicle muscle flap. It is not infrequent that the extension of the esophageal tumor is limited to the membranous trachea. In such instances, lateral resection of the membranous trachea is indicated if sufficient margins on each side are possible. Of the techniques for repairing the defect, we utilize the application of a pedicle flap of the latissimus dorsi muscle. On the basis of our experimental conclusions, lateral resection is indicated for patients in whom neoplastic involvement is limited to the membranous trachea.

CASE 4. A 75-year-old man with a carcinoma of the cervicothoracic esophagus underwent a subtotal esophagectomy, an extensive semicircumferential resection of the trachea, and an esophagogastrostomy. Through a partial midline sternotomy, the posterior wall of the trachea at the level of the thoracic inlet was resected, comprising a length of 8 tracheal rings. The extensive tracheal window defect was repaired by application of a pedicle flap of the latissimus dorsi. Postoperative endoscopy showed no leakage or stricture.

Complications

The most serious complication of combined tracheoesophageal resection is leakage of the tracheal anastomosis. We recommend that the pedicle flap of extrathoracic muscle always be placed over the tracheal anastomosis in order to avoid resultant mediastinitis. Other, nonfatal complications include paradoxical movement of the membranous trachea, impaired cough reflex, and recurrent laryngeal nerve palsy. All may lead to pulmonary complications.

REFERENCES

1. Kakegawa, T., Takeda, H., Iwamoto, M., et al.: Surgical treatment of esophageal cancer: in special reference to A₃ carcinoma of the esophagus, Jpn. J. Thorac. Surg. **33:**810, 1980.
2. Iizuka, T.: Surgical treatment for A₃ esophageal carcinoma, Jpn. J. Thorac. Surg. **33:**822, 1980.
3. Belsy, R.H.R.: Palliative management of esophageal carcinoma, Am. J. Surg. **139:**789, 1980.
4. Kawahara, H., Fujita, H., and Odagiri, S.: Combined resection of the thoracic aorta associated with esophagectomy for carcinoma of the esophagus, Rinsho Kyobu Geka **40:**1327, 1985.
5. Kawahara, H., Fujuta, H., Hidaka, M., et al.: Intrathoracic application of latissimus dorsi muscle flap for extended radical esophagectomy, J. Jpn. Surg. Soc. **85:**300, 1984.
6. Ohkubo, K., Hamada, M., Nishizawa, Y., et al.: Computed tomography of esophageal cancer: with special reference to the usefulness of PMG CT, Nippon Acta Radiol. **42:**740, 1982.
7. Adams, H.D., and van Geertruyden, H.H.: Neurologic complications of aortic surgery, Ann. Surg. **144:**574, 1956.
8. Akiyama, H.: Surgery for carcinoma of the esophagus, Curr. Probl. Surg. **17:**53, 1980.

Combined radical resection of adjacent organs involved by esophageal carcinoma

Discussion

Keyvan Moghissi

One of the significant developments in the surgical treatment of esophageal cancer is related to the technical advances that are being made to allow expansion of the indications for surgery and contraction of the criteria for patients' inoperability. It is in this context that Drs. Kawahara and Fujita's presentation is both exciting and instructive. They address themselves to two aspects of the local extension of the esophageal cancer, namely aortic and tracheal involvement. They rightly formulate the indications and selection of patients for combined radical resection of aortoesophageal and tracheoesophageal tumors.

Besides the obvious differences in techniques, there are a number of other relevant reasons for discussing the aortic and tracheal involvement of esophageal cancer separately. The first and foremost of these is that tracheal involvement by the cancer heralds an esophagotracheal fistula with all its distressing symptoms. Therefore, an operation that prevents this occurrence even without any expection of long-term survival is in our view a justified and worthwhile undertaking, because it will contribute to the amelioration of quality of life. But notwithstanding its prognostic consequences, aortic extension of an esophageal cancer does not per se affect the quality of life to the same extent as tracheal involvement. It therefore follows that there need to be more rigorous criteria of patient selection for combined radical aortoesophagectomy than for tracheoesophageal resection.

COMBINED AORTOESOPHAGEAL RESECTION

Involvement of the aorta by esophageal cancer is not an uncommon occurrence and accounts for unresectability of the tumor, and therefore inoperability, in a number of patients. The exact incidence cannot be precisely evaluated, since many patients with clinically inoperable cancer do not undergo surgical exploration that can ultimately and reliably indicate the true extent of the growth. Two autopsy studies[1,2] put the incidence of aortic involvement by esophageal cancer at 5% and 18%, respectively. However, these figures are not helpful for our discussion, because of the very nature of the material upon which the studies are based: (1) Not all patients with esophageal cancer who die undergo autopsy. (2) Not every esophageal cancer patient dies at the same stage of disease. (3) Both studies contain a heterogeneous group of cases—some with surgical treatment, others with radiotherapy, and yet a third group with no specific treatment.

Nevertheless, the incidence of aortic involvement in those patients who are surgically explored can be determined. In our series of 708 patients with carcinoma of the esophagus, the incidence of aortic involvement has been 7% among all patients who were surgically explored (about 90% of the total). Thus, 42 patients had aortic involvement by their esophageal cancer. Approximately one half of these had an unresectable tumor, or were inoperable because of reasons other than the aortic extension of the growth. Of the remaining, no patient was judged suitable for a radical aortoesophageal resection, although they had palliative resection of the esophageal tumor and reconstruction of the esophagus. It must, however, be pointed out that a careful retrospective study of these patients shows that, with our present understanding and experience, five patients could have had radical aortoesophageal resection. This means that, at most, 1% of our patients with carcinoma of the esophagus could have been offered aortoesophageal resection according to the criteria presented by Drs. Kawahara and Fujita. (We fully subscribed to these criteria.) These authors have obviously not discussed either the incidence of aortic involvement by esophageal cancer in their patients or the percentage of such patients who could be offered combined radical aortoesophageal resection. However, the fact that only four such resections are presented would suggest that only a small number of patients can benefit from this radical operation.

At the present time, I believe that there is a place for the operation of aortoesophageal resection, which should be kept in mind by all experienced esophageal surgeons, to be employed for suitable candidates. It is in order, however, to question a policy of extensive use of a surgical procedure that is aimed at a long survival without statistical justification of the probabilities of achieving that goal. It may therefore be worthwhile to suggest that those who embark on performing this radical operation should assure themselves that it achieves more than just palliation, and that there is a reasonable expectation of cure of the disease with a long-term survival of the patient.

What then of those who cannot be offered the radical resection but who are grossly dysphagic? Our experience suggests that (1) most patients with aortic involvement of esophageal cancer fall into this category and (2) many such cases are discovered only at thoracotomy. Under such circumstances we carry out a palliative resection of the esophagus and as much of the tumor as possible, with remnant esophagogastric anastomosis away from the area of growth of residual tumor on the aorta. More recently, since the introduction of Nd-YAG laser equipment in our department, we have applied extensive laser treatment to the area of the residual tumor and in some cases we have been able to fulgurate and vaporize all residual cancer. The long-term results of this will need evaluation.

COMBINED ESOPHAGOTRACHEAL RESECTION

Apart from postcricoid carcinomas, which are not the subject of this discussion, tracheal involvement by esophageal cancer is an uncommon occurrence. This reflects the lower incidence of carcinomas in the cervical and upper thoracic esophagus, where trachea and esophagus lie in intimate contact. In effect, carcinoma in these situations accounts for no more than 8% to 10% of all cases of esophageal cancer in western Eu-

ropean countries. In a series of 2400 patients with esophageal cancer, collected from 22 countries in Europe (excluding the United Kingdom), Giuli and Gignoux[3] found that only 5% of esophageal cancer occurred in the upper thoracic esophagus. In our own series of 708 esophageal cancer patients at Humberside Cardio-Thoracic Surgical Centre, the combined incidence of cervical and upper thoracic involvement was 10.5% of all cases. Among these, 20% had frank tracheal invasion.

Tracheal involvement by esophageal cancer in autopsy reports lies between 13% and 30% of all cases. These figures are subject to criticisms similar to those for aortic involvement by cancer of the esophagus. By far the most reliable indication of the incidence of tracheal involvement may be obtained from bronchoscopic examination, which is routinely undertaken by many surgeons, including me, in patients with cancer of the esophagus. One such study[4] of 525 patients put the incidence of tracheal involvement at 24% for cases of cervical and upper thoracic esophageal cancer, or 4.3% of all those with esophageal cancer. This is higher than in our series. We have found tracheal involvement in 15 patients, or 2% of all patients with cancer of the esophagus and cardia.

The management of carcinoma involving the trachea is controversial, and, like Drs. Kawahara and Fujita, we believe that combined resectional surgery should be undertaken when possible. There are good reasons to advance this view: (1) There is almost inevitable fistula formation following tracheal involvement by the tumor. (2) These high esophageal carcinomas are unsuitable for simple palliative procedures, such as intubation.

It must, however, be pointed out that in our experience combined resection with total clearance of tumor cannot be achieved in the majority of these patients. This is particularly true when the esophagotracheal tumor is situated at the inlet of the thorax or the root of the neck. It is mandatory, therefore, to investigate these patients meticulously, particularly with respect to the local extent of growth beyond the esophagotracheal mass.

It is also important not to lose sight, in some of these cases, of the possibility of the alternative and simpler surgery of colon bypass followed by radiotherapy.

Drs. Kawahara and Fujita presumably report no operative mortality and do not comment on long-term survival. Our experience with surgical treatment of seven patients with esophageal cancer and tracheal involvement can be summarized as follows: Two patients underwent colon bypass followed by radiotherapy. They survived 11 and 13 months, respectively. In two additional patients the tumor in the cervical esophagus infiltrated the trachea in proximity to the larynx without involving it. In these patients total laryngoesophagectomy with partial tracheal resection and a low permanent tracheostomy seemed the more satisfactory procedure than trying to preserve the larynx. Both these patients are alive, one 4 years and the other 6 months following operation. The remaining three patients had esophageal cancer involving the upper thoracic trachea and underwent esophagotracheal resection and a remnant esophagogastric anastomosis. The tracheal resection in these patients was partially circumferential, extending from 2 to 4 cm. The gap was bridged with a patch of Marlex mesh and pericardial graft.[5] One patient died 40 days postoperatively and the other two, 6 and 10 months after the operation.

These dismal results enforce the interest in radical resection advocated by Drs. Kawahara and Fujita only if one can rightly assume a long survival in some of their patients.

In conclusion, our general views on the management of tracheal involvement by the esophageal cancer can be best summarized as follows: (1) *Palliative* surgery should be offered to patients whose expectation of long survival is questionable because of the extent of tumor involvement. This may be accomplished with a bypass operation or incomplete resection of the tumor. (2) Radical resection of esophagotracheal carcinoma, followed by reconstruction, should be reserved for patients with a reasonable expectation of cure.

REFERENCES

1. Anderson, L.L., and Thomas, E.L.: Autopsy findings in squamous cell carcinoma of the esophagus, Cancer **50:**1587, 1982.
2. Mandard, A.M., Chasle, J., Marnay, J., et al.: Autopsy findings in 111 cases of esophageal cancer, Cancer **48:**329, 1981.
3. Giuli, R., and Gignoux, M.: Treatment of carcinoma of the esophagus: retrospective study of 2400 patients, Ann. Surg. **192:**44, 1980.
4. Choi, T.K., Siu, K.F., Lam, K.H., and Wong, J.: Bronchoscopy and carcinoma of the esophagus. I. Findings of bronchoscopy in carcinoma of the esophagus, Am. J. Surg. **147:**757, 1984.
5. Moghissi, K.: Tracheal reconstruction with a prosthesis of Marlex mesh and pericardium, J. Thorac. Cardiovasc. Surg. **69:**499, 1975.

CHAPTER 33 Surgical involvement in cooperative study protocols: experience of the OESO international group

Robert Giuli

The mediocrity of the therapeutic results observed from most of the isolated statistics on cancers of increasing incidence justifies a multidisciplinary approach to the very special problems presented by these patients. Efficiency in a project can be expected only in a multicenter study, guaranteed by the necessary statistics to perceive tendencies, eliminate hypotheses, or properly evaluate relationships between all observed facts.

In this context, and to approach these problems from the viewpoint of the daily experience of a specialized team, the Group OESO* was created in 1979 to establish a number of statistical studies on esophageal cancer. Its project was vast and required the intensive collaboration of motivated specialists from different countries to set up the various protocols and collect the data required. Four consecutive stages were programmed and these are the subject of this chapter.

THE PLAN

The first stage, which was the least restrictive for the participants, was a *retrospective* study, the results of which were presented during the September, 1979, meeting of the European Societies of Surgery and in *Annals of Surgery*.[1] This study gathered the largest number of resected tumors of the esophagus published to date and involved 2400 patients.

The tedium of filling out statistical cards, translated into five languages, from teams in 10 countries, was essential to the second stage of the program, a *prospective* study involving patients undergoing surgery. The results of this study were

*Organisation Internationale d'Etudes Statistiques pour les Maladies de l'Oesophage.

presented at the World Congress of the Group OESO, in 1984 in Paris.[2,3] The impetus was accelerated by the collective international and multidisciplinary structure of the established Group OESO and benefitted from the inclusion of renowned surgical teams from various countries. With such collaboration, the third stage of the program became possible.

This third stage involved setting up a study that was both *prospective* and *randomized*. This started in 1985. Necessary for the success of this study was the knowledge acquired during the earlier two stages of the Group OESO. The superb statistical assistance provided by the Department of Medical Statistics of the Gustave Roussy Institute in Villejuif, France, was abetted by the participation of the statistics team from the Memorial Sloan-Kettering Cancer Center in New York.

This project, presently in progress, is ambitious, bringing together personnel and information from 17 countries. It proposes to analyze simultaneously data gathered randomly from several groups of patients: those with surgery alone, those with surgery followed by radiotherapy, and those with surgery preceded and followed by chemotherapy. The number and the quality of the teams participating in this protocol allow limitation of the study to approximately 18 months. Brevity is necessary to preserve the enthusiasm of the teams.

The fourth stage, also in progress, is of enormous interest. It consists of an attempt at *prevention* by the randomized treatment of dysplasia, which long has been suspected as a predisposing pathologic condition. This protocol does not involve surgical teams. It was proposed by the Group OESO to certain centers of gastrointestinal

STAGE ONE

The first study by the group[1] has already presented interesting data concerning therapeutic trends. One of the first observations was that tumors of the upper third of the esophagus were no longer considered nonsurgical because of location. In 106 cases, the postoperative mortality was 31% and the 5-year survival rates were 14% (24-4*) and 21% (35-6).

Tumors in the middle third of the esophagus were suitable for statistical evaluation of long-term survival in 926 patients. The better prognosis of the *more extended esophageal resections* was clear. In 177 patients who had a limited resection with anastomosis below the aortic arch, the survival rate was less than 8% at 5 years (16-0), and, in this group, the operative mortality was 36%. Among 735 patients in whom the anastomosis was performed above the aortic arch, the operative mortality was lower (27%) and the overall survival at 5 years higher, 13% (16-10). When the resection was even more extensive and the anastomosis performed in the neck (84 patients), the operative mortality was similar (31%) but the long-term survival rate appeared better, 24% (40-8).

For tumors of the lower third of the esophagus (789), the mean 5-year survival rate (including postoperative mortality) was 17%. As in the case of the tumor situated higher, the breakdown of results of the various operations showed that the poorest results were found in association with low resection (13% [20-11] of 289), the prognosis improving when the anastomosis was high; the prognosis doubled with subtotal excision of the esophagus and replacement by colon with anastomosis in the neck (32% [49-14] of 61 patients). Similarly, emphasis was placed on the fact that, in carcinomas of the anatomic cardia (adenocarcinomas), there was a recognized need for extensive excision of the esophagus. It therefore seemed reasonable to include such tumors in the overall study. While the mean survival rate in such tumors (19% [24-14]) was only slightly higher than that for lesions of the middle third of the esophagus, it should be noted that the best 5-year results (46% [64-28] of 58 patients) were obtained following total gastrectomy with removal of more than 5 cm of esophagus.

In this set of statistics, involving patients operated upon in the late 1970s when resections without thoracotomy were not yet being done, the operative mortality seemed high, close to 30%. It became clear that the information for histologic classification of the different tumors was confusing. Overall assessment of long-term survival rates showed a more favorable prognosis for adenocarcinomas (518 cases), with a rate of 27% (34-20) at 5 years. By comparison, evaluation of the long-term survival rate of squamous cell carcinomas revealed a rather unusual finding. The most numerous "well-differentiated" squamous cell lesions (1155) were associated with the lowest long-term life expectancy (16% [19-12]). For "relatively undifferentiated" squamous cell carcinomas (425), the survival rate was higher (17% [22-12]), and similar to that of "undifferentiated" squamous cell carcinomas (163), reaching 25% at 5 years (39-11).

The prognostic value of the macroscopic appearance of the tumor was clear. The prognosis was most favorable when the tumor was fungating (22% [30-15]), intermediate in the case of ulcerated tumors (19% [24-14]), and poorest when the tumor was infiltrating (12% [18-7]).

In the evaluation of long-term survival rates, it was of interest to determine whether the length of the esophagus resected above the tumor had any influence. This parameter was recorded in centimeters up to 5 cm from the lesion. The number of high excisions decreased proportionately with the cephalad level of the carcinoma; high excision was accomplished in only 55% of the resections for carcinoma of the cardia. Histologic study of the site of esophageal transsection showed that, when histologic examination revealed tumor of the margin, in a large percentage (29%), the section had actually been made in a grossly healthy area, more than 4 cm from the tumor. This incidence was scarcely greater than that of invasion seen after section of the esophagus immediately adjacent to the carcinoma (24%).

A number of other surprising observations were made from analysis of these 2400 patients. The first concerns the poor prognosis for small tumors in comparison with large lesions. For those tumors with a diameter between 1 and 3 cm, there were no postoperative survivors at 5 years, regardless of cell type. As the size increased, long-term survival rates also increased, up to tumors of 4 cm, with these rates being invariably higher for adenocarcinomas (21% [30-12] and 53% [75-32]).* For tumors larger than 5

---

*Interval of confidence.

*The first percentage represents all patients undergoing operation and the second, those surviving surgery.

cm in diameter, the prognosis invariably decreased, with the same predilection in favor of adenocarcinomas. A possible interpretation of this phenomenon is provided in the T/N classification. In this comparison, which involves not the size of the tumor but its spread in terms of depth into the esophageal wall and into mediastinal lymph nodes, it may be noted that, although for stage T_3 the influence of the criterion N was negligible (13% [19-6] survival if N+ and 15% [19-11] if N−), it became dominant for the other T stages of tumor. The difference was substantial for T_2 tumors (25% [33-17] if N+ and 36% [47-26] if N−) and marked for tumors scored T_1 (0% at 4 years if N+ and 39% [64-14] if N−).

Other surprising observations were stated by Belsey[4] in his analysis of this set of statistics:

1. Absence of lymph node involvement was nevertheless associated with a local recurrence rate of 27%, 52% in the mediastinum and 35% in the esophagus.
2. With cervical lymph node involvement, paradoxically 33% of patients who underwent surgery were alive 5 years later.
3. Some of the earliest detected carcinomas had, after attempted curative surgery, been followed by return of the patient within 9 months riddled with metastases.

In short, to hazard a prognosis in any individual patient seemed virtually impossible despite preoperative staging.

STAGE TWO

We then felt it necessary to set up the basis for a *prospective* study. Other questionnaires, translated into five languages, were prepared to assemble data in areas that seemed of the greatest importance for the prognosis of these patients. In addition to the details of operative technique and pathologic study, the elements of preoperative endoscopy and preoperative, perioperative, and postoperative intensive care were also considered, as well as apparent correlations between the patient's nutritional and immune status and the development of postoperative complications. By this time participation in the Group OESO had increased, which made it possible to cross strictly European lines and include observations from Canada and Japan.

The results were presented during the first International Congress of the Group, in Paris in May, 1984.[2] Participants from 23 countries representing 10 different fields were asked to respond to a questionnaire including 135 items. Analysis of responses provided the following data.

The mortality for 790 patients undergoing resection was reported as 14.7%.

Resections without thoracotomy were done in 36 patients for tumors located between 20 and 34 cm from the dental arches. However, more than one patient in five was still operated on by a left thoracic approach. More than half of these were for tumors situated between 20 and 34 cm from the dental arches. Over 50% of the tumors situated between 25 cm and the cardia involved cervical approaches.

As in the previous observations, the tendency toward a *more extensive resection of the esophagus* was confirmed, with 215 total esophagectomies. Fifteen percent of these were performed for tumors of the lower third of the esophagus. In addition, 20 of the 22 tumors necessitating a circumferential pharyngolaryngectomy were felt to justify a combined thoracic and abdominal approach.

Even in cases of pharyngolaryngectomy, many patients underwent mediastinal and abdominal lymph node dissection; for carcinomas of the middle or lower third, the proportion of cervical lymph node dissections reached 10% (Table 33-1). However, despite a line of transsection more than 4 cm from the upper pole of the tumor, resection remained insufficient in 12.5% of cases (Table 33-2). *Early recurrences* occurred in 6% of patients in whom the line of transsection was histologically clear of tumor. This figure was multiplied by three in the presence of dysplasia (Table 33-3).

Analysis of the histologic data provided for this study confirmed *the inadequacies of the present classification* of tumors of the esophagus. Actually, if invasion of lymph vessels is less common than of blood vessels, and applies principally to moderately differentiated or relatively undifferentiated tumors, such invasion is found in 10% of "superficial" tumors. Moreover, 14% of purely mucosal tumors are associated with lymph node involvement; on the other hand, more than a quarter of those classified T_3 are free of such involvement. An absence of node involvement may coexist with macroscopic (32%) tracheobronchial invasion or with invasion of the lymph vessels (14%). There is no apparent statistical relationship between histologic cell type and the likelihood of tumor recurrence. Superficial tumors are not free of this risk (2% of 56 tumors classified T_{1b}). Finally, observations in this series, involving 71 superficial esophageal tumors (15 T_{1a} and 56 T_{1b}) have confirmed uncertainties in treatment. Lymph node dissection was carried out in the

TABLE 33-1. Lymph node excision

Postop. death Exc. − (%)	Exc. + (%)		22 CPL* (%)	54 upper third (%)	188 middle third (%)	425 lower third (%)	20 cardia (%)	16 total (%)
14	20	62 cervical	77	59	7	3		
16	14	534 mediastinal	23	41	90	75	60	62
18	14	589 coeliac	18	50	85	83	95	87
16	12	159 hepatic	4	22	16	25	30	25
14	16	175 splenic	9	11	19	30	35	19

From First Polydisciplinary International Congress of OESO: Cancer of the esophagus in 1984: 135 questions, answers compiled by R. Giuli, Paris, 1984, Editions Maloine.
*Circumferential pharyngolaryngectomies.

TABLE 33-2. Esophageal section (661)—histologic study

	Healthy	Neoplastic Permeation	Invasion	Dysplasia
	86%	5%	7.5%	1.5%
Healthy esophagus (average length)	6.9 cm	4.8 cm p- < 0.005	4.3 cm	3.4 cm

From First Polydisciplinary International Congress of OESO: Cancer of the esophagus in 1984: 135 questions, answers compiled by R. Giuli, Paris, 1984, Editions Maloine.

majority of cases (94%) of T_{1b}, and 7 of 15 patients underwent total esophagectomy for a T_{1a} tumor.

The information furnished by *nutritional parameters* led to the observation that, despite supplemental nutrition provided to 60% of patients, the clinical criteria for malnutrition (circumference of the arm, triceps skin thickness) showed no change. Similarly, the correlation coefficient between transferrin level and weight loss was not significant, and, despite alimentation techniques, no negative skin test (82 patients) ever became positive.

For a small number (19) of anergic patients, 66% had curative operations with uncomplicated postoperative course. By contrast, the degree of weight loss seemed to be statistically related to the operability of the tumor.

These different observations attest to the uncertainties still persisting in the diagnosis, classification, therapeutics, and prognosis of cancers of the esophagus. We continue to see in countries of high incidence an increasing number of patients with advanced tumor of the esophagus.

TABLE 33-3. Esophageal section—early recurrences

Healthy	Neoplastic Permeation	Invasion	Dysplasia
6%	25%	12%	18%
	p < 0.007		

From First Polydisciplinary International Congress of OESO: Cancer of the esophagus in 1984: 135 questions, answers compiled by R. Giuli, Paris, 1984, Editions Maloine.

STAGE THREE

Following this multicenter prospective study, from the impetus provided by these initial results and the international collaboration among specialists in disparate disciplines, it seemed appropriate to undertake the third stage of the OESO program: a truly therapeutic trial in a *randomized* fashion.

The goal of this therapeutic trial is to judge, in a statistically indisputable manner, the respective advantages of two therapeutic trials in comparison with surgical resection alone. Since cancer is still considered a disease in which surgery is the therapeutic mainstay, surgical resection would remain the reference arm of this study. For comparison, two other therapeutic modalities are considered—radiotherapy and chemotherapy.

The combination of radiotherapy with surgical resection is logical. A preliminary study of the results of such a combined approach led to the belief that the choice of preoperative radiation was not reasonable. On the other hand, *postoperative radiotherapy* at prophylactic doses of 45 Gy could reduce the local and regional recurrence rates and be effective for residual disease. This has been observed in other tumors. The effects of such treatment, performed under precise and reproducible conditions, are not yet known in cancer of the esophagus. This second arm of postoperative radiotherapy has therefore been selected by the Group OESO, beginning with radiation 6 to 8 weeks after surgery and extending 5 weeks, with 5 sessions per week of 1.8 Gy per treatment.

The third arm of this trial is *perioperative* chemotherapy. In this field, the experience of cancer centers such as Sloan-Kettering Center in New York is substantial. The protocol selected, therefore, was the one developed there by Kelsen. It consists, during the 2 months preceding surgery, of two cycles of cisplatin, eight of vindesine, and eight of bleomycin. Then, 6 to 8 weeks after surgical resection, a 22-week treatment of three cycles of cisplatin and 12 of vindesine is carried out. The proposed combination seems to answer desired prerequisites: an average of 50% responses, improvement of surgical resectability, and acceptable tolerance.

Even the experience of the Sloan-Kettering Center includes only 34 patients. This is the major problem of any study of this kind. The results are fragmentary, with only a *small number of patients* available as the basis for such a trial in any one therapeutic center.

On the other hand, with the number and quality of the teams participating in a therapeutic trial such as the group OESO, it may be possible to show that one of the treatments combined with surgery improves the 2-year survival by perhaps 10%. One hundred seventy patients would be needed in each arm—that is, a total of about 500 patients.

The constraints of such a trial are numerous. They require, from each team involved, a total acceptance of each detail of the protocol, not only in carrying out procedures but also in scrupulously recording data on the statistical cards devised. Despite these difficulties, including the pledge to a strict acceptance and observance of the protocol by the surgeon, the chemotherapist, and the radiotherapist of each team, explicit agreement for participation has been obtained from 39 teams representing 17 countries worldwide. These teams are from Europe (Germany, Belgium, Spain, France, Hungary, Italy, Poland, Turkey, Yugoslavia), from the Americas (United States, Brazil, Argentina, Chile), from the Mideast (Saudi Arabia, India), and from the Orient (Japan, China).

The randomization of the patients is done simultaneously at the Sloan-Kettering Center and the Gustave Roussy Institute, where a team of five specialists has been formed. This team carries out joint daily work consolidating the analysis of the cards as they are received, including verification and feeding into the computer.

In addition, two prognostic indexes will be tested as the different observations are received. The first is a *clinical classification,* which will attempt, by joining the clinical and nutritional parameters of each patient, to set up a numerical quotation with the assignment of a global score to each.

Reading of the principal publications leads one to note that the percentages of postoperative comications, of overall mortality, and of long-term survival vary greatly from one country to another, even from one team to another, without clear explanation. The use of such an index will permit the grouping of patients into precise categories, *within which* valid statistical comparisons can be carried out. The inclusion of Chinese, Japanese, American, and European teams allows comparisons of the clinical and nutritional conditions of patients operated on in different parts of the world. Such an analysis may lead to correlations, until now unsuspected, between the patient, his disease, and the treatment rendered.

The second prognostic index is a *histologic prognosis index.* Within the Group OESO, Appelman, a world authority on pathology of the esophagus, has been charged, in collaboration with an international group of pathologists he is heading, with developing such an index. The goal is to establish, for each patient, a global score that will make possible the determination, for each type of tumor operated on, of a prognostic factor based on real data and confirmed by subsequent developments. This index includes seven graduations and 12 different rubrics, associating macroscopic and microscopic aspects of the tumor. The evaluation of this index will be made by the two statistics centers. We hope to be able to propose, at the completion of this therapeutic trial, a *new classification system for tumors of the esophagus*.

For coordination in the exact interpretation of the histologic type of the tumors, Appelman, in his Ann Arbor laboratory, is centralizing the histologic data for each patient who undergoes surgery. He should receive and review about 12 slides per patient. For cases in dispute we anticipate discussion every 6 months, during a meeting of the pathologists of the special Group within the OESO.

A first evaluation of the results of this randomized trial might be expected when the randomization of the patients is complete, perhaps in 18 months.* This possibility corresponds to the dates of the Second International Congress of the Group OESO, in Paris, on May 21 to 23, 1987. That meeting was organized, as was the first Congress, with a precise questionnaire attempting to address problems raised by *benign lesions of the esophagus that predispose to esophageal carcinoma*, that is, caustic strictures, megaesophagus, peptic stenoses, and Barrett's esophagus. During this Congress a round table was conducted, assembling international pathologists to debate the elements of the *new pathologic classification* of esophageal cancers.

STAGE FOUR

Specialists agree that the solution to the problems posed by esophageal cancers resides primarily in their *prevention*. It has been clearly demonstrated by the Chinese that severe dysplasia of the esophagus is associated, in 9 to 12 years, with malignant degeneration in 66% of the cases.[5] In addition, it has been shown experimentally that

there is a favorable effect in the treatment of such lesions by carotenoids, substances of low toxicity, such as vitamin A, which improve dysplastic lesions or even make them disappear.

The Group OESO has therefore set up yet another therapeutic trial to test randomly in cases of dysplasia the effects of simple observation and *treatment by carotenoid substances*. This trial is presently in progress in the digestive endoscopy centers of five European countries.

CONCLUSIONS

The answers to all the many questions asked can only be found in statistical analysis, carried out by high-level professionals, of data carefully agreed upon beforehand. Only large numbers permit such statistical research, and only multicenter studies permit assembling such numbers. The Group OESO, with teams from Europe, Asia, and the Americas, make possible, for the first time, comparison of real data, which, hopefully, will provide answers to therapeutic decisions in the selection of specific treatments for patients with carcinoma of the esophagus.

REFERENCES

1. Giuli, R., and Gignoux, M.: Treatment of carcinoma of the esophagus: retrospective study of 2400 patients, Ann. Surg. **192**:44, 1980.
2. First Polydisciplinary International Congress of OESO: Cancer of the esophagus in 1984: 135 questions, answers compiled by R. Giuli, Paris, 1984, Editions Maloine.
3. Giuli, R., and Sancho-Garnier, H.: Diagnostic, therapeutic and prognostic features of cancers of the esophagus: results of the international prospective study conducted by the OESO Group (790 patients), Surgery, **99**:614, 1986.
4. Belsey, R.: Is it possible to talk of cure of carcinoma of the esophagus. In First Polydisciplinary International Congress of OESO: Cancer of the esophagus in 1984: 135 questions, answers compiled by R. Giuli, Paris, 1984, Editions Maloine, p. 382.
5. Huang, G.J.: What is the value of abrasive cytology in superficial Cancers? In First Polydisciplinary International Congress of OESO: Cancer of the esophagus in 1984: 135 questions, answers compiled by R. Giuli, Paris, 1984, Editions Maloine, p. 320.

*EDITOR'S NOTE: As of publication date, compilation of data is as yet incomplete.

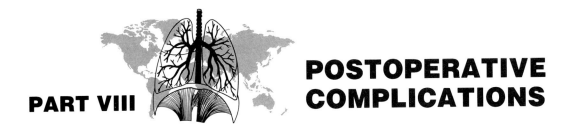

PART VIII — POSTOPERATIVE COMPLICATIONS

34 Immediate complications following esophageal surgery

E. Elman and Robert Giuli

The basis for comment on this subject is provided by data from the various studies of the Group OESO (see Chapter 33).

In the first study, a retrospective study published in 1980,[1] the operative mortality, for 2400 patients, was 30%. Its variations were minimal in relation to the location of the tumor, since it reached 31% for 106 tumors of the upper third, 31% for 926 tumors of the middle third, 30% for 789 tumors of the lower third, and 28% for 530 tumors of the cardia.

In the second study by this group, a prospective study done in 1984,[2] the operative mortality was clearly lower, but still reached 14.7% for 763 patients.

We have observed in this study that the fistula rate remained high (13.4%). The anastomotic fistulas were still significantly related to postoperative mortality. Punctate fistulas seemed to be frequent. Almost half of mediastinal abscesses developed in relation to a cervical anastomosis (see Table 34-1).

No difference was noted in the incidence of fistulas after mechanical or manual anastomosis done in a single layer (see Table 34-2). The use of automatic sutures was not as widespread as one might have thought. Stapled anastomoses were used 200 times in our set of statistics, with a total fistula rate of 10%, of which more than one quarter occurred before the fifth postoperative day. This incidence is approximately the same as for the 225 cases of single-layer manual anastomosis.

In the OESO series, the only statistically significant feature concerning the etiology of fistulas was the use of preoperative radiotherapy.

The incidence of fistulas was markedly lower than that observed in 1972 statistics,[3] when there were 95 fistulas in 415 esophageal resections (23%). The improvement during the interval may be credited to the fine semiabsorbable suture materials now in use throughout gastrointestinal surgery, much as they have been used in vascular surgery.

The peculiar anatomic features of the esophagus have been implicated in the genesis of complications—factors said to be beyond the control of the surgeon. Chief among these has been the greatly maligned esophageal blood supply. In actual fact, it must be pointed out that the esophagus has an excellent blood supply[4] and, indeed, that factors other than its poor innate perfusion must be responsible for postoperative esophageal leakage and fistula formation. From autopsy and intraoperative observations, it seems that the ischemic sloughing of structures anastomosed to the esophagus, rather than failure of esophageal blood supply itself, should be implicated in the genesis of leakage after esophageal reconstruction.

In fact, the most severe and preoccupying complications are pulmonary, some of which may be related to undetected anastomotic fistulas. With modern methods of management, anastomotic leaks should heal, yet 21% to 41% of patients with anastomotic complications die, usually from pulmonary complications. Overall these occur in 8% to 33% of the patients.[5,6] They include failure to cough and to clear secretions, pulmonary edema, atelectasis, tracheobronchitis, bacterial pneumonia, aspiration pneumonitis, empyema, pulmonary abscess, respiratory failure, and the acute respiratory distress syndrome requiring mechanical ventilatory support. Mortality following postoperative pulmonary complications ranges from 15% to 68%.[5,7]

Factors influencing postoperative pulmonary complications are numerous. It remains controversial whether these are significant factors, other than in the presence of clinical metastatic disease, concomitant disorders in elderly patients, palliative resections, or anastomotic leakage. However,

TABLE 34-1. Incidence of fistulas in relation to level of anastomosis

			Site of anastomosis		
Fistula	Pharynx	Neck	Apex of thorax	Above aortic arch	Below aortic arch
61 neck	4	57			
22 mediastinum		10	1	4	7
10 pleura		1	3	3	3

From First Polydisciplinary International Congress of OESO: Cancer of the esophagus in 1984: 135 questions, answers compiled by R. Giuli, Paris, 1984, Editions Maloine.

TABLE 34-2. Fistulas (103/769 = 13.4%) and type of anastomosis

	Single layer (225)	Two layers (321) p = 0.002	Mechanical (200)
Fistulas	9%	19%	10%
Punctate	72%	65%	62%
Large	17%	19%	24%
Loose separation	11%	16%	14%
		NS*	
Average time lapse (days)	8.1	8.8 NS	7.7
Early fistula (<5 days)	22%	50%	27%

From First Polydisciplinary International Congress of OESO: Cancer of the esophagus in 1984: 135 questions, answers compiled by R. Giuli, Paris, 1984, Editions Maloine.
*NS, Statistically not significant.

an increased incidence of pulmonary complications has been reported in patients over 60 years of age, when the tumor was located in the lower or middle third of the esophagus,[8] following preoperative bleomycin chemotherapy, after preoperative irradiation, with the use of an enriched oxygen mixture and large amounts of crystalloid fluid during anesthesia,[9] or after combined preoperative irradiation and extensive mediastinal surgery.[10] A similar increase in complications has been noted after left thoracophrenolaparotomy, compared with right thoracotomy and upper laparotomy[11]; after intraoperative endobronchial intubation with single-lung ventilation[12]; when a *total* esophagectomy was performed[6]; when ability to cough was reduced postoperatively[13]; following dissection of paratracheal lymph nodes; after damage to the vagus nerves; and subsequent to injury of the diaphragm.

It has been demonstrated that, after esophagectomy with gastric replacement through right thoracotomy and upper abdominal laparotomy, reduction of forced vital capacity does occur. Respiratory dysfunction is greater in duration and extent than that produced by either of these incisions alone.[14] On the other hand, a reduced incidence of pulmonary complications after esophagectomy has been reported following the use of a Swan-Ganz catheter for preoperative assessment of cardiopulmonary function and perioperative fluid management, following transhiatal esophagectomy without thoracotomy,[15] or after use of routine postoperative assisted ventilation with positive end-expiratory pressure (PEEP).[8]

Among the 790 patients studied by the OESO Group, 369 were documented to have pulmonary complications (46.7%). A past history of chronic bronchitis, preoperative radiotherapy, tracheobronchial invasion, endotracheal rather than endobronchial intubation, or severe hypoxemia during anesthesia was associated with a higher pulmonary complication rate (see Figs. 34-1 to 34-3).

Chronic obstructive pulmonary disease and restrictive pulmonary disease documented by spirometric tests, extent of esophageal resection, location of the surgical incision, systematic postoperative mechanical ventilation, use of PEEP, or monitoring of pulmonary capillary wedge pressure had no significant influence on the overall pulmonary complications. Similarly, transhiatal esophagectomy without thoracotomy was not as-

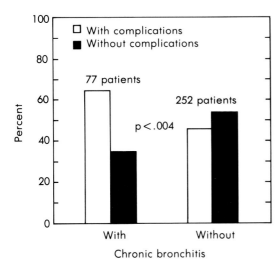

Fig. 34-1. Pulmonary complication rate in patients who have had chronic bronchitis.

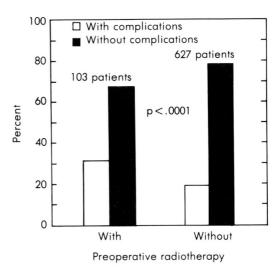

Fig. 34-2. Pulmonary complication rate in patients who have had preoperative radiotherapy.

sociated with a lower pulmonary complication rate than with conventional approaches.

Is it possible to prevent pulmonary complications? *Preoperatively,* careful assessment of pulmonary and cardiovascular function, nutritional status, and the presence of infection should be done. Patient education to ensure optimal postoperative pulmonary compliance is important, as is cessation of smoking, training in proper breathing by incentive spirometry, use of bronchodilators, and control of secretions or infection whenever indicated. Avoidance of radiotherapy is a prophylactic measure to reduce pulmonary complications (see discussion of Chapter 39).

Intraoperatively, use of prophylactic antibiotic therapy initiated before surgery seems mandatory in order to reach the peak plasma level at the time of esophageal resection. Reduction of duration of anesthesia and surgery; prevention of aspiration; control of secretions; use of assisted ventilation for both lungs, with large-volume flow rates and a well-humidified enriched oxygen mixture, except in the bleomycin-treated patient; use of intermittent hyperinflation of the lung if endobronchial intubation is performed; and reduction of single-lung ventilation time are all also of great importance. Similarly, providing fluid requirements, either by colloid or crystalloid solutions, slowly rewarmed and infused, guided by central venous pressure or pulmonary capillary wedge pressure monitoring, and avoiding transfusion therapy and hypothermia are appropriate guidelines recommended for any surgical procedure.

Postoperatively, incentive spirometry with patients in a semirecumbent position to prevent aspiration, continuous suction on pleural drains and gastric tubes, routine periodic fiberoptic bron-

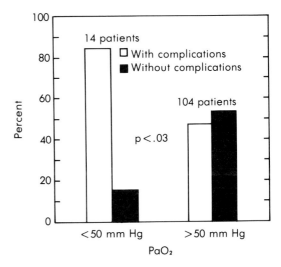

Fig. 34-3. Pulmonary complication rate according to PaO_2 during anesthesia.

choscopy, control of pain by epidural analgesia with morphine, and routine assisted ventilation are all advisable. Systemic antibiotic therapy is indicated, based on the sensitivity of bacteria obtained from blood and pulmonary cultures.

Although the rate of pulmonary complications is high and should be reduced, absolute avoidance of pulmonary complications after esophageal cancer is an unrealistic goal. Consider:

1. Even excluding pulmonary infections and emboli as causes of death, 19% of esophageal cancer patients die of respiratory failure.[16]
2. Pulmonary sepsis from aspiration of food and saliva is one of the primary symptoms of malignant esophageal obstruction.

3. Because there is no standard surgical treatment for carcinoma of the esophagus, some surgical procedures may carry a higher respiratory risk than others. Nevertheless, the choice of technique is still dependent on histologic findings, size, stage, and possibility of recurrence of the tumor rather than on the risk of complications. In our study, risk factors were a past history of chronic bronchitis, preoperative radiotherapy, tracheobronchial invasion, endotracheal intubation, and severe hypoxemia during anesthesia.

CONCLUSION

The accumulation of the results of the various world teams participating in the International Congress of the OESO yields a mean total operative mortality of approximately 10%, still quite far from the low figures (2% to 3%) published in large Chinese and Japanese series (Wu, Akiyama). It is likely that such differences depend not only on operative technique, but also perhaps on peculiar patient factors.*

The Group OESO has just started a randomized trial on cancer of the esophagus (see Chapter 33), assembling 39 teams from 17 countries in the world. This will enable us to place patients in strictly comparable categories and to evaluate the operative risk in a statistically consistent manner. In this way, differences that are evident in the reading of various partially published statistics can be explained, including adjusted operative mortality extending to several months after the procedure and proper classification of the patients in all published statistics. This should then enable us to determine a more accurate operative risk.

---

* EDITOR'S NOTE: The editors express concern that the incidence of anastomotic fistula (13.4%) and the postesophagectomy mortality rate (14.7%) derived from the 1984 OESO questionnaire may be accepted as a standard. Both statistics are high. It is possible to achieve a fistula rate of close to zero. A mortality of 2% to 5% is a not unrealistic goal.

REFERENCES

1. Giuil, R., and Gignoux, M.: Treatment of carcinoma of the esophagus: retrospective study of 2400 patients, Ann. Surg. **192**:44, 1980.
2. Giuli, R., and Sancho-Garnier, H.: Diagnostic, therapeutic and prognostic features of cancers of the esophagus: results of the international prospective study conducted by the OESO Group (790 operated patients), Surgery **99**:614, 1986.
3. Giuli, R., Estenne, B., and Lortat-Jacob, J.L.: La désunion des anastomoses oeso-gastriques dans la chirurgie des cancers de l'oesophage, Ann. Chir. **27**(6):567, 1973.
4. Payne, W.S.: The role of esophageal blood supply. In First Polydisciplinary International Congress of OESO: Cancer of the esophagus in 1984: 135 questions, answers compiled by R. Giuli, Paris, 1984, Editions Maloine, p. 222.
5. Postlethwait, RW., and Durham, C.: Complications and deaths after operations for esophageal carcinoma, J. Thorac. Cardiovasc. Surg. **85**:827, 1983.
6. Wilson, S., Stone, R., Scully, M., Ozeran, L., and Benfield, J.R.: Modern management of anastomotic leak after esohagogastrectomy, Am. J. Surg. **144**:95, 1982.
7. Demin, E.U., Stolyarov, V., and Volkov, O.: Primary complications after surgery for the cardio-esophageal region, Acta Chir. Scand. **148**:683, 1982.
8. Nakayama, K., and Kagegawa, T.: Latest management of pulmonary complications following esophageal surgery in Japan, Adv. Surg. Oncol. **4**:111, 1981.
9. Nygaard, K., Smith-Erichsen, N., Hatlevoll, R., and Refsum, S.B.: Pulmonary complications after bleomycin, irradiation and surgery for esophageal cancer, Cancer **41**:17, 1978.
10. Dunnick, N., Schwade, J., Martin, S., Johnston, M., and Glatstein, R.: Interstitial pulmonary infiltrate following combined therapy for esophageal carcinoma, Chest **81**:452, 1982.
11. Black, J., Kalloor, G.J., and Leigh-Collis, J.: The effect of the surgical approach on respiratory function after oesophageal resection, Br. J. Surg. **64**:624, 1977.
12. Bourgeois, R., Lassen, C., Guignard, J., Lemee, J., Freiermuth, C., and Langonnet, F.: Intubation selective versus intubation non-selective au cours de l'anesthésie pour resection de l'oesophage, Anesthésie et Réanimation **141**:72, 1984.
13. Sugimachi, K., Lleo, H., Natsuda, Y., Kai, H., Inocuchi, K., and Zaitsu, A.: Cough dynamics in oesophageal cancer: prevention of postoperative pulmonary complications, Br. J. Surg. **69**:734, 1982.
14. Bishop, D.G., and McKeown, K.C.: Postoperative hypoxemia: oesophagectomy with gastric replacement, Br. J. Surg. **66**:810, 1979.
15. Orringer, M.B.: Palliative procedures for esophageal cancer, Surg. Clin. North Am. **63**:941, 1983.
16. Ambrus, J.L., Mink, T.B., et al.: Causes of death in cancer patients, J. Med. **6**:61, 1975.

35 Complications of the anastomosis: leak and stricture

R. W. Postlethwait

ANASTOMOTIC LEAK

To restore alimentary tract continuity, any resection or bypass of the esophagus will require anastomosis of the esophagus or hypopharynx to the stomach, a greater-curvature gastric tube, colon, or jejunum. Dehiscence of the esophageal anastomosis is disproportionately frequent in relation to other gastrointestinal anastomoses.

Chassin[1] reviewed 13 reports totaling 2156 esophagogastric anastomoses. Leakage from the anastomosis occurred in 0% to 41%; the average was 10%. Of the 485 deaths occurring in patients with anastomotic leaks, the author estimated that about half were due to the leak. Ancona et al.[2] also reviewed the literature and found, in 2339 patients, anastomotic leak in 374, or 16%. They state that 47% of deaths were due to the leak. Huang et al.[3] reported 1572 resections, with 66 postoperative deaths. Anastomotic leak developed in 67, leading to death in 29. Thus, this complication caused death in 43.3% and was responsible for 43.9% of all deaths. We have reviewed the literature regarding patients who had cervical esophagectomy, transhiatal removal of the thoracic esophagus, and high esophagogastric anastomosis. Leak developed in 11.9% of 511 patients.

In Table 35-1, representative reports since 1981 are listed. Included are series from China and Japan. As far as could be determined, all were sutured anastomoses. Of the 5232 anastomoses, leak developed in 394, or 7.5%. The number of deaths attributed to this complication was infrequently noted; a reasonable estimate is between 25% and 50%. Anastomotic insufficiency thus is an important factor in the morbidity and mortality after these operations.

Reference should be made to the various ways of reporting anastomotic leaks. A number of authors note only major leaks, with or without recording those that are clinically unimportant and close within a few days. All leaks should be reported, subdivided if desired into the following categories: (1) no clinical manifestation, (2) spontaneous closure, (3) requiring reoperation, or (4) leading to death.

Causes

The usual detrimental factors listed are lack of serosa, impaired blood supply, excessive tension, faulty technique, malnutrition, residual carcinoma at line of resection, and preoperative irradiation.

1. On the basis of experiments performed a number of years ago,[18] we question the importance of the absence of the serosa. In dogs, the pressure causing anastomotic leak was identified after three types of anastomosis: end-to-end esophagus without resection, esophagus to gastric fundus after 4- to 6-cm resection, and end-to-end ileum without resection. Determinations were made immediately, at 6 hours, at 24 hours, and then at intervals to 12 days after operation. The esophageal anastomoses were equal to or stronger than the enteroenterostomies immediately and at all intervals up to 8 days. The esophagogastrostomy, early equally strong, decreased in strength at 4 days and did not attain equal strength until after 8 or 12 days. An interesting finding was the rapid sealing of the esophageal anastomoses by adjacent structures (mediastinal soft tissues, lung, pericardium) similar to the omentum in the abdomen.

2. The blood supply to the stomach, mobilized

TABLE 35-1. Anastomotic leak—sutured anastomoses

References	No. of patients	Post-operative death	Leak		Comment
			No.	Percent	
Huang et al. (1981)[4]	334	13	15	4.5	Preoperative irradiation
	736	22	27	3.7	No irradiation
Huang et al. (1981)[5]	43	6	6	13.9	Cervical anastomosis
	1305	49	46	3.5	Intrathoracic anastomosis
Lam et al. (1981)[6]	157	48	36	22.9	Pharyngogastric anastomosis
Ancona et al. (1982)[2]	193	?	29	15.0	
Lam et al. (1982)[7]	174	?	21	12.1	Resection
	34	?	18	52.9	Bypass
Maillet et al. (1982)[8]	271	45	17	6.3	
Wilson et al. (1982)[9]	123	?	12	9.8	
Conlan et al. (1983)[10]	71	?	17	23.9	Bypass
Launois et al. (1983)[11]	254	45	31	12.2	
Liu et al. (1983)[12]	319	?	12	3.7	
	114	?	1	0.9	Special technique
Xu et al. (1983)[13]	66	16	8	12.1	Upper third
	280	29	26	9.3	Middle
	318	22	18	5.7	Lower and cardia
Orringer (1984)[14]	100	6	5	5.0	Transhiatal
Pistolesi et al. (1984)[15]	57	?	9	15.8	
Gluckman et al. (1985)[16]	52	0	5	9.6	Free jejunal
Sugimachi et al. (1985)[17]	231	16	35	15.2	

for transposition into the thorax or neck, is from the right gastric and right gastroepiploic vessels. A number of injection studies have demonstrated the adequacy of the intramural vessels to the fundus. This is true also after excision of a portion of the lesser curvative, which usually is, or should be, done in operations for carcinoma. In the majority of patients, when the stomach is elevated into the thorax or neck, the fundus will appear adequately perfused, and when the incision is made for the anastomosis, brisk bleeding will be encountered. Why the blood supply should be compromised in some patients is not entirely clear. Atherosclerosis could be a factor, but more likely improper technique in dissection or gastric closure is at fault.

3. The amount of tension placed on the stomach should be considered relative to the level of the esophagogastrostomy, since the more proximal anastomoses are at increased risk of leak. Xu et al.,[13] for example, in a large series of patients reported leak in 12.1% for upper-third lesions, 9.3% for middle-third, and 5.7% for lower-third and cardia (see Table 35-1). Tension in esophagogastrostomy might be considered in more than the usual context—that is, motion during swallowing and the effect of gastric distention. Early in the experience with esophageal resection, surgeons emphasized the importance of suturing the fundus to firm tissue, such as the prevertebral fascia above the anastomosis, to avoid any tension on

the latter. In the average patient, the stomach will easily extend to the apex of the chest or the neck. Only with anastomosis to the hypopharynx will unrelieved tension occur. With each swallow, however, the esophagus shortens to a variable degree, and this is particularly important in the short cervical segment with anastomosis in the neck. Each swallow thus tugs on the anastomosis and essentially tends to pull the anastomosis apart. Should gastric distention occur, the stomach may act adversely through the increased intraluminal pressure or by the distracting force of the gastric wall.

4. Many ingenious methods of anastomosis have been described but no infallible techniques found. The basic principles do not differ from anastomoses in other portions of the gastrointestinal tract, although the esophagus is known to hold sutures less well. An interesting study in point was that of Tera and Aberg.[19] They determined the holding power of a single suture through the cut edge of the esophagus, stomach, duodenum, jejunum, ileum, colon, sigmoid, and rectum. The esophagus and sigmoid were the weakest, while the stomach and colon were the strongest.

A number of surgeons prefer a single-layer anastomosis; most utilize two layers. Our preference is the latter and involves two important components: a precise mucosal closure and a firm outer layer. Meticulous apposition of the mucosa is particularly important in esophagogastrostomy, since a mucosal gap invites infection and leakage. In a well-formed gastroenterostomy, the regenerative power of both stomach and small bowel epithelium will rapidly cover the defect. With esophagogastrostomy, gastric epithelium may extend rapidly, but the squamous epithelium of the esophagus is considerably slower to regenerate. The sutures may be interrupted or continuous, providing a purse-string effect is avoided for the latter. Knots should be within the lumen. The outer layer, preferably interrupted sutures, is through the muscularis propria and into the submucosa. The bites should be large enough to provide appreciable holding power.

Most of the available suture materials have been studied, without a consensus being reached. We prefer a synthetic absorbable suture for the inner layer and silk or a nonabsorbable synthetic multifilament material for the outer. Others have used sutures such as polypropylene and wire successfully. The technique of the anastomosis, however, is more important than the suture material.

Reinforcing or covering the anastomosis by a number of methods has been described. Although an inkwell type of anastomosis may not prevent reflux, it does provide reinforcement. Various degrees of fundoplication may be used. A pleural flap or intercostal muscle bundle will provide supportive coverage.

5. The adverse influence of malnutrition on wound healing has been known for many years, on the basis of animal experiments and clinical experience. Usually, patients with carcinoma of the esophagus will have lost considerable weight and present evidence of nutritional deficiency. Although enteral or parenteral feeding will bring improvement, restoration to normalcy may not be readily accomplished. In addition to the deleterious effect of malnutrition on wound healing, the compromising of immunologic response enhances the possibility of infection. An indirect relation of the state of nutrition and the risk in anastomotic healing is suggested by the stage of the disease at the time of operation. For example, Wilson et al.[9] had 18 anastomotic leaks after 72 palliative operations and only one after 95 potentially curative procedures. This is also shown in our experience: 34.6% leaks after bypass, 7.6% after palliative resection, and 3.7% after curative resection.

6. The presence of residual cancer at the anastomosis has been implicated in leakage. For example, Keighley et al.[20] after 50 adequate resections had four leaks with one death; 21 others had residual tumor at the anastomotic site, of whom 11 leaked and ten died.

7. Huang et al.[4] found no difference in the frequency of anastomotic leak after preoperative irradiation. After 334 resections in this group, 4.5% developed a leak. For 736 resections with no irradiation, 3.7% developed a leak. Presumably, the level of the anastomosis had been excluded from the treatment field. Lam et al.[6] reported 157 patients with carcinoma of the larynx, hypopharynx, or cervical esophagus who required pharyngogastric anastomoses. Sixty-two had irradiation and 37% leaked; of 95 without irradiation, 14% leaked, a significant difference. On the basis of this (and animal studies), irradiation does seem to adversely influence healing.

Stapled anastomosis

The availability of a dependable stapler for end-to-end or end-to-side anastomosis has led to its use by many surgeons. The principles already noted apply. Although the details of technique differ, the major component is precise apposition of the organs to be joined within the stapler. This is controlled by proper placement of the purse-string suture or sutures. When tied within the stapler, an adequate cuff of esophagus and stomach will be apposed for the anastomosis. After the stapler has been fired and removed, the integrity of the anastomosis must be checked. Tissue removed from the stapler should show two complete donuts; an incomplete ring of tissue indicates a defect in the anastomosis. External inspection and palpation through the gastrostomy provide needed assurance. Finally, colored saline may be injected into the lumen in the area of the anastomosis. Alternatively, air may be injected with saline filling the mediastinum. A small defect may be repaired; a large defect will usually need a new anastomosis.

Reinforcing sutures may be placed around the anastomosis. A fundus wrap may be used to cover the anastomotic area. The stapler should save time, but preparation for the anastomosis and placement of the purse string must be meticulous so that rather than time saved, the major advantage is a precise anastomosis.

The frequency of anastomotic leak, at least for early reports of small series, shown in Table 35-2, is less than that using suture technique. In the 484 patients reported, leak developed in 14, or 2.9%. Our experience[32] has been one leak in 60 patients, or 1.7%.

Diagnosis

Recognition of anastomotic leak is rarely a problem. Most anastomotic leaks become clinically evident within the first week and seldom develop after 14 days. A contrast barium swallow for radiologic examination is routinely obtained

TABLE 35-2. Anastomotic leak—stapled anastomoses

References	No. of patients	Post-operative death	Leak No.	Leak Percent	Comment
Dorsey et al. (1980)[21]	15	0	0	0	
Shahinian et al. (1980)[22]	12	0	0	0	
Fekete et al. (1981)[23]	45	6	1	2.2	
Graham et al. (1981)[24]	18	2	1	5.5	
Mills (1981)[25]	3	0	0	0	Bypass
Molina (1981)[26]	9	0	0	0	Cancer of cardia
Sannohe et al. (1981)[27]	20	0	2	10.0	
West et al. (1981)[28]	31	1	0	0	
Ancona et al. (1982)[2]	106	?	6	5.7	
Fabri and Donnelly (1982)[29]	30	2	0	0	
Huttunen et al. (1982)[30]	8	0	0	0	
Wilson et al. (1982)[9]	30	?	1	3.3	
Owen et al. (1983)[31]	47	?	1	2.1	Three gastric leaks
Hopkins et al. (1984)[32]	60	8	1	1.7	
Ferguson (1985)[33]	22	0	0	0	

between the fourth and seventh postoperative days. Drains are not removed until this study is obtained, confirming an intact anastomosis.

In the usual patient, frank anastomotic leak is suspected by a change in the character of the drainage, predominately to saliva and gastric secretions. A swallow of methylene blue–colored water or saline will appear in the drainage. Confirmation and some information as to the size of the leak are obtained with the swallow of contrast material (Fig. 35-1). Additional follow-up contrast radiologic or computed tomography (CT) studies are helpful in identifying undrained or inadequately drained areas.

Treatment

Because of many variables, a description of standard treatment will not be attempted, but the principles are (1) adequate drainage, (2) appropriate antibiotics, (3) gastric decompression, and (4) provision for nutrition. The last is of especial importance and may be satisfied by parenteral means, but a feeding jejunostomy often is preferable.

Assuming no other complications, the appearance of unusual drainage, most often from the anastomosis, should have its source identified. A leak from the stomach may be from the tacking sutures in the fundus, from the point of ligature of a short gastric vessel, or, most often, from the lesser-curvature closure. In our limited experience, these areas are more likely to close spontaneously than an equivalent leak at the anastomosis.

The size of the anastomotic deficit should be determined as accurately as possible, because this will influence the choice of treatment. This will vary from a pinpoint opening, to a partial dehiscence, or even to complete separation of the anastomosis. A small leak has a good possibility of closure, usually within 5 to 14 days. A major disruption, however, requires consideration of a second operation, for reanastomosis, for reinforcement and coverage, or for exclusion of the defect. An estimate of the size can be made from the amount of drainage, but more accurate information will be obtained by radiologic study. Occasionally a small, contained extravasation, without clinical manifestations, will be noted on the postoperative contrast study. Most of these will close, and no treatment is needed other than withholding oral intake.

Inberg et al.,[34] however, on the basis of their experience with 19 anastomotic leaks after 207 resections, state that immediate exploration should be performed to close or cover the area. A jejunostomy is also established.

The level of the esophagogastrostomy will influence treatment. Given defects of equivalent size, a leak in the neck is more likely to close than one in the mediastinum. This may in part be due to the ability to provide better drainage. The effect of movement (swallowing, respiration) is difficult to determine.

With few exceptions, the provision of adequate drainage is an obvious necessity. The main exception is the extravasation that may be appreciable in size but has remained well localized and

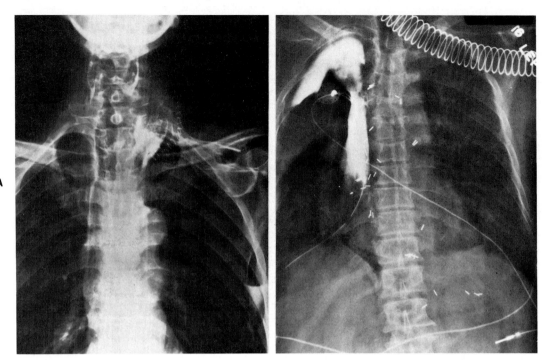

Fig. 35-1. A, Leak in neck from cervical anastomosis. **B,** Large intrathoracic leak that resulted in sepsis and death.

empties promptly back through the defect in the anastomosis. As long as the patient does not become septic, he or she may be followed by repeated contrast studies, with a reasonable possibility of closure.

The external drainage required will depend on the extent of the mediastinum and pleural cavity involved. A total empyema will need more extensive drainage than a localized collection. With drainage established, the patient must then be repeatedly examined, preferably by CT scan, to identify secondary loculations.

Finally, the development of an anastomotic leak unfortunately may be the precipitating event in a series of septic complications leading to death. The usual first involvement is pulmonary, requiring increasing efforts for respiratory support, and then multisystem failure. The logical solution is prevention, which in this context suggests prompt, vigorous, and appropriate treatment of the anastomotic deficiency.

ANASTOMOTIC STRICTURE

After resection of carcinoma of the esophagus, narrowing of the esophagogastric anastomosis may be a minor inconvenience, responding to one or two dilatations without further problem. In some patients, progression to a firm fibrous stricture requires multiple dilatations or even reoperation. In an unfortunate third group of patients, the stenosis is caused by recurrent carcinoma.

A number of authors describing the results of resection for carcinoma fail to note the frequency of anastomotic stricture. The following are representative recent reports, however. Owen et al.[31] reported radiologic evaluation in 31 patients 6 to 20 months after resection. Eight had benign strictures and seven tumor recurrence. Pistolesi et al.[15] after 57 resections had five patients with dilatable strictures, and three developed anastomotic recurrence of the tumor. Hennessy and O'Connell[35] reported 62 resections, with nine having anastomotic narrowing that responded to one or two dilatations. Eight patients developed dysphagia resulting from anastomotic recurrence. McKeown[36] had 48 deaths after 452 resections, so 404 patients were followed. Twenty-two strictures were classified as follows: fibrous, 12; due to esophageal ulcer, 1; postirradiation, 1; anastomotic recurrence, 6; and mediastinal recurrence, 2.

Orringer[14] reported six patients who developed a fibrous stricture after transhiatal esophagectomy. Gluckman et al.[16] reported an interesting group of 52 patients who had a free jejunal graft in the cervical region; six developed stenosis, two in the upper and four in the lower anastomosis. All responded to dilatation.

With utilization of the stapler, Shahinian et al.[22] had one easily dilatable stricture in 12 patients. West et al.,[28] in 31 intrathoracic stapled anastomoses, had four strictures, easily dilated, and one anastomotic recurrence. Graham et al.[24] used the stapler in 101 patients; 70 were esophageal transections for varices, the others resections. Stricture developed in 10, all responding to a single dilatation. Ferguson,[33] after 22 resections, had two strictures, both with use of the 25-mm cartridge, and none after using the 28- or 31.6-mm cartridge.

It had been our impression that stricture was more frequent after stapled anastomosis. Analysis of our series,[32] however, showed 9.4% after sutured and 13.3% after stapled anastomosis. The difference is not statistically significant.

Causes

When carcinoma appears at the anastomosis, this represents *persistence* of cancer rather than *recurrence*. Failure to obtain a normal proximal margin above the esophageal tumor has repeatedly been emphasized as avoidable. Although frozen section is not infallible, residual tumor is usually demonstrated by this technique. Through the years, this has led to increasing the acceptable length of palpable normal esophagus above and below the tumor, with 10 cm most frequently suggested. Some surgeons believe that subtotal or total esophagectomy is the advisable operation to avoid carcinoma at the proximal anastomosis.

Wound healing is a series of events, the major steps being formation of granulation tissue, deposition of collagen, contraction of myofibroblasts, and remodeling of the collagen. In an esophagogastric anastomosis, a defect in the closure, if only in the mucosa, is filled by granulation tissue, with more collagen formation and an increased likelihood of contraction to form a stricture. A similar adverse reaction may follow infection. The conditions may therefore be established by the technique of anastomosis. In addition, anastomotic leakage is acknowledged to predispose to stricture, although we know of no study devoted to this.

One unanswered question is why some strictures are soft, responding promptly to dilatation, while others progress to a hard fibrous stricture for which dilatation is difficult or impossible. The answer of excessive collagen deposition and contraction is probably correct but does not indicate why. Persistent low-grade infection may be a factor. In infants who have anastomosis for atresia, gastroesophageal reflux has been considered an important cause of persistent anastomotic stricture, and this may be a causative element too in the adult patient.

Because an anastomosis to the hypopharynx can be larger than one to the cervical esophagus, two groups of patients should have anastomosis at this level. After irradiation of the neck and after caustic injury, unrecognized intramural changes in the cervical esophagus predispose to eventual stricture.

Anastomotic narrowing after use of the stapler nearly always responds readily to dilatation. Although the studies of Polglase et al.[37] involved colorectal anastomoses in the dog, their findings should be applicable to esophagogastrostomy. The stapled anastomoses showed a 2- to 4-mm gap between the ends of the mucosa, which grossly appeared as "a flat circumferential ulcer." This would explain the frequency of stricture and the favorable results of treatment.

Diagnosis

The recognition of stricture presents no problem, since the radiologist with appropriate contrast study can accurately define the degree of narrowing (Fig. 35-2). The caveat is that tumor growing at the anastomosis must be excluded, which requires endoscopic examination. Should a cause be suspected such as reflux esophagitis or ulcer, esophagogastroscopy is again advisable.

Treatment

First, with reference to anastomotic recurrence of carcinoma, the few patients we have explored have not been resectable, because of the fixed extraluminal mass surrounding the anastomosis. This mass may be seen on plain x-ray films but should be more readily identified by CT scan. Irradiation therapy has provided only limited palliation; we have no experience with chemotherapy. Dilatation with or without endoesophageal intubation should provide some relief for the short period of remaining life. Laser treatment may be beneficial, but reports are limited (see Chapter 49).

After esophagogastrectomy, prior to discharge of the patient, a final barium swallow examination should be obtained to establish a baseline. In some patients, "sizing" of the anastomosis with Maloney bougies is advisable. The usual instructions regarding elevation of the head of the bed are given to minimize reflux of gastric contents.

As indicated previously, most strictures are easily dilated (Fig. 35-3). The problem arises in the firm fibrous stricture. For these, treatment must be individualized. Consideration must be given to the stage of the carcinoma as well as concomitant disease. Many patients are willing to accept monthly or even weekly dilatations to maintain a satisfactory, albeit not generous, lumen, which allows a soft diet. If the general condition of the patient is acceptable, resection and reanastomosis of a tight unyielding stricture may be considered.

Balloon dilatation, using balloons similar to those developed by Gruentzig for angioplasty, offers a promising alternative method. Lindor et al.[38] have described their experience in 111 patients with various types of upper digestive tract strictures. Eleven patients had a stricture after surgery for carcinoma of the esophagus. Although not stated, presumably these were esophagogastrostomies. Overall, the results were excellent in about 90%. These authors note that postoperative strictures responded as well as nonoperative strictures. They conclude this to be a safe, effective technique. The experience of our gastroenterologists has mainly been with benign strictures, but the results have been very satisfactory. Longitudinal cracking or splitting of the stricture may occur if dilatation is too vigorous.

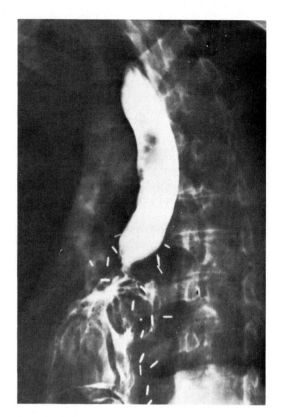

Fig. 35-2. Stricture after sutured anastomosis; improved with dilatation.

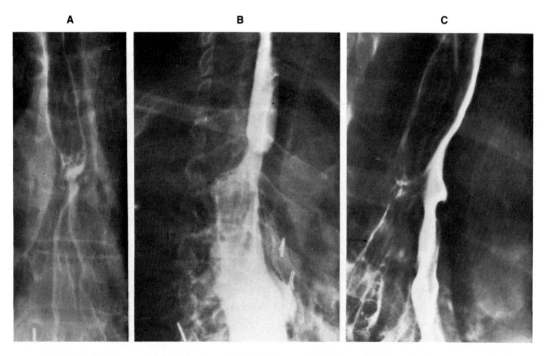

Fig. 35-3. A, Narrow stapled anastomosis. **B,** After one dilatation. **C,** Adequate lumen restored.

ADDENDUM

The preceding sections on anastomotic leak and stricture have considered mainly esophagogastrostomy. As noted, however, esophageal reconstruction or bypass may be accomplished with a greater-curvature gastric tube or a segment of colon or of jejunum. The principles regarding cause, diagnosis, and treatment are the same, although there are obvious differences. For example, the stomach nearly always remains viable, whereas the interposed colon will become necrotic in about 8% of patients. This indicates the more tenuous blood flow to and from the colon, and the increased possibility of anastomotic leak.

REFERENCES

1. Chassin, J.L.: Stapling technic for esophagogastrostomy after esophagogastric resection, Am. J. Surg. **136:**399, 1978.
2. Ancona, E., Bardini, R., Nosadini, A., Giunta, F., and Peracchia, A.: Esophagogastric anastomotic leakage, Int. Surg. **67:**143-145, 1982.
3. Huang, G.J., Wang, L.J., Liu, J.S., Cheng, G.Y., Zhang, D.W., Wang, G.Q., and Zhang, R.G.: Surgery of esophageal carcinoma, Semin. Surg. Oncol. **1:**74, 1985.
4. Huang, G., Gu, X., Zhang, R., Zhang, L., Zhang, D., Miao, Y., Wang, L., Lin, H., Wang, G., and Xiao, Q.: Combined preoperative irradiation and surgery in esophageal carcinoma: report of 408 cases, Chin. Med. J. **94:**73, 1981.
5. Huang, G., Zhang, D., Wang, G., Lin, H., Wang, L., Liu, J., Cheng, G., and Wang, X.: Surgical treatment of carcinoma of the esophagus: report of 1,647 cases, Chin. Med. J. **94:**305, 1981.
6. Lam, K.H., Wong, E.J., Lim, S.T.K., and Ong, G.B.: Pharyngogastric anastomosis following pharyngolaryngoesophagectomy: analysis of 157 cases, World J. Surg. **5:**509, 1981.
7. Lam, K.H., Cheung, H.C., Wong, J., and Ong, G.B.: The present state of surgical treatment of carcinoma of the oesophagus, J. R. Coll. Surg. Edinb. **27:**315, 1982.
8. Maillet, P., Baulieux, J., Boulez, J., and Benhaim, R.: Carcinoma of the thoracic esophagus: results of one-stage surgery (271 cases), Am. J. Surg. **143:**629, 1982.
9. Wilson, S.E., Stone, R., Scully, M., Ozeran, L., and Benfield, J.R.: Modern management of anastomotic leak after esophagogastrectomy, Am. J. Surg. **144:**95, 1982.
10. Conlan, A.A., Nicolau, N., Hammond, C.A., Pool, R., Nobrega, C.D., and Mistry, B.D.: Retrosternal gastric bypass for inoperable esophageal cancer: report of 71 patients, Ann. Thorac. Surg. **36:**396, 1983.
11. Launois, B., Paul, J.L., Lygidakis, N.J., Campion, J.P., Malledant, Y., Grosseti, D., and Delarue, D.: Results of the surgical treatment of carcinoma of the esophagus, Surg. Gynecol. Obstet. **156:**753, 1983.
12. Liu, K., Zhang, G.C., and Cai, Z.J.: Avoiding anastomotic leakage following esophagogastrostomy, J. Thorac. Cardiovasc. Surg. **86:**142, 1983.
13. Xu, L.T., Sun, Z.F., Li, Z.J., and Wu, L.H.: Surgical treatment of carcinoma of the esophagus and cardiac portion of the stomach in 850 patients, Ann. Thorac. Surg. **35:**542, 1983.
14. Orringer, M.B.: Transhiatal esophagectomy without thoracotomy for carcinoma of the thoracic esophagus, Ann. Surg. **200:**282, 1984.
15. Pistolesi, G.F., Lovisatti, L., Florio, F., Stella, P., Soregaroli, A., and Bergamo, I.A.: Radiological aspects of cancer of the esophagus, Int. Surg. **69:**41, 1984.
16. Gluckman, J.L., McCafferty, G.J., Black, R.J., Coman, W.B., Cooney, T.C., Bird, R.J., and Robinson, D.W.: Complications associated with free jejunal graft reconstruction of the pharyngoesophagus: a multiinstitutional experience with 52 cases, Head Neck Surg. **7:**200, 1985.
17. Sugimachi, K., Matsuzaki, K., Matsuura, H., Kuwano, H., Ueo, H., and Inokuchi, K.: Evaluation of surgical treatment of carcinoma of the oesophagus in the elderly: 20 years' experience, Br. J. Surg. **72:**28, 1985.
18. Postlethwait, R.W., Weinberg, M., Jenkins, L.B., and Brockington, W.S.: Mechanical strength of esophageal anastomoses, Ann. Surg. **133:**472, 1951.
19. Tera, H., and Aberg, C.: Tissue holding power to a single suture in different parts of the alimentary tract, Acta Chir. Scand. **142:**343, 1976.
20. Keighley, M.R.B., Moore, J., Lee, J.R., Malins, D., and Thompson, H.: Peroperative frozen section and cytology to assess proximal invasion in gastro-oesophageal carcinoma, Br. J. Surg. **68:**73, 1981.
21. Dorsey, J.S., Esses, S., Goldberg, M., and Stone, R.: Esophagogastrectomy using the autosuture EEA surgical stapling instrument, Ann. Thorac. Surg. **30:**308, 1980.
22. Shahinian, T.K., Bowen, J.R., Dorman, B.A., Soderberg, C.H., Jr., and Thompson, W.R.: Experience with the EEA stapling device, Am. J. Surg. **139:**549, 1980.
23. Fekete, F., Breil, P.H., Ronsse, H., Tossen, J.C., and Langonnet, F.: EEA stapler and omental graft in esophagogastrecomy: experience with 30 intrathoracic anastomoses for cancer, Ann. Surg. **193:**825, 1981.
24. Graham, H.K., Johnston, G.W., McKelvey, S.T.D., and Kennedy, T.L.: Five years' experience in stapling the oesophagus and rectum, Br. J. Surg. **68:**697, 1981.
25. Mills, S.A.: Use of EEA stapler for substernal esophagogastric anastomosis in palliation of esophageal carcinoma, J. Thorac. Cardiovasc. Surg. **82:**801, 1981.
26. Molina, J.E., Lawton, B.R., and Avance, D.: Use of circumferential stapler in reconstruction following resections for carcinoma of the cardia, Ann. Thorac. Surg. **31:**325, 1981.
27. Sannohe, Y., Hiratsuk, R., and Doki, K.: Single layer suture by manual or mechanical stapling technique in esophagojejunostomy after total gastrectomy, Am. J. Surg. **142:**403, 1981.
28. West, P.N., Marbarger, J.P., Martz, M.N., and Roper, C.L.: Esophagogastrostomy with the EEA stapler, Ann. Surg. **193:**76, 1982.
29. Fabri, B., and Donnelly, R.J.: Oesophagogastrectomy using the end-to-end anastomosing stapler, Thorax **37:**296, 1982.
30. Huttunen, R., Laitinen, S., Stahlberg, M., Mokka, R.E., Kairaluoma, M., and Larmi, T.K.: Experiences with the EEA stapling instrument for anastomoses of the upper gastrointestinal tract, Acta Chir. Scand. **148:**179, 1982.

31. Owen, J.W., Balfe, D.M., Koehler, R.E., Roper, C.L., and Weyman, P.J.: Radiologic evaluation of complications after esophagogastrectomy AJR **140:**1163, 1983.

32. Hopkins, R.A., Alexander, J.C., and Postlethwait, R.W.: Stapled esophagogastric anastomosis, Am. J. Surg. **147:**283, 1984.

33. Ferguson, C.M.: Esophagogastrostomy using the EEA stapling instrument, Am. Surg. **51:**223, 1985.

34. Inberg, M.V., Linna, M.I., Scheinin, T.M., and Vanttinen, E.: Anastomotic leakage after excision of esophageal and high gastric carcinoma, Am. J. Surg. **122:**540, 1971.

35. Hennessy, T.P.J., and O'Connell, R.: Surgical treatment of squamous cell carcinoma of the oesophagus, Br. J. Surg. **71:**750, 1984.

36. McKeown, K.C.: The surgical treatment of carcinoma of the oesophagus, J. R. Coll. Surg. Edinb. **30:**1, 1985.

37. Polglase, A.L., Hughes, E.S.R., McDermott, F.T., and Burke, F.R.: A comparison of end-to-end staple and suture colorectal anastomosis in the dog, Surg. Gynecol. Obstet. **152:**792, 1981.

38. Lindor, K.D., Ott, B.J., and Hughes, R.W., Jr.: Balloon dilatation of upper digestive tract strictures, Gastroenterology **89:**545, 1985.

Complications of the anastomosis: leak and stricture

DISCUSSION

Jean-Paul Witz

ANASTOMOTIC LEAK

Lowering the rate of anastomotic fistula and reducing its mortality are among the main advances in surgery for carcinoma of the esophagus. Discrepancies between large series are due to author interpretation in the reports. Systematic contrast swallow should be done on the seventh and fifteenth postoperative days and anytime there is an abnormal postoperative course. Any leak, even though blind, without clinical manifestation, and closing spontaneously, should be reported. In a retrospective study of 100 resections between 1982 and 1984, I observed 11% leaks: three blind, three very small, and five larger ones, with one death directly related to the fistula.

Causes

Causes are probably manifold, both local and general.

1. Blood supply to the extremity of the transplant (usually gastric tube, sometimes colon) is of prime importance. It may be difficult to appreciate in a gastric tube, and intraoperative verification by Doppler is helpful. Impedance of venous return, although rarely reported, seems to me to be a valid cause of vascular impairment and anastomotic leak, especially with the use of a colon replacement or in a cervical anastomosis. This may explain otherwise unexpected failures.

2. Undue tension of the anastomosis is not always admitted by the surgeon, but as Postlethwait states, "The more proximal anastomoses are at increased risk of leak." Like others, I have observed a twofold increase in the rate of leaks after cervical anastomosis. Shortening of the small segment of the esophagus during swallowing is also important. Gastric distention can and must be prevented by nasogastric tube drainage.

3. With regard to the methods of anastomosis and to suture material, every surgeon has his own particular technique, which he believes is the best (in his hands!). I use, whenever possible, a stapled anastomosis, because it may reduce the frequency of leaks.

4. It has been my experience that the presence of microscopic residual carcinoma at the suture line is related to leakage.

5. Preoperative irradiation, or previous irradiation for head and neck carcinoma, impairs healing.

6. The adverse influence of malnutrition or immunodeficiency is unquestioned. They are closely correlated to the extension and spread of the disease. Palliative resection in debilitated patients shows, as in other series, a much higher rate of leakage.

Diagnosis

As Postlethwait has stated, diagnosis is rarely a problem. The threat of a leak should be kept in mind until the fifteenth postoperative day, and drains should stay in place until the integrity of anastomosis is proved. The size of the leak is not always accurately evaluated by contrast swallow; thus we sometimes utilize direct endoscopic operation.

Treatment

Adequate drainage is the most important step in the treatment of the usual leak. Drainage outside the transplant should still be in place. I also use a double-lumen tube inside the transplant; one tube with holes facing the leak aspirates the saliva, and a second aspirates the gastric content. A small alimentary tube is placed in the proximal jejunum to complete parenteral nutrition. Jeju-

297

nostomy may be advisable in patients with larger leaks. Appropriate antibiotics are given.

Blind leaks require only observation.

A second operation, in my experience, is seldom essential unless it is for complete dehiscence or necrosis. Early reanastomosis is usually not possible or successful in an infected area. Inadequacy of drainage may also necessitate a second operation; coverage of the leak is then accomplished at the same time, in preference to attempted suture.

Anastomotic leak is rarely per se a cause of death. But in debilitated patients it appears to be the precipitating event in pulmonary or general septic complications, which in turn lead to death. Mortality in my series of patients with anastomotic leak has been 18%.

ANASTOMOTIC STRICTURE

Narrowing of the anastomosis may be "a minor inconvenience" for the patient, but it reproduces the main complaint for which he accepted the operation! The anastomotic stricture rate is reported in our country (France) to be between 10% and 15% (9.3% for my service). It appears to be higher after colonic transplant (20%) than after esophagogastric anastomosis, and higher after stapled anastomoses than after manual suture.

Causes

Almost 40% of the strictures are related to recurrence of carcinoma either at the suture line or in the adjacent mediastinum. For other strictures, predisposing factors may be irradiation, postoperative fistula (blind or clinical), impaired blood supply, and/or local infection.

Diagnosis

Contrast swallow and esophagoscopy provide the diagnosis in the majority of cases. CT scan is necessary to visualize mediastinal recurrence. In some cases the etiology is obvious only at operation.

Treatment

We have little to offer to our patients after recurrence. Jejunostomy is almost always necessary. Survival time is short, distant metastasis usually being associated with local recurrence.

For benign strictures a good functional result is often obtained after one or more dilatations. In case of failure, related to unusually hard strictures, a second operation may be considered if the patient is in good general condition and life expectancy is acceptable. Resection and reanastomosis are reported to give better results than plastic widening procedures.

36 Pulmonary complications

Shichisaburo Abo and Tamotsu Kudo

In recent years, the technique of surgery for esophageal cancer has improved significantly, and the operations being performed are relatively safe ones. Even in the circumstance of an aggressive approach to operations, as in this department (a rate of operation of 91% and a resectability of 100%), the operative mortality can be kept below 10%.[1] The improvement in operative results is achieved through refined operative skills and progress in preoperative and postoperative patient management. In order to improve further the operative results, it would be necessary to prevent postoperative complications. Among postoperative complications from operation for esophageal cancer, the primary category, both for morbidity and mortality, is pulmonary complications. Indeed, prevention and treatment of such complications is the foremost task today in the preoperative and postoperative management of the patient. Pulmonary complications are of various types and complicated disease profiles, but their specific features are brought to light through recent hemokinetic studies using the Swan-Ganz catheter plus measurements of extravascular lung water (EVLW). In this presentation, we report our concepts of the basis for pulmonary complications and how to prevent and treat them.

TYPES AND FREQUENCY OF PULMONARY COMPLICATIONS

Before we discuss pulmonary complications following operations for esophageal cancer, we must point out some confusion in the definition of the term. Some workers include pleural cavity complications in pulmonary complications, while others do not. In this report, in order to avoid confusion, only pulmonary parenchymatous disturbances are included, and pleural cavity complications such as hemothorax, pneumothorax, empyema, pleural effusions, and chylothorax are excluded.

Table 36-1 shows the reported incidence of postoperative parenchymatous pulmonary complications after esophagectomy. Nakayama and Kakegawa[2] reported total pulmonary complications in Japan during the period from 1974 to 1978. Their incidence was 17.5%, including pneumonia (51.0%), atelectasis (40.5%), acute respiratory distress syndrome (ARDS) (4.8%), and pulmonary edema (3.7%). Others reported incidences ranging from 5.8% to 28.1%. Mori et al.[5] reduced the incidence of pulmonary complications to 5.8% by monitoring the postoperative circulatory condition using the Swan-Ganz catheter and by postoperative ventilatory support.

TABLE 36-1. Frequency of pulmonary complications

Author	Nakayama and Kakegawa (1981)[2]	Tsuboi (1977)[3]	Watanabe et al. (1973)[4]	Mori et al. (1982)[5]	Postlethwait (1983)[6]
Rate	17.5% (601/3426)	16.3% (24/147)	28.1% (43/153)	5.8% (3/52)	13.4% (50/374)
Atelectasis	244	11	NR	1	NR
Pneumonia	306	7	NR	2	NR
Pulmonary edema	22	6	NR	NR	NR
ARDS	29	NR*	NR	NR	NR

*NR, Not reported.

The diagnostic criteria for reporting pulmonary complications have not yet been identified. For instance, there seems to be a difference of opinion about whether to regard minor changes on chest x-ray films as pulmonary complications.

ETIOLOGY OF PULMONARY COMPLICATIONS

The following outline shows what are presently considered causes for pulmonary complications after operations for esophageal cancer.

A. Preoperative factors
   1. The old patient, in general
   2. Impaired pulmonary function
   3. Concomitant disease, such as diabetes or chronic obstructive pulmonary disease
   4. Poor nutrition
   5. Cigarette smoking
B. Intraoperative factors
   1. Anesthesia
     a. Changes in bronchial secretion and defective expulsion mechanism
     b. Aspiration of gastric juice
   2. Operation
     a. Retraction of the lung
     b. Injury of the tracheal wall
     c. Injury of the vagus nerve and posterior pulmonary plexus
     d. Injury of the recurrent laryngeal nerve
     e. Bleeding
   3. Transfusion and fluid
     a. Microembolism
     b. Overinfusion
C. Postoperative factors
   1. Pain
   2. Aspiration of foreign material
   3. Infection
     a. Anastomotic leakage and empyema
     b. Sepsis resulting from intravenous hyperalimentation
   4. Overinfusion

Preoperative factors

Pulmonary function tests

Opinions are divided as to whether preoperative pulmonary function test results correlate with the incidence of postoperative pulmonary complications.

Watanabe et al.[4] reported that patients with a 1-second volume per body surface area ($FEV_{1.0}/m^2$) below 1.4 L/m^2 are likely to have postop-

catheter and by postoperative ventilatory support. erative respiratory insufficiency, while Murakami[7] and Doki et al.[8] reported correlations with 1-second rate (%$FEV_{1.0}$) and 0.5-second rate (%$FEV_{0.5}$), respectively. On the other hand, there are reports[2,9] that preoperative pulmonary function test results, whether showing restrictive or obstructive ventilatory disturbance, had nothing to do with the incidence of postoperative pulmonary complications. In our department, we have looked into the correlation between preoperative percent of normal vital capacity (VC) and percent of first-second forced expiratory volume ($FEV_{1.0}$) and the incidence of pulmonary complications in 191 patients subjected to esophageal cancer resection–reconstructive surgery. We recognized no correlation at all (see Fig. 36-1).

Reasons for these differences among reporters would be, first, that ordinary pulmonary function tests do not faithfully reflect the condition of the peripheral respiratory tract; second, that the surgical procedures employed differed from reporter to reporter; and, third, that the diagnostic criteria for pulmonary complications are not always the same.

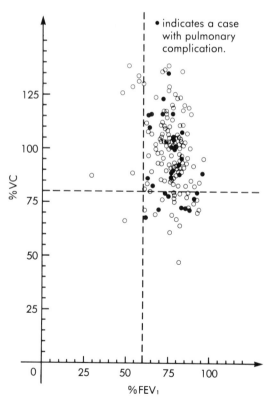

Fig. 36-1. Preoperative pulmonary function tests and pulmonary complications.

Predisposing factors

Postoperative pulmonary complications are said to increase with aging.[10] Elderly people often have diminished functional reserve capacities of heart, lungs, liver, and kidneys, and they not infrequently have complicating pulmonary diseases, such as emphysema and chronic bronchitis, or metabolic diseases, such as diabetes mellitus and hepatic functional deficiency. Especially in smokers, the incidence of pulmonary complications is high.[10,11] Moreover, a lowered nutritional state resulting from deficient oral intake depresses immunologic competence and weakens resistance to infection. Thus, many patients with esophageal cancer are thought to belong to a group at high risk for pulmonary complications.

Intraoperative factors

Endotracheal anesthesia and surgical procedures can both be important causes of postoperative pulmonary complications, especially with damage to the pulmonary rami of the vagus nerves resulting in increased secretion from the respiratory epithelium and difficulty in clearance by expectoration.

Postoperative factors

From the first postoperative day onward, patients tend to suffer from overhydration. This may actually begin during anesthesia. Also, infections can result in disseminated intravascular coagulopathy (DIC) or ARDS.

HYPOXEMIA AFTER THE OPERATION FOR ESOPHAGEAL CANCER

Patients with esophageal cancer who have undergone both thoracotomy and laparotomy suffer from more severe hypoxemia than those having been subjected to either of the two alone, with PaO_2 usually becoming lowest around the third postoperative day. Presently this hypoxemia following operation is often attributed to distribution imbalance in the ventilation-perfusion ratio resulting from microatelectasis and an increase in intrapulmonary shunts.[9,12]

In recent years, reports have been published on circulatory kinetics and lung water as unraveled by Swan-Ganz catheterization. In these reports, there is a tendency toward hypovolemia immediately after an operation for esophageal cancer but toward overhydration in and after 24 to 48 hours following operation.[3,13] With regard to the condition of wet lung after esophageal cancer operations, it is suggested that EVLW is increased early in the first postoperative day by the same mechanism as for permeability edema, but during the third or fourth postoperative day by the same mechanism as for high-pressure edema.[14]

As stated, after the operation for esophageal cancer obstruction of the peripheral respiratory tract results from retention of sputum, plus water retention in the pulmonary interstitium, which brings about a state more likely to form microatelectasis and consequent hypoxemia.

PROPHYLAXIS

On the basis of the condition of the patient with esophageal cancer before, during, and after the operation, we have put into practice a series of measures to prevent the pulmonary complications enumerated in Fig. 36-2.

Prior to operation, the patient is trained in breathing techniques and exercises. To improve any low nutritional state, infusion of high-calorie fluid is carried out. During and after the operation, care is taken to prevent aspiration.[11,15] From the latter half of the first postoperative day, an infusion is restricted and administration of a diuretic is started, to be continued to the third or fourth postoperative day. There is a report[5] recommending prophylactic artificial respiratory control during the operation and the first three postoperative days. We prefer endotracheal intubation only for pulmonary complications as measured by a PaO_2 less than 60 mm Hg or a $PaCO_2$ greater than 50 mm Hg ($FiO_2 = 0.4$). Then tracheostomy may be performed and, if still needed, mechanical ventilation (volumetric, with positive end-expiratory pressure [PEEP]) added. As an index of infused volumes, measurement of central venous pressure is utilized, but for exact examination of circulatory kinetics, monitoring is carried out with the insertion of the Swan-Ganz catheter. For control of postoperative pain, epidural analgesia is effective.

TREATMENT

The treatment of pulmonary complications after esophagectomy does not differ from treatment after operations for other diseases in the epigastric region.[5,11] Whatever the pulmonary complications, respiratory insufficiency must be treated with endotracheal intubation, and if necessary with mechanical ventilation via tracheostomy.

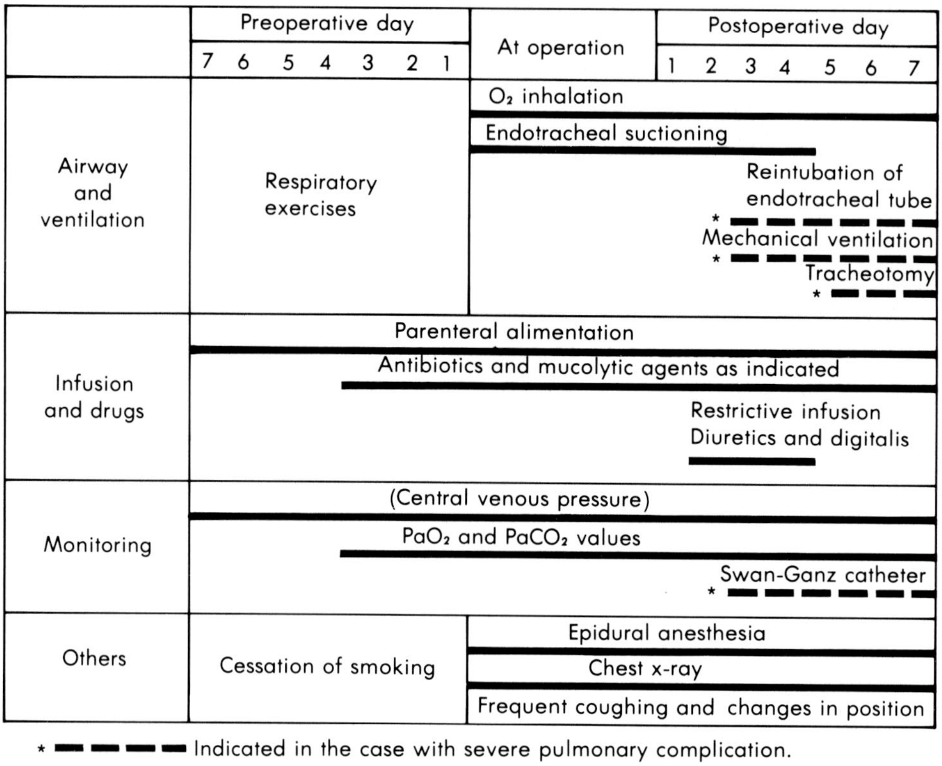

	Preoperative day							At operation	Postoperative day						
	7	6	5	4	3	2	1		1	2	3	4	5	6	7
Airway and ventilation	Respiratory exercises							O₂ inhalation							
								Endotracheal suctioning							
											Reintubation of endotracheal tube				
											* ▬ ▬ ▬ Mechanical ventilation				
											* ▬ ▬ ▬ Tracheotomy				
													* ▬ ▬ ▬		
Infusion and drugs		Parenteral alimentation													
		Antibiotics and mucolytic agents as indicated													
											Restrictive infusion Diuretics and digitalis				
Monitoring		(Central venous pressure)													
		PaO₂ and PaCO₂ values													
												Swan-Ganz catheter			
												* ▬ ▬ ▬ ▬ ▬		
Others	Cessation of smoking							Epidural anesthesia							
								Chest x-ray							
								Frequent coughing and changes in position							

* ▬ ▬ ▬ ▬ Indicated in the case with severe pulmonary complication.

Fig. 36-2. Diagram of the prophylactic measures and treatment of pulmonary complications.

Listed below are the essentials in the treatment of major pulmonary complications:

1. Atelectasis: frequent coughing, changes in position, and removal of intratracheal secretions by catheter suctioning via fibreoptic bronchoscopy
2. Pneumonia: administration of carefully selected antibiotics (especially effective against gram-negative bacilli) and improvement of nutrition
3. Pulmonary edema: administration of diuretics and cardiotonics, restriction of venous infusion, and monitoring of circulatory status with a Swan-Ganz catheter
4. ARDS: treatment of the causes that have triggered the onset of disseminated intravascular coagulopathy (DIC) and/or specific infection

culation are now better understood, and treatment progressing, thanks to the introduction of the Swan-Ganz catheter. There is still a group of conditions, such as ARDS, that have not been thoroughly elucidated.

In the future, defined diagnostic standards should be established for pulmonary complications, incidences of complications should be compared among various surgical procedures, and the requisite conditions should be set up for prophylactic artificial respiratory control when necessary. Further advances in the prophylaxis and treatment of pulmonary complications are desirable, because pulmonary complications are still the foremost cause of postoperative morbidity and mortality.

CONCLUSION

The types, prophylaxis, and treatment of pulmonary complications after operations for esophageal cancer have been outlined. With regard to hypoxemia and pulmonary complications specifically, the timing of postoperative overhydration has become clear. The details of pulmonary cir-

REFERENCES

1. Abo, S., and Kudo, T.: Esophagectomy combined with irradiation for carcinoma of the thoracic esophagus, Excerpta Medica, 1986. (In press.)
2. Nakayama, K., and Kakegawa, T.: Latest management of pulmonary complications following esophageal cancer surgery in Japan, Int. Adv. Surg. Oncol. **4**:111, 1981.
3. Tsuboi, M.: Studies on the postoperative pulmonary complications of the esophageal cancer, J. Jpn. Surg. Soc. **78**:223, 1977.

4. Watanabe, T., Kakei, M., et al.: Pulmonary complications after the operation in upper and mid-thoracic esophagus, J. Jpn. Surg. Soc. **74:**1136, 1973.

5. Mori, S., Murakami, K., et al.: Management of pulmonary complications following esophageal cancer surgery, Rinsho Kyobu Geka **2:**682, 1982.

6. Postlethwait, R.W.: Complications and deaths after operations for esophageal carcinoma, J. Thorac. Cardiovasc. Surg. **85:**827, 1983.

7. Murakami, T.: Studies on postoperative complications after surgery for esophageal cancer, Arch. Jpn. Chir. **47:**413, 1978.

8. Doki, K., Sannohe, Y., et al.: Studies on relation between the preoperative examination for the pulmonary function and the postoperative respiratory complications after surgical treatment of patients with esophageal cancer, J. Jpn. Assoc. Thorac. Surg. **28:**1525, 1980.

9. Sasaki, K.: A clinical study of pathophysiological mechanisms of postoperative prolonged hypoxemia resulting from the esophageal cancer surgery, J. Jpn. Assoc. Thorac. Surg. **26:**819, 1978.

10. Wightman, J.A.K.: A prospective survey of the incidence of postoperative pulmonary complications, Br. J. Surg. **55:**85, 1968.

11. Webb, W.R.: Postoperative pulmonary complications. In Artz, C.P., and Hardy, J.O., editors: Management of surgical complications, ed. 3, Philadelphia, 1975, W.B. Saunders Co., pp. 93-107.

12. Ando, N.: Studies on postoperative cardiopulmonary hemodynamics in patients with esophageal cancer as evaluated from various reconstructive procedures, J. Jpn. Surg. Soc. **79:**1426, 1978.

13. Motoki, R., Watanabe, K., et al.: Monitoring with Swan-Ganz catheter in the postoperative management of esophageal cancer, J. Jpn. Assoc. Thorac. Surg. **23:**717, 1975.

14. Ando, N., Obtaka, H., et al.: Studies on pre- and postoperative extravascular lung water changes in patients with esophageal cancer, J. Jpn. Surg. Soc. **84:**310, 1983.

15. Ong, G.B., La, K.H., et al.: Resection for carcinoma of the superior mediastinal segment of the esophagus, World J. Surg. **2:**497, 1978.

Pulmonary complications

DISCUSSION

Frigyes Kulka and István Pénzes

The causes of pulmonary complications following operations for cancer of the esophagus are complex, and yet most are not particularly related to the basic disease. In actual fact, it is only aspiration of ingested contents of the esophagus, occurring similarly in achalasia and diverticula, and eventual esophagotracheal or esophagobronchial fistula or a tumor compressing the trachea, that are specific complications of cancer of the esophagus.

In almost every case of cancer of the esophagus we find the following characteristic features: advanced age, moderate to great loss of body weight, difficulty at anesthesia because of chronic dehydration, and surgery requiring several hours, with two, and not uncommonly three, areas of the body explored.

Most of the pulmonary complications develop as a result of thoracotomy or thoracolaparotomy, or from concomitant disease and predisposing factors. These are hazards also in other fields of surgery. Elman et al.[1] have reported that among 790 patients undergoing surgery, 369 (47%) were documented to have pulmonary complications. A past history of chronic bronchitis, preoperative radiotherapy, tracheobronchial invasion, or severe hypoxemia during anesthesia was associated significantly with higher pulmonary complication rates. With patients at greater medical risk and with extended operations, the rate of pulmonary complications increases.

Among the preoperative risk factors, we attribute great significance to latent ventilatory and respiratory insufficiency, which must be recognized in time. Even in the absence of such latent disturbance, we make it compulsory for surgical candidates to undergo training in proper breathing and effective coughing. In the presence of manifest chronic obstructive pulmonary disease (COPD) every patient is taught breathing with the pressure-guided mask respirator. On the basis of favorable experience gained in large numbers of COPD patients subjected to thoracic surgery, we

emphasize that, by means of intermittent mask ventilator treatment, a considerable percentage of patients may be helped in overcoming the difficulties of the critical postoperative period. In a significant proportion of cases progression to respiratory failure can be prevented and ventilator support can be avoided. Drugs administered by nebulizer, patient concentration on the work of breathing, expiration against the highest resistance possible, and stimulation to cough and open small bronchi and alveoli all have a favorable effect. These favorable changes have been confirmed by blood gas analysis and by hemodynamic measurements.

Principal intraoperative risk factors include (1) inadequately chosen method of respiration (2) hypotension and hypoperfusion.

Many authors blame the intraoperative respiratory ventilation for many of the postoperative pulmonary complications. Efforts are concentrated on finding ways to avoid them. So, for example, unilateral endobronchial respiration is recommended to diminish aspiration, although in our opinion it merely makes the work of the surgeon easier but does not reduce the risk of aspiration. On the other hand, it increases the right-left shunt ratio and thus is a factor contributing to hypoxemia.

Ando et al.[2] and others continue mechanical respiratory support for 3 to 4 days after operation. Siewert et al.[3] prefer two-stage operation to the one-stage and have found that cardiopulmonary complications diminish. After the esophagectomy (first stage) the patient is maintained on mechanical respiratory support for 24 to 48 hours and then the reconstruction (second stage) follows.

We advocate the simplest endotracheal anesthesia and try to extubate the patient after the operation. Emphasis is placed upon postoperative physiotherapy and effective alleviation of pain. Only those patients in whom the thoracic cavity has been opened bilaterally stay on the respirator, and then only for a few hours.

Even after adequate preparation it is not uncommon that hypotension develops in the early stage of anesthesia, that it can be overcome only by considerable volume replacement, and that normotension can be maintained only in this way. We consider the fear of "overfilling" to be exaggerated. In the course of regular monitoring of the perioperative period by means of the Swan-Ganz catheter, we have found that the filling pressures of the right and left sides of the heart tend to be low rather than representing a hazard of overfilling.[4]

Even elderly patients with severe cardiorespiratory disease can be rendered "fit for operation" by means of adequate preoperative preparatory measures. On the other hand, during the perioperative phase stable circulation can be maintained only when fluids are given in "volumes required," because these patients characteristically develop hypovolemia. It seems advantageous and therefore desirable, not only from the surgical point of view, to provide sufficient fluid intake also during the postoperative period. In this way the possibility of postoperative thromboembolism and myocardial reinfarction can be reduced. It is a major advantage that bronchial secretions stay liquid and that the patients can expectorate easily when hydration is adequate. This is one of the most important factors in avoiding respiratory complications.

Hypovolemia may give rise to the low cardiac output syndrome, which, resulting in poor perfusion, may lead to anastomosis failure and ARDS. This ARDS is believed—erroneously, we think—to be "overfilling pulmonary edema." We believe that eventual "overfilling," and thus pulmonary edema, may be avoided if hypoxia is avoided. Hypoxia leads to an increase in capillary permeability. In addition to the administration of crystalloids, care is taken also to maintain normal oncotic pressure—for instance, by the administration of dextran.

The bulk of the postoperative risk factors can be traced to pathophysiologic events in conjunction with thoracolaparotomy: (1) decrease of the total (lung and chest wall) compliance; (2) decreases in VC and FEV_2, FRC, and V_T; (3) increase in oxygen utilization by the respiratory muscles; (4) increase of the V_D/V_T ratio; (5) postoperative hypoxemia; (6) inhibition of mucociliary clearance; and (7) abolition of the deep sigh reflex.

Further factors in pulmonary complications include silent aspiration, changes in cough mechanics, and pulmonary hypertension related to hypoxia, infection, or thromboembolism.

A cardiorespiratory state is seldom a contraindication to surgery. At the most, we take it into account when selecting the type of surgery to be performed. We do a transhiatal operation without thoracotomy when (1) FEV_1 is 600 to 800 ml, (2) VC is less than Sollwert 40%, (3) maximum breathing capacity (MBC) is less than 25 L, or (4) PaO_2 is less than 55 mm Hg and $PaCO_2$ is greater than 55 mm Hg.

In the postoperative period following thoracotomy, epidural administration of opiates relieves pain more effectively and advantageously than systemic administration.

The outcome of any respiratory complication is decisively influenced by any surgical complication. When leakage after an intrathoracic anastomosis occurs, recovery may be expected only when the mediastinitis can be relieved. In our opinion, reoperation is justified even when the patient is receiving ventilatory assistance.

We think the role of the vagus nerve in the etiology of the postoperative pulmonary complications is overemphasized. Operations are known in which spastic bronchitis, or "asthma," has improved after the vagus nerve and the pulmonary plexus have been sectioned. We claim, on the basis of evidence derived from more than 10,000 lung operations, that the eventual postoperative pulmonary complications were not related to transection of the vagus nerve. On the other hand, interference with the recurrent nerve may be the cause of severe respiratory complications resulting from swallowing dysfunction, aspiration, and difficulties in expectoration.

REFERENCES

1. Elman, A., Giuli, R., and Sancho-Garnier, H.: Risk factors of pulmonary complications following esophagectomy in carcinoma of the esophagus, Int. Eso. Week Abstracts **54**:46.
2. Ando, H., Shinozawa, Y., and Abe, O.: Necessity of postoperative artificial respiration in esophageal surgery, Int. Eso. Week Abstracts **52**:45.
3. Stewert, R., Adolf, J., and Bartels, H.: Cardiopulmonary function following transthoracic or transmediastinal esophagectomy, Int. Eso. Week Abstracts **56**:47.
4. Pénzes, I., et al.: The role of haemodynamic monitoring in the perioperative period, Anaesth. Intenziv Th. **14**:209, 1984.

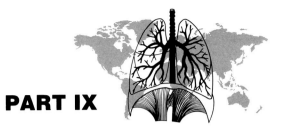

PART IX

THE ROLE OF OTHER THERAPEUTIC MODALITIES IN THE MANAGEMENT OF RESECTABLE DISEASE

Wei-bo Yin and Xian-Zhi Gu

Carcinoma of the esophagus remains a deadly disease for the majority of patients, despite improvement in the technique of surgery and radiotherapy. Surgery is the treatment of choice in the lower third, radiotherapy is preferred in the upper third, and a combination of preoperative irradiation and surgery may be the best for the middle third. Among 9571 patients admitted for treatment from 1958 to 1983 in the Cancer Institute, Chinese Academy of Medical Sciences, Beijing, only 1158 (12.1%) were treated by surgery alone; 741 (7.7%) were treated by preoperative irradiation plus surgery, 7462 (78.0%) by irradiation, and 210 (2.2%) by chemotherapy and/or other palliative measures. Surgery and radiotherapy are the two chief proved methods for the treatment of carcinoma of the esophagus.

PRINCIPLES

Radiotherapy is a local treatment. Its fundamental principle is to eradicate the cancer without undue damage to surrounding normal tissues. The primary objective is not only to keep the patient alive and tumor-free but also to restore his ability to work. At the very least, he should be able to take care of himself in his everyday life.

Carcinoma of the esophagus is usually of the squamous cell type with moderate radiosensitivity. When it is limited to the esophagus, the patient is a good candidate for permanent cure. But when the lesion extends beyond the muscular layer, extraesophageal extension is likely to occur. In the cervical region, invasion of the larynx, trachea, thyroid, or recurrent laryngeal nerve is possible. In the mediastinum, the tumor may invade the tracheobronchial tree, pleura, pericardium, recurrent laryngeal or phrenic nerves, or the large mediastinal blood vessels. Lymph node metastases are found in approximately 70% of patients subjected to postmortem examination.[1] The incidence is highest in patients with extensive or anaplastic tumors. Information regarding the distribution of lymph node metastases is important in the treatment planning. In general, a tumor of the upper-third segment metastasizes first to the paratracheal or carinal nodes, but the supraclavicular or lower jugular nodes may well be involved. Lesions of the lower two thirds tend to metastasize to lymph nodes in the mediastinum or epigastrium. Thirty percent of patients with squamous cell carcinoma of the esophagus have distant blood-borne metastasis at some time in the evolution of the disease. For these patients, only palliation can be achieved.

With no detectable metastasis and the lesion still limited to the mediastinum or the supraclavicular area, palliative treatment should be given to relieve symptoms and prolong life. Occasionally, long-term survival is obtained.[2]

The esophagus is surrounded by a number of organs including the spinal cord, trachea, and lung, of which the spinal cord is most vulnerable to radiation; it generally does not tolerate any dose beyond 40 Gy over 5 to 6 weeks. Higher doses are likely to cause radiation myelitis and hence paraplegia. The volume of pulmonary tissue irradiated should be strictly limited to prevent acute radiation pneumonitis and severe pulmonary fibrosis. In properly designed and performed radiotherapy with a curative dose, the trachea and spinal cord are usually spared as much as possible to avoid serious sequelae. To guard against complications, it is advisable to employ computed tomography (CT) and a computed treatment planning system (CTPS) in designing the therapy and a simulator in checking the design.

SELECTION OF PATIENTS

Indications. Patients with fair or good general condition, no supraclavicular lymph node metastases, lesions less than 7 cm in length, no serious obstruction, no severe chest or back pain, and no impending perforation are suitable for curative radiotherapy. Zhang et al.[3] reported the results in 130 patients for whom surgery was originally indicated but who, for medical or other reasons, were not operated upon but received radiotherapy instead. The 5-year survival rate of this series was 19%, which is encouraging. Although there has been no controlled trial of surgery against radiotherapy for "operable" cancers, such a trial would be both ethical and informative.

Radiotherapy is a definitive treatment, with milder reactions, lower risk, and less burden to the patient, as compared with surgery for carcinoma of the esophagus.

Palliative treatment. Supraclavicular lymph node metastasis can be palliated by radiotherapy and sometimes cure may be obtained.

Contraindications. Cachexia, signs of impending perforation, actual perforation, invasion of the trachea proved by bronchoscopy, stenosing lesions with severe obstruction, distant metastases, severe chest or back pain, and mediastinitis are contraindications.

TREATMENT

Preparation of patient. The patient should have some understanding about his illness, the goals of radiotherapy, possible reactions, and the management of these reactions. This prepares the patient for any possible discomfort and helps ensure completion of the treatment.

It is important to improve the general condition of the patient and to treat concomitant complications, maintain good oral hygiene, and provide high-protein, high-vitamin, and high-caloric diet.

External irradiation. Localization technique is as follows: Frontal and lateral barium esophag-

ograms are taken with the patient in the treatment position. A radiopaque ruler is placed on the skin surface for magnification correction. A surface contour is made at the level of the tumor center. Two sets of contours, one near the superior and the other near the inferior margin of the field are also prepared. The esophagus and spinal cord are marked on each contour chart for treatment planning, after which verification films are taken on a simulator.

Two to four fields are usually used, according to the treatment planning. 4-10 MV x-ray or telecobalt therapy is used for patients with carcinoma of the esophagus. To our knowledge, 8 or 10 MV x-ray is not superior to telecobalt in terms of survival rates.[4] Sometimes high-energy electron beam is useful if available, but it is by no means better than telecobalt[5] or 4-10 MV x-ray.

Intracavitary radiotherapy. Intracavitary radiotherapy for cancer of the esophagus has largely fallen into disuse since the introduction of supravoltage radiation. Yet in remote rural districts where access to external irradiation is difficult, it may still be valuable. The experience with 203 esophageal carcinoma patients treated by intracavitary radiation in Yaocun commune, Linxian county of Henan province, showed 88% marked improvement, and 8.4% (17 of 203) survived for over 5 years. Approximately half of the early cases with limited and superficial lesions were cured.[6]

RESULTS

Most of the results reported in China are from patients with advanced lesions. The survi-

TABLE 37-1. Results of radiotherapy for carcinoma of the esophagus in China

Institution and year	Radiation source	No. of patients treated	Five-year survival rate (%)
Field station, Linxian county, 1981 (unpublished data)	⁶⁰Co	79*	61 (83)†
Cancer Institute,[2] 1980	⁶⁰Co	3798	8.4
Loyang Third Hospital,[10] 1980	X-ray	266	12
Anyang Prefecture Hospital,[11] 1978	⁶⁰Co	3033	10
Shanghai Cancer Hospital,[12] 1978	⁶⁰Co	1034	16.8
Jiangsu Provincial Cancer Hospital,[13] 1978	⁶⁰Co	331	13.3
Xi'an Central Hospital,[14] 1975	⁶⁰Co	426	9.1
Linxian County Hospital,[15] 1981	⁶⁰Co, x-ray	1081	16.4
Xi'an Medical College,[16] 1974	⁶⁰Co	2310	9.3
Hobei Medical College,[17] 1981	⁶⁰Co	1245	8.3
Field station, Linxian county,[6] 1982	Intracavitary ⁶⁰Co	203	8.4

*Early lesion, less than 3 cm, superficial.

†Early lesion, inconspicuous on x-ray film.

TABLE 37-2. Prognostic factors in radiotherapy for esophageal carcinoma

	Five-year survival		
	No. of patients	Percent	p
Source			
Telecobalt	230/2613	8.8	
High-energy electron	49/642	7.6	>0.05
8-MV x-ray	17/171	9.9	
Age (yr)			
Under 39	18/203	8.9	
40-49	71/666	10.7	
50-59	123/1280	9.6	<0.01
60-69	63/1000	6.3	
Over 70	9/190	3.2	
Length of lesion (cm)			
5 or less	63/411	15.3	
5.1-7	108/1167	9.3	<0.005
7.1-9	80/1177	6.8	
9 or more	30/584	5.2	
Location of tumor			
Cervical	35/193	18.1	
Upper thoracic	86/727	11.8	
Midthoracic	149/2094	7.1	<0.001
Lower thoracic	11/325	3.4	
Obstruction			
Marked	37/627	5.9	
Moderate	168/1991	8.4	<0.001
Mild	65/600	10.8	
Clinical type			
Medullary	246/2960	8.3	<0.01
Fungating	29/387	14.4	
"Benevolent"	161/1615	10.0	<0.0001
"Malicious"	29/387	7.5	
Supraclavicular lymph node metastasis			
Positive	14/446	3.8	<0.01
Negative	262/2893	9.2	
X-ray appearance of tumor at end of radiotherapy			
Disappeared	72/402	19.7	
Almost disappeared	76/755	10.0	<0.01
Obvious residual tumor	126/1732	7.3	
No improvement, or progression	4/335	1.2	
Nominal standard dose (ret)			
Under 1600	11/343	3.2	
1600-1699	16/209	7.7	
1700-1799	30/387	7.8	
1800-1899	55/781	7.0	
1900-1999	75/795	9.4	
2000-2099	35/417	8.4	
Over 2100	29/407	7.1	
No. of fields			
3	32/244	13.1	
6	156/1815	8.6	

val data accumulated and listed in Table 37-1 are higher than those of Earlam and Cunha-Melo,[7] who reviewed 25 years' literature of 8489 cases before 1980, finding a 5-year survival rate of 6%.

Early carcinoma of the esophagus (i.e., car-cinoma in situ) was treated in the high-risk geographic areas. Fifty-two cases treated with telecobalt therapy gave 1-year, 3-year, 5-year, and 8-year survival rates of 100% (52 of 52), 88% (46 of 51), 73% (28 of 38) and 57% (17 of 30) respectively.[8] But according to Miao et al.,[6] for patients with these early carcinomas, the natural untreated 5-year survival rate was 78.3%.[9] The follow-up period for these patients should be longer, preferably up to 10 years.

PROGNOSTIC FACTORS

Many factors were found to affect the outcome of radiotherapy for carcinoma of esophagus. The most important ones are stage (length of lesion), clinical type, location of the primary lesion, age of the patient, and the amount of radiation, as shown in Table 37-2.

Stage (length of the lesion). The fact that the 5-year survival rate for early cancer was 73% demonstrates that length of the primary lesion affects survival.

Clinical type. In the clinicopathologic classification of esophageal carcinoma, there is a preponderance of medullary and fungating types of lesions, which lead to different survival rates after radiotherapy. Among patients with the type most commonly seen—medullary type—the prognosis is much better in the "benevolent" subtype (contour straight and rather smooth on esophagography) than in the "malicious" subtype (contour tortuous, indicating infiltration or adherence of carcinoma to surrounding tissues).

Location. Experience has shown that the higher the location of the lesion, the better the result of radiotherapy. Table 37-2 shows the validity of the results of patients with lesions between 5 and 7.9 cm in length, without supraclavicular lymph node metastasis, with no vocal paralysis, and nominal standard dose (NSD) between 1800 and 1999 ret. There is an obvious worsening in prognosis in radiotherapy from the upper toward the lower end of the esophagus.

Age. The treatment results are better in the 40 to 59 age group, poor for the patients over 60, and least favorable when the patients are over 70.

Technique. It is observed from Table 37-2 that choice of source of treatment is not very important. The response shown by barium meal is predetermined by the clinical type, stage, and location of the tumor. According to our analysis, if the tumor showed no change by barium meal at 40 Gy, it will not disappear even if the dose were increased to more than 70 Gy. It was also observed that the three-field technique is superior to the four- to six-field techniques, which conform to the experience of the Shanghai Cancer Hospital. This is probably due to the fact that in the four- to six-field irradiation, beam directioning, without being checked by a simulator, was not accurate. As to the optimum total dose, although our data do not show any difference in the range

of 50 to 80 Gy, the results are better at 60 Gy in 30 fractions over 6 weeks, as determined from the analysis of 1136 patients surviving over 5 years after radiotherapy[18] and also as reported by colleagues at Xi'an Medical College.[19]

X-ray appearance at the end of radiotherapy. The appearance of esophageal carcinoma shown by barium meal at the end of radiotherapy is important. The prognosis is always better in patients with complete disappearance of filling defect than in those with residual tumor or no change in the lesion.

CAUSES OF FAILURE

Local uncontrolled disease (residual tumor at conclusion of therapy as shown by x-ray) and recurrence after radiotherapy are the main causes of failure. Among 1334 patients in whom the causes of death were known, local uncontrolled disease, local recurrence, perforation, and massive hemorrhage constituted 85%. Distant metastasis, including supraclavicular lymph node involvement, accounted for only 10% of the deaths (see Table 37-3).

Yu et al.,[20] of the Cancer Institute, Chinese Academy of Medical Sciences, reviewed the results of a second course of radiotherapy for recurrent carcinoma of the esophagus after definitive radiation therapy. In all these patients, the lesion had either completely or almost completely disappeared. There were 81 patients who received a second course of treatment, and 137 patients received no treatment at all. The mean survival for the retreated group was 6.59 ± 4.66 months, and 4.51 ± 4.40 months for the untreated group.

COMPLICATIONS

Complications of radiotherapy for esophageal carcinoma include radiation myelitis with paraplegia, esophagitis, radiation pneumonitis, and mediastinal fibrosis. Radiation myelitis commonly occurs several years after treatment in patients whose spinal cord received more than 40 Gy in 30 to 35 fractions over 6 to 7 weeks. It is incurable. Hence, extensive irradiation of the spinal cord must always be avoided. The chief symptom of esophagitis is severe local pain, sometimes so distressing that the patient refrains from taking any food. Management includes temporary suspension of radiation, antibiotics, corticosteroids, and maintenance of parenteral nutrition. Esophagitis usually occurs after the dose has reached 40 Gy or after the end of treatment. It varies

TABLE 37-3. Failure and complications of radiotherapy for esophageal carcinoma

	No. of patients	Percent
Locally uncontrolled	641	48.0
Local recurrence	491	36.6
Perforation	43	3.2
Fatal hemorrhage	11	0.8
Postirradiation supraclavicular metastasis	75	5.6
Distant metastasis	60	4.5
Postirradiation second esophageal primary	6	0.5
Radiation myelitis	5	0.4
Others	2	0.2
TOTAL	1334	100.00

greatly in severity and its occurrence is difficult to predict. Radiation pneumonitis is not a risk when the three-field technique is used and each is no wider than 6 cm, but is likely to occur in ^{60}Co rotational therapy or in multiple-field techniques (18 or more fields) with orthovoltage radiation. Supravoltage irradiation causes mild mediastinal fibrosis, which appears as haziness in the mediastinal x-ray silhouette without giving rise to specific symptoms.

REFERENCES

1. Bloedorn, F.G., and Kasdorf, H.: Radiotherapy in squamous cell carcinoma of esophagus. In Clark, R.L., Cumley, R.W., Mcay, J.E., and Copeland, M.M., editors: Oncology 1970: proceedings of the Tenth International Congress, vol. 4, Chicago, 1971, Year Book Medical Publishers, pp. 111-120.

2. Yin, W.B., Zhang, L.J., Yan, Z.Y., Miao, Y.J., Yu, Z.H., Zhang, Z.X., Zhang, C.H., Wang, M., Li, G.H., Fan, L.Z., Zhang, L.N., Liu, Y.Y., Jiao, Y.Q., and Gu, X.Z.: Radiation therapy of cancer of esophagus: analysis of 3798 patients, Chin. J. Oncol. **2**:216, 1980. (In Chinese.)

3. Zhang, Z.F., Zhang, D.W., and Yang Z.Y.: Radiotherapy of carcinoma of esophagus. Tanjing Med. J. Oncol. [Suppl.] **2**:288, 1964. (In Chinese.)

4. Yin, W.B., Zhang, H.X., Zhang, L.J., Miao, Y.J., Zhang, Z.X., Wang, M., Gu, X.Z., Cao, D.X., Jia, C.Y., and Pu, L.N.: Use of simulator and 8 MV x-ray in the treatment of carcinoma of esophagus, Fourth National Congress of Radiology. (In Chinese.)

5. Yin, W.B., Zhang, L.J., Miao, Y.J., Yu, Z.H., Zhang, Z.X., Zhang, C.H., Wang, M., Li, G.H., Liu, Y.G., Jia, Y.W., and Gu, X.Z.: The results of high energy electron therapy in carcinoma of esophagus compared with telecobalt therapy, Clin. Radiol. **34**:113, 1983. (In Chinese.)

6. Miao, Y.J., Gu, X.Z., Hu, Y.M., Zhang, G.F., Gu, D.Z., Zhang, G.H., Yang, D.Y., Yui, W.M., and Zhang, C.L.: The intracavitary radiation of esophageal cancer, Chin. J. Oncol. **4**:45, 1982. (In Chinese.)

7. Earlam, R., and Cunha-Melo, J.R.: Oesophageal squamous cell carcinoma II. A critical review of radiotherapy, Br. J. Surg. **67**:457, 1980.

8. Xing, B.J., Fu, B.C., Qing, M.X., and Wu, J.J.: Radiotherapy of early carcinoma of esophagus, Fourth National Congress of Radiology. (In Chinese.)

9. Miao, Y.J., Li, G.Y., Gu, X.Z., and Chen, W.H.: Detection and natural progression of early oesophageal carcinoma: preliminary communication, J. R. Soc. Med. **74**:884, 1981.

10. Li, D.J., Yui, J.L., and Liu, X.P.: Orthovoltage x-ray therapy for esophageal carcinoma: report on 266 cases, Chin. J. Roentgenol. **4**:128, 1980. (In Chinese.)

11. Section of Radiotherapy Oncology, Shanghai Cancer Hospital: ^{60}Co teletherapy for esophageal cancer: analysis of 3033 cases, Henan Med. **4**:33, 1978. (In Chinese.)

12. Department of Radiation Oncology, Shanghai Cancer Hospital: Radiotherapy of esophageal carcinoma: report on 1034 cases, Cancer Res. Prev. Treat. **4**:46, 1978. (In Chinese.)

13. Jiangsu Cancer Prevention and Treatment Institute: Concentric oblique portal irradiation for cancer of esophagus, Chin. J. Roentgenol. **12**:105, 1978. (In Chinese.)

14. Section of Radiotherapy, Central Hospital, Xi'an City: ^{60}Co teletherapy for carcinoma esophageal: analysis of 426 cases, Cancer Res. Prev. Treat. **1**:28, 1975. (In Chinese.)

15. Department on Oncology, Xi'an Medical College Hospital: Radiotherapy for cancer of the esophagus: analysis of 2310 cases, Cancer Res. Prev. Treat. **3**:83, 1974. (In Chinese.)

16. Hou, F.X., Xui, Y.J., Ping, S.J., and Sha, Y.H.: Radiotherapy of cancer of esophagus in Linxian county: report on 1081 cases. In Symposium on radiology in Henan, 1981, pp. 84-88. (In Chinese.)

17. Wan, J, Zhang, D.A., Guo, B.Z., and Feng, S.Y.: ^{60}Co teletherapy for esophageal carcinoma: analysis of 1245 cases. In Monograph of Third National Symposium on Radiology, Beijing, 1981, p. 236. (In Chinese.)

18. The National Cooperative Group on Radiotherapy of Esophageal Cancer: Analysis of 1136 patients surviving for more than 5 years after radiation of cancer of the esophagus. In Monograph of Third National Symposium on Radiology, Beijing, 1981, p. 236. (In Chinese.)

19. Department of Oncology, Xi'an Medical College: Radiotherapy for cancer of esophagus: analysis of 2310 cases, Cancer Res. Prev. Treat. **3**:83, 1974. (In Chinese.)

20. Yu, Z.H., Miao, Y.J., Yin, W.B., and Gu, X.Z.: Retreatment of recurrent carcinoma of esophagus, Fourth National Congress of Radiology. (In Chinese.)

CHAPTER **38** Combined preoperative irradiation and surgery for esophageal carcinoma

Guo Jun Huang, Xian-Zhi Gu, Liang Jun Wang, Wei-Bo Yin, Ru Gang Zhang, Li Jun Zhang, Da Wei Zhang, Zhi Xian Zhang, Zheng Yan Wang, and Kan Yang

Results of treatment of carcinoma of the esophagus by either radiotherapy or surgery alone have not been wholly satisfactory. Reports on the combination of preoperative irradiation and surgery to improve treatment results for this malignancy have appeared more and more frequently during the past three decades. In 1960, Cliffton and associates[1] and Nakayama[2] reported independently the experiences with this combined treatment modality in 20 cases and 114 cases, respectively, with both coming to the conclusion that preoperative irradiation inhibited tumor growth and raised the resectability rate. Huang and associates[3] in 1962 reported 113 cases of esophageal carcinoma treated by this combined therapy, with a resectability rate of 70.8%, which was 12.4% higher than that of 161 cases treated at the same time period by surgery alone.

Subsequent reports by Akakura and associates in 1963,[4] Nakayama and Kinoshita in 1974,[5] Marks and associates in 1976,[6] Huang and associates in 1981,[7] and Parker and associates in 1982,[8] all indicated favorable results of this combined therapy in terms of resectability and long-term survivals as compared with the results of either radiotherapy or surgery alone.

The rationale for the combination of preoperative irradiation and surgery in the treatment of carcinoma of the esophagus is now widely, but not universally accepted. Its theoretic basis is as follows. Iatrogenic cancer cell dissemination at operation, with the possibility of metastasis and cancer implantation, is a recognized phenomenon. The cancer cells most easily disseminated during surgery are those in areas with a richer vascular supply, which are better oxygenated and more radiosensitive. Preoperative irradiation de-

vitalizes or sterilizes the cancer cells in these areas and thus reduces the risk of dissemination. The two common causes of surgical failure—namely, microscopic deposits of tumor cells not accessible to surgical resection and tumor invasion into adjacent vital organs—can be best controlled by preoperative irradiation. On the other hand, a bulky primary tumor usually contains large numbers of poorly oxygenated tumor cells, which are radioresistant and often the source of recurrence after radiotherapy. Surgery removes the primary tumor, not only eliminating the source of local recurrence but also rendering a high dose of preoperative irradiation unnecessary. It is therefore logical that by taking advantage of both preoperative irradiation and surgery in combination, better results can be achieved than by either modality alone.

This paper presents our experience with combined preoperative irradiation and surgery in two clinical studies, the first consisting of 408 selected patients treated from 1959 through 1976, preliminarily reported in 1981,[7] and the second of 83 of 160 randomized patients from 1977 through 1982. Patients who were primarily treated by radiotherapy but were later operated upon because of severe dysphagia, uncontrolled carcinoma, recurrences, and so on, were excluded from both studies.

STUDIES ON 408 SELECTED PATIENTS (1959-1976)[7]

The majority of patients selected for combined therapy in this study were those with carcinoma of the midthoracic esophagus and of poor or questionable resectability as evaluated on clinical grounds. As a result, there was a predominance of middle-third and stage III cases in this series.

During the same time period most patients with carcinoma more distally located, of more likely resectability as assessed clinically, were treated by surgery alone.

TNM staging

Postradiosurgical histopathologic staging of the 408 cases of the combined therapy group showed that 71.8% were stage III with extra-esophageal invasion and/or regional lymph node involvement and 9.8% stage IV with distant metastases. In only two cases, or 0.5%, was the carcinoma confined to only the mucosa and submucosa without lymph node involvement (stage I). In 73 (17.9%), the lesion involved the muscular layer but was confined to the esophagus with no evidence of lymph node metastasis (stage II). It is to be noted that preoperative irradiation may result in understaging at pathology the cases in which preexisting metastatic regional lymph nodes became cancer-free after irradiation.

Preoperative irradiation

In this study telecobalt was used in 310 (76.0%) and betatron in 69 (16.9%) cases. In the remaining 29 (7.1%) cases either a combination of the two sources or deep x-ray, occasionally in the early years, was used.

Most patients were irradiated 5 days a week with a tumor dose of 200 rad each day through anterior and posterior portals of 6 × 12 cm or 6 × 15 cm, depending on the tumor size. Table 38-1 shows the distribution of preoperative irradiation dosage in this study. In the later part of this study, the dosage was standardized to 4000 rad in each case.

The interval between completion of preoperative irradiation and surgery ranged from 2 to 3 weeks, averaging 17.4 days.

Surgical intervention

Resection of the esophageal carcinoma was usually done through the left thoracotomy approach, in the vast majority of cases using the stomach as a substitute. The overall resectability rate was 81.9% for the 408 cases (see Table 38-2). It can be seen that carcinoma of the middle third of the esophagus has the lowest resectability rate of all three segments, as is true with surgery of esophageal carcinoma without preoperative irradiation.

At operation the lungs and pleura were found to be little affected by preoperative irradiation. In some instances mild congestion and edema

TABLE 38-1. Distribution of preoperative irradiation dosage in 408 cases

Dosage (rad)	No. of cases	Percent
<2000	102	25.0
2100-3000	78	19.1
3100-4000	197	48.3
>4000	31	7.6
TOTAL	408	100.0

were seen over the irradiated mediastinal pleura. Usually there was some retraction and loss of luster of the mediastinal pleura overlying the tumor. Shrinkage of the tumor mass was noted in most cases. This was especially true in cases in which the postradiation esophagogram showed good radiation effects. Usually the tumor was smaller in size and softer in consistency, with ill-defined boundaries. In some cases the tumor had regressed so much that it was indeed difficult for the exploring fingers to locate exactly the lesion.

There were 15 deaths within 30 days of operation in the combined therapy group, an operative mortality of 3.4%. Thirteen of these deaths occurred in 334 resections, a resection mortality of 3.9%. In the 736 cases treated by surgery alone during the same time period, there were 22 (3.0%) operative deaths.

In the combined therapy group there were 15 postoperative anastomotic leaks among 334 resections, an incidence of 4.5%. The incidence of leakage of cervical anastomoses was 21% (5 of 24), and that of intrathoracic anastomoses was 3.2% (10 of 310).

There were 27 leaks among the 736 cases treated by surgery alone, an incidence of 3.7%.

It was estimated that in about one third of the cases treated by combined therapy, the site of esophageal anastomosis lay within the field of preoperative irradiation.

Pathologic studies

Changes in esophageal cancer brought about by preoperative irradiation were classified as mild, moderate, or marked. *Mild* reaction included those tumor specimens showing only minimal postradiation changes. The tumor showed no remarkable decrease in size, and its cells showed slight regression with keratinization and necrosis. *Moderate* reaction included those with appreciable decrease in tumor size. Microscopically, there was more marked regression of the tumor cells, which, however, were still distinguishable in discrete masses. *Marked* reaction included those in which the tumor mass had completely or nearly completely regressed. Mi-

TABLE 38-2. Resectability rates of 408 cases treated by combined therapy

Site of lesion	Operations	Resections	Resectability (%)
Upper third	27	26	96.3
Middle third	299	238	79.6
Lower third	82	70	85.4
ENTIRE GROUP	408	334	81.9

TABLE 38-3. Survival rates in 334 cases in the combined therapy group

Years after surgery	1	3	5	10	15
Resections	334	334	334	248	179
Survivors	260	135	113	57	32
Survival rate (%)	77.8	40.4	33.8	23.0	17.9

TABLE 38-4. Randomized study of combined preoperative irradiation and surgery versus surgery alone for carcinoma of the esophagus: analysis of 160 cases, 1977-1982

	Preoperative irradiation and surgery	Surgery alone
Resectability rate (%)	92.2 (79/83)	89.6 (69/77)
Thirty-day resection mortality (%)	3.8 (3/79)	4.3 (3/69)
Incidence of anastomotic leakage (%)		
Intrathoracic	0 (0/77)	1.7 (1/60)
Cervical	50 (1/2)	44 (4/9)
Incidence of lymph node metastasis (%)	21.5 (17/79)	30.4 (21/69)
Residual tumor at esophageal stump (%)	0 (0/79)	2.9 (2/69)
Five-year survival rate (%)	45.5 (10/22)	25.0 (4/16)

croscopic findings consisted of either total disappearance of tumor cells or only remnants of degenerated tumor tissue.

Of the 279 patients who had complete records, mild reaction was found in 87 (31.2%), moderate reaction in 90 (32.2%), and marked reaction in 102 (36.6%).

Pathologic studies of the resected specimens showed evidence of extraesophageal tumor invasion in 70.1% (230 of 328) and positive lymph node metastases in 34.3% (114 ot 332) of the cases.

Of the 736 patients treated by surgery alone, lymph node involvement was found in 321, or 43.6%.

Long-term survival rates

The 1- to 15-year survival rates in all 334 cases with tumor resection in the combined therapy group are shown in Table 38-3. The 5-year survival of 33.8% in this group was, however, not statistically different from that of 29.8% (205 of

689) of those treated during the same time period by surgery alone ($X^2 = 1.75$, $p > 0.05$).

It is to be noted that the criteria for case selection used in this study placed the group treated with combined therapy in an unfavorable prognostic situation as compared with the group treated by surgery alone. With this taken into consideration, the gratifying results obtained in the group treated by combined therapy may well be attributed to the merits of adjuvant preoperative irradiation.

STUDIES ON 160 RANDOMIZED PATIENTS (1977 to 1982)

To further verify the value of preoperative irradiation, a randomized study was started in 1977 for patients under 65 years of age with midthoracic esophageal carcinoma not exceeding 7 cm in roentgenographic length. In this study the linear accelerator was used for treatment almost exclusively, with a total dose of 4000 rad divided into 20 fractions over 4 weeks. Irradiation was given through anterior and posterior portals each 6 cm in width, covering the entire mediastinum from the upper border of the manubrium sterni to the xyphoid process.

This study included 160 patients eligible for analysis to the end of June, 1982. The combined therapy group consisted of 83 patients, 58 males and 25 females, with ages ranging from 28 to 65 and averaging 52.5 years. In the control group treated by surgery alone there were 77 patients, 53 males and 24 females, with ages ranging from 34 to 65, and averaging 52.4 years. The average lengths of tumors in both groups were the same, 5.2 cm.

The results, both early and late, as obtained by combined therapy versus those by surgery alone are shown in Table 38-4, which further illustrates the advantages of the former over the latter treatment modality.

The fact that the incidence of anastomotic leak in the combined therapy group is no higher than that in the group treated by surgery alone serves to indicate that preoperative irradiation at the recommended dosage has no untoward effects on esophageal healing, since in about half of the cases of the combined therapy group the esophageal anastomotic site was within the field of preoperative irradiation. The absence of residual tumor at the esophageal stump in the cases treated by combined therapy, as compared with the incidence of 2.9% in the control group, also indicates the tumoricidal effect of preoperative irradiation.

The lower incidence of lymph node metastasis in the combined therapy groups of both the selected patients and the randomized patients in the two clinical studies is best explained by sterilization of cancer cells and inhibition of new lymph node metastasis by the preoperative irradiation.

CONCLUSIONS

On the basis of our experiences with the two clinical studies, it may be concluded that the combination of preoperative irradiation and surgery in the treatment of carcinoma of the esophagus has advantages in promoting resectability and increasing long-term survival over surgery alone. With the recommended dosage and rest interval, preoperative irradiation has no untoward effect on healing of the irradiated esophagus, and poses no additional difficulty in surgical dissection. It is to be emphasized that this combined modality is especially indicated in more advanced cases of

midthoracic esophageal carcinoma with borderline resectability.

REFERENCES

1. Cliffton, E.E., Goodner, J.T., and Bronstein, E.: Preoperative irradiation for cancer of the esophagus, Cancer **13:**37, 1960.
2. Nakayama, K.: Combined surgical and radiation treatment for cancerous lesions with particular interest in prevention of recurrence (theoretical basis for the preoperative irradiation in the treatment of esophageal cancer). In Proceedings of the Japanese Cancer Association, 19th General Meeting, 1960, pp. 214-215.
3. Huang, G.J., Wong, J.Z., Liu, Y.Q., and Wu, H.: Preoperative irradiation for carcinoma of the esophagus: a report on the experiences of 113 cases, Shanghai, 1962, Shanghai Scientific and Technical Publishers, pp. 1-10.
4. Akakura, I., Nakamura, Y., and Kakegawa, T.: The combined treatment for carcinoma of the esophagus with radical resection and preoperative irradiation, Keio J. Med. **14:**145, 1963.
5. Nakayama, K., and Kinoshita, Y.: Surgical treatment combined with preoperative concentrated irradiation, JAMA **227:**178-181, 1974.
6. Marks, R.D., Jr., Scruggs, H.J., and Wallace, K.M.: Preoperative radiation therapy for carcinoma of the esophagus, Cancer **38:**84, 1976.
7. Huang, G.J., Gu, X.Z., Zhang, R.G., Zhang, L.J., Zhang, D.W., Miao, Y.J., Wang, L.J., Lin, H., Wang, G.Q., and Xiao, Q.L.: Combined preoperative irradiation and surgery in esophageal carcinoma: report of 408 cases, Chin. Med. J. **94:**733, 1981.
8. Parker, E.F., Gregorie, H.B., Prioleau, W.H., Jr., Marks, R.D., Jr., and Bartles, D.M.: Carcinoma of the esophagus: observation of 40 years, Ann. Surg. **195:**618, 1982.

CHAPTER 39 Excisional, radiational, and chemotherapeutic methods and results

Edward Frost Parker

The treatment of squamous cell carcinoma of the esophagus has involved dilatation, radiation, excision, or combinations thereof. More recently, chemotherapeutic and antibiotic regimens have entered the therapeutic arena, along with photo-kinetic (laser) beams applied endoscopically. When all else has failed or seemed impractical, endoesophageal prostheses have been implanted. All modalities have been used in varying sequences. No doubt, the manifold techniques have evolved because no single method has provided consistently good results. In fact, results have varied markedly in different countries[1] and in different parts of the same country.[2]

This further discussion will be limited to the squamous cell carcinoma, except for a rare primary adenocarcinoma. Adenocarcinoma arising in the cardia of the stomach and invading the terminal esophagus is considered a different disease. The fact that many aspects of its treatment involve many of the same principles is considered incidental.

The stage of the disease when first diagnosed is of paramount importance. When diagnosed in asymptomatic patients by microscopic examination of esophageal abrasive balloon brushings as practiced by the Chinese, it has been treated with great success by surgical excision alone.[3] We term such cases *localized* rather than early. "Early" is inaccurate because the temporal duration of the tumor is unknown, whereas "localized" implies absence of distant spread so that excision may be theoretically curative.

There is no comparable experience in the Western world. It is almost unknown to see an asymptomatic patient. Nearly all cases are advanced when first seen. Not only is there involvement of the muscular layer of the esophagus, but also there has been lymphatic spread, local and distant, in a high percentage of cases. There is great difficulty in assessing the extent of the tumor.

Complete assessment requires not only nonincisional procedures such as esophagoscopy and bronchoscopy, blood chemical analyses, standard x-ray films, computed tomography, and radioisotopic scans of bone and liver, but also such incisional procedures as celiotomy, mediastinotomy, and bilateral anterior scalene dissections to assess possible nodal or visceral involvement. In many cases, if not all, complete staging is impractical. It is understandable that there is no unanimity of opinion on optimal treatment.

Until the end of World War II, little was done in the way of therapy, except a feeding gastrostomy. Unfortunately, the ability to feed the patient did not alter the inexorable downhill course. Even the mortality from gastrostomy was high (17% to 25% in some series). Thereafter, we seldom used gastrostomy except as a temporary method of feeding in anticipation of reestablishment of the esophageal lumen by radiation, or following excision or bypass of the obstructing neoplasm.

The most frequently advocated methods of treatment in this country have been radiation and excision, or a combination of the two. Because of the differences in the ease of surgical access to the various levels, some have preferred to treat lesions in the upper half of the esophagus by radiation and those in the lower half by excision. However, it has been our opinion that there should be one best method of treatment applied to all, regardless of the level of the tumor. Until recently, we preferred the combination of preoperative radiation followed by excision if the patient was physiologically operable and the tumor technically resectable.

HISTORICAL EXPERIENCE

The rationale was based on observations[4] of 609 cases between 1940 and 1967. Seventy-six percent of the lesions were located in the upper

TABLE 39-1. Comparison of five series of patients with carcinoma of the esophagus, 1940-1975*

Reference	No. of patients	Operable disease	Resectable disease	Mortality	Two-year survivors
1940-1951[4]	170	56 (33)	30 (54)	17 (57)	1 (0.6)
1951-1957[4]	166	39 (23)	34 (87)	19 (56)	9 (5.4)
1957-1962[4]	135	30 (22)	21 (70)	3 (14)	11 (8.2)
1962-1967[8]	138	47 (34)	41 (87)	13 (32)	17 (12.3)
1967-1975[8]	300	116 (39)	90 (78)	18 (20)	23 (7.7)

*Numbers in parentheses are percentages. See text.

TABLE 39-2. Carcinoma of the esophagus: experience with treatments, 1980-1984*

Reference	Cases	Operable	Resectable	Mortality	Two-year survivors†
1980-1984[12]	129	55 (43)	39 (71)	5 (13)	11 (11)
Protocol group	89	43 (48)	31 (72)	3 (10)	8 (12.1)‡
Nonprotocol group	40	12 (30)	8 (67)	2 (25)	3 (9.4)§

*Numbers in parentheses are percentages.

† Among 98 patients seen between May, 1980, and October, 1982.

‡ One of the eight had megavoltage radiation therapy alone; chemotherapy and resection contraindicated.

§ One of the three had radiation alone.

and middle thoracic levels. The lower thoracic esophagus was involved in 15% and the cervical esophagus in only 7%. The majority of patients were in the sixth or seventh decades of life. Some degree of malnutrition was present in 87% when first seen. It is believed that the weight loss and weakness were not necessarily due to obstructive dysphagia or odynophagia alone. Approximately 40% had symptoms other than dysphagia as the presenting symptom. In many, weight loss antedated the onset of dysphagia. The tumors appeared to have a highly catabolic effect independent of, or in addition to, the malnutrition that follows the impaired ability to eat a normal diet. Most patients also manifested evidence of distant metastasis when first seen, or demonstrated serious complications of local extension, such as esophagobronchial or esophagotracheal fistula. In addition, many had associated diseases that affected operative risk adversely. In brief, the majority were poor operative risks.

1. *1940 to 1951.* In our initial study of 170 patients (Table 39-1),[4] our intent was surgical excision as the sole means of possible cure. Although there was good palliation among the survivors, the operative mortality was high and there was a single long-term survivor (15 years). Operability and resectability rates were low. Among the resectable cases, the resection was theoretically curative in fewer than half. Therefore, in spite of excellent palliation among survivors, we

abandoned this surgical approach because of its high mortality (57%). The malnutrition in most patients was considered to be the reason for poor results. We believed that this had to be corrected first in order to allow a reasonable chance of success with extensive operation requiring both celiotomy and thoracotomy and, in some cases, a cervical incision for anastomosis when excision extended to that level.

In Tables 39-1 and 39-2,[12] the operative cases are shown as a percentage of the entire series. The resectable cases are shown as a percentage of the operable. The mortality is shown as a percentage of the resectable. There were no deaths and no 2-year survivors in the 26 operable but nonresectable cases in the 1967 to 1975 series. The 2-year survivors are shown as a percentage of the patients in the entire series. If one wished to show the number of 2-year survivors as a percentage of the operable, or the resectable, or the survivors of resection, the figures could be made to look better. We think the method chosen is the most realistic.

2. *1951 to 1957.* It was logical that we turned next to radiation alone.[5] In this next series, radiation therapy was used in most, no matter how good an operative risk the patient appeared to be. The results were improved but still disappointing (see Table 39-1). Especially disappointing were the long-term results in 17 patients who appeared to be excellent operative risks with small localized tumors. The initial result was excellent, with res-

toration of the ability to swallow and reversal of the catabolic state. But 13 of these 17 patients died in approximately 12 months with local recurrence. Others had made similar observations. Many in this second series were inoperable, not because of the extent of tumor, but because of associated diseases or malnutrition alone. In these the results of theoretically curative irradiation were poor. On analysis of this series of 166 patients, it was clear that radiation as the sole potentially curative method had to be abandoned. However, in this second group there were two patients in whom esophagectomy was performed because of residual high-grade obstruction, with good long-term results. This led to the concept that the two methods might be combined. In other words, one could use radiation in all in whom it was tolerated, and thereafter resection while the patient was is an anabolic state with no evidence of residual radiation sickness. Others had observed that the combination of radiation and excision gave better results than either one alone.

3. *1957 to 1962.* In the third series, with preoperative radiation the operability and resectability rates were lower, reflecting the selection of better-risk patients. The mortality was 14%. The number of 2-year survivors increased again. The radiation therapy appeared to suppress tumor activity and decrease bulk. The ability to swallow was restored preoperatively in approximately 50% to 60% of the cases. Improvement in the nutritional state was clearly associated with decreased operative risk. At operation, the lesion at times could not be identified with certainty by inspection or palpation. In many, the operations were made easier because of residual edema in the tissue planes. However, in this third series, no matter how well the patient looked and felt, and no matter how normal the esophagogram might appear to be, microscopic examination of the surgical specimen showed residual carcinoma in 20 of 21 cases. The pathologic findings explained readily the high recurrence rate in cases treated by radiation alone and justified the addition of esophagectomy. Even though the disease was far advanced in many patients when first seen, it was clear that the possible merits of the combination should not be denied to those in whom it was applicable.

The radiation therapy[6] was megavoltage, 4500 rad in a period fo 3 to 4 weeks, delivered in 250-rad fractions. This dosage was chosen because it was known that spinal cord damage could result from a dosage of 5000 rad or more, and that 4500 rad was considered cancerocidal for microscopic disease. The indications for operation included a satisfactory nutritional state, improved strength and appetite, and stable or increasing weight. The

lesion should be less than 10 cm in length, with no evidence of invasion of the trachea or bronchi and no distant metastasis. The interval between completion of the radiation therapy and operation varied from 6 to 60 days. There was no established interval. There was no sense of urgency, and each case was considered individually. In a rare instance of esophagotracheal or esophagobronchial fistula, emergency operation for bypass and exclusion of the involved esophageal segment was performed.[7] The mortality in these cases was high, but in the survivors the palliation provided by averting a chronic suppurative bronchopneumonitis was most gratifying to the patient. The results of combined irradiation and resection are again seen in Table 39-1.

4. *1962 to 1967; 1967 to 1975.* After our experience with the 1957-1962 series of cases, in which the mortality was the lowest we had been able to attain and in which there was an increase in the number of 2-year survivors among patients who were amenable to treatment by radiation and excision, we continued the use of the same principles in another two series (1962 to 1967 and 1967 to 1975).[8] During these, we increased the length of the lesion amenable to resection from 8 to 10 to 12 cm (see Table 39-1).

Even though mortality in the 1962 to 1967 series had increased, we felt justified by the increase in the 2-year survival rate. (The survival statistics in the five series by method of treatment are shown in Table 39-3 by method of treatment.)

Additional observations in the 1967 to 1975 series concern mortality and survival. Among 15 patients having resection without preoperative megavoltage radiation therapy (MRT), there were six deaths (40%). In contrast, among 75 patients having resection following megavoltage therapy, there were 14 deaths (19%) (p = 0.10). The 2- and 5-year survival rates are shown in Table 39-4. Among 75 patients having resection following preoperative MRT, there was residual tumor in the surgical specimen in 65 (87%). There was no residual tumor in 10 cases, among whom there were two 5-year survivors (20%). Among the 65 patients with residual tumor in the surgical specimen, there were four (8%) 5-year survivors (p = 0.46).

PRESENT CONCEPTS OF COMBINED THERAPY

Analysis of the results of treatment in the 1967 to 1975 series failed to show improvement over the 1962 to 1967 series. Again a change was indicated. Reports of chemotherapy[9,10] as an adjunct to preoperative radiation and resection were

TABLE 39-3. Experience with carcinoma of the esophagus, by method of treatment

Reference	No. of patients	Method of treatment	Two-year survivors*	
1940-1951[4]	30	Resection alone	1	(3.3)
1951-1957[4]	17	MRT† alone	3	(17.6)
	61	MRT palliative	1	(1.6)
	5	Resection alone	1	(20)
	27	Resection palliative	2	(7.4)
	2	MRT + resection	2	(100)
1957-1962[4]	77	MRT alone	2	(2.6)
	21	MRT + resection	7	(33.3)
1962-1967[8]	70	MRT alone	2	(2.8)
	40	MRT + resection	11	(27.5)
1967-1975[8]	94	MRT alone	6	(6.4)
	15	Resection alone	2	(13.3)
	75	MRT + resection	15	(20)

*Numbers in parentheses are percentages.
†Megavoltage radiation therapy.

TABLE 39-4. Treatment methods for carcinoma of the esophagus—July, 1967, to July, 1975

Method	Cases	Two-year survival	Five-year survival
MRT alone	94	6 (6%)	1 (1%)
Resection alone	15	2 (13%)	1 (7%)
MRT + resection	75	15 (20%)	7 (10%)
All other cases	116	0	0
TOTAL	300	23 (7.7%)	9 (3.0%)

encouraging. Also, a report[11] of the treatment of cases of squamous carcinoma of the anus had indicated that any current change should include chemotherapy. A change in protocol was initiated in May, 1980, and continued in use for 4 years.[12] The chemotherapy consisted of mitomycin C, 10 mg as a bolus intravenous injection on day 1, and of 5-fluorouracil, 1000 mg per square meter of body surface area in 1000 ml of 5% glucose solution in distilled water given intravenously on each of days 1 to 4. The radiation treatment involved 3000 rad in 3 weeks with cobalt 60 or 6 MeV or greater with ports to cover the tumor and mediastinum 6 cm above and below the lesion. This therapy was considered preliminary to intended resection in all patients whose disease remained or became operable during or following the course of chemoradiation. Actually, in this and in previous series, we did not observe any patient who became operable after initial staging, unless the sole contraindication to operation was malnutrition and the patient's nutritional state could be restored to a satisfactory status by either enternal or parenteral feeding.

During the 4 years after May, 1980, 129 patients with primary carcinoma of the esophagus were seen, all squamous cell except one adenocarcinoma. Eighty-nine were entered into the protocol group; 40 were not. The operability, resectability, mortality, and 2-year survival rates are shown in Table 39-2. The operative mortality was lessened especially in the group treated according to protocol. If one combines the mortality statistics following resection from the 1967 to 1975 series and the 1980 to 1984 series, the mortality was 35% (8 of 23) in patients having no preoperative antineoplastic therapy and 16% (17 of 106) in those patients (75) having preoperative radiotherapy plus those (31) having preoperative chemotherapy and radiotherapy (p < 0.05).

There was one 2-year survivor among 33 patients having radiation therapy alone; one 2-year survivor among 12 patients having radiation and chemotherapy (without resection); seven 2-year survivors among 21 having "chemoradiation" and resection (33%); and two 2-year survivors among six patients having resection with no preoperative antineoplastic treatment (33%).

In patients having chemotherapy prior to resection, the percentage of surgical specimens

TABLE 39-5. Residual tumor in resected specimens after preoperative "chemoradiation" therapy

Year	No. of resections	Positivity
1980[12]	8	5
1981[12]	8	5
1982[12]	9	6
1983-1984[12]	6	4
TOTAL	31	20 (64%)

Among 3-year survivors, 1 specimen positive and 1 negative for residual tumors
Among 2-year survivors, 1 specimen positive and 1 negative for residual tumors
Among 1-year survivors, 2 specimens positive and 1 negative for residual tumors

showing residual carcinoma was 65% (20 of 31). This was a reduction from 87% (65 of 75) in our 1967 to 1975 series[8] with preoperative radiation and no chemotherapy (p < 0.025).

In view of the decreased radiation dosage in this last series, it is probably valid to attribute the lesser percentage of surgical specimens positive for carcinoma to the chemotherapeutic enhancement of the radiation effect in patients treated according to the protocol. But the absence of residual tumor in the resected specimen did not necessarily confer any improved chance for 2-year survival (see Table 39-5). In the patients who died, death was due to distant metastasis and not to local recurrence. However, after still another year's observation, there was distinctly longer survival in those in whom there was no residual tumor in the resected specimen. It was also disappointing that in several patients with presumed good prognoses, metastasis appeared in a shorter interval after resection than expected and in sites unusual for esophageal metastasis. This raised the possibility that the preoperative therapy, either chemotherapy or radiation therapy, or both, interfered in some manner with the resistance of the host to the carcinoma. A contrasting opinion has been expressed to the effect that intensive preoperative nutritional therapy feeds the tumor as well as the patient, and accounts for its aggressive growth and its early distant recurrence.[13]

WHERE TO?

As a result of our observations and those of others, it is apparent that the local tumor in the esophagus may be found to have been eradicated at the time of operation. It is clear that some better method of staging is needed in order to determine the possible need for resection if the patient can swallow normally.

Equally pertinent is the obvious need for methods of control of possible micrometastases. The majority of deaths after 2 and 5 years after resection are due to distant metastases rather than local recurrence. At the present time, in addition to continued trials of various combinations of therapy now in use, the potential for effective immunotherapy would seem to present the most promising means of cancer control, in both asymptomatic and symptomatic patients with either localized or extensive tumor.[14]

REFERENCES

1. Launois, B., Delarue, D., Campion, J.P., and Kerbaol, M.: Preoperative radiotherapy for carcinoma of the esophagus, Surg. Gynecol. Obstet. **153**:692, 1981.
2. Ellis, F.H., Gibbs, P., and Watkins, E., Jr.: Esophagogastrectomy, Ann. Surg. **198**:531, 1983.
3. Wu, Y.K., Huang, G.J., Shao, L.F., Zhang, Y.D., and Lin, X.S.: Progress in the study and surgical treatment of cancer of the esophagus in China, 1940-1980, J. Thorac. Cardiovasc. Surg. **84**:325, 1982.
4. Parker, E.F., and Gregorie, H.B.: Carcinoma of the esophagus: long-term results, JAMA **235**:1018, 1976.
5. Krebs, C., Neilsen, N., and Anderson, P.E.: Rotation treatment of cancer of esophagus, Acta Radiol. **32**:304, 1949.
6. Marks, R.D., Scruggs, H.J., and Wallace, K.M.: Preoperative radiation for carcinoma of the esophagus, Cancer **38**:84, 1976.
7. Fitzgerald, R.H., Bartles, D.M., and Parker, E.F.: Tracheo-esophageal fistulae secondary to carcinoma of the esophagus, J. Thorac. Cardiovasc. Surg. **82**:194, 1981.
8. Parker, E.F., Gregorie, H.B., Prioleau, W.H., Marks, R.D., and Bartles, D.M.: Carcinoma of the esophagus: observations of forty years, Ann. Surg. **195**:628, 1982.
9. Steiger, Z., Franklin, R., Wilson, R.F., Leichman, L., Seydel, H., Lol, J.F.H., et al.: Eradication and palliation of squamous cell carcinoma of the esophagus with chemotherapy, radiotherapy and surgical therapy, J. Thorac. Cardiovasc. Surg. **82**:78, 1981.
10. Bains, M.S., Kelsen, D.P., Beattie, E.J., and Martini, N.: Treatment of esophageal carcinoma by combined preoperative chemotherapy, Ann. Thorac. Surg. **34**:521, 1982.
11. Baroker, T.R., Nigro, N., Bradley, G., et al.: Combined therapy for cancer of the anal canal, Dis. Colon Rectum **20**:677, 1977.
12. Parker, E.F., Marks, R.D., Kratz, J.M., et al.: Chemoradiation therapy and resection for carcinoma of the esophagus: short-term results, Ann Thorac. Surg. **40**:121, 1985.
13. Fisher, J.E.: Adjuvant parenteral nutrition in the patient with cancer (editorial), Surgery **96**:578, 1984.
14. Ettinghauser, S.E., Mule, J.J., and Rosenberg, S.A.: Immunotherapy of lung micrometastases from a murine sarcoma with recombinant interleukin-2: mechanism of action, Surg. Forum **36**:390, 1985.

DISCUSSION—Chapters 37 to 39

Robert Guili

This discussion is based on results registered by the Group OESO in studies published since its creation in 1979; these OESO studies are detailed in Chapter 33 and may be compared with discussions in Chapters 37 to 39.

INITIAL STUDY (1980)

The first of the studies, using 2400 cases and published in 1980, was retrospective and did not lead to *definite* conclusions.[1] Radiotherapy was given most frequently in cases of infiltrating tumors (270 patients). These were the only lesions in which a favorable effect of such treatment could be detected (21%, 29-13*). The influence of preoperative or postoperative radiotherapy on the course of the neoplastic disease was assessed in relation to the size of the tumor. It was the small- and medium-size tumors (less than 4 cm in diameter, 164 of 207 and 72 of 100) that were irradiated, with the apparent aim of enhancing the results of complete surgical excision. When less than 3000 cGy, preoperative or postoperative radiotherapy was of no value. Indeed, the recurrence rate and metastases under such circumstances showed values higher than in other assessments (87%). In contrast, beyond 3000 cGy and in particular when given after surgery, radiotherapy appeared to influence both recurrence (36%) and metastasis (30%) rates. In this context, a study of reoperation led to no particular conclusion concerning recurrence.

Comparison was also made of the histologic appearance of resected lymph nodes, both for all patients and for those who had undergone preoperative radiotherapy. Adenocarcinomas were associated with the highest lymph node involvement (74% of 585 patients). In approximately one quarter of patients, these lymph nodes were situated in the mediastinum. It was in such patients, despite the poorest theoretical response to irradiation, that a relative decrease was seen in lymph node involvement after treatment (64% of 28 pa-

tients treated). In contrast, while the overall invasion rate in squamous cell carcinomas was somewhat lower (63% in 1882 patients), preoperative radiation did not produce any detectable improvement (61% for 589 patients). The percentage of surgical excisions showing macroscopic invasion was the same as in those patients who had not undergone radiotherapy (44% of 254 patients).

In an attempt to define the influence of irradiation on the carcinoma according to site, the following conclusions may be drawn. Radiotherapy was used in the upper third of the esophagus in 72 patients and appeared to be somewhat effective. This effect was nevertheless tangible only in a small number of patients (14%), in whom both preoperative and postoperative treatment was given. The 5-year survival rate was 46% (84-8). In the other cases (86%), preoperative (25%, 49-0) or postoperative (35%, 63-6) radiotherapy had no evident effect.

Five hundred ninety-four tumors of the middle third were irradiated, usually (62%) before surgery. Long-term results, evaluable only in those patients who survived, failed to reveal any improvement (20%, 26-13).

No improvement was noted with radiotherapy of the lower third of the esophagus, as far as long-term prognosis was concerned, in 306 patients. Preoperative irradiation was used in 57% of patients, with the best long-term survival rate being 29% (40-18).

Forty-eight patients with a tumor of the cardia were irradiated; usually this treatment was reserved for patients with a poor prognosis. The majority (64%) underwent radiotherapy before operation; among these there were no survivors at 4 years. Postoperative irradiation (52%) did not yield a better result, only 10% (29-0). The level remained lower than the mean rate for postoperative survival in all patients with tumors of the cardia (27%).

When lymph node involvement was present, radiotherapy was not associated with any im-

---

*Interval of confidence.

TABLE 1. Preoperative radiotherapy* and postoperative complications

Complications	103 XR+†		627 XR−
	Rate (%)		
None	32	p < 0.0001	57
Fistula	20	p < 0.005	12.6
Alveolar syndrome	50	p < 0.0001	25.5
Interstitial syndrome	15	p < 0.05	6
Overall pulmonary complications	32	p < 0.005	20
Assisted ventilation	85.5	p < 0.0005	50

*Patients, 103 (13.6%); average dose, 36 Gy + 22; number of sessions, 15.
†*XR*, Radiotherapy.

TABLE 2. Use of preoperative radiotherapy by stage and histology

	No.	XR+ 92	XR− 642
		NS	
T_{1a}	15	13%	87%
T_{1b}	56	5%	95%
T_2	206	14.5%	85.5%
T_3	457	12%	88%
		NS	
Squamous cell, well differentiated	258	8%	92%
Squamous cell, moderately differentiated	147	27%	73%
Squamous cell, poorly differentiated	127	19%	81%
Adenocarcinoma	173	1% p < 0.001	99%

provement in long-term prognosis. Whether it was given preoperatively or postoperatively, use of irradiation showed no benefit in comparison with nonirradiated patients (22%, 26-16). Indeed, the long-term postoperative survival rate of treated patients was poorer, whether treatment was preoperative (12%, 23-1) or postoperative (11%, 23-0). Such findings suggest the lack of efficacy of radiation treatment in this series.

SECOND SERIES (1984)

The second study was prospective and included 790 patients. Results were published after the First Polydisciplinary International Congress of OESO, which was held in Paris in 1984.[2] In this study 103 patients treated with radiotherapy before surgery were compared to 627 nonirradiated patients. The risk of postoperative fistula development and/or pulmonary complications after such treatment was identified. Percentages were highly significant (see Table 1).

For squamous cell carcinoma neither the stage of the tumor nor the histologic differentiation played any role in the use of preoperative radiotherapy. In contrast, adenocarcinomas virtually never received preoperative radiotherapy (see Table 2).[2]

Finally, with a follow-up period of 24 months, there was no statistical difference favoring preoperative radiotherapy. Survival medians are the same (see Table 3).[2]

In an assessment of treatment, including parameters such as type of anastomosis, organ used for replacing the esophagus, location of the carcinoma, surgical approach, and location of the anastomosis, preoperative radiotherapy was the only element associated with a higher percentage of fistulas than was found in the control group (see Table 4).[2]

Postoperative radiotherapy was only rarely used in patients who had been irradiated before operation. It was primarily indicated for tumors in which the prognosis was apparently the worst (macroscopic invasion of the mediastinum,

TABLE 3. Survival with and without preoperative radiotherapy

	6 months	12 months	18 months	24 months
XR + (56) (median: 5.6 months ± 1.1)	46% (60-32)	26% (38-13)	15.5% (26-4)	12% (22-1)
XR − (102) (median: 6 months ± 1.6)	50% (61-38)	35% (48-21)	22% (36-8)	13% (29-0)

TABLE 4. Preoperative radiotherapy and fistula development

XR + 103	XR − 651
20%	12.6%
	$p < 0.005$

TABLE 5. Use of postoperative radiotherapy*

	Indications		
	Macroscopic invasion	**Lymph nodes positive**	**Surgeon's impression**
XR +	41%	71%	14%
XR −	30%	59%	21%
		$p = 0.01$	

*Postoperative XR, 139 (average dose, 50 Gy ± 25; average duration, 7 weeks); both preoperative and postoperative XR, 13.

lymph node metastases, and unfavorable impression as determined by the surgeon) (see Table 5).[2]

OESO CONFERENCE (1984)

At the OESO multidisciplinary congress in Paris in 1984, radiotherapy was the subject of numerous discussions relating to questions posed by physicians of different specialties. The various teams could not reach unanimity.

The data reported by Pearson[3] do not seem to be corroborated by others. He believes that primary treatment by radiotherapy *only* should be considered for patients with no demonstrable distant metastases, with primary tumors no more than 9 cm in length, and without invasion of the trachea or bronchi. If a cylindrical volume 15 cm long and 6.5 cm in diameter is irradiated, he believes it will include more tissue circumferentially than can be removed by an esophagectomy.

A minimum tumor dose of 5000 cGy in 20 fractions in 28 days must be given. In his experience, treatment mortality is less than 1%. Of 401 patients irradiated, 186 (46%) survived a year; 70 (17%), 3 years; and 54 (13%), 5 years. Moreover, the 54 long-term survivors who had only radiotherapy constitute a particularly fortunate group from the functional point of view. Most are euphagic, regain normal weight, and retain normally functioning larynx, lungs, cardia, and stomach. Half of them have trouble with stricture.

In a randomized study presented at the same congress, Husemann[4] compared, in controlled groups, resection alone versus resection either with radiation or with radiation plus chemotherapy consisting of cisplatin and bleomycin. In this study postoperative mortality increased in correlation with preoperative therapy—from 31% in the control group, to 40% for radiation, to 47% in the combined treatment. The high mortality was most often the result of functional lung disorders. The rate of resected esophageal tumors

TABLE 6. Results of combined preoperative irradiation and surgery for carcinoma of the esophagus (China)

Authors	Years of study	No. of cases	Resectability (%)	Resection mortality (%)	Survival year after surgery	Percent survival after 5 years
Huang et al.	1959-1976	408*	81.9	3.9	5	31.6% (67/212)
	1965-1974	200*			10	21.9% (39/178)‡
Shao et al.					5	40.5% (81/200)
Zhang et al.	1972	210*	90.5	2.6	5	40.8% (20/49)
Huang et al.	1977-1982	83†	95.2	3.8	5	45.5% (10/22)

*Nonrandomized.
†Randomized.
‡These figures are for 10 years after surgery.

with a potential for cure by gross observation seemed to improve with preoperative therapy, but overall rates showed no statistical difference in comparison with the control group.

The Chinese experience presented by Huang[5] was important because of the large number of patients included. In a first study, based on 408 patients given preoperative irradiation, it was shown that the incidence of anastomotic leak was not significantly different from that of the group treated by surgery alone, even if the esophageal anastomotic site was located within the field of preoperative irradiation. However, the 5-year survival rate was not statistically different from that of the control group. (See also Chapter 38.)

To verify further the effects of preoperative irradiation, Huang presented a randomized study, started in 1977, of patients under 65 years of age who had middle-third esophageal carcinomas not exceeding 7 cm in length. These patients were randomized into two groups—one treated with combined preoperative irradiation and surgery, and the other with surgery alone. The study included 160 patients, to the end of June 1982, with a resectability rate of 95.2% in the irradiation group (79 of 83) compared with 89.6% (69 of 77) for the surgery-alone group. Similarly, the 5-year survival was 45.5% for the radiation group (10 of 22) and 25% for the surgery group (p = 0.1). From these results, it does seem that preoperative irradiation promotes both resectability and long-term survival for patients with carcinoma of the esophagus. This has also been reported by other Chinese teams (see Table 6).

ADDITIONAL STUDIES

In addition to these studies, it seems that two relatively recent randomized studies attest to the difficulty of forming an opinion on the value of preoperative radiotherapy.

The first, published in 1981,[6] reports the results of a randomized study involving 124 patients treated between 1973 and 1976. The preoperative radiation regimen was 40 Gy administered over 8 to 12 days, surgery being performed within 8 days following completion of radiation. Only patients with middle-third and distal-third lesions were included in the study. The resection rates of those receiving preoperative radiation and those going directly to surgery were similar (67% versus 70%). There was also no difference in operative mortality in either arm of the trial. Most disappointing were the mean and long-term survival rates. When the operative mortality was excluded from the analysis, the average survival rate was only 4.5 months for patients receiving preoperative radiation and 8.2 months for those treated with surgery alone. Five-year survival was also similar: 11.5% for those in the surgical arm and 9.5% for those receiving preoperative radiation therapy.

The second randomized study, sponsored by the European Organization for Research on Treatment of Cancer (EORTC), was started in 1976.[7] The treatment plan involved randomization of patients to either 3300 rad of radiation, given over 12 days and followed by surgery, or to surgery alone. At the time of the preliminary report, 160 patients had been followed for at least 1 year. The resection rate was 74.5% and was similar for the two groups. The operative mortality was 19.5%, and was also similar. At the time of this analysis, there was no difference in survival.

It seems, therefore, that although a number of studies have suggested that radiotherapy has a beneficial effect on the resection rate and the short-term survival, these hypotheses have not been confirmed by these two recent randomized trials. Furthermore, in the studies using higher radiation doses,[8] there is an increased risk. In addition to the operative mortality, 4 of the 40 patients in this series died after irradiation of 50 to 60 Gy given over 7 weeks.

CONCLUSIONS

These facts explain the Group OESO decision to start an international randomized therapeutic trial on the possible advantages of treatments associated with surgical resection. It has seemed preferable to turn toward the possible advantages of *postoperative* radiation for tumors of the esophagus. This would be designed to improve survival by reducing the frequency of local and/or regional recurrence, which occurs in 30% to 50% of patients and is responsible for death, since there is then no effective salvaging treatment. For postoperative radiotherapy to have the maximum chance of success, an adequate dose is required—that is, neither too high, risking complications, nor too low, risking ineffectiveness.

In the protocol of the Group OESO, now underway, after potentially curative surgery, radiotherapy is started 6 weeks after the operation, or 8 weeks in the case of postoperative complications. It is administered in doses of 45 Gy over 5 weeks with each week including five sessions of 1.8 Gy each. The total dose is therefore administered over 25 sessions and 35 days.

The histologically precise nature of the excised tumor is said to have importance in the results of radiotherapy applied after surgery. In this trial, particular attention is given to the careful interpretation of the histologic slides. Within the Group OESO, a subgroup of international pathologists was organized under Appelman (Ann Arbor, Michigan) to centralize in his laboratory all the pathology slides of each patient undergoing tumor resection.

This therapeutic trial involves the participation of 39 teams from 17 countries in Europe (nine), America (four), the Near East (two), and the Far East (two). Randomization is done among three arms: (1) surgical resection alone, (2) surgery plus postoperative radiotherapy, and (3) surgery plus perioperative chemotherapy. A global 500 patients will have data centralized simultaneously at the Institute Gustave Roussy in Villejuif, France, and at the Memorial Sloan-Kettering Cancer Center in New York. The first presentation of results is expected at the Second International Congress of the Group OESO, in May, 1987, in Paris.

REFERENCES

1. Giuli, R., and Gignoux, M.: Treatment of carcinoma of the esophagus: retrospective study of 2400 patients, Ann. Surg. **192:**44, 1980.
2. First Polydisciplinary International Congress of OESO: Cancer of the esophagus in 1984: 135 questions, answers compiled by R. Giuli, Paris, 1984, Editions Maloine.
3. Pearson, J.G.: Should radiotherapy be considered? In First Polydisciplinary International Congress of OESO: Cancer of the esophagus in 1984: 135 questions, answers compiled by R. Giuli, Paris, 1984, Editions Maloine, p. 33.
4. Husemann, B.: In other cases, surgery can be envisaged: Pre-operative radiotherapy or chemotherapy. In First Polydisciplinary International Congress of OESO: Cancer of the esophagus in 1984: 135 questions, answers compiled by R. Giuli, Paris, 1984, Editions Maloine, p. 56.
5. Huang, G.J.: In other cases, surgery can be envisaged: pre-operative radiotherapy or chemotherapy. In First Polydisciplinary International Congress of OESO: Cancer of the esophagus in 1984: 135 questions, answers compiled by R. Giuli, Paris, 1984, Editions Maloine, p. 59.
6. Launois, B., et al.: Pre-operative radiotherapy for carcinoma of the esophagus, Surg. Gynecol. Obstet. **153:**690, 1981.
7. European Organization for Research on Treatment of Cancer, Gastrointestinal Tract Cooperative Group: Pre-operative radiotherapy for carcinoma of the esophagus: results of a prospective multicentric study. In DeMeester, T.R. and Skinner, D.B., editors: Esophageal disorders, pathophysiology and therapy, New York, 1985, Raven Press, pp. 367-371.
8. Doggett, R. and Guernsey, J.: Combined radiation and surgical treatment of the thoracic esophagus: final report, Front. Radiat. Ther. Oncol. **5:**147, 1970.

CHAPTER 40

Preoperative chemotherapy in epidermoid carcinoma of the esophagus

David Kelsen

Several recent reviews have confirmed the dismal prognosis for patients with esophageal cancer, even when disease appears to be limited to the local-regional area—that is, T_{1-3}, $N_X M_0$. With either surgery or radiation therapy alone, these reviews indicate that 1-year survival was less than 20%; at 5 years, only 4% to 6% of patients were still alive.[1,2] The major reason for the failure of conventional therapy to cure a larger percentage of patients may be seen from the results of several autopsy series. Anderson and Ladd, and Bosch et al., have demonstrated that, in Western patients, esophageal cancer is widely disseminated within a short time of initial diagnosis (a median of 4 months from diagnosis to autopsy in Anderson and Ladd's series).[3,4] Although, in both autopsy studies, residual local disease was found in a substantial number of patients, in only a few patients was this the only site of cancer; the majority had lung, liver, nodal, adrenal, or other sites of distant spread.

Thus, symptomatic Western patients appear to have more extensive, widespread cancer at the time of diagnosis than, for example, asymptomatic Chinese patients found during mass screening programs. While esophagectomy alone yields high cure rates in the latter, treatment directed only at the esophagus and periesophageal tissues appears doomed to failure in most Western patients.

The concept of neoadjuvant systemic chemotherapy in this disease has both theoretical and practical grounds. Preoperative (or preradiation) chemotherapy allows an early attack on both the primary tumor and metastatic disease. Since resection is frequently difficult because of lateral tumor spread, preoperative therapy may, in responding patients, increase the resection rate. Using treatment prior to surgery allows an in vivo assessment, in both individuals and in groups of patients, of the effectiveness of a drug or drug combination, aiding in the selection of postoperative therapy.

Although the hypothesis that neoadjuvant chemotherapy improves resection rates and survival is attractive, it remains very much a theory. There have now been 11 studies reported in which chemotherapy alone has been given prior to a planned surgical procedure. With one exception, these studies have involved combination chemotherapy in which the heavy metal cisplatin is the common denominator.[5-15] Most (but not all) of these regimens have demonstrated antitumor activity in patients with advanced, metastatic disease. Chemotherapy in this patient population is palliative in nature, and the measurements of drug effectiveness have been objective tumor response rates and durations of response. In a number of neoadjuvant trials, both patient populations were studied concurrently; that is, the trials included patients with local-regional and extensive (metastatic) cancer. All of these initial studies are single-arm, feasibility trials.

An example of one such study is an early trial from Memorial Hospital of the Memorial-Sloan Kettering Cancer Center. In this phase II program, a total of 68 evaluable patients were treated with cisplatin, vindesine, and bleomycin.[5] Twenty-four patients had metastatic or recurrent cancer; they received chemotherapy alone. The remaining 44 patients had local-regional disease, and were treated in a multimodality program involving chemotherapy prior to planned surgery and/or radiation. One or two cycles of chemotherapy were given prior to the definitive local-regional treatment. Response to chemotherapy for patients with local-regional disease was assessed by serial barium esophagrams, repeat endoscopy, and most

329

importantly, by surgical staging in the operative group. Details of response criteria have been described previously; complete response to chemotherapy required that no viable tumor be found by pathologic examination of the resected primary tumor and lymph nodes, and that no visceral disease be present.[16] The overall response rate (complete and partial) for all 68 patients was 53%.

Of the 44 patients with local-regional disease, 34 were treated prior to planned surgery, and 10 prior to planned radiation. All preoperative patients underwent exploration; 28 (82%) had resectable disease. In general, those patients who had responded to chemotherapy were more likely to have resectable disease then were those who did not respond. In a nonrandomized trial, it is very difficult to assess the impact on resection rates of a given preoperative regimen. One factor that may give some indication of the ability of such an approach to increase the ease of resection is downstaging of the primary tumor (that is, drop of at least one stage when compared with the pretreatment clinical stage). In this study, downstaging was seen in 30% of patients. Three patients had no residual tumor in the resected esophagus, and two additional patients had residual carcinoma in situ only. This suggests an impact on primary tumor bulk of substantial magnitude.

Operative morbidity did not appear to be increased. All patients in this study underwent modified Ivor Lewis procedures. Ten patients had major but nonfatal complications.[17] Three had pulmonary dysfunction (atelectasis or pneumonia), one of whom required prolonged ventilatory support. Cardiac arrhythmias that were brief in duration were seen in six patients. One patient had an anastomotic leak, and two patients required dilatation of an anastomotic stricture. The overall treatment-related mortality was 8.8%: two postoperative deaths and one drug-related death. The median duration of survival for all 34 patients was 16.2 months; 23% were alive more than 3 years after start of therapy.

Although chemotherapy-associated toxicities were tolerable, they were substantial and should not be underestimated. In spite of aggressive antiemetic regimens, nausea and vomiting were seen in almost all patients; alopecia was universal. Vindesine, an investigational vinca alkaloid, produced a mild-to-moderate peripheral neuropathy in 50% of patients. More serious toxicities included renal damage (peak serum creatinine > 2.5/100 ml) in 19%, and significant myelosuppression. Leukopenia was the dose-limiting factor in this regimen, with a median white blood cell count nadir of 1900/mm.[3]

Similar results have been seen with other preoperative regimens. For example, two investigators have used cisplatin-vindesine-bleomycin in a neoadjuvant setting. Schlag et al., using a modified schedule, treated 23 patients prior to surgery. The response rate was 43%; toxicities included substantial leukopenia, nausea and vomiting, and alopecia. Eighteen patients had resectable disease; the operative mortality was 19.2%.[7]

Roth et al., at the National Cancer Institute, have reported the preliminary results of an ongoing randomized trial in which patients undergo immediate surgery or received preoperative and postoperative chemotherapy in addition to surgery. The response rate to cisplatin-vindesine-bleomycin was 44%; toxicities were similar to those seen in the Memorial Sloan-Kettering study. Operative morbidity and mortality were similar in the two arms. Survival data were not yet available.[18]

In other trials using cisplatin-containing regimens, tumor response rates range from 30% to 60%; resection rates in most studies range from 60% to 90%. General chemotherapy toxicities are similar to those described above, with some regimens (such as those including a 5-fluorouracil infusion) causing more mucositis and somewhat less leukopenia.[8-9]

Two studies that point out the potential for unusual risks and the need for very close collaboration between medical oncologist, surgeon, and anesthesiologist have been reported. Schlag et al., as noted above, treated a group of 23 patients with a bleomycin-containing regimen prior to surgery. At the beginning of their study, no attempt was made to control the oxygen concentration (FiO_2) given during the surgical procedure. Two patients developed severe postoperative pulmonary failure. Thereafter, the FiO_2 was kept below 30%, and there was careful monitoring of fluid replacement. No further cases of pulmonary failure were seen.[7] In the second trial, published in abstract form from the University of Illinois, 15 patients received preoperative therapy with a regimen including mitomycin and bleomycin. Both bleomycin and mitomycin are potential pulmonary toxins. In the University of Illinois study, a 45% operative mortality was seen (10). Earlier studies at Memorial Sloan-Kettering with testicular cancer patients had demonstrated that, once having received bleomycin, patients had an increased risk of developing severe pulmonary dysfunction following surgery.[19] The key factor appears to be exposure to a high FiO_2 during and after surgery. If the FiO_2 is kept below 30% and there is careful monitoring of fluid replacement, there appears to be no increased incidence of an acute respiratory distress syndrome. The study of Schlag et al. would support this observation.

An increased risk of pulmonary damage following esophageal surgery is not limited to patients who have had prior exposure to chemotherapy. Dunwick and co-workers reported severe and fatal pulmonary failure following use of radiation plus miconidazole given prior to esophagectomy. In their study, four of seven patients receiving 4000 rad of radiation given in twice-weekly 400-rad doses prior to exploration developed a picture of acute respiratory distress, usually within 24 to 72 hours of surgery, exactly as seen in the testicular cancer patients having received bleomycin. At postmortem examination, histologic changes of organizing alveolitis, interstitial fibrosis, and dilatation of interstitial and subpleural lymphatics were seen diffusely throughout the lung, even in areas that had not received radiation. An additional group of 24 patients treated with the same radiation regimen without surgery did not develop this picture.[20]

The use of concurrent chemotherapy and radiation will be discussed in detail in Chapter 41. However, a similar increased risk of severe pulmonary toxicity has been seen using this approach, in spite of careful control of factors such as the FiO_2. It may well be that after use of a combination of two pulmonary toxins (radiation and chemotherapy), and especially when the chemotherapeutic agents also act as radiation sensitizers, any exposure to increased oxygen at surgery is hazardous.

The neoadjuvant chemotherapy trials reported to date have demonstrated that objective tumor shrinkage can be obtained in approximately 40% to 50% of patients with local-regional disease, with substantial but acceptable toxicities. When chemotherapy is given as a single modality (without concurrent radiation), there appears to be no increase in operative morbidity or mortality. However, whether this approach will result in improved resection rates and survival is not yet known. Carefully performed, randomized control trials are needed to answer this question. A number of such studies are currently underway or are being planned. Almost all of them use a cisplatin-containing combination. Whether "maintenance" (postoperative) chemotherapy is useful is also not known; this is a separate question that also must be addressed. Until these studies have *proved* that the neoadjuvant approach is worthwhile, it remains an investigational technique and should not be used in a nonstudy setting.

REFERENCES

1. Earlam, R., and Cunha-Menlo, Jr.: Oesophageal squamous cell carcinoma: a critical review of radiotherapy, Br. J. Surg. **67:**457, 1980.
2. Earlam, R., and Cunha-Menlo, J.: Oesophageal squamous cell carcinoma: a critical review of surgery, Br. J. Surg. **67:**381, 1980.
3. Anderson, I., and Ladd, T.: Autopsy findings in squamous cell carcinoma of the esophagus, Cancer **50:**1587, 1982.
4. Bosch, A., Frias, Z., Caldwell, W., et al.: Autopsy findings in carcinoma of the esophagus, Acta Radiol. Oncol. **18:**103, 1979.
5. Kelsen, D.P., Hilaris, B., Coonley, C., et al.: Cisplatin, vindesine and bleomycin chemotherapy of local-regional and advanced esophageal cancer, Am. J. Med. **75:**645, 1983.
6. Coonley, C., Bains, M., Kelsen, D.P., et al.: Cisplatin-bleomycin in the treatment of esophageal carcinoma: a final report, Cancer **54:**2351, 1984.
7. Schlag, P., Hermann, R., Fritze, D., et al.: Preoperative chemotherapy in localized cancer of the esophagus with cisplatinum, vindesine, and bleomycin. In Wagner, D., Blijhan, G., Smeets, J., and Wils, J., editors: Primary chemotherapy in cancer medicine, New York, 1985, Alan R. Liss, Inc., p. 253.
8. Carey, R., Choi, N., Hilgenberg, A., et al.: Preoperative chemotherapy (5FU-DDP) as initial component in multimodality treatment program for esophageal cancer, Proc. ASCO. **4:**78, 1985.
9. Shields, T.W., Rose, S.T., Hellerstein, S.M., et al.: Multimodality approach to treatment of carcinoma of the esophagus, Arch. Surg. **119:**558, 1984.
10. Kulka, L., Ladd, T., McGuire, W., et al.: Multimodality therapy of squamous carcinoma of the esophagus (abstract), Proc. ASCO AACR **22:**449, 1981.
11. Fukimaki, M., et al.: Role of preoperative administration of bleomycin and radiation in the treatment of esophageal cancer, Jpn. J. Surg. **5:**48, 1975.
12. Kelsen, D.P., Coonley, C., Hilaris, B., et al.: Cisplatin, vindesine, and methyl-glyoxal bis (guanylhydrazone) chemotherapy of esophageal cancer, Cancer Treat. Rep., 1986. (In press.)
13. Gennis, M., Forastiere, A., Orringer, M., et al.: Trial of cisplatin, methylglyoxal bis (guanylhydrazone) and Velban in squamous cell and adenocarcinoma of the esophagus (abstract), Proc. ASCO **4:**85, 1985.
14. El-Akkad, S., Amer, M., and Kerth, W.: Combined chemotherapy, surgery and radiation therapy for esophageal cancer (abstract). In Proceedings of the 13th International Cancer Congress, 1983.
15. Forestiere, A., Patel, H., Hankins, J., et al.: Cisplatin, bleomycin and VP-16-213 in combination for epidermoid carcinoma of the esophagus, Proc. ASCO **2:**123, 1983.
16. Kelsen, D.P., Heelan, R., Coonley, C., et al.: Clinical and pathological evaluation of response to chemotherapy in patients with esophageal cancer, Am. J. Clin. Oncol. **6:**539, 1983.
17. Bains, M., Kelsen, D.P., Beattie, E.J., et al.: Treatment of esophageal carcinoma by combined preoperative chemotherapy, Ann. Thorac. Surg. **34:**521, 1982.
18. Roth, J.A., Pass, H.I., Flanagan, M.M., et al.: Randomized trial of pre- and postoperative cisplatin, vindesine, and bleomycin (DVB) chemotherapy in epidermoid carcinoma of the esophagus. Proceedings of the 14th International Congress of Chemotherapy. (In press.)
19. Goldiner, P., Carlon, G., Cuitkovic, E., et al.: Factors influencing postoperative morbidity and mortality in patients treated with bleomycin, Brit. Med. J. **1:**1664, 1978.
20. Dunwick, N., Schnade, J., Martin, S., et al.: Interstitial pulmonary infiltrate following combined therapy for esophageal carcinoma, Chest **81:**453, 1982.

CHAPTER 41 Concurrent chemotherapy and radiation therapy for squamous cell cancer of the esophagus

Zwi Steiger

Since squamous cell carcinoma of the esophagus treated with a single conventional cancer therapeutic modality carries a poor prognosis, studies have been undertaken to combine these modalities with an aim of improving the results. In the past, attempts to cure cancer of the esophagus were directed toward the primary growth and the lymph-bearing area. A larger, more radical operation was supposed to be more effective in achieving this goal. This approach, although valid in theory, by itself is futile in cancer of the esophagus. The surgical concept of a wide excision cannot even be accomplished in cancer of the esophagus. The proximity of vital organs obviates it. In addition, most patients presenting with cancer of the esophagus have nonresectable disease because of local invasion of the tumor and either overt or occult metastatic disease. The addition of radiation and chemotherapy to surgery to facilitate eradication of tumor at the primary site and chemotherapy for the assumed existing metastatic disease is logically sound. Certain chemotherapeutic agents have also been shown to have radiosensitizing properties and, when given concomitantly with radiation, add a new dimension to the control of the primary tumor by reducing the size of the tumor, reducing the extent of local invasion, and thereby increasing the resectability rate.

THE WAYNE STATE UNIVERSITY EXPERIENCE

In a pilot study done in the early seventies at Wayne State University and the Detroit Medical Center, seven patients with advanced squamous cell cancer of the esophagus were treated with repetitive courses of mitomycin C, 5-fluorouracil, and radiation. All seven had marked symptomatic relief from dysphagia.

From the experiences of this study a protocol was developed that consisted of a continuous infusion of 5-fluorouracil, 1000 mg/m²/day, on days 1 through 4 and days 29 through 32. Mitomycin C, 10 mg/m², was given as an intravenous bolus injection on day 1. Radiation of the lesion was started on day 1. A total of 3000 rad was given in 15 fractions of 200 rad daily on days 1 to 5, 8 to 12, and 15 to 19. Radiation ports included 5 cm of the esophagus on either side of the tumor. The width of the port was 8 cm.

Esophagectomy was performed in suitable patients 3 to 4 weeks after completion of the chemotherapy and radiotherapy. The esophagectomy was performed by either standard Ivor Lewis approach (using a laparotomy and right thoracotomy) or a transhiatal esophagectomy without thoracotomy and anastomosis of the fundus of the stomach to the cervical esophagus. Only patients with biopsy-proved squamous cell carcinoma of the esophagus were eligible. The prestudy workup included esophagography, triple endoscopy, chest x-ray film, tomography of the lungs, bone and liver scans, SMA-17, CEA, and creatinine determinations, pulmonary functions tests, and arterial blood gas determinations.

The initial 55 patients who received 5-fluorouracil with mitomycin C were divided into two groups. In group I were patients who during workup had no evidence of locally advanced or metastatic disease and had no medical contraindications to surgery. Thirty patients were in this group. Twenty-five patients did not meet the eligibility criteria and were placed in group II and treated with palliative intent. From the first group, 23 patients had the esophagus resected. Sixteen had an Ivor Lewis approach, and seven had a transhiatal resection. Nine of these twenty-three patients (39%) had no residual local disease. Subclinical metastatic disease was found in five patients. Three of the 23 (13%) patients died postoperatively. Another four died soon after the 30-day postoperative period from sepsis. Six patients with residual disease received postoperative chemotherapy and radiation therapy. All six developed recurrence, two with local and four with disseminated disease. The patients with subclinical metastases in the liver or celiac and paracardial nodes also received further therapy. The postoperative complications were higher in the thoracotomy group. These included contained anastomotic leaks (two), wound infection, pleural effusion, and respiratory insufficiency. In the nonthoracotomy group the complications were anastomotic leak in the neck, recurrent laryngeal nerve injury, respiratory insufficiency, and anastomotic stricture. The combined chemotherapy and radiation therapy was well tolerated. The median survival was 16 months. Four (17.3%) patients from this group survived 5 years.

The 25 patients in group II did not meet the criteria for curative intent as outlined in the protocol. Ten patients had no surgical procedure and died at 2 to 52 weeks, two because of local recurrence and three with disseminated disease. Five patients had Celestin tubes inserted because of persistent dysphagia, three had bypass procedures, and four had palliative esophageal resections. One had repeat dilatations and two had exploratory laparotomies. The median survival in this group was 16 weeks. [1]

In a subsequent study, the mitomycin C was replaced with cisplatin. This was done when cisplatin was found to be effective against squamous cell cancer. It was given as an intravenous bolus on days 1 and 29 at 100 mg/m^2. The rest of the protocol remained the same including radiation treatment. There were 21 patients in this pilot project. All patients completed the preoperative treatment course. Two patients declined the proposed operation; 19 patients had surgery. Four patients were found to have nonresectable tumors and had palliative bypass operations. Fifteen patients had resections of the esophagus with curative intent. In five of the 15 (33%) no cancer was found in the resected esophagus and lymph nodes. An additional two patients had no tumor in the esophagus, but had tumor in the celiac nodes. Postoperatively, the remaining eight patients with tumor found in the resected esophagus

received radiation therapy. The two patients with positive celiac nodes and no cancer in the esophagus received radiation to a portal covering these nodes. Patients without any cancer in the resected specimen received no further therapy. Three (15.9%) patients died postoperatively. Two additional patients died soon after the postoperative period. The median survival for the 21 patients was 18 months; for the 15 who had esophagectomy after preoperative treatment, the median survival was 24 months. Each of the five patients who did not have residual disease in the resected specimen survived 24 months. Three survived 48, 50, and 56 months. One of them developed another primary in the lung.

Of the ten patients with tumor in the pathologic specimen, one is free of disease at 60 months, four died of local recurrence, three have local and distant disease, and two have distant disease only. [2]

THE SOUTHWEST ONCOLOGY GROUP EXPERIENCE

The Southwest Oncology Group (SWOG)[3] adopted the Wayne State University protocol, with a reduction of the cisplatin dose to 75 mg/m^2. The study was done between April, 1981, and March 1984. One hundred two out of 106 evaluable patients completed the radiation and chemotherapy; 84% of the patients were males. Of the tumors in which measurements were recorded, 34 were less than 5 cm in length and 50 were larger. The majority of patients experienced toxicity in the form of nausea and vomiting. Four patients had life-threatening myelosuppression. Of the 102 patients completing the radiochemotherapy, in 14 the disease progressed prior to the surgery. Eleven refused surgery, and six were considered poor risks. Of 71 who had the operation, 16 had nonresectable disease, 13 had a palliative resection, 24 had residual disease in the resected esophagus, and 18 had no disease in the resected specimen. Seven (11%) died postoperatively. The median survival for the 71 patients having surgery was 14 months, and for those with complete response to the preoperative chemotherapy and radiotherapy, 32 months. Of the 106 evaluable patients, 21 remain alive. [3]

EVALUATION OF THE STUDIES

These three studies have flaws, and the combined modality approach has drawbacks. The number of patients is small, and none of the studies is randomized. The data can be compared only with historical series. Toxicity in the form of nausea and vomiting, mucositis, and myelosuppression is a problem, always unpleasant but usually tolerated. There is also an increased risk of developing adult respiratory distress syndrome postoperatively, which may be due to damage of the alveolar cells by the combination of the chemotherapy and radiotherapy, to a high FiO_2, and to manipulation of the lungs during surgery. The delay of surgery in patients who did not respond to treatment is expensive, and precious time is wasted in handling the tumor. Compensation in the form of a complete response (although not always a sure prognostic sign for long-term survival) of 39%, 41%, and 47% is a reason for some optimism. The disappearance of dysphagia is also a reason for rejection of further treatment by some patients. At surgery there is a downstaging of the extent of the disease, and tumors initially considered nonresectable may become resectable. The esophagus at surgery often feels normal, and the resection becomes technically easier.

The operative risk of esophageal resection remains high, and the answer to the question of whether patients who have responded completely to the chemoradiation therapy should be advised to have surgery is not easy to answer. This question arises at this juncture because some patients who responded completely and did not have resection of the esophagus had recurrence of the disease in the form of distant metastases only. Had surgery been performed, it could not have improved survival and might even have shortened it by an operative mortality. If there are factors present that increase the risk of surgery in the patient with a complete clinical response as seen by a normal barium swallow, endoscopy and biopsy, and computed tomography, esophagectomy is not advised. However, residual undetectable malignant cells under the mucosa can be a source for recurrence and metastatic disease. Resection should be recommended in patients with no medical contraindications. In good-risk patients with residual local disease who have completed two cycles of chemotherapy and received 3000 rad, resection of the esophagus is recommended. Increasing the radiation dose to 5000 rad with further chemotherapy and witholding surgery in these patients is now being tried. Patients with obvious metastatic disease with a partial or complete response, in whom dysphagia is relieved, can continue with their medical management. The immediate survival and the 2- and 3-year survival (35.7% and 19%) are better than in our past experience. The 5-year survival (11.6%)

is also better than in the past but, however, remains low.

REVIEW OF THE LITERATURE

Recently, a number of investigators have written of their clinical trials investigating the role of chemotherapy and radiotherapy as surgical adjuncts for patients with squamous cell cancer of the esophagus. Fujimaki and associates reported on a group of 46 patients treated with bleomycin followed by ^{60}Co irradiation. An esophagectomy was carried out 5 to 21 days after completion of their radiation. Effective histologic results were seen in 85% of the resected specimens.[4]

Werner reported on the use of methotrexate as a radiosensitizing agent, given intravenously once a week for 3 weeks. This was followed with 2000 rad directed to the primary tumor. Surgery was performed 3 weeks after completion of radiotherapy. Of 491 patients with squamous cell cancer of the esophagus, 93 were selected for this study. Of the 93 patients 55 (59.1%) had the operation. The operative mortality was 14.5%. Thirty-one percent had no gross and 27% no histologic evidence of tumor in the resected specimen. The range of survival was 3 to 60 months, with an average of 26 months. Pulmonary toxicity was not described.[5]

Miller et al. reported on preoperative cisplatin, cisplatin with 5-fluorouracil, and cisplatin with vinblastine. Radiation was given postoperatively. Eighteen of 20 patients completed the study. In 11 patients tumor regression was seen, but in none was the primary tumor completely eradicated by preoperative chemotherapy. Fourteen survived 1 year, and 11 survived for 12 to 24 months.[6]

Soga et al. treated 109 patients with bleomycin and radiation preoperatively, achieving a remarkable 32.2% 5-year survival.[7]

Parker and colleagues did not find any advantage by adding chemotherapy to the preoperative radiation. They used a combination of mitomycin C, 5-fluorouracil, and 3000 rad, and found the resectability rate to be the same as when preoperative radiation was used alone. The percentage of resected specimens showing residual tumor decreased. However, the absence of any residual tumor in the resected specimen has not conferred any improved chance of long-term survival. The 2-year survival of 33% (7 of 21) was about the same as in their previous series of patients, treated with 4500 rad in 3 weeks and resection without chemotherapy.[8]

Adelstein el al. found the combination of chemotherapy and radiation to be risky and abandoned it. They treated eight patients with 5-fluorouracil, cisplatin, and methotrexate, with 3000 rad given simultaneously. Two patients had complete remission and, six had partial remission. Five patients developed adult respiratory distress syndrome; three of them died.[9]

Nygaard et al. also found that bleomycin combined with radiation preoperatively carried an increased risk of serious pulmonary problems. They suggested using a smaller dose of bleomycin and a technique of irradiation with the least exposure of the lungs.[10]

Andersen et al. also found no advantage to preoperative bleomycin and radiation as compared with preoperative radiation alone.[11]

In a study in which surgery was withheld, Engstrom et al., treated 13 patients with stage I or II squamous cell carcinoma and three with adenocarcinoma of the esophagus, using a combination of 6000 rad in 30 fractions concomitantly with mitomycin C and 5-fluorouracil. The therapy was well tolerated. Thirteen had either x-ray or endoscopic clearance of intraluminal tumor by 3 months after therapy. However, patients had mild to moderate residual narrowing of the esophagus, and five patients had severe stricture (three associated with recurrent disease) requiring dilatation or gastrostomy tube feeding. The disease-free survival range was 2 to 40 + months, with a median greater than 22 months. This combined modality was well tolerated and produced satisfactory local control of esophageal cancer.[12]

Byfield et al. reported favorable responses using 5-fluorouracil and radiation, resulting in relief of dysphagia with acceptable toxicity.[13]

In a prospective randomized study Kolarič et al. treated 31 patients with inoperable cancer of the esophagus with a combination of bleomycin and adriamycin and a combination of these agents and radiation. The response rate in the first group was 19% and in the latter 60%. Three patients in the latter group had a complete response, and the average duration of the remission in these was 11 months. Although the number of patients was relatively small, the advantage of combining chemotherapy and radiation therapy was evident.[14]

Earle et al., in a controlled randomized Eastern Cooperative Oncology Group study using bleomycin and radiation, found that bleomycin did not contribute favorably to palliation or survival. Treatment results were discouraging.[15]

Resbeut el al. used vincristine, methotrexate, folinic acid rescue, and cisplatin, followed with radiation. One month after the end of radiation therapy, 43% showed a partial response and 32% a complete response. The median duration of the response was 8 months. The median survival for responders was 12.9 months and 5.9 months for nonresponders.[16]

Abitbol reported using 5-fluorouracil, methotrexate, and cisplatin, and 6000 rad. Eight of nine patients had achieved an objective response, with five having a complete response. Three were alive at 3.5, 6, and 20 months. All responding patients were able to swallow solid foods, except for one with an esophageal stricture. The regimen was found to be feasible and provided local control of the disease.[17]

Thus, despite some negative reports, there seems to be convincing evidence that combining two or more chemotherapeutic agents with radiotherapy can eradicate local tumor in a large number of patients, with improved palliation or resectability and increased disease-free intervals and survival.

REFERENCES

1. Franklin, R., Steiger, Z., Vaishampayan, G., Asfaw, I., Rosenberg, J., Loh, J., Hoschner, J., and Miller, P.: Combined modality therapy for esophageal squamous cell carcinoma, Cancer **51**:1062, 1983.
2. Leichman, L., Steiger, Z., Seydel, H.G., Dindogru, A., Kinzie, J., Toben, S., Mackenzie, G., and Shell, J.: Preoperative chemotherapy and radiation therapy for patients with cancer of the esophagus: a potentially curative approach, J. Clin. Oncol. **2**:75, 1984.
3. Poplin, E., Leichman, L., Seydel, H.G., Steiger, Z. and Flemming, T.: Combined therapies for squamous cell carcinoma of the esophagus: a Southwest Oncology Group study (SWOG-8037). (Unpublished data.)
4. Fujimaki, M., Soga, J., Wada, K., Kawaguchi, M., Maeda, M., Sasaki, K., Omori, Y., and Muto, T.: A new chemotherapy as a preoperative treatment for esophageal cancer surgery. In proceedings of the VIIth International Congress of Chemotherapy, Prague, 1971, pp. 643-646.
5. Werner, I.D.: Multidisciplinary approach to the management of carcinoma of the oesophagus, Digestion **16**:284, 1977.
6. Miller, J.C., McIntyre, B., and Hatcher, C.R., Jr.: Combined treatment approach in surgical management of carcinoma of the esophagus: a preliminary report, Ann. Thor. Surg. **40**(3):289, 1985.
7. Soga, J, Fujimaki, M., Tanaka, O., Sasaki, K., Kawaguchi, M., and Muto, T.: Analysis of preoperative combined bleomycin and radiation therapy for esophageal carcinoma, World J. Surg. **7**:230, 1983.
8. Parker, E.E., Marks, R.D., Jr, Kratz, J.M., Cheikhouni, A., Warren, E.T., and Bartless, D.M.: Chemoradiation therapy and resection for carcinoma of the esophagus: short term results, Ann. Thorac. Surg. **40**(2): 121, 1985.
9. Adelstein, D., Snow, N., Sharan, V., Horrigan, T., Hines, J., Carter, S., Crum, E., Schacter, L., and Mendelsohn, H.: Postoperative respiratory failure after preoperative chemotherapy and mediastinal radiation for

esophageal cancer, Proc. Ann. Meet. Am. Soc. Clin. Oncol. **3:**135, 1984.

10. Nygaard, K., Smith-Erichsen, N., Hatlevoll, R., and Refsurm, S.B.: Pulmonary complications after bleomycin, irradiation and surgery for esophageal cancer, Cancer **41:**17, 1978.

11. Andersen, A.P., Berdal, P., Edsmyr, F., Hagen, S., Hatlevoll, R., Nygaard, K., Ottosen, P., Peterffy, P., Kongsholm, H., and Elgen, K.: Irradiation, chemotherapy and surgery in esophageal cancer: a randomized clinical study—the first Scandinavian trial in esophageal cancer, Radiother. Oncol. **2(3):**179, 1984.

12. Engstrom, P., Coia, L., Paul, A.: Non-surgical management of stage I and II esophageal carcinoma, Proc. Am. Soc. Clin. Oncol. **4:**91, 1985.

13. Byfield, J.E., Barone, R., Mendelsohn, J., Frankel, S., Quinol, L., Sharp, T., and Seagren, S.: Infusional 5-fluorouracil and x-ray therapy for nonresectable esophageal cancer, Cancer **45:**703, 1980.

14. Kolarič, K., Maričič, Z., Roth, A., and Dujmovič, I.: Combination of bleomycin and adriamycin with and without radiation in the treatment of inoperable esophageal cancer, Cancer **45:**2265, 1980.

15. Earle, J.D., Gelber, R.D., Moertel, C.G., and Hahn, R.G.: A controlled evaluation of combined radiation and bleomycin therapy for squamous cell carcinoma of the esophagus, J. Radiat. Oncol. Biol. Phys. **6:**821, 1980.

16. Resbeut, M., Le Prise–Fleury, E., Ben-Hassel, M., Goudier, M., Morice-Rouxel, M.F., Douillard, J.Y., and Chenal, C.: Squamous cell carcinoma of the esophagus: treatment by combined vincristine-methotrexate plus folinic acid rescue and cisplatin before radiotherapy, Cancer **56:**1246, 1985.

17. Abitbol, A., Straus, M.J., Franklin, G., Billet, D., Sullivan, P., and Morgan, R.E.: Infusional chemotherapy and cyclic radiation therapy in operable esophageal and gastric cardia carcinoma, Am. J. Clin. Oncol. **6:**195, 1983.

CHAPTER **42** **Hyperthermia treatment effective for patients with carcinoma of the esophagus**

Keizo Sugimachi, Hidemasa Matsufuji, and Hidenobu Kai

The use of hyperthermia to treat clinical malignant lesions has gained increasing interest. Hyperthermia combined with chemotherapy and radiotherapy seems to have a synergistic effect on malignant lesions.[1,2] The major problem limiting wide application of diathermy is the difficulty in heating tumors deeply located in tissues.

After several years of continued research on various designs and extensive experiments on laboratory animals, we have designed an apparatus. This apparatus has capacitive-type heating with a radio frequency at 13.56 MHz and is equipped with a pair of endotract electrodes and an extracorporeal electrode.[3]

We have also devised hyperthermia combined with chemotherapy and irradiation (HCR therapy) for treating malignant lesions of the esophagus as an adjunct to surgery.[4] In order to clarify the effect of hyperthermia, a cooperative study of 13 university hospitals of Japan was undertaken.[5] The clinical results show HCR to be a promising modality for treating carcinoma of the esophagus.

PATIENTS

One hundred and fourteen patients with primary esophageal carcinoma underwent hyperthermia treatment using the Endoradiotherm 100A* (ERT 100A) (Fig. 42-1). These patients were divided into two groups, based on resectability of the esophageal carcinoma. Group A included 64 patients, all of whom underwent subtotal esophagectomy after preoperative hyperthermia with or without chemotherapy and radiation. Group B included 50 patients, all of

whom had a nonresectable carcinoma and who underwent HCR therapy alone or were given hyperthermia combined with chemotherapy or irradiation.

In the 64 group A patients, with a resectable esophageal carcinoma, preoperative hyperthermia was given for 3 weeks at 3 or 4-day intervals, to a total of six times, in the range from 42° to 44° C for 30 minutes. In the 50 in group B, esophagectomy was impossible because of far-advanced carcinoma or poor general clinical status. Combined therapy was continued as long as possible. The average doses of irradiation and hyperthermia were 46.6 Gy and 12.5 times, respectively.

As for chemotherapy, bleomycin, cisplatin, and FT-207 were the agents mainly prescribed and were selected by the attending physicians in each institute.

Clinical efficacy, based on tumor regression determined by esophagograms and endoscopic findings, was assessed according to the guidelines for clinical and pathologic studies of solid tumors.[6] Histologic studies of the resected specimens were based on specific defined criteria.[7]

RESULTS

Tumor regression was evaluated by esophagograms in surgical cases, and the total response rate was 51.7% (complete response in 4 of 58; partial response in 26 of 58) (see Table 42-1). For nonresectable cases, the total response rate as evaluated by esophagograms was 70.5% (complete response in 10 of 44; partial response in 21 of 44).

However, the objective total response rate as evaluated by endoscopic findings in group A pa-

*Kureha Chemical Industry Co., Ltd., Tokyo, Japan.

337

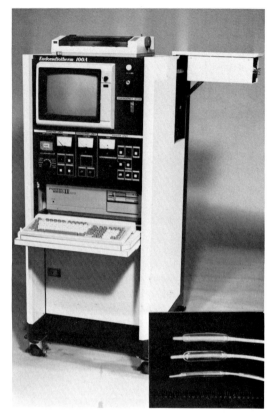

Fig. 42-1. The Endoradiotherm 100A unit and *(inset)* the endotract electrodes for radiofrequency.

tients was 75.4% (complete response in 11 of 57; partial response in 32 of 57). The efficacy as evaluated by endoscopic findings in cases of group B was complete response in 15 of 47 (31.9%) and partial response in 25 of 47 (53.2%), the total response rate being 85.1%.

As to the histopathologic study of resected specimens, the therapy given to those in whom viable neoplastic cells were completely destroyed was defined as "markedly effective" (Ef$_3$),[7] and that for patients in whom most of cancer cells were extensively damaged, despite the presence of some viable cells, was defined as "moderately effective" (Ef$_2$). For all others, the therapy was categorized as "ineffective" (Ef$_1$).

In 64 group A patients, there was a marked effect (Ef$_3$) in 13 (20.3%), a moderate effect (Ef$_2$) in 31 (48.4%), and no effect (Ef$_1$) in 20 (31.3%).

DISCUSSION

Basic studies have clarified that hyperthermia has an antitumor effect. Whether or not hyper-

thermia will serve as an effective treatment against cancer depends entirely on a device capable of heating an appropriate anatomic site to an appropriate temperature, together with the development of techniques capable of accurately measuring the temperature distribution in the region.

We have devised the ERT 100A for treating esophageal carcinoma. The setup consists of a flexible "endotract electrode" with thermosensors, and an extracorporeal electrode. The endotract electrode, with a small surface area, is a slender cylinder inserted into the esophagus through the oral cavity; the extracorporeal electrode, with a large surface area, is placed directly on the chest wall of the patient. In case of radiofrequency capacitive coupling, the RF wide electrode on the body surface concentrates the electromagnetic flux near the intraluminal applicator because of differences in the surface area between these electrodes.

To date, a total of 114 patients with carcinoma of the esophagus have been treated with hyperthermia, using this heating system. In patients from whom the carcinoma of the esophagus was excised, we have confirmed histopathologically that all viable cancer cells were completely destroyed in 13 out of 64 cases (20.3%). Most of the cancer cells in 31 other patients (48.4%) were extensively damaged.

In contrast Iizuka et al.[8] stated in their cooperative report that preoperative combined therapy with 45 mg of bleomycin and 30 Gy of ^{60}Co given to 79 patients resulted in complete destruction of cancer cells in seven (8.9%), and in 37 (46.8%) the cancer cells were extensively damaged.

The ERT 100A, involving use of an endotract antenna, is available for treating other types of malignancies, such as colorectal carcinoma or carcinoma of the uterine cervix. Further related clinical studies are underway using this inexpensive, easy-to-apply equipment for treating malignant tumors. The results that have been presented in this interim report may lead toward more potent treatment of deeply located malignant tumors.

SUMMARY

Hyperthermia combined with irradiation and chemotherapy has significantly enhanced the antitumor effects of the latter two modalities. The Endoradiotherm 100A system induced no severe

TABLE 42-1. Objective responses

Modality	Complete response	Partial response	No change	Progressive disease
Evaluated by esophagogram				
Group A* (58 cases)	4 (6.9%)	26 (44.8%)	28 (48.3%)	0
Group B* (44 cases)	10 (22.7%)	21 (47.7%)	12 (27.3%)	1 (2.3%)
Evaluated by endoscopy				
Group A† (57 cases)	11 (19.3%)	32 (56.1%)	14 (24.6%)	0
Group B‡ (47 cases)	15 (31.9%)	25 (53.2%)	7 (14.9%)	0

*Evaluation was impossible in 6 cases each.
†Evaluation was impossible in 7 cases.
‡Evaluation was impossible in 3 cases.

side effects in patients with carcinoma of the esophagus.*

REFERENCES

1. Manning, M.R., Cetas, T.C., Miller, R.C., Oleson, J.R., Conner, W.G., and Gerner, E.W.: Clinical hyperthermia: results of a phase I trial employing hyperthermia alone or in combination with external beam or interstitial radiotherapy, Cancer **49**:205, 1982.

2. Hahn, G.M.: Potential for therapy of drugs and hyperthermia, Cancer Res. **39**:2264, 1979.

3. Sugimachi, K., et al.: Endotract antenna for application of hyperthermia to malignant lesions, Gann **74**:104, 1983.

4. Sugimachi, K., et al.: Preoperative hyperthermo-chemoradiotherapy effective for carcinoma of the esophagus, J. Surg. Oncol. **27**:199-204, 1984.

5. Sugimachi, K., et al.: Hyperthermia for patients with esophageal carcinoma: a multi-institutional interim report, J. Jpn. Soc. Cancer Ther. (In press.) (With English abstract.)

6. Koyama, Y.: Hexylcarbamoyl-5-fluorouracil (HCFU) masked 5-fluorinated pyrimidine, Cancer Treat. Rev. **8**:147, 1981.

7. Japanese Society of Esophageal Diseases: Guidelines for the clinical and pathological studies on carcinoma of the esophagus, Jpn. J. Surg. **6**:69, 1976.

8. Iizuka, T., et al. (Co-operative clinical study group for esophageal carcinoma): Preliminary report on multidisciplinary treatment for esophageal carcinoma, Jpn. J. Clin. Oncol. **10**:215, 1980.

*EDITOR'S NOTE: This report is indeed *interim*. Hyperthermia has been used with or without chemotherapy, but no attempt has been made to distinguish the results. As with all adjuvant therapy, there is a need for randomized studies so that the contributions (or lack thereof) of each element in the protocol can be assessed. Dr. Sugimachi reports that he soon will have "sufficient cases to evaluate the effectiveness of hyperthermia only" (letter of January 21, 1988).

CHAPTER 43

Postoperative long-term immunochemotherapy

Kaichi Isono, Shoichi Onoda, and Takenori Ochiai

It has been observed that the immunologic status of esophageal cancer patients is depressed as a result of both age and malnutrition. In addition, it becomes profoundly depressed by standard therapy: surgical operation, radiation, and/or chemotherapy. Therefore, using immunotherapy for immunodepressed esophageal cancer patients seems rational. We have introduced immunotherapeutic drugs such as PSK, CWS, and bestatin for treatment of esophageal cancer, beginning in 1975. This chapter describes the immunotherapeutic and chemotherapeutic drugs used for treatment of esophageal cancer and the results of their clinical use.

ADJUVANT AGENTS USED FOR ESOPHAGEAL CANCER TREATMENT
Immunotherapeutic agents

Immunotherapeutic agents include PSK, CWS, and bestatin.

PSK. PSK is a protein-bound polysaccharide extracted from mecelia, CM101. It contains 18% to 38% protein, and its molecular weight is approximately 100,000. Given by mouth, it may return the depressed immunologic status to a normal level and shows a host-mediated anticancer effect. Following various basic experiments, it was introduced clinically.[1] It was reported that negative skin tests of the patients were changed to positive and that patient survival rates were improved.

CWS. CWS was first prepared from the cell wall of *Mycobacterium* by Yamamura et al.[2] They showed that the cell wall fraction of the bacilli, a residue after removal of protein and lipid, contains an immunopotentiating activity. The substance was designated as cell wall skeleton (CWS). Later, they found that the CWS of *Nocardia rubra* has effects similar to those of the

CWS of *Mycobacterium*. Culturing *Nocardia* is somewhat easier than culturing *Mycobacterium*, and therefore CWS of *Nocardia* has been applied clinically.

Bestatin. Bestatin was first discovered by Umezawa et al.[3] It is a low-molecular-weight substance whose activity is to modify the immunologic capacity of the patient. The mechanism of action of bestatin is that by binding with aminopeptidase-B leucine aminopeptidase of the cell membrane of immunocompetent cells, it changes the nature of cell membranes and modifies immunologic responses. It was reported that bestatin augments the delayed type of skin reactions, NK cell activity, and interleukin II production. An antitumor effect was also demonstrated.

Chemotherapeutic agents

Chemotherapeutic agents used include bleomycin, peplomycin, and cisplatin.

Bleomycin. Bleomycin (BLM) is an anticancer antibiotic prepared by Umezawa et al.[4] from *Streptomyces verticillis*. The mechanism of the anticancer effect of BLM is by amputation of DNA chains and inhibition of DNA synthesis. It is usually given to patients intravenously or intramuscularly in physiologic saline solution. BLM is also used in various oil emulsion, ointment, suppository, and solid forms. It is indicated only for squamous cell carcinoma and malignant lymphoma.

Peplomycin. Peplomycin (PEP) is a derivative of BLM and has a structure of a dehydration bond of carbonic acid and *N*-(3-aminopropyl)-2-phenethylamine. Its anticancer activity is stronger than that of BLM. The side effects of PEP are similar to those of BLM, but pulmonary fibrosis is less frequent than with BLM.

Cisplatin. Cisplatin (CDDP) was discovered by B. Rosenbery at the University of Michigan in 1965. Clinical research has been conducted by the U.S. National Cancer Institute. This agent has strong anticancer effects but also frequent nephrotoxicity. CDDP is considered cytotoxic by virtue of its bindings of DNA.

CLINICAL EFFECT OF PREOPERATIVE COMBINED IMMUNOCHEMOTHERAPY

Nakayama et al.[5] and Cliffton[5a] attempted to improve resectability and patient survival rate of esophageal cancer patients by providing preoperative radiation. Since that time we have performed preoperative combined therapy as routine treatment in our department. The results of preoperative combined therapy have been categorized in degrees of effectiveness.[6] "Highly effective" indicates that no live cancer cells are found in the specimen histologically. "Slightly effective" and "ineffective" mean that live cancer cells are present in less than one third and more than one third, respectively, of the specimen.[7] With preoperative combined therapy, highly effective findings were present more often than the other categories.

The best way to observe the effect of preoperative immunochemotherapy on the cancer cells is study of the specimen taken at the surgical operation. Soon after BLM was introduced clinically, we set up a protocol in which 120 to 300 mg of BLM was given preoperatively and the specimen was observed histologically to evaluate the effect of BLM. Slightly effective results were found in 20% and ineffective results in 80% of cases. There were no highly effective results with BLM alone. Pulmonary fibrosis was a troublesome side effect of BLM and prevented use of BLM alone preoperatively. A new protocol of combination of preoperative radiation and BLM was developed. In this protocol, the dose of BLM was reduced to 75 to 100 mg, 7.5 to 10 mg/day given intramuscularly, to minimize pulmonary fibrosis. PEP later replaced BLM, at 5 mg/day.

The immunotherapeutic agents, PSK, CWS, and bestatin, were introduced to clinical use in 1975, 1976, and 1978, respectively, and a new protocol was devised as a preoperative combined therapy of radiation with immunochemotherapy (Fig. 43-1).

The first protocol of radiation alone, the second protocol of radiation plus chemotherapy, and the third protocol of radiation plus immunochemotherapy were performed in the patients during the same period. Comparison of the clinical results of the three protocols was not made by strictly controlled methods but by historical study. Radiation alone was given to 93 patients, and its effective rate was 45%. Radiation plus chemotherapy was given to 57 patients, and its effective rate was 70%. Radiation plus immunochemotherapy was given to 56 patients, and its effective rate was 73%; highly effective findings were as high as 30%, compared with 13% and 23% for the other groups (see Table 43-1). These results indicated that radiation and chemotherapy plus immunotherapy produced the best preoperative treatment results for esophageal cancer.

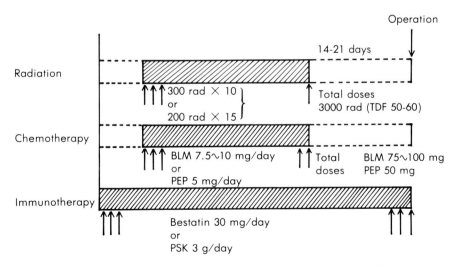

Fig. 43-1. Protocol of preoperative combined treatment for esophageal cancer.

TABLE 43-1. Effect of preoperative therapy for primary lesion of esophageal cancer (TDF $\geq$ 50), 1968-1985, Department of Surgery, Chiba University

	No. of cases	Not effective or slightly effective	Effective	Highly effective
Radiation (TDF $\geq$ 50)	93	51 (55%)	30 (32%)	12 (13%)
Radiation + chemotherapy	57	17 (30%)	27 (47%)	13 (23%)
Radiation + chemotherapy + immunotherapy	56	15 (27%)	24 (43%)	17 (30%)
Bleomycin alone (120-300 mg)	10	8 (80%)	2 (20%)	0

IMMUNOCHEMOTHERAPY IN COMBINED POSTOPERATIVE TREATMENT

It is generally accepted that there is a limited effectiveness of anticancer drugs when patients have a large mass of primary tumor in esophageal cancer. Greater effectiveness might be expected after a large tumor mass is reduced by surgery. In these cases postoperative combined therapy with anticancer drugs has been applied.

Effect of bestatin

A randomized clinical study was performed in a cooperative fashion in 20 institutions in Japan, from June, 1980, through March, 1982, to evaluate the effect of bestatin on the survival rate of esophageal cancer patients.[8] The patients were allocated either to a bestatin-treated group or to a non-bestatin-treated group by a double-blind method. Bestatin was started postoperatively, 30 mg/day, and continued as long as possible. Statistical differences in the patient survival rate curves of all observation periods between the two treatment groups were tested by generalized Wilcoxon test (GW) and Cox-Mantel test (CM), and statistical differences at each postoperative point in time were calculated by Greenwood method (G). Patient survival rates for all resectable cases were not statistically different between the two groups by GW, and they were slightly different by CM (see Fig. 43-2). When comparison was made in the patients receiving preoperative therapy, a statistical difference of both survival rate curves was seen by GW (see Fig. 43-3) and also at 4, 6, 7, and 8 postoperative months by G.

Preoperative radiation or chemotherapy suppressed lymphocyte counts, B cell counts, PHA blastogenesis, and PPD skin test, and increased T cell counts.[9] Bestatin had a favorable effect in these immunosuppressed cases and increased patient survival.

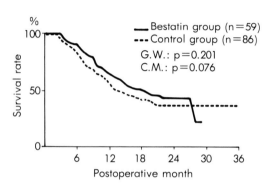

Fig. 43-2. Survival rates of postoperative esophageal cancer patients treated with bestatin (Japanese multicenter study).

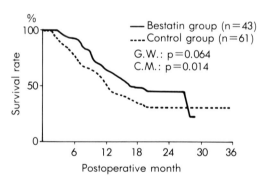

Fig.43-3. Survival rates in patients treated with bestatin and receiving preoperative treatment (Japanese multicenter study).

The effect of bestatin on the patient survival rate was compared in early, intermediate, and advanced stages. The "early" stage meant that cancer was confined within the adventitia of the esophagus and lymph node metastasis was limited to the regional nodes. The "intermediate" stage

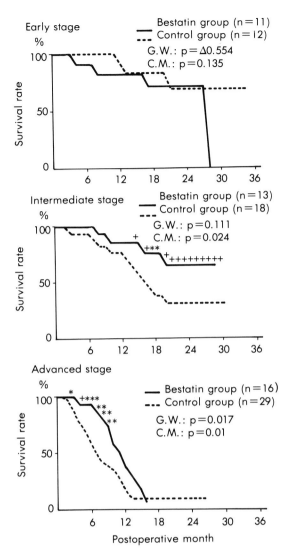

Fig. 43-4. Survival rates for patients treated with bestatin, according to stage of esophageal cancer (Japanese multicenter study).

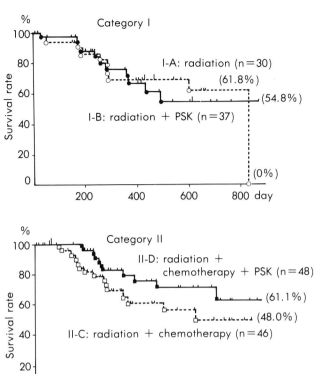

Fig. 43-5. Patient survival rates in Japanese Krestin Study Group. Of a total of 171 patients entering trial, 161 reported here (10 patients dropped out or died of other disease). Follow-up rate, 99.4%.

meant that cancer expanded beyond the adventitia and/or lymph node metastases were present outside of regional nodes and that both of them were curatively resected. The "advanced" stage meant that cancer invaded other organs, or that lymph node metastases were not completely removable, or that blood-borne metastasis was observed. Bestatin was effective in the intermediate and advanced stages (see Fig. 43-4).

Both the immunologic status and the nutritional status were depressed by advanced cancer. Bestatin was helpful in improving the general status of immunosuppressed patients.

Effect of PSK

It has been obvious that the depressed immunologic capacity of esophageal cancer patients is further compromised by radiation. A multicenter clinical trial has also been done to evaluate PSK in these patients.[10]

In the trial, the patients were divided into one of four treatment groups. The patients of group IA received postoperative radiation alone, the patients of group IB received radiation and PSK, the patients of group IIC received radiation and chemotherapy, and the patients of group IID received radiation, chemotherapy, and PSK. Eligibility criteria for inclusion in the study were as follows: more than 2000 rad of radiation; administration of PSK, 3 g/day, for more than 3 months; and more than 45 mg of BLM or 600 mg/day of tegafur for more than 3 months. The trial continues in progress. The observation period is rather short so far. However, a trend has been observed by statistical testing by Kaplan-Meier method (see Fig. 43-5) of the effectiveness

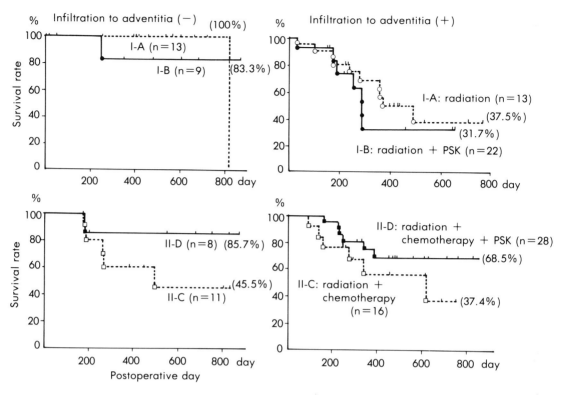

Fig. 43-6. Survival rates of patients with and without cancer infiltration to the adventitia of the esophagus (Japanese Krestin Study Group).

of PSK. The results showed that survival rates at 800 days were 61.8% in IA, 54.8% in IB, 48.0% in IIC, and 61.1% in IID. the survival rate for patients receiving radiation and chemotherapy (IIC) was the poorest. The result indicated that treatment with radiation and chemotherapy was insufficient because they depress the general condition or immunologic status of the patient. The importance of immunotherapy was indirectly suggested by this result.

Patient survival was measured in relation to infiltration to the adventitia or lymph node metastasis. In both situations, the patients receiving radiation and chemotherapy had the poorest survival rates. Administration of PSK as immunotherapy improved the survival rates (see Figs. 43-6 and 43-7).

Immunotherapy and long-term results

The data shown in Figs. 43-2 to 43-7 were the results of multicenter cooperative study. Patient background factors, such as operative procedures and postoperative care, are slightly different among the institutions. In addition, observation periods of the studies are not yet long enough. In light of these facts, the results obtained in our

department will be described as a single-center trial.

Curative resection cases. Postoperative immunotherapy for curative resection cases (in which removal of primary cancer and regional lymph nodes is completely performed) is a form of adjuvant therapy. Should undectable cancer cells be left at a microscopic level, treatment with anticancer drugs could be capable of inhibiting growth of the residual cancer cells.

At the Department of Surgery, Chiba University, a total of 137 esophageal cancer patients underwent curative resection in the 11 years between 1975 and 1985. The 5-year survival rate for 71 patients who did not receive postoperative immunotherapy was 27.3%, and that for 66 patients receiving postoperative immunotherapy, such as PSK, bestatin, or CWS, was 37.4%. The difference was statistically significant ($p < 0.05$) (see Fig. 43-8).

Even in the curative resection cases, many patients died from recurrent carcinoma. In these cases of relapse, the periods between operation and relapse and between relapse and death were 17.4 months and 11.8 months for the immunotherapy group (28 cases) and 14.2 months and 4.1 months for the non-immunotherapy group (21

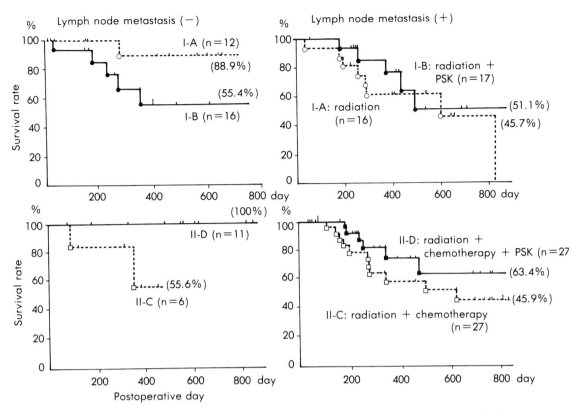

Fig. 43-7. Survival rates of patients with and without lymph node metastasis (Japanese Krestin Study Group).

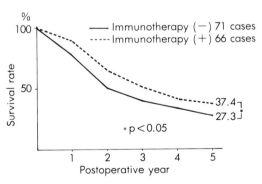

Fig. 43-8. Immunotherapy and survival rates of patients with resectable esophageal cancer (curative resection cases), 1975 to 1985, Department of Surgery, Chiba University.

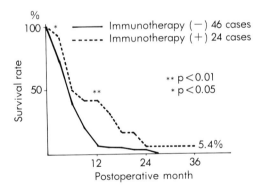

Fig. 43-9. Immunotherapy and survival rate of patients with resectable esophageal cancer (noncurative resection cases), 1975 to 1985, Department of Surgery, Chiba University.

cases). These results show that postoperative immunotherapy was effective in prolonging both the interval before relapse and the survival time after relapse.

Noncurative resection cases. We have already stated that bestatin was effective in advanced cases. In noncurative resection cases, immuno-

therapeutic agents, including bestatin, PSK, and CWS, brought similar results. With the use of immunotherapy, the 1-year survival rate improved from 5.1% to 41%. However, the 2-year survival rate was only 5.4%, even in the immunotherapy group. This illustrates a limitation of effectiveness of immunotherapy (see Fig. 43-9).

Present status of postoperative chemotherapy

Bleomycin was introduced clinically with much expectation in 1968. However, the effectiveness for squamous cell carcinoma of the esophagus was less than for the squamous cell carcinoma of the skin. In addition to side effects of fever, liver dysfunction, and alopecia, a major problem with pulmonary fibrosis was reported. For that reason BLM is no longer used for long-term adjuvant therapy.

At a present time, BLM is used for preoperative combined therapy or for postoperative short-term treatment only.

Peplomycin was expected to be more effective than BLM and to have fewer side effects, especially the pulmonary fibrosis. However, it proved not so effective as BLM, and side effects also occur. Therefore, it has not been used for long-term treatment either.

Cisplatin has a potent anticancer effect. However, because of severe side effects, such as nephrotoxicity, nausea, and myelosuppression, introduction to clinical use was delayed. Recently, it has been used for advanced malignant cases and for noncurative resection cases, with much careful attention to its side effects. It is too early to evaluate the effectiveness of CDDP at the present time.

Recently, new drugs have been receiving consideration in clinical trials, and drugs that had been regarded as ineffective for squamous cell carcinoma have been reevaluated. Combined treatment with tegafur, which is effective for adenocarcinoma, is as effective as BLM when they are used with radiation.[11] In our multicenter PSK trial, tegafur was used alternately with BLM, and the results in the group receiving either BLM or tegafur are better than the results in the other treatment group.

CONCLUSIONS

1. With the addition of immunochemotherapy, the effectiveness of preoperative radiotherapy has improved.
2. Postoperative immunotherapy has prolonged both the period between operation and relapse and the survival period after relapse.
3. An effectiveness of immunochemotherapy has been observed in advanced cases.
4. Anticancer chemotherapeutic agents effective for esophageal cancer have major side effects and are not appropriate for long-term adjuvant therapy.

REFERENCES

1. Ito, K.: Krestin, Cancer and chemotherapy **4**:425, 1977. (In Japanese.)
2. Azuma, I., et al.: Anti-tumor activity of cell wall skeltons and peptidoglycolipids of mycobacteria and related microorganisms, Gann **65**:493, 1974.
3. Umezawa, H., et al.: Bestatin, and inhibition of aminopeptidase B, produced by actinomyces, J. Antibiot. **29**:97, 1976.
4. Umezawa, H., et al.: New antibiotics, bleomycin A and B, J. Antibiot. **19A**:200, 1966.
5. Nakayama, K., et al.: Preoperative radiation for esophageal cancer. GEKA **22**:325, 1960. (In Japanese.)
5a. Cliffton, E.E., Goodner, J.T., Bronstein, E.: Preoperative irradiation for cancer of the esophagus, Cancer **13**:37, 1960.
6. Isono, K., et al.: Preoperative radiation for esophageal cancer and patient outcome, Surgical Treatment **30**:245, 1974. (In Japanese.)
7. Japanese Society for Esophageal Diseases: Guide lines for the clinical and pathologic studies for carcinoma of the esophagus, Jpn. J. Surg. **6**:79, 1976.
8. Sato, H., et al.: Effect of bestatin on primary tumor and prognosis in patient with esophageal carcinoma, J. Jpn. Soc. Cancer **19**(10):2312, 1984.
9. Saito, T., et al.: Factors of suppression of cellular immunology in esophageal cancer patients, J. Jpn. Soc. Clin. Surg. **47**:1, 1986. (In Japanese.)
10. Esophageal Cancer Krestin Study Group: Effect of Krestin on esophageal cancer, J. Jpn. Soc. Cancer Ther. **20**:1704, 1985. (In Japanese.)
11. Co-operative Clinical Study Group of Esophageal Carcinoma: Preliminary report on multidisciplinary treatment for esophageal carcinoma, Jpn. J. Clin. Oncol. **10**:215, 1980.

DISCUSSION—Chapters 40 to 43

Michael Burt and Manjit S. Bains

Standard therapy for esophageal carcinoma has been surgery or radiation therapy. Surgical resection has yielded 5-year survival rates of 0 to 21%[1]; curative radiation therapy, 0 to 20%.[2] In general, 5-year survival rates in the Western hemisphere have been under 10% whether treatment has been surgery or radiation therapy, or both. Because the outlook for patients with localized esophageal carcinoma has historically been less than satisfactory by standard treatment methods, investigators have attempted to combine standard surgical resection with preoperative and/or postoperative adjuvant therapy. The adjuvant therapy has included chemotherapy, radiation therapy, immunotherapy, or hyperthermia, either alone or in combination.

PREOPERATIVE CHEMOTHERAPY

Memorial Sloan-Kettering Cancer Center has investigated the use of preoperative chemotherapy followed by surgical resection in patients with operable squamous cell carcinoma of the esophagus.[3-8] The report by Dr. Kelsen (Chapter 40) in this volume summarizes the experience with preoperative chemotherapy and surgery. Similar reports are summarized in Table 1. Almost all investigators are utilizing a cisplatin-based regimen in their preoperative chemotherapy protocols. After completion of chemotherapy, the operability rates range from 59% to 100%. Of greater note are the resectability rates of 35% to 90%, with most of the series in the range of 70% to 80%. These data, however, are not dissimilar from the data presented by Earlham and Cunha-Melo in their collective review of surgery for 83,783 patients with squamous cell carcinoma of the esophagus.[14] Their review determined an overall operability rate of 58% and an overall resectability rate of 39%. Therefore, 66% of operable patients were resected.*

Survival advantages from preoperative chemotherapy may or may not materialize as the

series noted in Table 1 are analyzed with passage of more time. Dr. Kelsen has reviewed the data from Memorial Sloan-Kettering Cancer Center; the median duration of survival for all 34 patients was 16.2 months. This appears to be slightly better than the 10- to 12-month median survival with surgery alone,[14] but the number of patients does not allow a definitive answer.

PREOPERATIVE CHEMOTHERAPY AND RADIATION

The results of five series of patients with squamous cell carcinoma of the esophagus treated preoperatively with chemotherapy and radiation therapy are summarized in Table 2. Dr. Steiger reviews the experience at Wayne State University in Chapter 41. Two such studies are included in Table 2.[16,18] He then summarizes the Southwest Oncology Group study of 106 patients treated utilizing the Wayne State University protocol, but with a reduction of cisplatin dose from 100 to 75 mg/m². Of 102 patients completing preoperative therapy, 71 (70%) were deemed operable. Of these, 77% (55 of 71) were resectable, with an operative mortality of 11%. The median survival for the 71 patients undergoing surgery was 14 months. These results are comparable to two published Wayne State University reports,[16,18] with operability following preoperative chemotherapy and radiation therapy in the range of 70% to 90% and resectability rates of 70% to 100%. In the previous study with 5-fluorouracil and cisplatin,[18] the median survival was 18 months in the 21 patients studied. With a large number of patients, Dr. Steiger reports a median survival of 14 months in the 71 patients undergoing surgery.

• • •

It appears from Tables 1 and 2 that the results of preoperative chemotherapy alone and with preoperative radiation therapy are similar with regard to resectability, mortality, and survival rates. Although it is difficult to compare the results of these studies with surgery or radiation therapy alone,

---

*EDITOR'S NOTE: The reader is advised to look critically at the Earlham–Cunha-Melo data.

TABLE 1. Preoperative chemotherapy

Drug*	No.	Operable No. (%)	Resectable No. (%)	Mortality No. (%)	Median Survival (mo)
CDDP–5-FU[9]	24	22 (92)	19/24 (79)	1/22 (5)	NS
CDDP-Bleo[8]	34	34 (100)	26/34 (76)	4/34 (11)	10
Bleo[10]	19	NS	10/19 (53)	1/10 (10)	NS
CDPP–5-FU[11]	17	10/17 (59)	6/17 (35)	0/6 (0)	NS
CDPP-Bleo-VDS[6]	34	34/34 (100)	28/34 (82)	3/34 (9)	18.5
CDPP-VDS-MFBG[12]	14	13/14 (93)	12/14 (86)	1/12 (8)	NS
CDPP* (5-FU or VBL)[13]	20	18/20 (90)	18/20 (90)	1/18 (6)	NS

*CDDP, Cisplatin; 5-FU, fluorouracil; bleo, bleomycin; VDS, vindesine; VBL, vinblastine; MGBG, mitoguazone; NS, not stated.
†Two treated with 5-FU, three with VBL.

TABLE 2. Preoperative chemotherapy and radiation therapy

Drug*	Radiation (rad)	No.	Operable No. (%)	Resectable No. (%)	Treatment Mortality (%)	Survival (mo)
MTX[15]	2000	93	55/93 (59)	NS	14	26†
5-FU–MITO[16]	3000	30	23/30 (77)	23/23 (100)	17	12‡
Bleo[17]	3000	65	38/65 (58)	24/38 (63)	12	6‡
Bleo[10]	3000	68	NS	48/68 (71)	12	NS
5-FU–CDDP[18]	3000	21	19/21 (90)	15/19 (79)	27	18‡

MTX, Methotrexate; 5-FU, fluorouracil; Mito, mitomycin C; bleo, bleomycin; CDDP, cisplatin; NS, not stated.
†Mean.
‡Median.

it does not appear that preoperative therapy has greatly affected survival in patients with localized squamous cell carcinoma of the esophagus. One may argue that preoperative chemotherapy with or without radiation therapy must still be considered experimental.

PREOPERATIVE HYPERTHERMIA

Drs. Sugimachi, Matsufuji, and Kai (Chapter 42) report a novel preoperative modality for patients with primary esophageal carcinoma—the use of hyperthermia with or without chemotherapy and radiation therapy. Utilizing radiofrequency energies by means of a slender electrode placed into the esophagus and a larger electrode placed on the chest, they generate hyperthermia of the esophagus, although no temperature measurements are reported.

Sixty-four patients with operable carcinoma of the esophagus underwent this protocol, receiving hyperthermia for 3 weeks at 3- to 4-day intervals. Chemotherapy included bleomycin, cisplatin, and FT-207 at the discretion of the attending physician. The dosages of drugs are not stated, nor is the amount of preoperative radiation therapy. For this group the total response rate was 52% when evaluated by esophagogram and 75% when evaluated by endoscopic findings. Histologic examination of resected specimens in this group revealed completely destroyed carcinoma in 20%. A second group, consisting of 50 patients deemed nonresectable, demonstrated similar roentgenographic and endoscopic response rates.

Although this modality has potential benefit for patients with localized esophageal carcinoma, the data currently presented do not allow analytic dissection of the effects of hyperthermia versus those of chemotherapy and radiation. In addition, we do not have data demonstrating a survival benefit from this form of preoperative therapy. More appealing is the use of this modality as palliation in those patients with inoperable carcinoma of the esophagus. Again, however, we do not know whether the effects demonstrated by esophagograms or endoscopy are secondary to hyperthermia or to the chemotherapy and radiation therapy.

POSTOPERATIVE LONG-TERM IMMUNOCHEMOTHERAPY

Drs. Isono, Onoda, and Ochiai (Chapter 43) report experience with both preoperative and postoperative immunochemotherapy. In a preoperative study they demonstrated complete eradication of viable carcinoma cells in 13% of those receiving preoperative radiation therapy (3000 rad), 23% of those with radiation plus chemotherapy (bleomycin or peplomycin), and 30% of those with radiation therapy, chemotherapy, and immunotherapy (PSK or bestatin). Although sterilization of tumor by preoperative therapy and then proceeding to resection has theoretical advantages, there are no conclusive data that this translates into long-term survival.

The authors relate their experience at the Department of Surgery, Chiba University, in the evaluation of 137 patients with esophageal carcinoma after a curative resection in the 10 years between 1975 and 1985. Seventy-one patients received no further therapy, with a 5-year survival of 27.3%. Sixty-six patients received postoperative immunotherapy (PSK, bestatin, or CWS), with a 5-year survival of 37.4%, a significant difference ($p < 0.05$). Although it appears that postoperative immunotherapy may improve long-term survival, the two groups of patients may not be comparable, which is often the case with retrospective analyses. The authors admit that their data were extracted from a larger multicenter operative study and therefore may not be controlled for patient characteristics. However, the marked difference in 5-year survival between the two groups deserves further investigations to determine if postoperative immunotherapy is efficacious and, if so, which agents are best.

REFERENCES

1. Cukingnan, R.A., and Carey, J.S.: Carcinoma of the esophagus, Ann. Thorac. Surg. **26:**274, 1982.
2. Hancock, S.L., and Glatstein, E.: Radiation therapy of esophageal cancer, Semin. Oncol. **11:**144, 1984.
3. Kelsen, D.P., Cvitkovic, E., Bains, M., et al.: Cis-dichlorodiammineplatinum (II) and bleomycin in the treatment of esophageal carcinoma, Cancer Treat Rep. **62:**1041, 1978.
4. Kelsen, D.P., Ahuja, R., Hopfan, S., et al.: Combined modality therapy of esophageal carcinoma, Cancer **48:**31, 1981.
5. Kelsen, D.P., Bains, M., Chapman, R., et al.: Cisplatin, vindesine, and bleomycin (DVB) combination chemotherapy for esophageal carcinoma, Cancer Treat Rep. **65:**781, 1981.
6. Bains, M.S., Kelsen, D.P., Beattie, E.J., Jr., et al.: Treatment of esophageal carcinoma by combined preoperative chemotherapy, Ann. Thorac. Surg. **34:**521, 1982.
7. Kelsen, D., Hilaris, B., Coonley, C., et al.: Cisplatin, vindesine, and bleomycin chemotherapy of local-regional and advanced esophageal carcinoma, Am. J. Med. **75:**645, 1983.
8. Coonley, C.J., Bains, M., Hilaris, B., et al.: Cisplatin and bleomycin in the treatment of esophageal carcinoma: a final report, Cancer **54:**2351, 1984.
9. Carey, R.W., Hilgenberg, A.D., Wilkins, E.W., et al.: Preoperative chemotherapy followed by surgery with possible postoperative radiotherapy in squamous cell carcinoma of the esophagus: evlauation of the chemotherapy component, J. Clin. Oncol. **4:**697, 1986.
10. Fujimaki, M., Soga, J., Karoogluchii, M., et al.: Role of preoperative administration of bleomycin and radiation in the treatment of esophageal cancer, Jpn. J. Surg. **5:**45, 1975.
11. Shields, T.W., Rosen, S.T., Hellerstein, S.M., et al.: Multimodality approach to treatment of carcinoma of the esophagus, Arch. Surg. **119:**558, 1984.
12. Kelsen, D.P., Fein, R., Coonley, C., et al.: Cisplatin, vindesine, and mitoguazone in the treatment of esophageal cancer, Cancer Treat. Rep. **70:**255, 1986.
13. Miller, J.I., McIntyre, B., and Hatcher, C.R.: Combined treatment approach in surgical management of carcinoma of the esophagus: a preliminary report, Ann. Thorac. Surg. **40:**289, 1985.
14. Earlham, R., and Cunha-Melo, J.R.: Oesophageal squamous cell carcinoma: a critical review of surgery, Br. J. Surg. **67:**381, 1980.
15. Werner, I.D.: The multidisciplinary approach in the management of squamous cell carcinoma of the esophagus, Front. Gastrointest. Res. **5:**130, 135, 1979.
16. Franklin, R., Steiger, Z., Vaishampayan, G., et al.: Combined modality therapy for esophageal squamous cell carcinoma, Cancer **51:**1062, 1983.
17. Andersen, A.P., Berdal, P., Edsmyr, F., et al.: Irradiation, chemotherapy, and surgery in esophageal cancer: a randomized clinical study, Radiother. Oncol. **2:**179, 1984.
18. Leichman, L., Steiger, Z., Seydel, H.G., et al.: Preoperative chemotherapy and radiation therapy for patients with cancer of the esophagus: a potentially curative approach, J. Clin. Oncol. **2:**75, 1984.

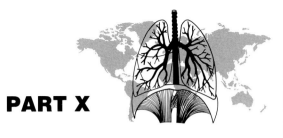

PART X

PALLIATIVE MANAGEMENT OF ADVANCED (NONRESECTABLE AND INOPERABLE) DISEASE

CHAPTER 44 The relative merits of definitive radiotherapy and palliative resection

Noah C. Choi

The natural history of carcinoma of the esophagus has not been altered by current therapeutic methods, and therefore any reported cure rate over 10% is a reflection of patient selection rather than improved therapeutic factors.[1,2] Because so few patients, except a small subset with early-stage carcinomas (T_1 lesion), can expect long-term survival, the primary therapeutic objective is palliation, with cure being an important but secondary goal. It has not been a simple matter to achieve even a sustained palliation of dysphagia that will last more than 6 months by either surgery or radiation. The tragic death of a patient as a result of palliative procedures becomes tolerable only if it is balanced by a very appreciable expectation of gain in improved survival. Recent advances in the frontier of preoperative therapy with a combination of multidrug chemotherapy and radiation or multidrug chemotherapy alone have been encouraging, and improved survival for even advanced locoregional carcinoma (T_2, T_3, and N_1 lesions) might be obtainable in the near future.[3-6] The management of esophageal carcinoma will undergo major revision over the next 5 to 10 years, and therefore a brief discussion of the role of radiation for this carcinoma is timely and necessary.

Surgery for esophageal carcinoma is judged incomplete, according to the definition of an operation for cancer, if there are nonresectable vital structures in immediate contact with the esophageal wall, thus precluding the resection of enough normal tissue to make a clean margin. This anatomic restriction for a radical cancer operation, coupled with a high operative mortality rate (15% to 20%), has allowed radiation to be a better therapeutic alternative for the upper two thirds of the esophagus.[7] However, radiotherapy has its own limitations. The long term survival ($\geq$5 years) rate has been only 5% to 10%, even with the maximum tolerable dose of radiation of 6000 to 6600 cGy, although a sustained palliation of dysphagia has been appreciated by the majority of patients. Approximately 60% to 70% of these patients, even after definitive radiotherapy, continue to have persistent uncontrolled or recurrent locoregional carcinoma leading to recurrent dysphagia. Biologic reasons for this poor control of locoregional carcinoma with radiation include the fact that the carcinoma is large and contains a high component of hypoxic tumor cells, the limited tolerance of intrathoracic vital structures to radiation, and the patient's poor general condition. Autopsy studies, before the era of definitive treatments, indicated that an inverse relationship was noted between the length of the esophagus involved by the carcinoma and the potential curability.[8] When the carcinoma was 5 cm or less in length, it was localized in approximately 41% of patients, locally advanced in 23%, and distantly metastasized in 36%. When the size of the carcinoma exceeded 5 cm, as determined by pathologic examination, the carcinoma was localized in only 10% of patients, locally advanced in 14%, and distantly metastasized in 76%. On the basis of these autopsy data, there is still a 10% to 24% chance of a potential long-term survival after locoregional treatments, even for patients with a carcinoma longer than 5 cm.

It is not necessary to separate the goals of management into palliation and cure on the basis of the carcinoma size alone, inasmuch as these two objectives can be integrated into a plan of management that may accomplish both without one compromising the other.[9] For example, radiotherapy can achieve both goals if the radiation

A   B   C

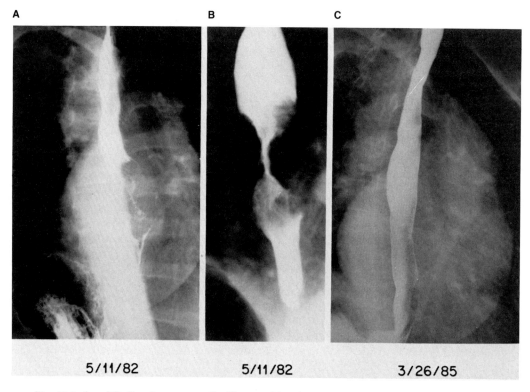

5/11/82   5/11/82   3/26/85

Fig. 44-1. A and **B,** Esophagograms of a 53-year-old patient with a large squamous cell carcinoma at the middle third of the esophagus causing a marked obstruction. Operation was not performed because of a severe metabolic disorder. **C,** A repeat esophagogram 34 months after 6400 cGy shows a complete remission of the lesion and a return of the esophageal patency.

dose and treatment volume are tailored according to the patient's tolerance (see Fig. 44-1).

DEFINITIVE RADIOTHERAPY ALONE

Radiotherapy offers sustained relief of malignant obstruction of the esophagus in the majority of patients (60% to 70%), even when attempted cure fails. There is no treatment-related mortality. More than half (59%) of a series of 51 patients who received definitive radiotherapy for non-resectable carcinoma at the Massachusetts General Hospital manifested improvement in the ability to swallow for a period that equalled two thirds of their remaining lifespans.[10] The study from Edinburgh by Pearson also showed that radiotherapy is very effective in relieving dysphagia at all three anatomic levels of the esophagus.[7] The long-term survival tends to be better for females than for males. Radiotherapy fares better than surgery for lesions in the upper two thirds of the esophagus, but surgery is better for the lower one third of the esophagus. Even with the maximum

tolerable dose to intrathoracic vital structures, definitive radiotherapy for a locally advanced large carcinoma is still attended by a local failure rate of 60% to 70%.

PREOPERATIVE RADIOTHERAPY AND SURGERY

Preoperative radiation has been studied extensively for advanced locoregional squamous-cell carcinoma of the esophaghus (T_2 and T_3 lesions) in an attempt to improve the resectability and cure. One such trial is a study reported by Katlic and Grillo at the Massachusetts General Hospital (1965 to 1970).[11] Forty patients were included in the study protocol, which consisted of three stages: (1) a substernal colon bypass to establish the patients's swallowing ability,[12] (2) 4500 cGy at daily fractions of 200 to 250 cGy, 5 days a week, to the carcinoma and mediastinum, and (3) if there was no evidence of distant metastases or irresectability, block excision of the entire intrathoracic esophagus and the adjacent medi-

A   B   C

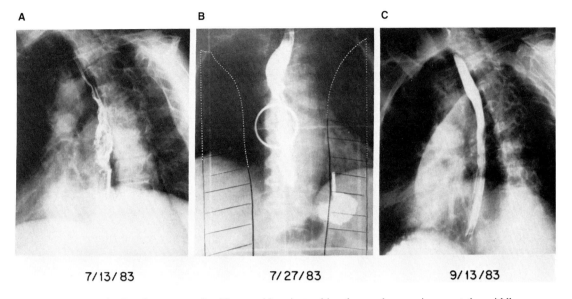

7/13/83   7/27/83   9/13/83

Fig. 44-2. A, Esophagogram of a 66-year-old patient with a large adenocarcinoma at the middle third of the esophagus. A combined treatment of preoperative radiation and surgery was planned. **B,** An anteroposterior simulation film, 2 weeks after, for an anteroposterior-posteroanterior parallel opposed approach (preoperative) shows the large ulcerated lesion and the treatment volume outlined by individually tailored cerrobend blocks. **C,** A repeat esophagogram, 3 weeks after 3600 cGy, shows a dramatic regression of the lesion and a good restoration of the esophageal patency. Surgery was not performed, because pulmonary metastases developed in the interim.

astinal tissue, including the subcarinal lymph nodes. Only 16 patients eventually needed radical esophagectomy, and only one of these was living free of disease at 5 years after a completion of the three stages. Other groups have reported similar poor results after preoperative radiation for locally advanced carcinoma of the esophagus. Patients with adenocarcinoma of the esophagus also have been treated with preoperative radiation in an attempt to convert a nonresectable carcinoma to a resectable one. Good palliation, however, can be achieved for adenocarcinoma of the esophagus even when the curative attempt fails (see Fig. 44-2).

SURGICAL SALVAGE FOR LOCAL FAILURE AFTER DEFINITIVE RADIOTHERAPY

When the failure rate is as high as 60% to 70% with current definitive radiotherapy for locoregional carcinoma of the esophagus, surgical salvage can appropriately be questioned for recurrent esophageal obstruction. If such a procedure is contemplated, demonstrable distant metastases should not be present, and the patient's general condition should be acceptable. A patient with

the potential to withstand operation should be followed closely with a view to salvage by resection should local recurrence develop. Such surgery is technically more difficult than esophageal resection in an unirradiated patient. The majority of the patients who suffer local recurrence after definitive radiotherapy for nonresectable carcinoma are not suitable for surgery. Indeed, in a large series of patients treated by Pearson, only a few patients could be salvaged by surgery.[13]

NEW TRENDS IN PROSPECT

Innovative approaches are being sought to improve the dismal outcome of the current treatment for patients with advanced carcinoma of the esophagus. An exploration for a potential synergism of concurrent radiation and drugs is an interesting and potentially rewarding approach. Leichman and associates used cisplatin and 5-fluorouracil, both known to have a radiosensitizing effect, and radiation as preoperative therapy.[3,14,15] There were 21 patients who were initially included in this trial, but two refused surgery, leaving 19 for survival analysis. Five (26%) of these 19 patients had had no residual carcinoma at the time of surgery. Each of these five patients survived for 24 months or longer. Two of the five died of apparently unrelated disease, whereas the other three remain alive without evidence of recurrent disease at 30, 33, and 39 months. A drawback of concurrent chemotherapy and radiation is a potential increased toxicity. Although 5 of 19 patients died in the postoperative period in the pilot study, the operative mortality rate was reduced to 9.8% (8 of 86) by subjecting only patients with resectable carcinoma to surgery in a subsequent and extended trial of the same study design by the Southwest Oncology Group and the Radiation Therapy Oncology Group.[4] A significant finding was a complete remission rate of 25% (22 of 86), both clinically and histologically, at the time of the esophagectomy. It has also been suggested that patients who have achieved complete remission might be spared esophagectomy.

Preoperative multidrug chemotherapy alone also has achieved a significant regression of the carcinoma, and it might be able to convert a nonresectable tumor to a resectable one. One such trial is a pilot study from the Massachusetts General Hospital in which two cycles of cisplatin plus 5-fluorouracil are given before the esophagectomy. After operation, radiation (5000 cGy) is given to the tumor bed and the adjacent mediastinum if the regional lymph nodes are involved or the resection margins are positive.[5] Thirty-one patients have participated in this study since August 1981. The carcinoma was resected in 81% of patients, with an operative mortality of 10%. Complete clinical remission, as judged by the esophagogram, computed tomography of the chest, and inspection at the time of surgery, was achieved in 45% of patients. However, only 5% of patients showed no evidence of carcinoma by microscopic examination. The projected median survival time is 16.5 months, with the long-term survival rate still to be determined. Kelsen and associates at the Memorial Hospital (New York) also have explored the role of preoperative chemotherapy by employing cisplatin plus bleomycin initially and cisplatin plus bleomycin and vindesine later.[6] Postoperative radiotherapy was given at 400 cGy twice weekly for a period of 4 weeks for patients with stage III lesion (T_3 or N_1). After one or two cycles of chemotherapy, downstaging of the primary lesion was seen in 33% of the patients. In 3 of 34 patients, no residual carcinoma was found in the resected specimen. The overall treatment-related mortality was 9%. For the entire group, the median survival was 16.2 months, and the 24-month survival was 26%.

A combination of drugs (cisplatin and 5-fluorouracil) and radiation is most promising for nonresectable squamous cell carcinoma of the esophagus. Palliative resection can be employed for patients with a dramatic response to this approach and with a good general condition. For this combined treatment, the radiation dose should be kept at 4000 to 4400 cGy, at which level no increased radiation-related operative mortality is expected. With this innovative approach, patients with even locally advanced esophageal cancer can be treated with more cautious optimism than ever before.

REFERENCES

1. Earlam, R., and Cunha-Melo, J.R.: Esophageal squamous cell carcinoma. I. A critical review of surgery, Br. J. Surg. **67**:381, 1980.
2. Earlam, R., and Cunha-Melo, J.R.: Esophageal squamous cell carcinoma. II. A critical review of radiotherapy, Br. J. Surg. **67**:457, 1980.
3. Leichman, L., Steiger, Z., Seydel, H.G., et al.: Preoperative chemotherapy and radiation therapy for patients with cancer of the esophagus: a potentially curative approach, J. Clin. Oncol. **2**:75, 1984.
4. Leichman, L., Steiger, Z., Seydel, H.G., and Vaitkevicius, V.K.: Combined preoperative chemotherapy and radiation therapy for cancer of the esophagus: the Wayne State University, Southwest Oncology Group and Radiation Therapy Oncology Group experience, Semin Oncol **11**:178, 1984.
5. Carey, R.W., Hilgenberg, A.D., Wilkins, E.W., and Choi, N.C.: Preoperative chemotherapy followed by surgery with possible postoperative radiotherapy in squamous cell carcinoma of the esophagus: evaluation of the chemotherapy component, J. Clin. Oncol. **4**:697, 1986.
6. Kelsen, D., Bains, M., Hilaris, B., and Martini, N.: Combined modality therapy of esophageal cancer, Semin. Oncol. **11**:169, 1984.
7. Pearson, J.G.: Radiation therapy for carcinoma of the esophagus. In Choi, N.C., and Grillo, H.C., editors: Thoracic oncology, New York, 1983, Raven Press, pp. 303-325.
8. Fleming, J.A.C.: Radiotherapy in cancer of the thoracic oesophagus, Thorax **2**:206, 1947.
9. Burdette, W.J.: Palliative operation for carcinoma of cervical and thoracic esophagus, Ann. Surg. **173**:714, 1971.
10. Langer, M., Choi, N.C., Orlow, E., Grillo, H.C., and Wilkins, E.W., Jr.: Radiation therapy alone or in combination with surgery in the treatment of carcinoma of the esophagus, Cancer. **58**:1208, 1986.
11. Katlic, M., and Grillo, H.C.: Carcinoma of the esophagus. In Choi, N.C., and Grillo, H.C., editors: Thoracic oncology, New York, 1983, Raven Press, pp. 279-301.
12. Wilkins, E.W., Jr., and Burke, J.F.: Colon esophageal bypass, Am. J. Surg. **129**:394, 1975.
13. Pearson, J.G.: The value of radiotherapy in the management of squamous esophageal cancer, Br. J. Surg. **58**:794, 1971.
14. Douple, E.B., and Richmond, R.C.: Enhancement of the potentiation of radiotherapy by platinum drugs in a mouse tumor, Int. J. Radiat. Oncol. Biol. Phys. **8**:501, 1982.
15. Byfield, J.E., Barone, R.M., Mendelsohn, J., et al.: Infusional 5-fluorouracil and x-ray therapy for nonresectable esophageal cancer, Cancer **45**:703, 1980.

The relative merits of definitive radiotherapy and palliative resection

DISCUSSION

Julius L. Stoller

What you should put first in all the practice of our art is how to make the patient well; and if he can be made well in many ways, one should choose the least troublesome.

Hippocrates (460?-377? BC)

Let's begin with a provocative statement: Regardless of histology or treatment *symptomatic* carcinoma of the esophagus and cardia of the stomach is for all practical purposes an incurable disease. This statement is neither novel nor original. However, its tacit acceptance is a prerequisite for a rational approach to the understanding of carcinoma of the esophagus and cardia as it presents itself to us in industrialized countries.

The personal experiences of almost every reader can give the lie to "the statement," because there are individuals who have presented with symptomatic disease and have, in one way or another, defeated that maxim. But these are sporadic events, and taken in an overall context, only about 5% of those symptomatic at presentation can hope to survive 5 years and probably less than half of that number are truly "cured."[1,2] Even more troubling are the hints that biologic predetermination may have more to do with these results than therapeutic intervention that physicians or surgeons might choose. In one series, nine of 135 patients survived in a range of 2 to 17 years.[3] In seven of these nine cases, resection inadequate for cure was documented! Two patients of my own are a further illustration. In 1970 I resected an adenocarcinoma of the cardia by means of a standard left thoracoabdominal approach and an esophagogastrectomy. A large, palpable lymph node was included with the specimen. Pathologic examination showed this node to be entirely replaced by tumor. This was rightly regarded as a very bad prognostic finding, and yet as late as 1983, 13 years later, the patient was alive and his only problem was a benign esophageal stricture, which had been present and dilatable for many years. At a diagnostic rigid esophagoscopy in another hospital the second patient had his tumor perforated by alligator biopsy forceps. This complication was recognized within a few hours, and the perforated tumor was closed by thoracotomy and suture. Some weeks later I performed a standard Lewis-Tanner procedure. Perforation of a gastrointestinal tract tumor may diminish any expected prognosis by as much as 50%. Nevertheless, this man remains free of disease after 9 years.

But what of our colleagues who believe that "the statement" is negative, defeatist, and more importantly, simply not true? Sporadic publications and presentations seem to indicate that in some centers at least, better results can be achieved.[4,5] These speak out boldly in the medical and surgical literature in spite of criticisms concerned with selection and with follow-up protocols. Such details may be important because it is likely that small differences in protocol produce diverging results. But even with that caveat and with the use of techniques and protocols not materially different from those being used in the centers reporting unusually good survival figures, duplication has been unusual. What can this mean? Frankly, one has no answer, but, in any event, if the mass of surgeons and radiotherapists around the world cannot regularly repeat the "good results" pattern, then for most patients such "results" cannot make much difference. It is neither desirable nor logistically possible for every patient in the industrialized world with *symptomatic* carcinoma of the esophagus to present himself at the one or two centers where he might be led to hope for a better result.

One recognition must be given to the emphasis of the word "symptomatic." When dysphagia supervenes in malignant esophageal disease, a late stage has been reached in the process. The importance of symptoms is emphasized by examining the literature from northern China.[6-8] The high incidence of squamous carcinoma of the esophagus there makes mass population screening studies worthwhile. The results of surgical treatment of these presymptomatic tumors produce astonishing 5-year survival rates of the order of 90%. But one interesting study revealed that 23 patients refused treatment after the diagnosis of asymptomatic squamous cancer had been made.[8] These patients were followed and 78.3% survived 5 years! Further, it was clear that once symptoms did develop, patients behaved exactly as though they had been diagnosed in European and North American industrialized countries. In short, their conditions deteriorated rapidly. The responsibility for our impotence against this disease must surely rest with this insurmountable reality: when cancer of the esophagus and cardia becomes symptomatic, it is already three minutes until midnight.

Treatment presents another frustration. The en bloc resection prescription, which affords some success in other gastrointestinal cancer surgery, has little meaning for the esophagus. One cannot contemplate a true en bloc resection in the mediastinum because it is not a structure but rather a collection of organs connected by areolar tissue and lymphatic vasculature. The radiotherapist has similar problems in that he or she must not inflict damage on surrounding vital structures and it would be in no one's interest for him or her to cause a slough of the esophagus! In addition, almost always cells may be found well beyond the treatment field. Add to this advanced age and infirmity from other degenerative diseases and perhaps some might think that my "provocation" is at most a mere whisper.

Once we accept as a working framework the concept of practical incurability (see Table 44-1), we should ask ourselves what treatment can be offered to provide maximum palliation. Adopting such a regimen will not affect the small number of 5-year survivors. The word "palliation" is in common use in the literature of carcinoma of the esophagus and cardia, but it has rarely been defined. This is because it is an abstract concept. But it must be defined for this disease and indeed for the many other incurable conditions that we are forced to treat in this era of advancing longevity. Visick[9] has shown that a score system for assessing results can be valuable. His technique is widely quoted in the European surgical literature relating to peptic ulcer. The idea is based on the concept attributed to Lord Kelvin that "it is only when you can attach numbers to something that you can begin to understand it." In other words, science is measurement. In 1977 an attempt was made to assess whether radiotherapy alone or surgery alone gave better palliation in squamous cancer of the esophagus.[10] In that retrospective study (Table 44-2) it was perhaps not surprisingly discovered that no answer was possible, because data that would have allowed such a score system as shown in the box on p. 359 was developed and applied prospectively. So far two studies have been published using this system as a way of assessing results. In a study of extrathoracic bypass procedures[11] it was possible to see graphically how surviving patients had fared. Using the score system, the second study suggested[12] that there is no major difference in the palliation achieved by radiation alone and surgery alone using current standard techniques. If more rigorous testing of this proposition bears it out, then one can hardly offer surgical resection, since the morbidity and mortality of radiotherapy is certainly less. Surgical resection is preferred for *adenocarcinoma* of the cardia and lower third of the esophagus because radiotherapy is certainly to be rated as a poor second.

Measurements of palliation and, by implication, of the quality of life are still in their infancy. The perfect test is not yet developed. However, interest in the concept is growing by geometric progression. On the other hand, most publications of the results of esophageal cancer surgery or other treatment show that the authors still report results only in terms of survival and recurrence.[13]

TABLE 44-1. Survival 6 months to 5 years*

	Treatment			
Survival (year)	Surgery alone	Radiotherapy alone	Surgery and radiotherapy	Other
0.5	14	11	11	2
1	10	4	4	1
2	5	2	2	1
3	4	1	1	0
4	3	0	0	0
5	1	0	0	0

From Stoller, J.L., Samer, K., Toppin, D.L., et al.: Can. J. Surg. **20**:454, 1977.

*12 untraced at 5 years.

TABLE 44-2. Swallowing status of 127 patients with esophageal cancer at separation from hospital

Diet	Treatment				Total (and %)
	Radiotherapy alone	Surgery alone	Surgery and radiotherapy	Other	
Nil	0	7	4	1	12 (9.4)
Liquids	13	4	4	1	22 (17.3)
Soft foods.	17	4	8	0	29 (22.9)
All foods	8	9	1	0	18 (14.2)
Inadequately recorded	15	6	7	18	46 (36.2)

From Stoller, J.L., Samer, K., Toppin, D.L., et al.: Can. J. Surg. **20**:454, 1977.

PLEASE MARK CORRECT ANSWERS (X)

A. Swallowing
  1. Nil—not even saliva . . . . _____ (0)
  2. Clear fluids only . . . . _____ (15)
  3. Blenderized diet. . . . . _____ (25)
  4. Most soft food . . . . _____ (35)
  5. Any food . . . . _____ (45)
B. Pain (whether or not related to swallowing)
  1. Yes—always present . . . . _____ (0)
  2. Yes—sometimes present . . . . _____ (5)
  3. No . . . . _____ (40)
  (If 1 and 2, answer)
  1. Severe . . . . _____ (0)
  2. Moderate—responds poorly to meds . . . . _____ (10)
  3. Moderate—responds to meds . . . . _____ (20)
  4. Mild—needs no regular treatment . . . . _____ (25)
C. Sleep   D. Leisure
  1. Poor . . . . _____ (0)   1. None . . . . _____ (0)
  2. Moderate—responds   2. Reduced to sedentary
     poorly to meds . . . . . . _____ (2)   inactive leisure . . . . . . _____ (3)
  3. Moderate—responds   3. As pretherapy, only
     to meds . . . . _____ (4)   slightly reduced. . . . . . _____ (4)
  4. Normal . . . . _____ (6)   4. As before therapy. . . . _____ (5)
E. Work status—has level of work activity been reduced (including housework)?
  1. No . . . . _____ (4)
  2. Yes . . . . _____ (0)
  (If yes, answer below)
  Current work activity
  1. Not working . . . . _____ (0)
  2. Light work—part-time. . . . . _____ (2)
  3. Lighter work—full-time . . . . _____ (3)
  4. Previous or equivalent part-time . . . . _____ (3)

Stoller, J.L., and Cox, D.: Unpublished material.

Table 44-3 shows some of the available tests listed in a recent review of the subject.[14] Perhaps a quality-of-life index that is oriented to a single disease may be easier to evaluate since one knows the major symptoms suffered by the patient during and following the disease and its treatment. It then remains to weight suitably various factors so that the score reflects the actual clinical situation. A study of this aspect of cancer of the esophagus and its treatment is currently being mounted at the University of British Columbia.[15] In this study it is hoped to test the reliability and validity of the score system outlined in the box above. The development of some objective system of this na-

TABLE 44-3. Quality-of-life tests

Test	Administrator	No. of categories	No. of questions	Average time to complete	Approximate time to score	Reliability	Validity
Karnofsky Performance Status Scale	Clinician	1	10	1 min	30 sec	Poor	Good
Linear Analogue Self-Assessment	Patient	4	25	2 min	Lengthy	Very good	Good
QL-Index	Clinician or patient	5	15	1 min	30 sec	Good	Good
Cancer Inventory of Problem Situations	Patient	21	131	18 min	10 min	Very good	Good
Psychological Adjustment to Illness Scale	Clinician or patient	7	45	20-30 min 15-20 min	10 min	Very good	Good
Hospital Anxiety and Depression Scale	Patient	2	14	2 min	2 min	Good	Good

Data from Clark, A., and Fallowfield: J. R. Soc. Med. **79:**165, 1986.

ture will be very important for future patients. New techniques are being developed, such as Selectron (see Chapter 45, p. 362) delivery of radiation and transhiatal esophagectomy without thoracotomy. These methods are unlikely to change the overall prognosis, and if they are to have any serious meaning, future publications will be required to tell us something about the quality of life that has been achieved. Anecdotal descriptions of palliation as "good" or "acceptable" will no longer suffice. With some sort of numerical index we should be able to compare treatment techniques between different centers. Whether the score system I have outlined here is used, or some totally novel approach, matters little. Whatever method is chosen, it must be suitably validated and shown to be reproduceable and in keeping with everyday clinical experience. Assignment of a numerical value to treatment outcome is an idea that is growing in importance. Even in centers that report enviable 5-year survival rates, the fact remains that most patients still do not do well. For that group, too, it will certainly be important to know if "the cure" has been better or worse than the disease.

REFERENCES

1. Earlham, R., and Cunha-Melo, J.R.: Esophageal squamous cell carcinoma. I. A critical review of surgery, Br. J. Surg. **67:**381, 1980.
2. Earlham, R., and Cunha-Melo, J.R.: Esophageal squamous cell carcinoma. II. A critical review of radiotherapy, Br. J. Surg. **67:**457, 1980.
3. Belsey, R., and Hiebert, C.A.: An exclusive right thoracic approach for cancer of the middle third of the esophagus, Ann. Thorac. Surg. **18:**1, 1974.
4. Pearson, J.G.: Value of radiotherapy in management of esophageal cancer, Am. J. Roentgenol. Radium Ther. Nucl. Med. **105:**500, 1969.
5. Nakayawa, K, Yanagisawa, F., Nabeya, K., et al.: Concentrated preoperative irradiation therapy, Arch. Surg. **87:**1003, 1963.
6. Coordinating Group for Research on Esophageal Cancer, Linhsien County, Honan: Early diagnosis and surgical treatment of esophageal cancer under rural conditions, Chin. Med. J. **2:**113, 1976.
7. Linxian (Henan): Esophageal cancer control committee, Esophageal Cancer Research **2:**6, 1975.
8. Yanin, M., Guangyi, L., Xianzhi, G., and Wenhong, C. Detection and natural progression of early esophageal carcinoma: preliminary communication, J.R. Soc. Med. **74:**884, 1981.
9. Visick, A.H.: Study of failures after gastrectomy (Hunterian lecture), Ann. R. Coll. Surg. Engl. **3:**266, 1948.
10. Stoller, J.L., Samer, K., Toppin, D.L., et al.: Carcinoma of the esophagus: a new proposal for the evaluation of treatment, Can. J. Surg. **20:**454, 1977.
11. Stoller, J.L.: Preliminary results of bypass surgery for unresectable strictures of the esophagus, Am. J. Surg. **139:**654, 1980.
12. Stoller, J.L., and Brumwell, M.L. Palliation after operation and after radiotherapy for cancer of the esophagus, Can. J. Surg. **27:**491, 1984.
13. McPeek, B., Gilbert, J.P., and Mosheller, F.: The end result quality of life. In Bunker, J.P., Barnes, B.A., and Moshell, F., editors: Costs, risks and benefits of surgery, New York, 1977, Oxford University Press, p. 172.
14. Clark, A., and Fallowfield, L.J.: Quality of life measurements in patients with malignant disease: a review, J.R. Soc. Med. **79:**165, 1986.
15. Stoller, J.L., and Cox, D.: Unpublished material.

45 Brachytherapy for inoperable cancer of the esophagus and cardia

Keith Michael Pagliero and Christopher Giles Rowland

Intracavity irradiation is a recent addition to the spectrum of possible therapy for carcinoma of the esophagus.[1,2] The idea, however, is not new, radium bougienage having been pioneered in Toronto, Canada, some 25 years ago.[3] Results then indicated a worthwhile response, but the technique was abandoned because radiation exposure, both to the patient and to other patients and staff, was so uncontrolled that the dangers outweighed the benefits. Recent advances in technology have urged us to review the situation. Considerable success in safety has recently been achieved with brachytherapy, for carcinoma of the cervix in particular. The virtual elimination of the risks has been achieved by the afterloading of radioactive materials in specially screened rooms. Exposure to radiation has, therefore, been confined to the patient. In addition, during the years that have elapsed since radium bougienage, knowledge of the properties of various radioactive substances has resulted in the selection of ones that achieve good treatment dosage at the target with a reduction of scatter in tissues where exposure is undesirable.

CHOICE OF PATIENT

Presently we have used brachytherapy only for palliation of the symptoms of esophageal cancer. The term "palliation" needs to be qualified. Belsey[4] has described "cure" in this awesome condition as a "fortunate accident," so that any treatment could be considered palliative. However, the majority of surgeons will strive to achieve these few "cures" by resection, since apart from one highly selected series of cases treated with external beam radiotherapy,[5] not as yet reproduced by any other group, no other form of treatment has resulted in a worthwhile incidence of long-term survival.

By palliation, we refer to the treatment of those patients who, because of advanced disease with local extension or metastatic involvement, are unlikely to survive more than 12 months. This definition excludes patients in whom this state of affairs is discovered only after surgical exploration. In these it is our practice in most cases to perform palliative resection or bypass. The definition, however, includes a group of patients in whom the disease is technically curable by resection but the general condition of the patient prohibits major surgery.

ALTERNATIVES

Similar patients have been treated in the past by laparotomy and intubation with Celestin tubes.[6] Such treatment is not without its problems, and more recently endoscopic intubation has proved to be a somewhat safer procedure.[7] Dissatisfaction with the morbidity and mortality of intubation has prompted other workers to investigate the use of laser vaporization of tumors with or without photosensitization or chemotherapy.[8] Others use simple esophageal bougienage.[9]

THE TECHNIQUE
Assessment of the lesion

Initially, fiberoptic esophagoscopy is performed and the diagnosis confirmed histologically. Occasionally it is necessary to dilate the esophagus sufficiently to allow passage of the endoscope (35 French gauge) in order to visualize the full extent of the disease. Dilatation greater than this is not encouraged. The modest dilatation achieved in those with severe dysphagia, however, is often enough to allow patients to nourish themselves adequately in preparation for whatever treatment is subsequently advised. At the time of this initial investigation opportunity is taken to assess the extent of the disease clinically and with computed tomography, ultrasound screening, and other investigations as indicated. If there is evidence of spread to the liver, scalene nodes, or other distant metastases, we treat by brachytherapy. In the incurable situation of tracheobronchial involvement, we advise surgical bypass or intubation in preference to brachytherapy.

At the same time, patients are assessed for general fitness and suitability for major surgery. The criteria that render any patient operable or inoperable defy accurate definition. In the borderline case, judgment must be left to the individual surgeon.

The equipment

The Selectron is a remote afterloading system developed by Nucletron of Holland. A six-channel Selectron low-dose-rate machine was installed in Exeter in 1982; it uses 48 ^{137}Cs sources, each of 40-mCi activity. In principle, a microprocessor controls the pneumatic transfer of the sources down a flexible tubing into previously inserted "applicators." If, for instance, staff were to enter the treatment room, the sources are automatically and rapidly driven back into a special safe, thus eliminating staff exposure.

The applicator

We have designed a flexible applicator (Fig. 45-1) of 8-mm external diameter that may be introduced into the esophagus over an Eder-Puestow guide wire. The actual insert tube that transfers the sources is placed and locked within this external tube. During positioning of the applicator under fluoroscopy, an insert of dummy marker pellets is used. For treatment the insert tube transfers the sources to the terminal 13 cm of the applicator. If, however, a decision is made to treat the whole esophagus, a second and shorter insert tube is used following the first so as to allow a treatment length of up to 26 cm.

The insertion

We have used general anesthesia, primarily because of the availability of anesthetists and their preference for this form of management. However, simple sedation and local anesthesia have been used occasionally and quite satisfactorily and are obviously more cost effective. With the use of fluoroscopy, the upper and lower extents of the tumor are defined endoscopically and on the screen showing where to position the applicator accurately. A guide wire is passed into the

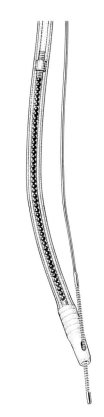

Fig. 45-1. Applicator threaded onto esophageal guide wire.

stomach and the endoscope removed. The applicator is then passed to the desired position straddling the tumor (Fig. 45-2). In longer tumors the applicator is placed to treat the lower extent first, and a second insert tube is placed to treat more proximal disease later. The applicator position is maintained by fixation to a simple face mask (Fig. 45-3) strapped to the patient's head. This face mask contains a reinforced insert in case the patient should choose to chew the applicator! The patient is then transferred back to the Selectron suite for treatment.

The treatment

The patient is observed throughout the course of treatment by closed-circuit television. If any difficulty arises, staff are free to enter the room without radiation hazard. The Selectron automatically reprograms itself with regard to treatment times.

THE DOSE

In the study we chose to use all 48 cesium sources to give a relatively high dose rate. We

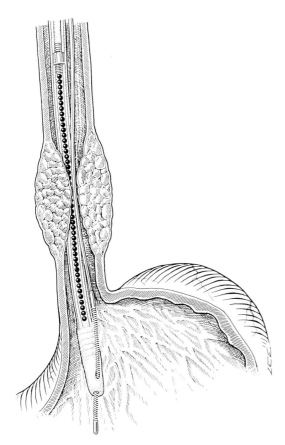

Fig. 45-2. Applicator containing radiopaque marker pellets straddling esophageal tumor.

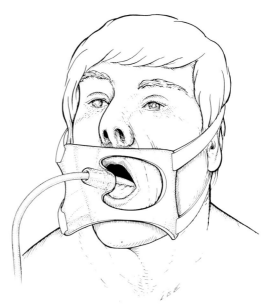

Fig. 45-3. Face mask to fix the position of the applicator.

also used a fairly high single-dose fraction because we believed that this gave us a better chance of obtaining tumor response; thus a dose of 1500 cGy at 10 mm off central axis was chosen (giving approximately 3500 cGy at the surface). This was given in 1.14 hours as a 12-cm line source. The target volume is thus represented by a cylinder 2 cm in diameter and 13 cm in length.

We believed that this high-dose single fraction was justified in these patients inasmuch as we were aiming at rapid palliation. With this dose, more abnormal tissue side effects might be anticipated, but we felt this was not important in view of short anticipated patient survival. In fact, so far we have observed very few abnormal tissue side effects with this treatment.

RESULTS

Seventy-two patients were treated, with an age range of 47 to 93 years (median age, 76 years). Exactly one half were male. They exhibited a variety of lesions both in position and length (see Tables 45-1 and 45-2).

The indication for palliative Selectron treatment was, in 26 patients (36%), evidence of distant metastasis; in three patients (4%), anastomotic recurrence following previous esophagogastrectomy; and in 43 patients (60%), medical unfitness for major surgery.

Patients were required to tolerate the applicator in the mouth and esophagus for almost 1 hour (in a few cases 2 hours, when long lesions required a double application). Three patients refused to complete the treatment. One had 60% of the required dose and is included in the study. A further 12 found the treatment unpleasant, but 57 took it in stride.

Hospital stay (Fig. 45-4) was short, 70% of patients leaving the hospital within 3 days. Stays of longer duration were not so much the result of the procedure but for social reasons, such as the elderly patient living alone. Four of seven patients hospitalized for more than 2 weeks had had laparotomy immediately before treatment.

The study also includes supplementary treatment in a number of cases (see Table 45-3). External beam radiotherapy prior to Selectron therapy implies a failure of the former treatment. External beam radiotherapy after Selectron therapy was used in nine selected patients who had achieved a good response to brachytherapy and who, at 6 weeks, showed no evidence of metastatic disease and were then considered sufficiently robust to undergo such a course. Seven

TABLE 45-1. Histology versus site of lesion*

	Squamous cell carcinoma	Adenocarcinoma	Others	All
Involving body of esophagus	28	8	1	37
Involving cardia only	6	15	0	21
Involving cardia and stomach	3	7	2	12
TOTAL	37	30	3	70

*Two patients referred from another hospital—histology not known.

TABLE 45-2. Median tumor lengths in centimeters (macroscopic appearance)

	Squamous cell carcinoma	Adenocarcinoma	Others
Involving body of esophagus	5	4	2
Involving cardia only	9	7	—
Involving cardia and stomach	10	10	2
Any site	6	7	2

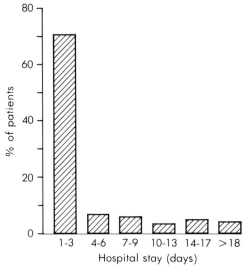

Fig. 45-4

TABLE 45-3. Treatment given in addition to Selectron (in 36 of 72 patients)

Treatment	Cases	Percent
External beam radiotherapy		
Before Selectron	5	7
After Selectron	9	12
Repeat Selectron	7	10
Intubation	15	21

patients were retreated with the Selectron after an initial good response was marred by a recurrence of tumor. In 15 cases we resorted to intubation either when there was poor initial response or when tumor recurred early. In four of these cases death was directly attributable to intubation.

Symptomatic assessment was made by a general practitioner not attached to our department of thoracic surgery or oncology. Documented improvement in swallowing occurred in a high proportion of cases regardless of the site, length, or histology of the tumor. This improvement was often maintained, suggesting that the "bougienage" effect of the applicator was not a major con-

tribution. The actual incidence of "response" may have been higher, since not all patients complained of dysphagia prior to treatment.

Not all patients responded, and in several dysphagia returned at various times, illustrated graphically in Fig. 45-5 (squamous cell carcinoma) and Fig. 45-6 (adenocarcinoma.). Dysphagia was graded as follows: 0, unable to swallow saliva or liquids; 1, able to swallow liquids only; 2, able to swallow pureed or minced food; 3, eating normally.

In one case recurrent dysphagia resulted from a benign stricture considered most likely to be due to irradiation. All other recurrences were due to tumor regrowth.

All patients underwent a pretreatment barium swallow, but a follow-up barium at 6 weeks was done in only 14 cases. In 12 out of 14 a marked objective response was seen (Fig. 45-7).

Survival is recorded in Fig. 45-8, showing less than half of the patients alive at 6 months but some still alive at 1 year.

Side effects were few. Of the 69 patients undergoing the full treatment, two suffered sore throat, two esophagitis, five epigastric pain, and

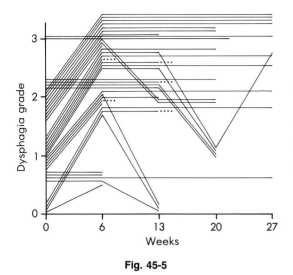

Fig. 45-5

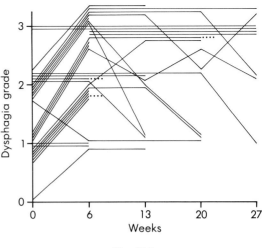

Fig. 45-6

one nausea and diarrhea. One patient is thought to have developed a radiation stricture that responded to simple bougienage. There was no hospital mortality. One patient was, however, readmitted early with a tracheoesophageal fistula at the site of the treated tumor, which was undoubtedly due to treatment, and subsequently died from this complication. This patient was known to have endotracheal tumor prior to treatment, but our naive expectation that brachytherapy would merely create an esophageal channel without causing a fistula was proved wrong.

DISCUSSION

This is a pilot study. It has been tempered a little by a certain understandable mistrust on our part, so that, as in the cases treated by post-Selectron external beam radiotherapy, we have altered course to traditional forms of treatment in the considered interests of the patients, perhaps a little earlier than necessary. Nevertheless, we can say that the designed method of afterloading has proved reliable and has a high degree of patient tolerance. There is undoubtedly a response in many patients, as measured by improvement in symptoms and roentgenographic or endoscopic appearances. This was to be expected in view of Rider and Mendoza's original experience.[3] We have chosen symptomatic dysphagia as our index of benefit. It is the cardinal complaint of most patients and has proved the most relevant feature in the patient's comprehensive follow-up assessment. We might have employed a more detailed assessment[10] but faced the problem of following an elderly, often frail or cachectic, population

scattered widely in rural parts of the United Kingdom. When possible and in the majority, we relied on personal interviews, but several patients were assessed by reference to relatives or family physicians, sometimes after the patient's death. We believed, therefore, that in the context of this study a broad assessment of these simple catagories of dysphagia (graded from 0 to 3) was the most meaningful. This is not to deny the importance of other parameters of well-being. However, it seems that the state of the cancer and the patient's age and frailty were more important factors in this respect than the treatment.

The radiation dose chosen, despite consultation and careful consideration, was ultimately an educated guess. We were pleasantly surprised and pleased to find that it achieved a therapeutic response with a minimum of complications. The one case in which death was expedited by a tracheoesophageal fistula has led us to avoid Selectron treatment when there is tumor involvement of both the esophagus and the tracheobronchial tree. Clearly, more work needs to be done to determine an optimum dose that will give a maximum therapeutic response without the side effects that have been described by Hishikawa et al. using combined external beam radiotherapy and intracavity irradiation.[11]

It could be argued that the initial modest dilatation to 35 French gauge to allow endoscopic inspection is a contributory factor. Undoubtedly this does cause a same-day improvement that is encouraging to the patient, but our own experience of simple bougienage does not match that of Heit et al.[9] We believe that the dilatation we have achieved would be of short-term benefit only.

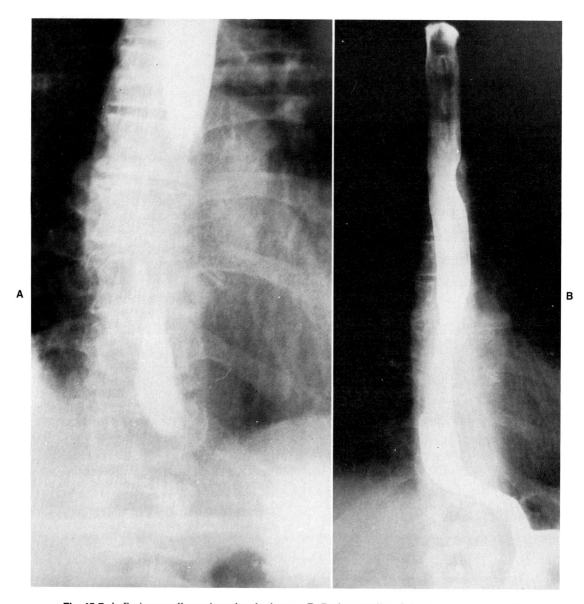

Fig. 45-7. A, Barium swallow prior to brachytherapy. **B,** Barium swallow following symptomatically successful brachytherapy.

The survival figures seem to be better than those for a similar group of patients whom we had previously treated by intubation[12] and were enhanced by a zero hospital mortality. Improvement in survival was not primarily our aim but is a welcome benefit that is presumably due to the active treatment of the disease process rather than the passive bypass of a tube. Indeed, patients have survived 1 year following a single application of the Selectron.

The early results of this treatment have led us to employ Selectron therapy in preference to intubation. Selectron treatment, however, does not

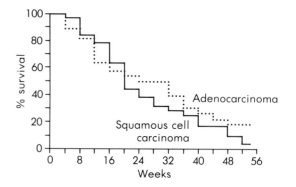

Fig. 45-8

preclude any form of subsequent palliative treatment, and indeed one fifth of our patients were ultimately intubated. Complications of intubation were frequent (48%) and often severe, whereas our Selectron patients suffered only temporary minor discomforts. The single most significant advantage of Selectron therapy was in the management of patients whose mental capacity was reduced. An intelligent, alert patient with an indwelling esophageal tube and a good set of teeth can eat virtually normally. Unfortunately, many of our patients were both edentulous and unable to comprehend the importance of choosing their diet carefully. Among patients we treated by intubation many became blocked at some time and required emergency admissions. In the entire Selectron series there was not a single case of emergency admission for dysphagia.

The hospital stay was extremely short, which is important to patients destined to survive only a few months. Such early discharge from hospital cannot be achieved in operative interventions such as palliative bypass or intubation. Even laser therapy may require two or three sessions and is, therefore, more time consuming.

Where Selectron fits into the spectrum of management is at present debatable. Palliative bypass has been advocated[13] and has our support. Indeed, we resect or bypass twice as many patients as we treat conservatively. However, this particular group of patients studied was considered unsuitable for this form of management. We eagerly await reports of laser vaporization with or without photosensitization, which is generating enthusiasm at the present time. Such excellent results have been achieved in other forms of cancer with chemotherapy that it is to be hoped that a significant breakthrough may be forthcoming in the field of esophageal cancer.

For the time being, however, we believe that our happy initial experience and those of others[14] suggest a real place for intracavity irradiation in the treatment of esophageal carcinoma. It merits further evaluation, particularly in regard to fractionation and its integration with external beam radiation and/or surgery.

We also want to reduce the cost of cancer management and believe that, by reducing hospital inpatient time, outpatient transport costs, and the community services, this can be achieved. This we hope to investigate further in our ongoing studies.

REFERENCES

1. Rowland, C.G., and Pagliero, K.M.: Intracavity irradiation in palliation of carcinoma of oesophagus and cardia, Lancet **2**:981, 1985.
2. Hishikawa, Y., et al.: Early esophageal carcinoma treated with intracavitary irradiation, Radiology **156**(2):519, 1985.
3. Rider, W. and Mendoza, R.: Some opinions on the treatment of cancer of the esophagus, Am. J. Radiol. **105**:514, 1969.
4. Belsey, R.: Is it possible to talk of cure of carcinoma of the esophagus? In First Polydisciplinary International Congress of OESO: Cancer of the esophagus in 1984: 135 questions, answers compiled by R. Giuli, Paris, 1984, Editions Maloine, pp. 382-386.
5. Pearson, J.G.: The present status and future potential of radiotherapy in the management of esophageal cancer, Cancer **39**:882, 1977.
6. Celestin, L.R.: Permanent intubation in inoperable cancer of the esophagus and cardia, Ann. R. Coll. Surg. Engl. **25**:165, 1959.
7. Atkinson, M., et al.: Tube introducer and modified Celestin tube for use in palliative intubation of esophagogastric neoplasm at fibreoptic endoscopy, Gut **19**:669, 1978.
8. Fleischer, D.F., et al.: Endoscopic Nd:YAG laser therapy for carcinoma of the esophagus: a new palliative approach, Am. J. Surg. **143**:180, 1982.
9. Heit, H.A., et al.: Palliative dilatation for dysphagia in esophageal carcinoma, Ann. Intern. Med. **89**:629, 1978.
10. Stoller, J.L., et al.: Carcinoma of the oesophagus: a new proposal for the evaluation of treatment, Can. J. Surg. **20**:454, 1977.
11. Hishikawa, Y., et al.: Esophageal ulceration induced by intracavitary irradiation for esophageal carcinoma, Am. J. Radiol. **143**(2):269, 1984.
12. Unruh, H.W. and Pagliero, K.M.: Pulsion intubation versus traction intubation for obstructing carcinomas of the esophagus, Ann. Thorac. Surg. **40**(4):337, 1985.
13. Stoller, J.L.: Preliminary results of bypass surgery for unresectable strictures of the esophagus, Am. J. Surg. **139**:654, 1980.
14. Stoller, J.L., et al.: Intracavity irradiation for oesophageal cancer, Lancet **2**:1365, 1985.

Brachytherapy for inoperable cancer of the esophagus and cardia

DISCUSSION

Albino D. Flores

Rowland and Pagliero[1] have generated a renewed enthusiasm for the use of intracavitary irradiation in the palliative treatment of advanced cancer of the esophagus and cardia.

Intracavitary irradiation is a well known and proven radiotherapy modality technique. Intracavitary irradiation alone and/or together with external beam irradiation has been a standard conventional treatment for early cancer of the cervix and body of the uterus.[2] Significant progress has occurred in recent years in regard to radiation protection for the patient and for the personnel handling the radioactive materials.

1. Radium, which was initially used for interstitial and intracavitary irradiation, has been completely replaced by safer, leak-proof radioactive materials, such as ^{137}Cs, ^{60}Co, and ^{192}Ir.
2. Radioactive elements with much higher specific activity than radium (cesium, cobalt, iridium) have reduced significantly the treatment time, which was several days when radium was used.
3. The introduction of remote afterloading systems to handle high-intensity radioactive materials has eliminated the unnecessary radiation exposure and improved safety for the staff.

The obvious advantages of intracavitary irradiation (brachytherapy) are as follows:

1. The radiation dose is higher to the tumor than to adjacent normal tissues.
2. Radiation sources can be placed and removed easily.
3. The anatomy is preserved.
4. The radiation exposure to staff is avoidable.

The dosimetry provided by a 10-cm linear source, as for the esophagus, is shown in Fig. 45-9. From this illustration we can see that although the dose for the intraluminal esophageal mucosa is adequate, the short distance from the radioactive material to the tumor (4 mm) does not permit an adequate dose of radiation in depth to the periesophageal region.

DEFINITION OF PALLIATIVE TREATMENT

Palliation means the toning down, mitigation, or lessening of the disease process or complaint. At our institution the use of palliative treatment is reserved for those patients who have an incurable disease either because of disease extent or because of precarious general health. The specific intent of the palliative treatment is to mitigate or improve the major symptoms these patients have and/or delay possible related complications resulting from the disease. This treatment should be simple, have specific aims, be lacking in morbidity and, of course, mortality, and be of short duration in order to allow these patients to remain outside the hospital as long as possible so that they can enjoy the relatively short life span they have.

RATIONALE FOR COMBINED INTRACAVITARY AND EXTERNAL IRRADIATION IN CANCER OF THE ESOPHAGUS AND CARDIA

The radiobiologic effect on the tumor is directly proportional to the amount or dose of radiation given. The tolerance of the normal tissues limits the amount of radiation that can be safely given without introducing complications (therapeutic ratio). The tolerance of critical organs adjacent to the esophagus—spinal cord, lung, mediastinum, and heart—limits the amount of radiation that can be safely given by external beam irradiation to the esophageal malignancy. This fact may lead to persistent disease. The addition of intracavitary to external beam irradiation is

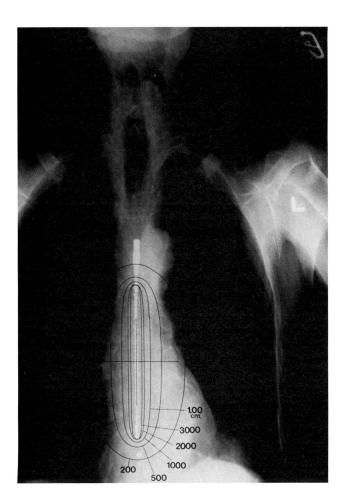

Fig. 45-9. Isodose distribution for intracavitary irradiation with ^{137}Cs.

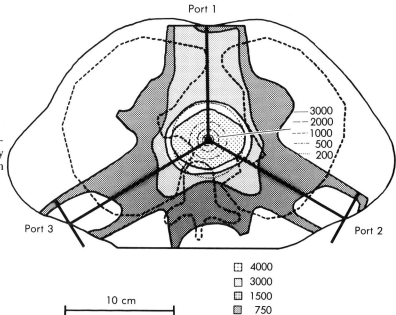

Fig. 45-10. Isodose distribution of combined intracavitary irradiation and external beam radiotherapy.

attractive for the esophagus, since the more exophytic, hypoxic, necrotic intraluminal disease is irradiated to higher doses by the intracavitary treatment without affecting the adjacent normal tissues and the external irradiation providesa better dose in depth to the most peripheral, better oxygenated, probably more sensitive portion of the esophageal malignancy (see Fig. 45-10).

MATERIALS AND METHODS

At the Cancer Control Agency in Vancouver, British Columbia, all patients are staged clinically and radiographically. Barium-swallow roentgenography, CT scanning, fiberoptic upper gastrointestinal endoscopy, and bronchoscopy are performed in all cases of esophageal carcinoma to define the disease extent. Only patients who have direct disease extension into the trachea and bronchial mucosa are excluded; otherwise, all other patients are considered suitable to receive the combined treatment. Bulging of the tracheal or bronchial mucosa without frank invasion is not a contraindication for the protocol study.

TECHNIQUE PROCEDURE

The placement of the esophageal bougie for intracavitary irradiation, in our institution, is a simple outpatient procedure done only under local anesthesia (lidocaine spray) and mild sedation (diazepam, 5 to 10 mg, or lorazepam, 2 mg):

1. After the local anesthesia a soft rubber bougie (F24 or F26) is passed to the stomach (80% of patients) or to the level of the stricture (20% of patients) in order simply to allow the patient to adapt to the inconvenience.
2. The rubber tube is then removed, and a 260-cm Teflon-coated guide wire (included in 60 cm of an F8 to F10 cut-end feeding tube) is guided to the stomach under fluoroscopy (Fig. 45-11).
3. The cut-end feeding tube is removed, and the esophageal stricture dilated to F32 by a balloon dilator for 2 minutes if required (Fig. 45-12).
4. The balloon dilator is removed, and the esophageal bougie containing dummy markers for intracavitary treatment then is placed and secured in the desired position under fluoroscopy (Fig. 45-13).
5. The patient is moved to the treatment room, where by remote control the radioactive ele-

ments (40 pellets of ^{137}Cs) are moved from the container to esophageal bougie.

The standard treatment time for all patients is 1½ hours during which they read or watch television (Fig. 45-14). A cylinder of tissue 2 cm in diameter and 10 cm in length is treated in this manner to 1500 cGy in 1½ hours. The esophageal bougie is usually removed by the nurse, and the patient goes home. The patient starts a course of external beam radiotherapy as an outpatient. Three fields (one anterior and two posterior obliques) are used, and a cylinder of tissue $5 \times 6 \times 16$ cm is treated to 4000 cGy in 15 treatments in 3 weeks at 100 SAD isocentre. For patients potentially resectable (lower esophagus and cardia) the external beam radiotherapy consists of only 3000 cGy in ten fractions in 2 weeks, the operative procedure being arranged 1 week after the last treatment.

All patients are seen monthly for the first year, and a computer form to assess their quality of life is filled out on each occasion (data sheet and self-rating scales).

TREATMENT RESULTS AND COMPLICATIONS

From March, 1985, to March, 1986, 75 patients have been treated at our institution with this combined treatment modality. Sixty-three of these patients are evaluable for a preliminary analysis of tolerance to this combined treatment and of palliation of swallowing for at least 3 months. The clinical distribution of all patients according to the TNM classification is shown in Table 45-4. Eleven, or 17%, of the patients already had distant metastasis at presentation but are included in the analysis. Two patients with lower esophageal squamous cell carcinoma classified as $T_2N_0M_0$ were treated because their overall general conditions and ages were considered unsuitable for a surgical treatment. Similarly, six patients with $T_2N_0M_0$ in the cardia were treated, one because of associated cirrhosis and portal hypertension, one for recurrent disease after esophagectomy, one after exploration showed inoperability (worse surgical staging), and three as preoperative irradiation prior to planned esophagectomy.

The remainder of patients had tumors in the upper esophagus or midesophagus (11 and 22, respectively) or had clinically inoperable cancers in the lower third or cardia (8 and 14, respectively).

A total of 11 patients were surgically explored before the combined treatment. Four patients were explored after the combined treatment; three

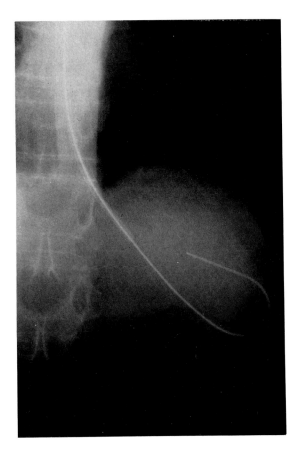

Fig. 45-11. Guide wire to stomach.

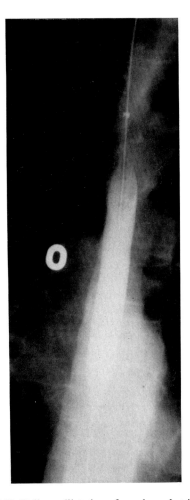

Fig. 45-12. Balloon dilatation of esophageal stricture.

of them were actually resected, although one had abdominal carcinomatosis.

Response to treatment was assessed in relation to palliation of the dysphagia (see Table 45-5). The patient was considered improved if there was either complete restoration of swallowing ability for solids or partial restoration (ability to swallow soft or blenderized foods). If the patient was able to swallow only liquids or required dilatation immediately or during the first 3 months of treatment, the treatment was considered a failure.

Only five (7%) patients required dilatations immediately after treatment. Thirty-nine (62%) patients had complete restoration of their swallowing ability for all types of foods. Most patients (58 [92%]) had initial improvement lasting at least 3 months. Nineteen (30%) of them later required, however, some form of dilatation to maintain this status. There was no mortality related to the procedure. One patient died 3 months after the intracavitary irradiation as a consequence of possible radiation-induced pneumonitis. This was a patient treated for recurrent disease 6 months after initial radical external beam irradiation (4500 cGy

in 3 weeks) who already had well-documented chronic pulmonary disease. The complication clearly was unrelated to the intracavitary treatment but possibly related to the external beam therapy. Radiation esophagitis, although common, was mild in most patients (58 [92%]), did not interfere with their nutrition and was of short duration (2 to 3 weeks). The radiation esophagitis was moderate or severe in five cases, requiring dilatations and analgesics in all of them. The dysphagia in all these cases was, however, superimposed on and confused with progression of the malignancy; in only one case did the dysphagia persist to death, at 4 months.

Of all patients, 67% (31 of 46) are still alive at 6 months and 25% (6 of 24) are alive 1 year or more after the combined treatment.

In 16 patients the intracavitary irradiation was given for recurrent disease after initial external irradiation. In 47 patients the intracavitary irra-

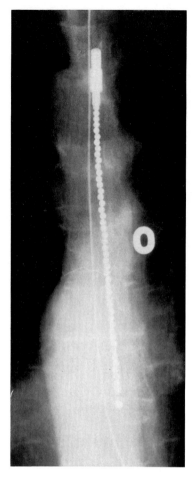

Fig. 45-13. Esophageal bougie with dummy sources.

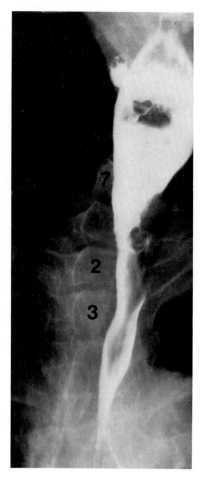

Fig. 45-15. Patient before combined treatment.

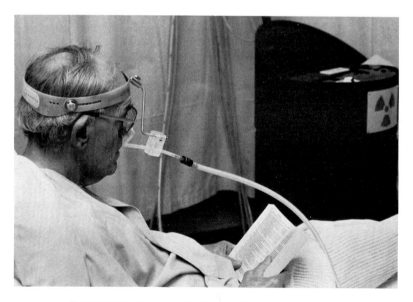

Fig. 45-14. Patient receiving intracavitary treatment.

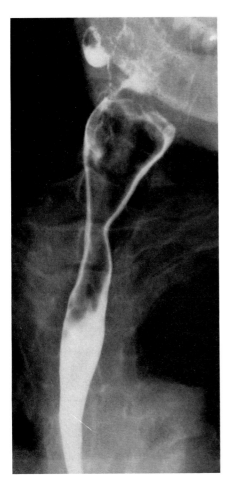

Fig. 45-16. Patient after combined treatment.

diation preceded external beam radiotherapy.

Twenty-eight out of 38 (73%) patients without distant metastasis (M_0) are still alive 3 to 13 months after the combined treatment.

Of the 14 patients with $T_2N_xM_o$ status, only two have died with disease (one was treated for recurrence after esophagectomy and one died 10 months after treatment with local disease). Twelve of the 14 (85%) patients are still alive after 3 to 13 months, without apparent clinical disease (see Figs. 45-15 and 45-16).

DISCUSSION

Cancer of the esophagus and cardia is almost always advanced when first diagnosed. Early detection is extremely rare in North America, and the Chinese experience with the early asymptomatic patient[3] may be an outstanding exception that we do not see in British Columbia or in the Western world, where most patients are diagnosed with dysphagia and already advanced and incurable disease. Operations for adenocarcinoma of the cardia or squamous cell carcinoma of the lower third of the esophagus have a lower operative mortality than for the middle or upper thirds. The overall survival is equally poor, however, in the two histologic entities, both having similar patterns of failure.

As shown by a review of the literature[4] patients receiving external beam radiotherapy alone have a probable survival at 1 year of 18%, at 2 years 8%, and at 5 years 6%. Similar results are obtained with surgery;[5] out of 100 patients, 58 will be explored and 39 resected, but only 26 will

TABLE 45-4. Distribution of patients with cancer of esophagus and cardia according to TNM classification

	N_0	N_1	N_2	N_3	M_1	Totals
T_1	—	—	—	—	—	—
T_2	12	1	—	1	—	14
T_3	27	4	—	7	11	49
TOTALS	39	5	—	8	11	63

TABLE 45-5. Results of treatment

Site	No. of cases	Histology	Response to therapy		
			Complete	Partial	Poor—need for dilatations
Upper esophagus	11	Squamous cell carcinoma	7	4	—
Midesophagus	22	Squamous cell carcinoma	10	10	2
Lower esophagus	10	Squamous cell carcinoma	6	2	2
Cardia	20	Adenocarcinoma	16	3	1
TOTALS	63		39 (62%)	19	5
				92%	

TABLE 45-6. Patterns of failure: autopsy findings in 112 patients (among 483 patients with carcinoma of esophagus and cardia)

	No. of patients
Local disease	93 (83%)
Liver	59
Lung	39
Bone	12
Adrenals	8
Brain	5
Other	35

TABLE 45-7. Causes of death in the same series

	No. of cases
Pneumonia (aspiration, fistula)	349 (82%)
Cerebrovascular accident	32
Bleeding	15
Suicide	5
Postoperative complications	23

leave the hospital with the tumor excised. Eighteen percent of patients treated by surgery survive 1 year, 9% for 2 years, and 4% for 5 years.

There has never been a randomized control study to compare radiation and surgery for similar cases, and it is unlikely that such a scientific exercise will be acceptable to the patient. One has to wonder, even if randomization is possible, given the similar long-term results, whether such a trial is ethical and should be encouraged in view of the wide disparity related to morbidity and mortality that exists between these two treatment arms.

At our hospital, during the decade of 1970 to 1980, we have seen 483 patients with carcinoma of the esophagus and cardia; 401 (83%) had tumors larger than 5 cm, and in 288 (60%) the disease had already extended beyond the esophageal wall. Eighty-nine patients (18.8%) had distant metastasis when first seen. An analysis of the pattern of failure in these cases (see Table 45-6) shows that most patients die with persistent disease at the primary site and the cause of death is usually aspiration pneumonia resulting from obstruction caused by the persistent cancer in the esophagus (see Table 45-7).

The overall 5-year survival rate at our institution was 9.8% for all patients treated by conventional external beam radiotherapy. The 5-year survival is so low in most institutions[4,5] that cure is considered an unusual curiosity. Some[6,7] believe that palliative treatment only should be the main goal of treatment.

The main aim and intent of a palliative treatment differs significantly among authors, but while some degree of morbidity to treatment may

be acceptable, it is entirely unjustified to accept a "palliative treatment" that has a potential risk equal to perioperative mortality.

For the majority of patients with cancer of the esophagus and cardia, the aim of treatment should be an improvement of the quality of life as it relates to their ability to swallow. The simplicity of the intracavitary irradiation, the convenience of the short treatment time, and the radiation safety provided by the remote afterloading system make this treatment ideal for a palliative situation as in cancer of the esophagus. The addition of external beam radiotherapy improves dose at depth to the most peripheral, better oxygenated portion of the esophageal disease and makes this combination a most promising treatment for this disease at all sites.

CONCLUSIONS

1. Irradiation with intracavitary high-intensity ^{137}Cs is an easy, quick, and efficient way to restore the ability to swallow in patients with cancer of the esophagus and cardia.
2. Intracavitary irradiation when combined with external beam radiotherapy is an acceptable, tolerable treatment with low morbidity.
3. The potential benefits of this combined treatment for esophageal cancer at all levels need to be explored as a *palliative treatment* in all cases, as a *potentially curative* treatment in the upper esophagus, and as an *adjuvant* preoperative treatment in the lower esophagus and cardia.

REFERENCES

1. Rowland, C.G., and Pagliero, K.M.: Intracavitary irradiation in palliation of cancer of the esophagus and cardia, Lancet **2**:981, 1985.
2. Fletcher, G.: Cancer of the uterine cervix (Janeway Lecture, 1970), Am. J. Roentgenol. Radium Ther. Nucl. Med. **3**:225, 1971.
3. Yanjim, M., Guangyi, Xianzhi, G., and Wenheng, C.: Detection and progression of early esophageal carcinoma: preliminary communication, J.R. Soc. Med. **74**:884, 1981.
4. Earlam, R., and Cunha-Melo, J.R.: Esophageal squamous cell carcinoma. II. A critical review of radiotherapy, Br. J. Surg. **67**:457, 1980.
5. Earlam, R., and Cunha-Melo, J.R.: Esophageal squamous cell carcinoma. I. A critical review of surgery, Br. J. Surg. **67**:381, 1980.
6. Hawkins, J.R., Cole, R.N., Attar, S., and McLaughlin, J.S.: Carcinoma of the esophagus: experience with a philosophy for palliation, Ann. Thorac. Surg. **23**:400, 1977.
7. Belsey, R., and Hiebert, C.A.: An exclusive right thoracic approach for cancer of the middle third esophagus, Ann. Thorac. Surg. **18**:1, 1974.

CHAPTER 46 Surgical palliation: esophageal resection— a surgeon's opinion

F. Henry Ellis, Jr.

Long-term survival after any form of therapy for carcinoma of the esophagus and cardia is discouraging, so all treatment modalities must be considered palliative. Only when early diagnosis becomes possible will survivorship be improved appreciably. Survivorship is poor because well over 50% of patients with this disease have distant metastases by the time of treatment. Symptoms do not develop until late in the course of the disease, for complete encirclement of the esophagus with tumor usually must occur before symptoms of esophageal obstruction develop. That the disease is potentially curable is evident from the Chinese experience with endoscopic screening of asymptomatic patients in an endemic area. Such techniques can identify early lesions, and treatment can be administered promptly. A Chinese study[1] reported a resectability rate of 100% and a 5-year survivorship of 90% in cases diagnosed early in this way. This approach to early diagnosis would probably not be cost-effective in most of the Western world, where the incidence of the disease is low.

Accepting that most treatment for carcinoma of the esophagus and cardia is palliative, one should select a modality that satisfies certain criteria. It should be applicable to most patients, be accompanied by low death and morbidity rates, and permit the patient to return promptly to a meaningful life with relief of preexisting symptoms. In my opinion, resection best fits these requirements. Adjunctive therapy, either preoperative radiotherapy or radiotherapy combined with chemotherapy, has not yet been shown to have a sufficiently beneficial impact on survivorship to justify the added time, expense, and morbidity involved.

SURGICAL RESECTION
Reported results

The role of resection in the treatment of carcinoma of the esophagus and cardia is often challenged because of low operability and resectability rates and high hospital death rates. This pessimistic view is supported by a recent review of the literature by Earlam and Cunha-Melo.[2] This report disclosed a resectability rate of 67% for all patients operated on, with a hospital death rate of 33.3% for those resected and an overall 5-year survival rate of 4%. In my opinion, these data are derived from outdated information and do not reflect current results. Data from several large series of patients reported in recent years from different parts of the world are presented in Table 46-1 and show the wide variation in reported results. The report of Wu and Huang[5] from the People's Republic of China probably reflects current practice more accurately. In the recent experience of a number of Chinese hospitals, the resectability rate was 81%, the hospital death rate was 6%, and the 5-year survival rate was 25%.

Personal experience

Because of the wide variation in reported results, one ultimately must rely on personal experience in selecting therapy. Table 46-2 summarizes the Lahey Clinic experience with carcinoma of the esophagus and cardia between January, 1970, and January, 1986. The overall operability rate was 81.3%. The remaining data concern only those patients who underwent operation on the thoracic surgical service. The aggressiveness with which surgical resection was performed is indicated by the resectability rate of 87.9%. Nodal involvement, liver metastases, and

375

TABLE 46-1. Recently reported results of surgery for cancer of the esophagus and cardia

Series	Place	No. of patients	Operability (%)	Resectability (%)*	Hospital deaths (%)	Five-year survival (%)†
Cederqvist et al.[3] 1978	Sweden	986	15	45	37.5	15
van Andel et al.,[4] 1979	Holland	328	42	61	21.0	21
Wu and Huang,[5] 1979	China	818	Not stated	81	5.6	25
Griffith and Davis,[6] 1980	England	513	Not stated	41	12.0	15
Giuli and Gignoux,[7] 1980	Europe	2,400	Not stated	Not stated	30.0	14
Earlam and Cunha-Melo,[2] 1980	(Literature review)	83,783	58	67	33.3	16
Akiyama et al.,[8] 1981	Japan	354	Not stated	59	1.4	35
Ellis et al.,[9] 1983	United States	209	80	89	1.3	22
Skinner,[10] 1983	United States	181	66	80	11.0	18
Orringer,[11] 1984	United States	100	Not stated	Not stated	6.0	17‡
Bertelsen et al.,[12] 1985	Denmark	364	82	64	25.0	15
Galandiuk et al.,[13] 1986	United States	238	71	50	7.0	15

*Percentage of patients operated on.

†Percentage of patients surviving resection.

‡Four-year survival.

TABLE 46-2. Operations* for carcinoma of the esophagus and cardia at Lahey Clinic from 1970 to 1986

	No. (%)
Total patients	385
Number of operations	313 (81.3%)
Operations reviewed	271
Resection	238 (87.9%)
Hospital deaths	5 (2.1%)
Other procedures	33
Celestin tube	16
Miscellaneous	17
Hospital deaths	4 (12.1%)

*Includes only patients having operation on the thoracic surgical service.

even occasionally lung metastases did not constitute contraindications to resection. In fact, in 16.8% of patients the procedure was truly palliative rather than curative in that tumor was knowingly left behind. Five patients died within 30 days of operation, for a hospital death rate of 2.1%. Cardiovascular problems accounted for all of the deaths—three myocardial infarctions, one pulmonary embolus, and one cardiac arrest.

Surgical technique

Various techniques have been advocated to restore continuity of the alimentary tract after esophagogastrectomy. I prefer, when possible, to perform an esophagogastrostomy regardless of the level of the tumor. A left thoracotomy is employed for lesions of the lower esophagus and cardia, and more than one half of the tumors were so located (see Fig. 46-1). Either a combined abdominal incision and right thoracotomy (Fig. 46-2) or transhiatal esophagectomy with cervical esophagogastrostomy is used for lesions at higher levels (Fig. 46-3). When the stomach is not available, a colon interposition procedure employing the left colon is preferred (Fig. 46-4). When laryngectomy must be performed concomitantly with resection of a cervical esophageal lesion, radiotherapy is the preferred alternative. When palliation is the goal of surgery and long-term survival is in doubt, I do not believe that depriving a patient of speech qualifies as a palliative procedure. Furthermore, radiotherapy has a higher success rate in managing lesions of the cervical esophagus than it does for other levels.

Results of resection

My associates and I have reported[14] the results for some of the patients listed in Table 46-2. Major complications prolonging hospitalization developed in 27 patients. Seven patients had anas-

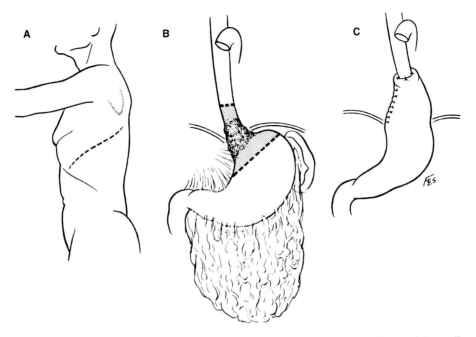

Fig. 46-1. Technique of esophagogastrectomy and esophagogastrostomy for carcinoma of the cardia. **A,** Site of incision. **B,** Extent of resection *(shaded area).* **C,** Completed esophagogastrostomy.

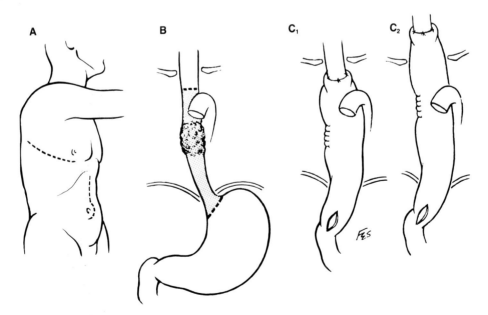

Fig. 46-2. A, Combined abdominal incision and right thoracotomy for lesions of the upper thoracic esophagus. **B,** Extent of resection *(shaded area).* **C₁,** Esophagogastrostomy can be performed in the chest. **C₂,** If submucosal spread is great, a cervical anastomosis through a third incision can be performed. (From Ellis, F.H., Jr.: Surg. Clin. North Am. **60:**273, 1980.)

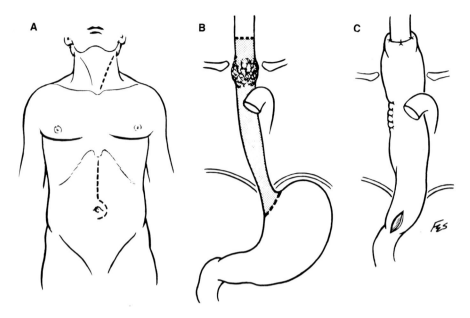

Fig. 46-3. For esophagectomy without thoracotomy, the patient is in the supine position. **A,** Upper midline and left cervical incision *(broken lines)* are made. **B,** Extent of resection *(shaded area)* is shown. **C,** Completed anastomosis. (From Ellis, F.H., Jr.: Surg. Clin. North Am. **60**:275, 1980.)

tomotic leaks, two of which were intrathoracic. Other complications included subphrenic abscess (five patients), gastrointestinal obstruction (five patients), respiratory failure (five patients), and miscellaneous complications (five patients). An additional 10% of patients had minor complications. In the absence of major complications or staged operations, the average hospital stay was 13 days. Most important, dysphagia was successfully relieved in 81.2% of those patients whose ability to swallow could be assessed.

Although palliation may be the main goal of therapy, continued efforts to improve survival are essential. The adjusted survival rate of patients after resection was 16.3% at 5 years, and the median survival time was 17.3 months (see Fig. 46-5). The effect of staging on survival is shown in Fig. 46-6. Five-year survival was 36.6% for patients with stage I disease, 31.1% for stage II, 8.3% for stage III, and none for stage IV. Comparison of curative and palliative resection showed no 5-year survivors among those who underwent palliative resection, with a median survival time of 7 months (see Fig. 46-7), nearly twice that of untreated patients. The 5-year survival of patients having a curative resection was 19% with a median survival time of 20.5 months. Thus, esophagogastrectomy not only provides excellent palliation at relatively low risk but also offers the best opportunity for cure of any of the available forms of therapy.

ALTERNATIVE SURGICAL TECHNIQUES

As indicated in Table 46-2, patients in whom tumor was found to be nonresectable for technical reasons underwent a variety of procedures in an effort to relieve dysphagia. The most common of these was the use of the Celestin tube, a technique of traction intubation that has had wide application throughout the world for nonresectable lesions of the esophagus and cardia. It is particularly applicable for lesions in the lower esophagus and cardia. The tube, which is passed perorally by the anesthesiologist, is retrieved by the surgeon through a gastrostomy and fixed firmly in position with a nonabsorbable suture. Such complications as dislodgment, hemorrhage, perforation, and obstruction may be anticipated in some patients. A death rate of 18% has been reported[15] after this procedure. The overall hospital death rate for various miscellaneous palliative procedures performed at the Lahey Clinic was 12.1%, with most of the death occurring in patients undergoing traction intubation with the Celestin tube.

An alternative approach for the patient whose lesion is found to be nonresectable for technical reasons is peroral or pulsion intubation after the patient has recovered from the exploratory procedure. A variety of tubes have been developed for this purpose, including the Atkinson, Celestin, and Tytgat tubes with flanged upper ends to

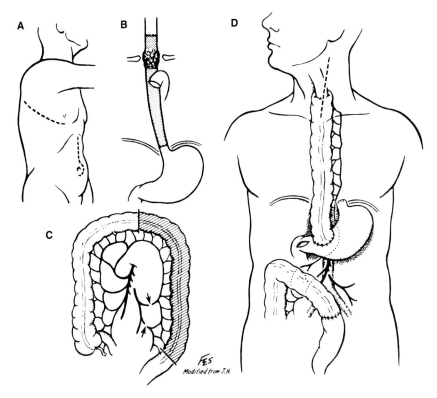

Fig. 46-4. Esophagectomy with interposition of antiperistaltic segment of left colon. **A,** Incisions used in performance of esophagectomy, cervical esophagogastrostomy, pyloromyotomy, and gastrostomy. **B,** Extent of esophageal resection *(shaded area).* **C,** Preparation of segment of left colon *(shaded area)* for interposition based on middle colic artery. Note sites of vascular interruption *(arrows),* which maintain the integrity of the vascular arcade. **D,** Completed operation. (From Ellis, F.H., Jr.: Surg. Clin. North Am. **60:**277, 1980.)

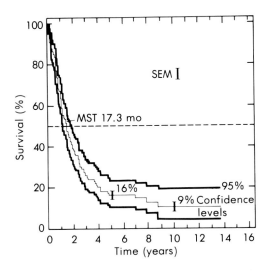

Fig. 46-5. Adjusted survival rates for patients surviving resection for carcinoma of esophagus and cardia at Lahey Clinic Medical Center—January, 1970, to July, 1984. *SEM,* Standard error of mean; *MST,* median survival time. (From Ellis, F.H., Jr., Gibb, S.P., and Watkins, E., Jr.: Can. J. Surg. **28:**494, 1985.)

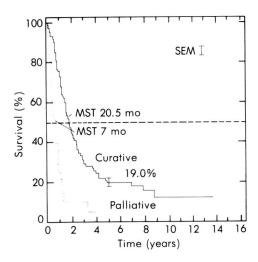

Fig. 46-6. Adjusted survival rates according to stage of disease for patients surviving resection for carcinoma of the esophagus and cardia at Lahey Clinic Medical Center—January, 1970, to July, 1984. *SEM,* Standard error of mean; *MST,* median survival time. (From Ellis, F.H., Jr., Gibb, S.P., and Watkins, E., Jr.: Can. J. Surg. **28:**494, 1985.)

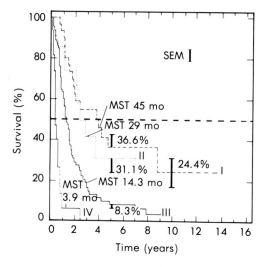

Fig. 46-7. Adjusted survival rates for patients surviving curative and palliative resection for carcinoma of the esophagus and cardia at Lahey Clinic Medical Center—January, 1970, to July, 1984. *SEM,* Standard error of mean; *MST,* median survival time.

help maintain position. A recent review of the experience in Great Britain[16] with the use of these tubes disclosed that perforations occurred in 9% of patients, 8% of the tubes became blocked, 10% became dislodged, and the procedure was accompanied by a death rate of 4.5%. Whether traction or pulsion intubation is used, total palliation of dysphagia is not often achieved, for the patient is usually restricted to a mechanically soft diet to minimize the tube blockage.

For nonresectable lesions of the cardia, a side-to-side esophagogastrostomy leaving the carcinoma in place, as originally proposed by d'Allaines and associates in 1949,[17] can provide excellent palliation with a reasonably low hospital death rate. For lesions at a higher level in the thoracic esophagus, particularly those that may involve such adjacent structures as the tracheobronchial tree, an operation first performed by Kirschner in 1920[18] may provide useful palliation in selected cases. As originally described, the operation consisted of thorough mobilization of the stomach and Roux-en-Y drainage of the intraabdominal esophagus followed by presternal placement of the stomach to facilitate a cervical esophagogastrostomy after transection of the cervical esophagus and suture closure of its distal end. This procedure was later revived by Ong,[19] and those who employ it now do not drain the esophagus but merely exclude it from the alimentary tract. This procedure has also been modified by positioning the stomach substernally or by performing an intrathoracic anastomosis prox-

imal to the nonresectable tumor. Orringer's experience[20] with 37 such procedures proved disappointing, however, for nine deaths (24%) and several major complications occurred. Satisfactory palliation with this bypass was achieved in only 25% of the survivors. Therefore, it should be used sparingly and only under very special and optimum circumstances.

Feeding gastrostomy or jejunostomy provides no palliation, in that neither restores the swallowing mechanism. Such procedures may be justified occasionally only as a temporary measure between stages of a reconstructive procedure, such as a colon interposition, or to maintain nutritional status in a patient who must undergo radiotherapy in anticipation of the ultimate resumption of normal alimentation.

ACKNOWLEDGEMENT

I am grateful to Dr. David M. Shahian and Dr. Peter Maggs for permission to include patients operated on by them on the thoracic surgical service.

REFERENCES

1. Coordinating Group for Research on Esophageal Cancer, Linshein County, Henan: Early diagnosis and surgical treatment of esophageal cancer under rural conditions, Chin. Med. J. **2:**113, 1976.
2. Earlam, R., and Cunha-Melo, J.R.: Oesophageal squamous cell carcinoma. I. A critical review of surgery, Br. J. Surg. **67:**381, 1980.
3. Cederqvist, C., Nielsen, J., Berthelsen, A., and Hansen, H.S.: Cancer of the oesophagus. II. Therapy and outcome, Acta Chir. Scand. **144:**233, 1978.
4. van Andel, J.G., Dees, J., Dijkhuis, C.M., Fokkens, W., van Houten, H., de Jong, P.C., and van Woerkom-Eykenboom, W.M.: Carcinoma of the esophagus: results of treatment, Ann. Surg. **190:**684, 1979.
5. Wu, Y.-K., and Huang, K.-C.: Chinese experience in the surgical treatment of carcinoma of the esophagus, Ann. Surg. **190:**361, 1979.
6. Griffith, J.L., and Davis, J.T.: A twenty-year experience with surgical management of carcinoma of the esophagus and gastric cardia, J. Thorac. Cardiovasc. Surg. **79:**447, 1980.
7. Giuli, R., and Gignoux, M.: Treatment of carcinoma of the esophagus: retrospective study of 2,400 patients, Ann. Surg. **192:**44, 1980.
8. Akiyama, H., Tsurumaru, M., Kawamura, T., and Ono, Y.: Principles of surgical treatment for carcinoma of the esophagus: analysis of lymph node involvement, Ann. Surg. **194:**438, 1981.
9. Ellis, F.H., Jr., Gibb, S.P., and Watkins, E., Jr.: Esophagogastrectomy: a safe, widely applicable, and expeditious form of palliation for patients with carcinoma of the esophagus and cardia, Ann. Surg. **198:**531, 1983.
10. Skinner, D.B.: En bloc resection for neoplasms of the esophagus and cardia, J. Thorac. Cardiovasc. Surg. **85:**59, 1983.

11. Orringer, M.B.: Transhiatal esophagectomy without thoracotomy for carcinoma of the thoracic esophagus, Ann. Surg. **200**:282, 1984.

12. Bertelsen, S., Aasted, A., and Vejlsted, H.: Surgical treatment for malignant lesions of the distal part of the esophagus and the esophagogastric junction, World J. Surg. **9**:633, 1985.

13. Galandiuk, S., Hermann, R.E., Gassman, J.J., and Cosgrove, D.M.: Cancer of the esophagus: the Cleveland Clinic experience, Ann. Surg. **203**:101, 1986.

14. Ellis, F.H., Jr., Gibb, S.P., and Watkins, E., Jr.: Overview of the current management of carcinoma of the esophagus and cardia, Can. J. Surg. **28**:493, 1985.

15. Saunders, N.R.: The Celestin tube in the palliation of carcinoma of the oesophagus and cardia, Br. J. Surg. **66**:419, 1979.

16. Bennett, J.R.: Intubation of gastro-oesophageal malignancies: a survey of current practice in Britain, 1980, Gut **22**:336, 1981.

17. d'Allaines, F., Dubost, C., and Galley, J.J.: Oesophago-gastrostomies palliatives sans résection dans les cancers de l'oesophage et du cardia, J. Chir. **65**:289, 1949.

18. Kirschner, M.A.: Ein neues Verfahren der Oesophago-plastik, Arch. Klin. Chir. **114**:606, 1920.

19. Ong, G.B.: The Kirschner operation: a forgotten procedure, Br. J. Surg. **60**:221, 1973.

20. Orringer, M.B.: Substernal gastric bypass of the excluded esophagus: results of an ill-advised operation, Surgery **96**:467, 1984.

CHAPTER **47** Surgical palliation in obstructing lesions— intrathoracic bypass procedures

Attila Vörös, Janos Kiss, and Frigyes Kulka

Being incapable of making the patient tumor-free, surgical palliation has the aim of diminishing complications caused by the tumor, if possible for as long as the patient lives. It has to abolish as quickly as possible the inability to take nourishment and also must prevent further progression of pulmonary complications. Thereby the quality of life may be improved and survival may be prolonged.

The above requirements are met differently by the various methods of palliation. In our opinion the best palliation is resection. When the tumor cannot be removed and the life expectancy and condition of the patient make it feasible, the so-called bypass may be the method of choice. In advanced conditions, endoprosthesis and the nutrient catheter-pharyngostomy may be chosen from among the surgical procedures.

PATIENTS AND METHODS

In the period January 1, 1973, to December 31, 1985, 813 patients, aged 26 to 82 years, were treated for tumors of the esophagus and gastroesophageal junction at the First Department of Surgery, Postgraduate Medical School, Budapest, Hungary (see Table 47-1).

The extent and site of the tumor were determined by chest x-ray film and double-contrast barium meal radiography, esophagoscopy, and, when justified, also by submucography, and, in cases of esophageal tumors involving the upper and middle parts, by tracheobronchoscopy. The diagnosis was confirmed in every case by preoperative histologic studies. In addition to the routine laboratory tests, cardiologic and respiratory function tests were also done.

Resection was the method of choice even when the tumor invaded adjacent tissues. Feasibility of

resection was ascertained in the first place on the basis of tracheoscopic evidence. When no tumorous infiltration was visible in the pars membranacea, resection was attempted. Palliative removal of the tumorous esophagus eliminates the possibility of tracheoesophageal fistula formation.

Resection is ruled out when esophagorespiratory fistula has developed and when the tracheobronchial tree shows tumorous infiltration. In such cases we resort to the bypass procedure. We have chosen this operation even when the mediastinum was extensively invaded by the tumor (Fig. 47-1). However, when the bypass is chosen, the patient must be in a satisfactory condition to tolerate it.

The bypass procedure was chosen in 32 cases of tumor of the esophagus and gastroesophageal junction (see Table 47-2). This type of surgery was done in 17 cases because of the presence of esophagorespiratory fistula and in 12 cases because of neoplastic infiltration of the tracheobronchial system or extensive invasion of the mediastinum. In three cases a large tumor at the gastroesophageal junction had to be bypassed because of adherence to the aorta and crura of diaphragm. Prior to operation the hematologic, fluid, and electrolyte status of the patient was corrected and intensive physiotherapy introduced to diminish the risk of pulmonary complications. When it was feasible, peroral pretreatment with topical antibiotics, such as powdered metronidasol-neomycin, was employed. Since it was time-consuming, no effort was made to improve the alimentary condition of the patient.

In cases of gastroesophageal junction tumors, jejunum was used, and, in lower- and middle-part esophageal tumors, whole stomach and less frequently colon, were used for the bypass.

Tumors of the gastroesophageal junction are

TABLE 47-1. Total number of patients with carcinoma of the esophagus and gastroesophageal junction admitted to the First Department of Surgery, Postgraduate Medical School, Budapest, Hungary, 1973 to 1985

	No. of patients (%)	No. of deaths (%)
Total admissions	813 (100)	119
Not operated on	101 (12.4)	12
Operated on	712 (87.6)	107
Operated-on patients	712 (100)	107 (15)
Exploration	131 (18.4)	37 (29.1)
Gastrostomy	18 (2.5)	4 (22.2)
Endoprosthesis	91 (12.8)	15 (16.5)
Catheter pharyngostomy	4 (0.6)	— —
Bypass	32 (4.5)	6 (18.7)
Resection	436 (61.2)	45 (10.3)

operated on through a left thoracolaparotomy. When explorative laparotomy proves the tumor not to be removable and the patient is suitable for bypass (no peritoneal carcinomatosis, ascites, or extensive liver metastases and the general condition of the patient is satisfactory), a Roux-en-Y loop is made from the first jejunal loop. The jejunal loop is led into the chest through an opening created separately in the diaphragm, and a side-to-end esophagojejunostomy is done in the tumor-free part of the esophagus (Fig. 47-2).

When possible, we use stomach for esophageal bypass. When there is an esophagorespiratory fistula, the distal esophageal stump is closed blindly, because the patient can expectorate any discharge accumulating in the closed esophageal part. When there is no fistula, the remaining esophageal segment should be properly drained.

The operation begins with median laparotomy. The stomach is mobilized. Subsequently, blood supply to the stomach is provided by the right gastroepiploic and right gastric arteries. After mobilization of the duodenum with Kocher's maneuver, pyloromyotomy is performed. When there is no esophagorespiratory fistula, the stomach is divided with a GIA stapler, leaving behind a small gastric stump below the esophagogastric junction. A Roux-en-Y loop is made from the first jejunal loop. The tip of the Roux-en-Y loop is closed. The gastrojejunal anastomosis is made over the jejunostomy tube leading into the esophagus. Around the catheter the jejunal and gastric walls are coapted merely with 4 to 5 seromuscular stitches, without a true anastomosis (Fig. 47-3).

The decompressing drain is removed in about a fortnight.

From a left cervical incision the esophagus is exposed, closed aborally with a TA 55 stapler, and divided. A retrosternal tunnel is created for the bypass.

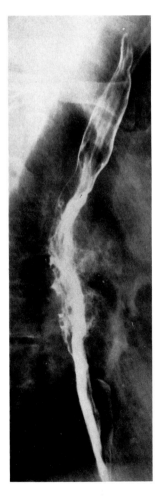

Fig. 47-1. Barium esophagram showing extensive middle third carcinoma invading structures including the carina and main bronchi.

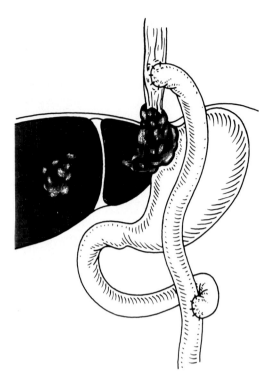

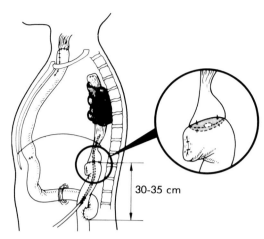

Fig. 47-3. The draining gastrojejunal anastomosis made over the decompressing jejunostomy catheter.

Fig. 47-2. Diagram of bypass of unresectable carcinoma at gastroesophageal junction. The Roux-en-Y loop is anastomosed end-to-side of esophagus.

TABLE 47-2. Bypass for carcinoma of the esophagus and gastroesophageal junction (First Department of Surgery, Postgraduate Medical School, Budapest, Hungary)*

		Esophagus	
	Gastroesophageal junction	With esophagotracheal or esophagobronchial fistula	Without fistula
Gastric			1‡
With drainage	—		8
Without drainage	—	10 (3)†	
Jejunal	3	—	—
Colonic	—	7 (3)	3

*Total number of patients, 32; deaths, 6 (18.7%).

†Deaths in parentheses.

‡Intrapleural esophagofundostomy (right thoracic approach).

TABLE 47-3. Complications of bypass procedures in 32 patients

	No. of patients	Deaths
Anastomotic leakage	3	0
Pneumonia and respiratory failure	6	6
Pneumonia	4	0
Wound infection	5	0

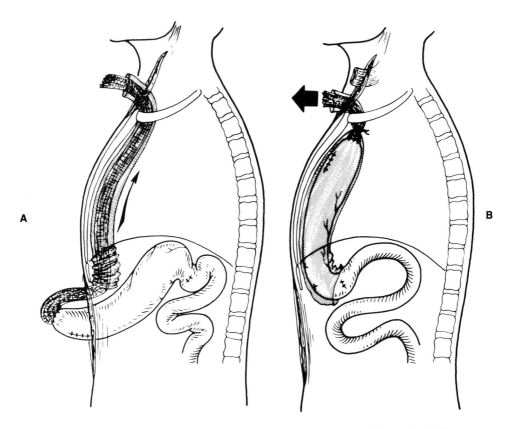

Fig. 47-4. The technique of passing the stomach through the retrosternal tunnel. **A,** The gauze-containing plastic sheath is passed down tunnel and the gauze sutured to the gastric fundus. **B,** The stomach is drawn upward within the plastic sheath.

The following method is used to handle the gastric or colonic segment:

A thin-walled plastic sheath, with a strip of gauze in it, is pulled into the retrosternal tunnel by means of an instrument and thread. The gastric fundus is fixed to the strip of gauze. The plastic sheath is tied firmly onto the strip of gauze with a strong thread. The plastic-sheathed stomach is pulled up through the retrosternal tunnel to the neck. The advantage of the method is that during pulling up, traction is exerted on the plastic sheath, which protects at the same time the stomach and its nutrient blood vessels against tear and crushing by adjacent tissues (Fig. 47-4). The esophagogastric anastomosis is created with one-layer, interrupted, monofilament atraumatic steel-wire sutures.

In the presence of an esophagorespiratory fistula the aboral (distal) end of the esophagus is closed blindly. Immediately above the gastroesophageal junction the muscular wall of the esophagus is incised circularly, and the mucosa is closed by ligation and then divided. Over the mucosal stump the muscular layer is closed with interrupted stitches.

Bypass with a colon segment is the most strenuous procedure for the patient. This is the method of choice when the stomach cannot be used for the bypass (for instance, because of previous gastric resection). An isoperistaltic left colon segment is most often used, receiving its blood supply from the left colic artery. Anatomic reasons may make it necessary to use an isoperistaltic right colonic segment, supplied by the middle colic artery. This bypass is placed retrosternally also. The colon segment is pulled up in the same way as described for the bypass with stomach. When there is an esophagorespiratory fistula, the esophagus is closed and divided above the gastroesophageal junction, as described. When there is no fistula the esophagus is closed over a decompressing jejunostomy catheter inserted into its lumen via the gastroenterostomy (Fig. 47-5). This can be removed 2 weeks later.

Most of the postoperative complications were pulmonary (see Table 47-3). Six of our esopha-

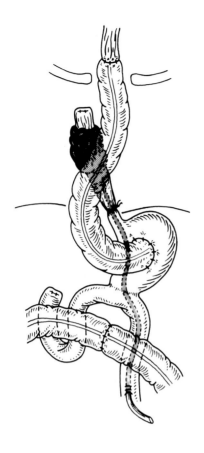

Fig. 47-5. Colon bypass, used in the situation of prior gastrectomy, with decompressing jejunostomy catheter placed retrograde through the gastrojejunostomy into the ligated esophagus (not used in cases of esophagorespiratory fistula).

gorespiratory fistula patients died of complications of aspiration. Suture dehiscences in the cervical anastomosis healed spontaneously.

DISCUSSION

In cases of progression of nonresectable esophageal tumors the complaints can be relieved by the bypass operation. This eliminates obstruction, the hazard of aspiration, and the sequelae of a potential esophagorespiratory fistula. It does not fundamentally prolong survival.

Sharing Akiyama's opinion[1] in principle, we think that the so-called bypass procedure is justified in the following cases:

1. There is severe dysphagia, and esophagorespiratory fistula formation is imminent.
2. The tumor has spread extensively into its surrounding structures.
3. Esophagorespiratory fistula is present.

The general condition of the patient should be carefully assessed, and the localization and extent of the tumor should be precisely determined in every case.

From the point of view of function, the Roux-en-Y loop is the best for use in bypass. However, for anatomic reasons, it can be used only in 90% to 95% of cases.

In 1965 Belsey[2] reported on 105 cases of esophageal bypass with colon, including 12 cases of palliative bypass performed because of tumor. Mortality and morbidity rates are higher when the colon is used instead of the stomach. Therefore it should be performed on the basis of absolute indication only (e.g., after gastric resection).

The gastric bypass operation placed retrosternally by high gastric division was described in 1974 by Akiyama and Hiyama.[3] We think this is the best method today for retrosternal bypass of the esophagus. Mannell,[4] Angorn and Haffejee,[5] and Conlan et al.[6] employ postoperative irradiation of the tumorous esophagus following retrosternal bypass with stomach.

Bypass of a tumorous esophagus is contraindicated when there is insufficient length of esophagus above the tumor in the cervical region for anastomosis, when there are distant, disseminated metastases, or when the expected survival is compromised by the poor nutritional status or associated disease of the patient.

In 1984 Gignoux and Segol[7] reported on the evidence obtained from 18 teams. The data indicated that the need for bypass operations was low, that the stomach had been used most frequently for bypass, and that the average survival was 7 to 9 months.

The majority of surgeons share the view that simpler, one-stage operations should be given preference in palliative surgery, since survival is so short.

CONCLUSION

Successful, uncomplicated esophageal bypass operations abolish dysphagia and diminish the hazard of pulmonary complications.

REFERENCES

1. Akiyama, H.: Surgery for carcinoma of the esophagus. In Current problems in surgery, vol. 17, Chicago, 1980, Year Book Medical Publishers, pp. 54-120.
2. Belsey, R.H.: Reconstruction of the esophagus with left colon, J. Thorac. Cardiovasc. Surg. **48:**205, 1965.
3. Akiyama, H., and Hiyama, M.: A simple esophageal bypass operation by the high gastric division, Surgery **75:**674, 1974.
4. Mannell, A.: Carcinoma of the esophagus. In Current problems in surgery, vol. 19, Chicago, 1982, Year Book Medical Publishers, pp. 554-648.
5. Angorn, B., and Haffejee, A.A.: Retrosternal gastric bypass for the palliative treatment of unresectable esophageal carcinoma, S. Afr. Med. J. **64:**901, 1983.
6. Conlan, A.A., Nicolaou, N., Hammond, C.A., Pool, R., de Nobrega, C., and Mistry, B.D.: Retrosternal gastric bypass for inoperable esophageal cancer: a report of 71 patients, Ann. Thorac. Surg. **36:**396, 1983.
7. Gignoux, M., and Segol, P.H.: Palliative surgical treatment for carcinoma of the esophagus, Int. Surg. **69:**257, 1984.

CHAPTER 48 The malignant tracheoesophageal or bronchoesophageal fistula

Andrew Alan Conlan

The anatomic proximity of the upper and middle portions of the intrathoracic esophagus to the membranous posterior wall of the trachea and left main bronchus has critical implications for patients with either primary esophageal or airway cancer. The intimate anatomic relationship reflects the common embryologic derivation of the trachea and esophagus following partition of the primitive foregut tube. The covert but rapid local extension of esophageal cancer to involve the adjacent tracheobronchial tree is usually complete before clinical presentation of the patient. Midesophageal carcinoma is the commonest site of occurrence of the tumor, and airway invasion is the prime cause of nonresectability. Airway infiltration is commonly silent, diagnosed by x-ray studies and confirmed at bronchoscopy. X-ray findings of tracheal stripe thickening, a retrotracheal mass with sinus tract formation, represent grades of tumor progression with necrosis. These findings have prompted the term "evolving fistula" or "potential fistula." Once cancerous infiltration and replacement of the membranous airway wall has occurred, two outcomes are possible:

1. Slowly progressive airway infiltration, causing few initial symptoms but ultimately bronchial and bronchocarinal obstruction syndromes. These are recurrent lung infections with copious bronchial secretions often aggravated by frequent aspiration. This sequence is modified by radiation therapy.
2. Esophagorespiratory fistula formation.

An analysis of x-ray abnormalities of the retrotracheal area in 102 patients with midesophageal cancer showed 63 with evidence of tumor involvement of the airway. An esophagorespiratory fistula developed in 22% of patients in this group.[1] It would appear that in the patient population with esophageal cancer in the United States, about 5% will develop tracheoesophageal fistulas.[2-4] In the endemic areas of South Africa, up to 18% of patients will develop and present initially with malignant esophagorespiratory fistulas.[5]

Malignant esophagorespiratory fistulas can be classified as follows:

A. Spontaneous
   1. Esophageal carcinoma
   2. Bronchogenic carcinoma
   3. Tracheal carcinoma
   4. Lymphoma of mediastinal nodes
B. Iatrogenic
   1. Post–radiation therapy
   2. Laser tumor resection
   3. Endoesophageal intubation
   4. Post–esophageal instrumentation
   5. Postchemotherapy

Malignant esophagorespiratory fistulas occur most frequently with primary esophageal carcinoma. Primary tracheal cancer, which is subject to the same local anatomic relationships, infiltrates the adjacent esophagus early. Approximately 15% of these patients develop fistulas.[2] Bronchogenic carcinoma is a rare cause of fistula but may give rise to this from either main bronchus. A fistulous communication with a small-order peripheral bronchus may occur, particularly between the right lower lobe and the esophagus. This latter occurrence may present as a chronic and refractory lung abscess syndrome.[2-4] Lymphoma of the subcarinal or mediastinal nodes or the esophagus itself is a rare cause of malignant fistula. However, it presents severe management problems in a potentially long-lived and even curable patient.

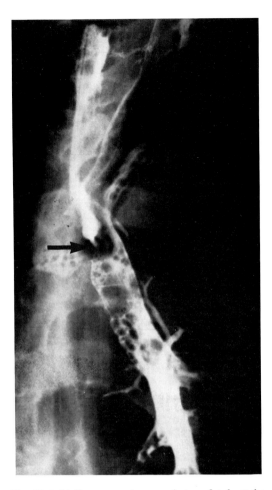

Fig. 48-1. Malignant esophagorespiratory fistula at the origin of the left main bronchus.

LOCATION AND DIAGNOSIS OF AIRWAY FISTULA FORMATION

The term "malignant tracheoesophageal fistula" is used to cover all locations of airway fistulas. "Esophagorespiratory" is perhaps a better term. A survey of reported fistulas in the literature would indicate that 65% are tracheoesophageal in position, 30% are bronchoesophageal, and the remaining 5% involve a small-order bronchus or what seems to be the periphery of a lobe.[2-4]

Approximately half of patients with upper esophageal and midesophageal cancer fistulas will develop them spontaneously. It is significant that the remaining 50% occur during or after radiation therapy, and the role of radionecrosis is at least contributory. Sixteen of 27 cases of esophagorespiratory fistula resulting from cancer that were reported by Little et al.[3] occurred either during or following radiation therapy. The caus-

ative role of radiation is difficult to prove, but it is contributory.[2-4] Fistula formation is now increasingly reported after laser resection or esophageal tumors. The risk is increased when laser resection is combined with radiation or chemotherapy.

The diagnosis of a fistula is a clinical one, but confirmation and localization must be sought with a modified, small-volume, upper gastrointestinal contrast study. Bronchography contrast medium gives superior visualization and is an isotonic aqueous solution that is quickly eliminated. Small volumes are appropriate. Aspiration of contrast medium must be distinguished from esophagorespiratory fistulas, especially in patients with vocal cord palsy. A left bronchocarinal fistula is shown in Fig. 48-1.

The occurrence of a fistula between an infiltrated airway and a cancerous obstructed esophagus is disastrous. Most patients rapidly deteriorate as a result of gross and repetitive pulmonary aspiration. Fulminant gram-negative or anaerobic bronchopneumonia supervenes, often with lung abscess formation. The underlying abnormality is essentially irreversible and nonresectable for either cure or palliation. An important fact is that, even when the disease is locally advanced, two thirds of patients will not have extrathoracic disease.[2,3] The cause of rapid clinical decline and death is unrelieved aspiration, severe infection, and respiratory failure. In the absence of generalized metastases, palliation of the local disease offers scope for worthwhile intervention with the prospect of a lengthy period of comfortable existence. Without intervention the natural history of a malignant esophagorespiratory fistula is death in approximately 4 weeks.

TREATMENTS
Supportive treatment and enterostomy

Included with standard supportive therapies are the operations of gastrostomy or jejunostomy alone, and cervical esophagostomy or salivary duct ligation alone. These operations performed in the setting of supportive care measures do not have a significant impact on the central problem. They contribute to the maintenance of nutrition and the partial treatment of ongoing esophagopulmonary aspiration and possible gastroesophageal reflux. Reports of their use confirm their lack of value when employed singly, and they incur a surprising operative mortality.[2,4,6]

Important aspects of general supportive therapy are:

1. Suspension of all oral intake and the com-

mencement of intravenous fluid replacement and nutritional maintenance (total parenteral nutrition)

2. Vigorous treatment of respiratory infection with broad-spectrum antibiotics and physical therapy

3. Minimization of potential reflux with an elevation of the head of the bed

The optimization of patient condition will lead to the early selection of candidates for a meaningful surgical intervention. Conversely, there is a role for the responsible relinquishment of invasive surgical care methods in patients who are preterminal with extensive bronchopneumonia and respiratory failure unresponsive to the above measures.

Endoesophageal intubation

The concept of siting a soft tubular prosthesis across the defect appears to present a minimal therapeutic intervention, with a potential for worthwhile palliation. Endoesophageal tubes can be inserted by a push-through technique (Livingstone-Procter), which requires esophagoscopy and esophageal dilatation. X-ray control increases safety. The pull-through technique (Celestin tube) requires a laparotomy to control endoesophageal instrumentation. The latter tube is longer, disrupts the esophagogastric sphincter, and is fixed to the stomach wall. Successful siting of the endo-esophageal prosthesis should direct oral intake past the tamponaded fistula. The Johannesburg experience (see Chapter 51), however, is disappointing. Occlusion of the fistula is frequently incomplete, with ongoing repetitive aspiration. We believe this is due to tumor necrosis and enlargement of the fistula as a result of tube pressure. Hospital mortality in our institution is 28%.

A hospital mortality of 25% to 35% for push-through tubes, and 30% to 64% for pull-through tubes, is reproduced in large South African series.[5,7] It appears to be unavoidable and is due to perforation, pulmonary aspiration, bronchopneumonia, respiratory failure, and sepsis. The formidable postdischarge incidence of tube-related complications—lumen obstruction, reflux and aspiration, tube displacement, bleeding, recurrent pneumonia, and pain—detracts further from this therapeutic choice. Tube function in Third World patients is disappointing and reflects poor patient compliance with efforts to reduce tube obstruction and minimize reflux and aspiration.

Despite the hospital mortality and the short-coming in performance, endoesophageal tubes allow 75% of patients with malignant esophago-respiratory fistula to leave the hospital. The toll of tube-related complications thereafter results in a relentless and quick attrition of the survivors.

Mean survival after discharge is 2.2 months, and 50% of patients discharged will be readmitted for tube-related complications.

Surgical therapy

The disease, though local, is nonresectable for either cure or palliation, with very few exceptions. Cases have been reported of patients undergoing combination esophagectomy and lobectomy, or esophagectomy and sleeve bronchocarinal resection.[8] The more usual surgical approach is one that isolates the cancerous fistula by disconnection of the intrathoracic esophagus, with either immediate or delayed esophageal bypass.[8-12]

Initial esophageal isolation and exclusion

The use of cervical esophagostomy and esophagogastric interruption (by division and suture, ligation, or stapler division) with feeding jejunostomy follows sound surgical principle. Tube drainage of the isolated esophageal segment to the neck or the abdominal wall has sometimes been added. This concept of fistula isolation and defunction halts ongoing aspiration and allows infection to be controlled and treated. In addition, patient nutrition can be maintained and the cancer can be staged. Following clinical stability, gastrointestinal continuity can be restored.[2,3]

Little et al.[3] reported seven patients who underwent defunctioning and esophageal segment drainage. Only one patient ultimately achieved oral intake with an extracorporeal tube. The remaining six had poor palliation (four) and fair palliation (two) but no sustained restoration of gastrointestinal function. The mean survival from fistula formation was 17 weeks. Schreiber and Pories[13] reported four patients who underwent esophageal exclusion and gastrointestinal reconnection with an extrathoracic tube bypass system, and good palliation is reported by the authors. Martini et al.[2] report 12 patients who had esophageal exclusion only as initial therapy, with good palliation of symptoms, but they do not specify how many went on to successful reconstruction.

Duranceau and Jamieson[4] summarized 37 patients from the literature treated by esophageal exclusion and record a hospital mortality from 17% to 50%. Surviving patients received good palliation of symptoms, but few went on to successful gastric or intestinal bypass and restoration of oral intake. It thus appears that the staging of esophageal exclusion and subsequent reconstruction is associated with appreciable mortality and morbidity and ultimate failure to achieve esophageal bypass in most patients. The surgical approach

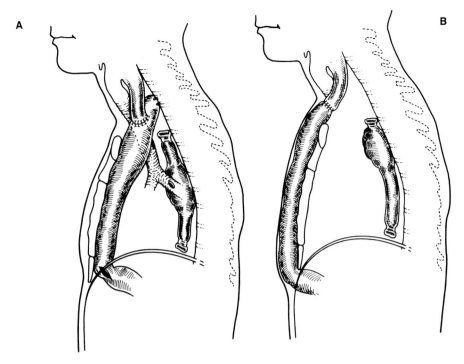

Fig. 48-2. A, Retrosternal placement of the stomach. **B,** Presternal placement of the stomach, thus avoiding a high esophageal carcinoma.

practiced at the Department of Thoracic Surgery in the Johannesburg teaching hospitals has been disconnection of the malignant fistula and concomitant reconstruction of gastrointestinal tract continuity with retrosternal gastric bypass. This surgical policy is reported by others,[2,3,8-10,12-15] the only difference being choice of visceral substitute—stomach, jejunum, or colon.

Retrosternal gastric bypass

Retrosternal gastric bypass (RSGB) is the bypass procedure most commonly used for malignant esophagorespiratory fistula. The esophagus is transected above tumor at the thoracic inlet and just below the diaphragmatic hiatus and abandoned. The fistula is thus effectively defunctioned. Gastrointestinal continuity is restored with the use of the stomach in the retrosternal position. The stomach can be brought presternally to the neck if a high esophageal tumor needs to be avoided. These positions are shown in Fig. 48-2. The simplicity of RSGB and the reliability of the stomach, with a short operating time, make this procedure popular. RSGB has been done more than 150 times for malignant and benign esophageal disease by the Department of Thoracic Surgery during the period from 1979 to 1986. No gangrene of the stomach occurred.

Technical considerations. The general principles of RSGB have been thoroughly reported.[9-12] The operation has been modified to expedite completion. The whole stomach in simple isoperistaltic form is used rather than tube formation. The lesser curve is resected to remove the lymphatic sump of the middle and lower esophagus. The use of staplers (T55, T30, GIA) expedites esophageal closure and lesser-curve transection. Cautery division of omentum between arterial branches is done so that formal ties are used only for vascular pedicles. The vagus nerves are divided to gain 3 cm of esophageal lengthening. The intraabdominal esophagus is transected between two applications of the stapler (T55). The crus of the diaphragm is used to cover the esophageal staple line. Pyloromyotomy rather than pyloroplasty is done when the pylorus is perceived to be scarred, small, or spastic. The duodenum and the head of the pancreas are mobilized. The left subphrenic space is now routinely drained (23F intercostal drain) because of the incidence of subphrenic collections and sepsis. The substernal tunnel is commenced by opening the subxiphoid space. This completes the abdominal section of the operation (duration: about 40 minutes).

The cervical operation can be commenced by

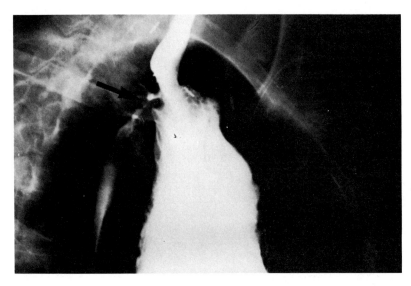

Fig. 48-3. Fistula formation between the cervical esophagogastric anastomosis and the excluded esophageal segment.

a second surgeon, which greatly expedites the whole procedure. The cervical esophagus is transected between two stapler applications (T30). Gentle blunt manual dissection from the abdominal incision up the anterior mediastinum close to the sternum, with the lungs deflated, forms the tunnel. Four fingers should pass from the retrosternal space into the neck. The retromanubrial space is bluntly enlarged leftward behind the clavicle. This guarantees ample room for the stomach in the thoracic inlet. Manubrial and clavicular resection have not been necessary. The stomach is passed through this tunnel to the neck and anchored to the prevertebral fascia, and a single-layer esophagogastric anastomosis is done. Intraoperative pneumothorax is checked by x-ray film.

Esophageal segment leakage syndromes. The clinical practice of esophageal abandonment has been followed by mucocele formation in the excluded esophagus. This is in general a benign occurrence. Drainage of the defunctioned segment was and is practiced by anastomosis to a jejunal loop.[8,12] However, an excessive leakage rate and increased postoperative morbidity have encouraged the deletion of this operative step.[9,11,13] After RSGB for malignant esophagorespiratory fistula, the segment drains into the tracheobronchial tree. Subsequent radiotherapy may enlarge the fistula and guarantee complete drainage.

No confirmed reports of leakage syndromes from the isolated segment after RSGB for airway fistula have been reported. This presumably reflects adequate segment drainage. We suspect that segment leakage is related to tension buildup and poor healing and sloughing of staple lines. We have observed and treated segment leakage syndromes in approximately 4% of patients undergoing RSGB for unresectable carcinoma.

CERVICAL SINUS SYNDROME. Cervical sinus syndrome presents as cervical purulent discharge refractory to adequate drainage. The anastomosis is intact on repeated contrast study. Sinugraphy through the discharging neck wound demonstrates a track leading to the isolated esophageal segment. We have allowed patients to drain chronically with a cervical mucous fistula.[3]

FISTULA FORMATION. Fistula formation is a serious occurrence. A communication is established between the posterior wall of the esophagogastric anastomosis and the isolated segment (Fig. 48-3). It prohibits oral intake, but it responds to management by conservative methods. These are suspension of oral intake and initial total parenteral nutrition followed by several weeks of nutritional maintenance given through a soft small-bore Silastic nasoenteral feeding tube. This allowed closure of the fistulous connection to occur in four patients. Weekly small-volume contrast studies monitored the healing process (Fig. 48-4). This type of fistula formation would doubtless have serious consequences in a patient with a malignant esophagorespiratory fistula, because of aspiration.

DISTAL ESOPHAGEAL STUMP LEAKAGE. Sloughing of the distal esophageal segment staple line and leakage present as left subphrenic sepsis. Lower thoracic and upper abdominal CT scans

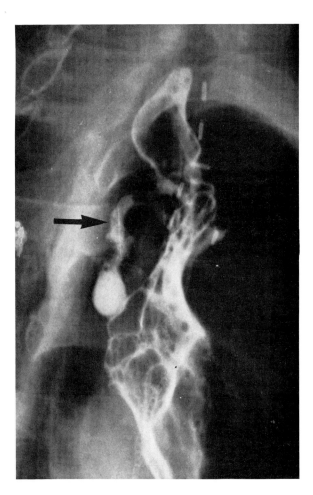

Fig. 48-4. Reduction of a fistulous tract to a diverticulum during nasoenteral nutritional maintenance. Closure occurred later.

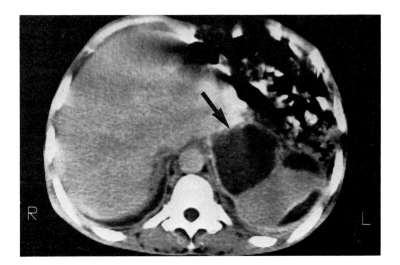

Fig. 48-5. A left subphrenic abscess located by CT anterior to the spleen. Smaller perisplenic collections are present.

are valuable for the diagnosis and definition of pleural and subphrenic sepsis (Fig. 48-5). Current policy at our unit is to drain prophylactically the left subphrenic space. If there is minimal postoperative drainage, the tube is removed about day 5. Conversely, continued drainage from this tube is an indication to retain it, and sinugraphy often demonstrates filling of the excluded segment of esophagus. This tract closes by granulation as the tube is advanced out.

Results of RSGB for malignant esophagorespiratory fistula. The presence of esophagorespiratory fistulas dramatically reduces the effectiveness of surgical bypass procedures.[8,9,12,15] RSGB can be performed with good results (hospital mortality: 9% to 11%) for patients with airway invasion. Patients with malignant airway fistula incur a higher mortality and often chronic unrelieved morbidity. In the Johannesburg series[9] 18 patients underwent RSGB for malignant esophagorespiratory fistula present for at least 4 weeks. Nine patients received assisted ventilation postoperatively from 48 hours to 3 weeks. Six of these patients underwent tracheostomy. Five patients developed anastomotic leakage, but the leaks closed in three. Nine patients died in hospital from severe bronchopneumonia and respiratory failure. Two of these patients had cervicomediastinal sepsis resulting from anastomotic leakage. Three patients reported in the hospital mortality figure died at 4, 4½, and 6 weeks postoperatively. They had healed, their fistulas were isolated, and they were eating normally. Discharge was not possible, because of poor social circumstances and clinical inanition. They suffered from chronic pneumonitis. Thus, only 8 of 18 patients left the hospital free of infection and respiratory symptoms. They were eating normally and survived from 1½ to 7 months, with a mean survival of 3½ months.

Wong et al.[12] reviewed RSGB in 142 patients, of whom 18 had malignant airway fistula. Overall mortality for the group was 41.5%, but mortality was 61.1% for those with fistulas. The principal cause of death was respiratory failure (72.9%). Anastomotic leaks occurred in 47.2%, but most healed. Wound infection occurred in 22%. Mean survival was 5 months. The authors acknowledge the increased mortality in these patients with advanced malignant disease but note the high mortality of other procedures with less palliative potential. Smaller series of gastric bypass procedures for malignant airway fistula have been reported, with good results and excellent palliation.[4,10,13,14] Mean survival was from 5 to 7 months.

Alternate intestinal esophageal substitution

Jejunum and colon are other choices as visceral esophageal substitutes after fistula disconnection. They take longer to prepare and apply than stomach. Extensive dissection and multiple anastomoses are required, blood supply is variable, they pose specific problems (e.g., redundancy, herniation, and strangulation.) There seems no specific advantage to retaining the stomach as a capacitance chamber in patients whose life expectancy is about 6 months. Functional problems are common with colon but rare when the stomach is used as a conduit.

Jejunal interposition. The Hong Kong surgical group has an extensive experience. Ong and Kwong[8] reported on nine patients with malignant airway fistulas managed by double jejunal bypass. They used a long loop of jejunum placed presternally to connect the cervical esophagus to the stomach. A second jejunal loop drained the excluded intrathoracic esophagus and stomach by Roux-en-Y arrangement. Four of the nine patients died in the hospital of bronchopneumonia and respiratory failure. Hospital mortality was 44%, and mean patient survival was 3½ months. The authors reported excellent palliation of symptoms.

Ong et al.[15] reported a further 18 patients who underwent jejunal-loop bypass and gastric fundoplication for nonresectable intrathoracic esophageal cancer. Only three patients had malignant fistulas. A long jejunal loop again gave continuity between the cervical esophagus and the stomach. The gastric fundus was then plicated about the terminal esophagus to control reflux. Five of the 18 patients died (27.8%) of pneumonia and respiratory failure. Jejunal gangrene occurred in one patient. Mean survival was 3½ months. One of the three patients with airway fistulas died. Wong et al.[12] note a 3.8% incidence of gangrene in 212 jejunal interpositions.

Colon interposition. The use of isoperistaltic colon to restore gastrointestinal continuity after fistula exclusion is reported by several authors. Martini et al.[2] report 10 patients who were successfully reconstructed using colon. There was no operative mortality, and palliation was excellent, provided esophagogastric division had been done to prevent reflux. Little et al.[3] report five patients with malignant airway fistulas who had colon interposition and defined three as having good function but two as having fair or poor function. There was no operative mortality. Several smaller series of patients have been reported and summarized.[4] The procedure as applied carried a low operative mortality, with good palliation in the patients chosen.

Surgical comment

The problem of treatment selection for patients hospitalized with malignant airway fistula is difficult. The presence of established bronchopneumonia, which is indicative of a fistula of significant duration, is probably best managed by endoesophageal intubation or esophageal exclusion without reconstruction. It must be accepted that there is an unavoidable baseline mortality for any therapeutic intervention in this patient group. Those who improve following fistula exclusion can be considered for esophageal visceral bypass. Surgical isolation of the fistula and concomitant visceral bypass should be done for patients with recent fistula formation and a good performance status. Patients developing fistulas during radiation or chemotherapy, or following laser resection or endoscopic mishap, should come to early surgery. Retrosternal gastric bypass has been frequently employed and in selected patients gives excellent palliation and a good functional result. There is no surgical procedure that can be used in all patients suffering from malignant airway fistulas. Appropriate staging of fistula exclusion and visceral reconstruction offers the best prospect of optimizing the conditions of marginal surgical candidates.

REFERENCES

1. Daffner, R.H., Postlethwait, R.W., and Putman, C.E.: Retrotracheal abnormalities in esophageal carcinoma: prognostic implications, Am. J. Roentgenol. **130**:719, 1978.

2. Martini, N., Goodner, J.T., D'Angio, G.J., and Beattie, E.J.: Tracheoesophageal fistula due to cancer, J. Thorac. Cardiovasc. Surg. **58**:319, 1970.

3. Little, A.G., Ferguson, M.K., Demeester, T.R., Hoffman, P.C., and Skinner, D.B.: Esophageal carcinoma with respiratory tract fistula, Cancer **53**:1322, 1984.

4. Duranceau, A., and Jamieson, G.G.: Malignant tracheoesophageal fistula, Ann. Thorac. Surg. **37**:346, 1984.

5. Angorn, I.B.: Intubation in the treatment of carcinoma of the esophagus, World J. Surg. **5**:535, 1981.

6. Petrovsky, B.V., Perelman, M.I., Vantsian, E.N., and Bagirov, D.M.: Palliative and radical operations for acquired esophagotracheal and esophagobronchial fistulas, Surgery **66**:463, 1969.

7. Hegarty, M.M., Angorn, I.B., Bryer, J.V., Henderson, B.J., Le Roux, B.T., and Logan, A.: Palliation of malignant esophago-respiratory fistulas by permanent indwelling prosthetic tube, Ann. Surg. **185**:88, 1977.

8. Ong, G.B., and Kwong, K.H.: Management of malignant esophagobronchial fistula, Surgery **67**:293, 1970.

9. Conlan, A.A., Nicolaou, N., Delikaris, P.G., and Pool, R.: Pessimism concerning palliative bypass procedures for established malignant esophagorespiratory fistulas: a report of 18 patients, Ann. Thor. Surg. **37**:108, 1984.

10. Mannell, A., and Plant, M.: The management of malignant oesophago-airway fistulae, Aust. N.Z. J. Surg. **53**:31, 1983.

11. Roeher, H.D., and Horeyseck, G.: The Kirschner bypass operation: a palliation for complicated esophageal carcinoma, World J. Surg. **5**:543, 1981.

12. Wong, J., Lam, K.H., Wei, W.I., and Ong, G.B.: Results of the Kirschner operation, World J. Surg. **5**:547, 1981.

13. Schreiber, H., and Pories, W.: External diversion for palliative treatment of malignant tracheoesophageal of bronchoesophageal fistulas, Am. J. Surg. **131**:775, 1976.

14. Skinner, D.B.: Esophageal reconstruction, Am. J. Surg. **139**:810, 1980.

15. Ong, G.B., Lam, K.H., Lim, S.T.K., and Wong, J.: Jejunal loop bypass and fundoplication for malignant esophagobronchial fistula, Surg. Gynecol. Obstet. **154**:165, 1982.

DISCUSSION—Chapters 46 to 48

Zwi Steiger

Although the majority of patients with carcinoma of the esophagus have advanced disease, there still exists a need for a therapeutic intervention to relieve the dysphagia. Since palliative surgery carries high mortality and morbidity, the role of surgery is being debated. The preceding three chapters, from three different parts of the world, confirm the fact that relief of dysphagia resulting from cancer of the esophagus can be done effectively with an acceptable morbidity and mortality. Our approach to this challenging problem is essentially the same, with a few minor variations.

The question as to the choice of surgical procedure to perform is dictated by the general condition of the patient.

In a patient whose general condition is satisfactory and who appears to be able to tolerate an operation of greater magnitude, a palliative resection or bypass is the procedure of choice. Most of the time the improvement in the general condition of the patient can be accomplished by preoperative hyperalimentation using a feeding jejunostomy or a central venous line.

Palliative resection of the obstructing carcinoma through the transhiatal route,[1] bringing the stomach through the posterior mediastinum into the neck and anastomosing the proximal esophagus to the fundus of the stomach, is gaining acceptance. The advantages of this procedure are that there is no need for changing the patient's position during the operation and that the anastomosis is done in the neck. The chest is not opened. The procedure is usually well tolerated by most patients. In the event of an anastomotic leak, the leak is localized in the neck and does not have the grave prognosis of a leak in the chest. The drawback of this procedure is that part of the operation is done blindly and unrecognized bleeding from an injured azygos vein or aorta or tearing of the trachea can occasionally occur. Arrhythmias and hypotension from compression of the heart and aorta during the blunt dissection have occasionally been reasons for abandoning the procedure and performing the traditional Ivor Lewis[2]

procedure. This operation requires two separate incisions, one in the abdomen for mobilization of the stomach and performing a pyloroplasty and the second, a right thoracotomy, resecting the esophagus and anastomosing the proximal esophagus to the fundus of the stomach. The procedure takes longer and is not suitable for lesions in the upper third of the esophagus. A jejunostomy is added for feeding in the immediate postoperative period.

When the primary tumor is not resectable, we circumvent[3] the tumor, again using whenever possible the stomach through the Ivor Lewis method, leaving the gastroesophageal junction intact and either anastomosing the fundus of the stomach to the esophagus side-to-side above the tumor or, more commonly, transecting the esophagus, closing the distal end, and anastomosing the proximal end to the fundus of the stomach. In nonresectable lesions of the upper third of the esophagus, the esophagus is left in place and the stomach brought substernally into the neck and anastomosed to the cervical esophagus.[4] We do resect the left sternoclavicular junction to provide more room for the fundus of the stomach. We have left the bypassed esophagus closed on both ends, but usually we drain the distal esophagus with the help of a large Foley catheter brought out in the right subcostal area. The tube is removed in 2 or 3 weeks when the drainage ceases.

In lesions of the gastroesophageal junction that are not resectable, the fundus of the stomach is brought into the left chest and anastomosed above the tumor to the esophagus, again either using the side-to-side technique or transecting the esophagus, closing the distal end, and anastomosing the fundus to the proximal end as described by Johnson and Clagett.[5]

When the patient's condition is poor, there are few options available, the simplest one being repeated dilatation of the tumor to permit passage of some food and saliva. This method has limited effectiveness, and we use it in advanced disease, in patients who are not relieved of dysphagia after receiving radiation therapy, and in patients with advanced carcinoma of the cervical esophagus. The procedure is done under fluoroscopic guidance. A guidewire is passed through the biopsy channel of the flexible esophagoscope and the dilatation performed with the Eder-Puestow dilators. Dilatation may also be accomplished by passing Jackson dilators through the rigid esophagoscope.

Another simple method for some alleviation of the discomfort of an obstructing carcinoma of the esophagus, again used in patients whose conditions are poor, is insertion of a prosthetic tube, by either the pulsion or the traction method. The prosthesis serves as a stent across the obstructing tumor. The advantage of this tube is the rapidity and simplicity of its insertion, but morbidity and operative mortality are high.[6] The high operative mortality may be partially due to the fact that the procedure is usually reserved for the patient who is in poor condition and who would not tolerate a major intervention. We have had a number of perforations of the esophagus with the pilot probe to which the tube is fixed and pulled into the stomach. We have had tube migration, erosion into the aorta, and perforation of the esophagus and stomach. The tube that crosses the gastroesophageal junction results in incompetence of this junction, with constant reflux. There is a need for a change in the patient's diet, and the patient must sleep in a semi-sitting position. We add a pyloroplasty to the procedure to facilitate gastric emptying. We have practically abandoned the use of these tubes and use them only in patients whose prognosis is most grave.

The combination of feeding enterostomy and esophagostomy requires constant care and is not well accepted by the patient. It is used mainly as a temporizing procedure to relieve aspiration in the patient with a totally obstructed esophagus, to improve his respiratory status, and to augment his nutritional status. When the procedure is done for palliation, it is important to construct the esophagostomy low in the neck, so that an extracorporeal conduit can be used to connect the esophagostomy and gastrostomy, the method that Torek used for his patient so effectively for many years.[7] We were never able to teach a patient to use it.

In malignant respiratory esophageal fistulas the problem of dysphagia is aggravated by the continuous contamination of the respiratory tract with saliva. The surgical palliation again depends on the general condition of the patient. If the condition is good, then substernal bypass of the fistula is indeed the best palliation. The excluded esophagus can safely be closed on both ends, or again a large Foley catheter can be inserted into the distal end of the excluded esophagus for drainage. Anastomosing the distal end of the esophagus to a Roux-en-Y jejunal loop is ideal but time-consuming.

When the patient's condition is poor, cervical esophagostomy, feeding jejunostomy, and gastrostomy are preferred. When the fistula is small, occasionally a prosthetic tube may occlude the fistula and alleviate dysphagia. On a few occasions, after bypassing and excluding the fistula, we have administered radiation and chemotherapy with the hope that the lesion will become resectable. So far we have not been able to accomplish this.

The number of our patients requiring palliative resection of the esophagus has been decreasing since we started using chemotherapy and radiation therapy for carcinoma of the esophagus. This combined treatment has relieved the dysphagia in about one third of the patients and obviated any need for surgery. The cost-effectiveness of this mode of treatment has not been calculated. Many of our patients opt for this alternative mode of therapy. A stricture occurring at the site of the primary tumor can be dilated. Palliative resection is then reserved only for the patient who does not respond to such treatment and remains obstructed.

REFERENCES

1. Orringer, M.B., and Sloan, H.: Esophagectomy without thoracotomy, J. Thorac. Cardiovasc. Surg. **76**:643, 1978.
2. Lewis, J.: Surgical treatment of carcinoma of the esophagus with special reference to a new operation for growths of the middle third, Br. J. Surg. **34**:18, 1946.
3. Steiger, Z., Nickel, W.O., Wilson, R.F., and Arbulu, A.: Improved surgical palliation of advanced carcinoma of the esophagus, Am. J. Surg. **135**:782, 1976.
4. Orringer, M.B., and Sloan, H.: Substernal gastric bypass of the excluded thoracic esophagus for palliation of esophageal carcinoma, J. Thorac. Cardiovasc. Surg. **70**:836, 1975.
5. Johnson, C.L., and Clagett, O.T.: Palliative esophagogastrostomy for inoperable carcinoma of the esophagogastric junction, J. Thorac. Cardiovasc. Surg. **60**:269, 1970.
6. Saunders, N.R.: The Celestin tube in the palliation of carcinoma of the esophagus and cardia, Br. J. Surg. **66**:419, 1979.
7. Torek, F.: The first successful case of resection of the thoracic portion of the esophagus for carcinoma, Surg. Gynecol. Obstet. **16**:614, 1913.

CHAPTER 49 Laser therapy as palliation for advanced, nonresectable carcinoma

Richard B. McElvein

The results of treatment of patients with esophageal carcinoma have been generally poor using conventional methods, including surgery, radiation therapy, and chemotherapy. Unfortunately, many patients present with advanced disease and are not suitable candidates for definitive treatment.[1,2]

A variety of forms of palliation have been used, including chemotherapy, radiation therapy, incomplete resection, bypass, exclusion, dilatation, and insertion of prosthetic tubes to maintain a lumen. These methods have been used singly and in combination by a number of authors, generally with poor results.

A new modality, laser energy, has become available in recent years and has been applied to esophageal carcinoma for palliation, with encouraging results.

LASER PHYSICS

"Laser" is an acronym for "light amplification by stimulated emission of radiation." The first effective laser was developed by Maiman in 1960, and since that time a wide variety of laser devices have been developed and used in many applications.[3] In medicine, three lasers have been found to be effective, each having its own advantages and disadvantages. The carbon dioxide laser, operating in the 10.6-nm range, is produced from a mixture of carbon dioxide, nitrogen, and helium gas and emits an invisible light that may be focused and directed by means of tubes and mirrors.

The Nd:YAG (neodymium:yttrium-aluminum-garnet) laser emits radiation in the 1.06-nm range and is derived from a crystal matrix stimulated with a flash lamp. The Nd:YAG laser produces a beam that can be transmitted through flexible fibers.

The argon laser is derived from ionized low-pressure argon gas excited electrically and emits a beam operating in the 0.458-nm range. This can also be passed through flexible wave guides.

The tissue interactions of lasers vary with the wave length of the laser, the color of the tissue, and the composition of the tissue. For example, the carbon dioxide laser beam is absorbed in water, with a rapid rise in temperature to 100° C producing steam with a resultant mechanical and chemical disruption of tissues. The argon laser beam is absorbed by red pigment in tissues, and energy is released when the beam strikes red tissues. Absorption of Nd:YAG laser energy is independent of water content and color.[4]

The power of the laser (measured in watt-seconds), the focus or spot size, the absorption and reflection, scattering, the blood supply of the tissue, and thermal density of the tissue are all variables that affect the end result of laser interaction.

LASER USAGE

The carbon dioxide laser has been used sporadically for esophageal carcinoma, but it is limited by the lack of a suitable flexible wave guide to direct the carbon dioxide laser beam.

The argon laser has been used in a few patients, but, because of its low power density as compared with the Nd:YAG laser, its use has not been pursued.

The Nd:YAG laser has been used by surgeons in many parts of the world. Although there has been no large dominant series, collective experience indicates that this laser shows promise in providing acceptable esophageal palliation.

Patient acceptance of laser therapy is high. Some of its effectiveness as compared with other palliative procedures results from the fact that there is no incision and no general anesthetic. The lesion is treated under direct vision, and major complications have been few.

PATIENT SELECTION AND EVALUATION

The selection of patients as candidates for endoscopic laser therapy has been variable. As with any new therapy, the majority of patients have been deemed nontreatable by other modalities. The goal of laser therapy is palliation of dysphagia, odynophagia, pain, and bleeding, in addition to providing an improved lumen of the esophagus so that the patient may swallow and have a better quality of life. These goals seem achievable by our current techniques using laser energy.

The majority of patients who have had laser treatment have been markedly debilitated with asthenia and weight loss; almost all have had nearly complete or complete obstruction of the esophagus. They have had demonstrable local invasion or distal metastases and have been thought untreatable by other means.

Patients undergoing Nd:YAG laser therapy have been evaluated by an esophagogram and esophagoscopy with biopsy to prove malignant disease. They have had computed tomography (CT) of the thorax and abdomen demonstrating unresectable disease and/or the presence of liver metastasis, or they have had chest x-ray films, pulmonary function studies, and liver function studies indicating severe physiologic impairment. The selection of laser treatment is generally made after all other avenues have been discarded.

TECHNIQUE

Under topical anesthesia, a flexible fiberoptic esophagoscope is passed into the esophagus to the level of the obstruction. If a suitable lumen is present, the instrument is insinuated distally through the tumor. Laser treatment is then commenced in retrograde fashion. If the instrument cannot be passed through tumor, the laser treatment is commenced proximally, down the esophagus. Passing a guide wire is an aid in indicating the true lumen, so that laser treatment can be directed in the axis of the esophagus, rather than perpendicular to the wall, which would increase the risk of perforation.

The initial reaction of the malignant tissue to the Nd:YAG laser is a white circular burn. With continued application of laser energy, there is cavitation with charring and production of smoke, which can be aspirated through the endoscope. The process is continued until tissue destruction obscures the field of vision; at this point the procedure is terminated. It then can be repeated at intervals until the desired effect is achieved.

RESULTS

Fleischer and Kessler[5] have reported on the use of the Nd:YAG laser in 14 patients with squamous cell carcinoma of the esophagus, who required a mean of 5.3 treatments in an average of 11.6 days with a mean energy level of 24,394 watt-seconds. The initial treatment was usually followed by a second treatment in 48 hours, when necrotic debris was aspirated and additional tissue destruction carried out. Concomitant dilatation of the esophagus was performed. The lesions averaged 8.2 cm in length. These authors noted mild fever and leucocytosis with some substernal pain in several patients. One patient, who had had previous radiation therapy, developed a tracheoesophageal fistula, which was successfully treated with an endoluminal prosthesis. Another patient developed a perforation of the esophagus requiring surgical drainage. The mean survival from the initiation of treatment was 14 weeks.

Mellow et al.[6] treated 11 patients with the Nd:YAG laser, all of whom had squamous cell carcinoma of the esophagus with marked weight loss and long lesions (approximately 8 cm). The patients were treated every other day with 90 to 100 watts of power, for a median number of 3.3 treatments. The median survival was 17 weeks, with one complication of a tracheoesophageal fistula.

Krasner and Beard,[7] from the United Kingdom, also using the Nd:YAG laser, treated nine patients, using 100 watts of power in bursts of 0.5 to 1.0 seconds, for a median treatment energy level of 2950 watt-seconds. These authors used an average of three treatments, given every 2 to 4 weeks. The mean survival was 15.8 weeks, with a range of 3 to 39 weeks. There were two deaths as a result of complications—one following tube insertion with perforation and the other from a perforation in a 91-year-old woman.

Agrawal et al.,[8] again using the Nd:YAG laser, reported their experience in New Orleans with 21 patients averaging 63 years of age. These authors used 80 to 100 watts of power administered in 1-second bursts for a mean treatment of 4215 watt-seconds. Their patients were treated an average of 5.8 sessions over 11.2 days. Agrawal et al. were able to achieve a usefully patent lumen of the esophagus in 20 of the 21 patients, with a mean survival of 11 months.

CONTACT PROBES

The initial application of Nd:YAG laser energy was with a fiber placed, and energy applied, at a distance of 1 to 2 cm from the malignant tissue. If the original fibers came into contact with tissue, they became fouled and inoperative. The development of contact laser fibers has allowed greater precision in the application of the energy. A synthetic sapphire tip, attached to the end of the Nd:YAG fiber, serves as a hot probe that can be applied directly to the tissues through the esophageal lumen, presumably with better energy application and greater safety.[9]

HEMATOPHORPHYRIN DERIVATIVES

The development of photosensitizing agents in the form of hematophorphyrin derivatives (HpD) has provided another means of treating esophageal carcinoma with lasers.

Hematophorphyrin derivatives are prepared from blood treated with various concentrations of acids and the resultant material purified. Injected into the patient, the hematophorphyrin derivative is uniformly distributed through all the tissues of the body but is selectively retained in malignant tissue and rapidly excreted from normal tissue. This leaves a photosensitive agent within tumor substance, which can be activated by laser light to provide singlet oxygen and destruction of malignant tissue.[10]

The activation of the HpD can be carried out with both the Nd:YAG laser and the argon laser. This technique does not depend upon thermal destruction of tissue by high energy levels but instead is dependent on the activation of the hematophorphyrin derivative by a laser light.

McCaughan et al.[11] have used a tunable argon dye laser operating in the 630-nm range in 16 patients who have been treated with intravenous injection of 2 mg/kg of Photofrin II (HpD). (See also Chapter 50.) Topical anesthesia and a flexible instrument are used, with the argon laser directed to the tumor by means of a flexible fiber. McCaughan et al. have been able to apply the laser to the surface of the tumor or, in some instances, pass the fiber into the lumen distally to provide

circumferential activation of the HpD. The initial treatment is performed 48 hours after injection of the HpD and is repeated in 3 days, then as necessary in a month, and then every 2 to 3 months. McCaughan et al. have found a patient median survival of 6.5 months, with improved survival of 8.1 months in patients with a high Karnofsky score. Three complications have occurred—one sterile effusion not requiring therapy and two strictures responding to dilatation. One of the stricture of patients is a long-term survivor.

COMBINED THERAPY

Endoscopic laser therapy for esophageal carcinoma has been combined with other treatment methods. Ghazi and Nussbaum[12] have treated six patients, principally with an Nd:YAG laser. Five of these patients had laser treatments followed by dilatation and insertion of a prosthesis. One patient had a pretreatment respiratory fistula, which was successfully treated with the laser and placement of a prosthesis. Ghazi and Nussbaum used treatment of 4000 to 6000 watt-seconds, given in 1-second bursts every other day, and have had survival ranging from 1 to 18 months. Two complications have occurred—one of bleeding, which was controllable, and one pneumoperitoneum, which did not require therapy.

Lambert et al.[13] have used laser therapy in conjunction with chemotherapy consisting of 5-fluorouracil and cisplatin along with radiation therapy. They divided their 43 patients into groups and found that those patients with T_3 lesions had a 20% 12-month survival.

The complications of combined laser therapy include fever, leucocytosis, abdominal pain, perforation, and bleeding. Some of these complications may be independent of the treatment, since they are common complications of the basic disease.

SUMMARY

At first blush, it appears that laser therapy for advanced esophageal carcinoma may be effective in prolonging quality and, perhaps, length of life. The treatment affects only the internal luminal disease and does, in the main, provide a patent alimentary canal.

There are many unanswered questions about laser therapy: the appropriate energy levels, the interval between treatments, the number of treatments, and whether continuous or pulsed laser energy is more effective.

At this time, laser endoscopy is in its infancy but does show promise of helping those unfortunate patients who present late in their disease with obstruction and otherwise untreatable esophageal cancer.

REFERENCES

1. Earlam, R., and Cunha-Melo, J.R.: Oesophageal squamous cell carcinoma. I. A critical review of surgery, Br. J. Surg. **67**:381, 1980.
2. Earlam, R., and Cunha-Melo, J.R.: Oesophageal squamous cell carcinoma. II. A critical review of radiotherapy, Br. J. Surg. **67**:457, 1980.
3. Polanyi, T.G.: Physics of surgery with lasers, Clin. Chest Med. **6**:179, 1985.
4. Sliney, D.H.: Laser-tissue interactions, Clin. Chest Med. **6**:203, 1985.
5. Fleischer, D., and Kessler, F.: Endoscopic Nd:YAG Laser therapy for carcinoma of the esophagus: a new form of palliative treatment, Gastroenterology **85**:600, 1983.
6. Mellow, M.H., Pinkas, H., et al.: Endoscopic therapy for esophageal carcinoma with Nd:YAG laser: prospective evaluation of efficacy, complications and survival, Gastrointest. Endosc. **29**:165, 1983.
7. Krasner, N., and Beard, J.: Laser irradiation of tumours of the oesophagus and gastric cardia, Br. Med. J. **288**:829, 1984.
8. Agrawal, N.M., Akdamar, K., Godiwala, T., and Ertan, A.: Nd:YAG laser treatment of cancer of the esophagus, Clin. Res. **34**:214A, 1986.
9. Ell, C., Hochberger, J., and Lux, G.: Clinical experience of non-contact and contact Nd:YAG laser therapy for inoperable malignant stenoses of the oesophagus and stomach, Lasers Med. Sci. **1**:143, 1986.
10. Dougherty, T.J.: Photodynamic therapy, Clin. Chest Med. **6**:219, 1985.
11. McCaughan, J.S., Williams, T.E., and Bethel, B.H.: Palliation of esophageal malignancy with photodynamic therapy, Ann. Thorac. Surg. **40**:113, 1985.
12. Ghazi, A., and Nussbaum, M.: A new approach to the management of malignant esophageal obstruction and esophagorespiratory fistula, Ann. Thorac. Surg. **41**:531, 1986.
13. Lambert, R., Sabben, G., et al.: Laser in the non-surgical treatment of squamous cell cancer in the esophagus, Lasers Surg. Med. **5**:191, 1985.

CHAPTER 50 Palliation of esophageal malignancy with photodynamic therapy

James S. McCaughan, Jr., and Thomas E. Williams, Jr.

Most physicians who manage patients with cancer of the esophagus know the agony and frustration these unfortunate people suffer because of their disease or well-intentioned therapeutic endeavors. The medical literature contains many reports of chemotherapy, ionizing radiation, surgical resections, bypasses, exclusions, dilatations, prosthetic insertion, and combinations of these techniques, which attest to the inadequacy of our treatment techniques. Regardless of the form of therapy, we generally obtain less than a 4% 5-year survival rate.

Earlam and Cunha-Melo's report[1] indicates that at least as many as 60% of patients with newly diagnosed esophageal carcinomas are candidates for palliation only. Chemotherapy and/or ionizing radiation provides some relief, but the tumor frequently recurs with obstruction in less than 6 months.

Although recent reports indicate that rates of resectability are rising (Finley et al.,[2] 68%; Ellis,[3] 89%), the incidence of celiac node involvement (83%) seen in the resected patients contained in the report of Finley et al. further emphasizes that most of our efforts must, of necessity, be directed toward palliation. Given a mean life expectancy of only 2.5 to 5 months for this age group of patients with esophageal cancer, it is clear that good palliation must (1) relieve obstruction and (2) have a low mortality risk. Various current reports indicate the mortality risk for palliative surgical resection to be 1.7% to 6.7%, and intraluminal tube palliation 1.5% to 22.6% (most older reports give mortality risks in the 15% to 30% range for both forms of palliation). Unfortunately, many intraluminal tubes become obstructed by food, dislodge from their positions, or erode through the esophagus and cannot be used for high lesions.

We believe that photodynamic therapy to patients previously injected with hematoporphyrin derivative or Photofrin II to photosensitize the tumors provides suitable relief of obstruction at a low mortality risk. It has the further advantage of being performed in an outpatient setting, thereby providing these patients with more time at home during their remaining days.

In 1978, Dougherty et al.[4] reported success in treating cutaneous and subcutaneous malignancies with photodynamic therapy. Since then the basic premise that malignancies presensitized with hematoporphyrin derivative can be selectively destroyed by exposing them to light has been confirmed by many investigators. Melanomas of the choroid plexus,[5] head and neck cancers,[6] bladder tumors,[7] gastric cancer,[8] female genital tract tumors,[9] primary skin cancers,[10] lung cancers,[11,12] and other tumors have been treated.[13]

The sensitizer hematoporphyrin derivative (HpD)—or its more purified form, Photofrin II—when given intravenously, disseminates to malignant and normal cells, but clears more rapidly from the nonmalignant tissue. After 48 to 72 hours there is a differential concentration of sensitizer between the tumor cells and the adjacent normal tissue. When 630 ± 2 nm light (red) is directed onto the tumor area, the sensitizer absorbs the light energy to produce a photochemical reaction. One proposed mechanism of action may be the production of singlet oxygen, which destroys the tumor cells. Since there is less sensitizer remaining in the normal tissue, little or no reaction occurs in it.

In the past 3 years we have treated 190 patients with this form of therapy. This report summarizes the results obtained from 60 treatments to 25 patients with malignancy involving the esophagus; 48 injections of sensitizer were used.

TECHNIQUES

All of these patients had received, refused, or were ineligible for conventional surgery, chemotherapy, or ionizing radiation therapy. Some also previously had received Nd:YAG laser therapy and dilatation. Their ages ranged from 54 to 88; 21 were male, four were female. The cell types of the various tumors are shown in Table 50-1.

Two to 6 days after injection of the sensitizing agent, the tumor areas were photoradiated with light delivered through quartz fibers inserted through the biopsy channel of a fiberoptic esophagoscope for periods of time depending on the length of the tumor (up to 90 minutes). Topical anesthesia and intravenous sedation were used, with the patient awake and responsive. The electrocardiogram, blood pressure, and pulse rate were continuously monitored and nasal oxygen administered. The 630-nm light was generated by a 20-watt argon laser (Spectra Physics model 171) pumping a tunable dye laser (Spectra Physics model 375) circulating rhodamine-B or kiton red dye. The light was directed onto the surface of the tumor, or the fiber was inserted directly into the tumor interstitially by straight-cut or cylinder diffusing fiber tips.

Esophagoscopy and biopsy were repeated 2 to 3 days after treatment, and retreatment was performed at that time if indicated. Esophagoscopy and biopsy were also performed 1 month after treatment and then every 2 or 3 months or as needed.

Since most of these patients had end-stage cancer of the esophagus or stomach or other severe medical problems, an attempt was made to evaluate the effect of the treatment on the quality of life as well as the length of survival. The parameters used were body weight, swallowing ability, Karnofsky Performance Status (KPS), and an esophageal grading (EG) system, which assigns a numerical grade for each of the following: (1) pain (whether or not related to swallowing), (2) swallowing ability, (3) sleep quality, (4) leisure activity, and (5) work status (including housework). The maximum grade is 100.

RESULTS
Survival

The average survival of all 25 patients was 6.8 months, with four patients alive 5, 6, 17, and 25 months after their first treatments. The average survival of those who died was 5.5 months, with a range of 3 weeks to 19 months.

The average survival for 21 patients with an initial Karnofsky Performance Status greater than 30 was 7.8 months, while four patients with an initial KPS of 30 or less survived an average of 1.3 months.

Cause of death

Eighteen patients died from generalized disease, one from gastrointestinal hemorrhage from the tumor, one from myocardial infarction, and one from pneumonia resulting from aspiration of gastric tube feedings resumed 2 days after treatment of what previously had been a complete esophageal obstruction. (See Tables 50-1–50-3.)

Quality of survival

One month after the initial treatment, the average KPS increased from 58 to 68, the esophageal grade from 58 to 76, and the weight from 141 to 142 pounds. Most of the improvement was due to increased swallowing ability.

The four patients who died within 1 month had a KPS of 40 or less, and all were completely obstructed. However, their average esophageal grade increased by 28 points, and two were able to eat a soft diet and two were able to drink liquids at the time of their deaths.

Except for the two patients who had pretreatment tracheoesophageal fistulas (no. 186, and no. 188) and one who had a subsequent cervical esophagostomy (no. 20), all (including seven with complete obstruction) were able to swallow at least liquids at the time of their deaths.

Unfortunately, patients who were mechanically able to swallow food lost their desire to eat as anorexia developed because of their disease.

The average minimum diameter of the esophagus, as estimated by esophagoscopy, increased from 5 mm to 11 mm at 1 month.

Fig. 50-1 (patient no. 27) shows a squamous cell cancer almost completely obstructing the lumen of the esophagus and its appearance 2 months after photodynamic therapy, at which time he was able to eat a regular diet and had gained 17 pounds of weight. Fig. 50-2 shows his esophagogram before and 2 months after treatment.

Fig. 50-3 (patient no. 24) shows a patient who was completely obstructed from adenocarcinoma and the reaction 2 days and 2 months after treatment.

Status of survivors

Presently, four patients are able to eat at least a soft diet. Two patients have residual disease. One patient has recurrent disease at 17 months. One patient, no. 99 (Fig. 50-4), has no evidence of disease at 25 months.

TABLE 50-1. Summary patient data

No.	ARS*	Diagnosis	Site (cm)	LG (cm)	#INJS	#RXS	Dose range (joules)	D OP (mm)	D OP (mm) 1 mo	Mo LX	Cause of death/status
014	88WM	Esop, melanoma	31-38	7	5	5	420-680 (CS)	8	13	19	DOD
020	54WM	Esop, SQ	25-32	7	2	2	420-700 (CS)	4	8	8	DOD
024	64WM	Esop, AD	38-48	10	4	4	420-630 (CS)	0	12	11	Myocardial infarction
027	61BM	Esop, SQ	35-42	7	2	2	630 (CS)	7	14	6	DOD
029	75WM	Esop, AD	30-36	8	1	2	630 (CS)	5	13	3	DOD
031	58WM	Esop, stom, AD	40-45	6	2	2	540 (TS); 600 (TS); 600 (TI)	11	14	3	DOD
036	71WF	Esop, SQ	26-38	12	1	3	420 (CS)	8	13	10	DOD
049	65WF	Esop, AD	35-42	8	1	1	420 (CS)	0	8	1	Aspirated gastric tube feeding
055	70BM	Esop, SQ	18-25	7	1	1	600 (TS); 700 (TI)	2		0.6	DOD
073	88WM	Esop, AD	18-?		1	1	1200 (TI); 420 (CS)	0	8	4.5	DOD
099	69WM	Esop, melanoma	38-40	2	2	2	420-730 (CS)	NL	NL	25	Alive/NED
105	68WM	Esop, AD	34-45	11	4	6	420-840 (CS)	8	14	11	DOD
110	58WM	Esop, stom, AD	28-40	11	2	2	450-900 (CS)	10	13	3	GI hemorrhage
132	68WM	Esop, AD	20-35	22	4	5	600 (CS); 600 (CS) 3150 (TI); 2100 (TI) 2040 (TI)	8	13	10	DOD
134	67WF	Esop, SQ	30-42	10	1	2	540 (CS)	3		0.6	DOD, prior PNC
138	75WM	Esop, SQ	29-39	2	2	3	540-600 (CS)	NL	14	17	Alive, rec dis
139	55WM	Esop, SQ	17-21	4	3	5	450-720 (CS)	7	12	9.5	DOD
142	64WM	Esop, SQ	25-35	16	1	2	300 (CS); 2340 (TS)	4		1	DOD
162	72WM	Esop, SQ	18-23	5	1	1	500 (CS)	5		1.5	DOD
172	69WM	Esop, stom, AD	35-40	5	2	2	445-700 (CS)	6	10	6	Alive, resid dis
173	58WM	Esop, SQ	12-26	8	1	2	400-600 (CS)	0	8	3.5	DOD
175	72WF	Esop, SQ	27-30	3	1	1	400-500 (CS)	8	9	5	DOD
180	68WM	Esop, AD	28-40	12	2	2	400-500 (CS)	4	12	5	Alive, resid dis
186	57WM	Esop, SQ	17-25	8	1	1	400-700 (CS)	2	8	2.5	DOD, TEF
188	59WM	Esop, SQ	17-23	6	1	1	600 (CS)	6	10	2.5	DOD, TEF

*ARS, age, race, sex; Esop, esophagus; stom, stomach; SQ, squamous cell carcinoma; AD, adenocarcinoma; site (cm), number of centimeters from teeth; LG, length of tumor; #INJS, number of injections of photosensitizer; #RXS, total number of treatments; CS, cylinder fiber, surface irradiation; TS, straight-tip fiber, surface irradiation; TI, straight-tip fiber, interstitial irradiation; D OP (mm), minimum diameter of opening in millimeters; D OP (mm) 1 mo, minimum diameter of opening 1 month after treatment; Mo LX, months from first treatment to time of last examination and/or death; cause of death/status, cause of death/status of patients still alive; NL, not listed; DOD, Died of disease; NED, no evidence of disease; TEF, tracheoesophageal fistula.

TABLE 50-2. Clinical benefit

No.	Diet	Diet (1 mo)	Diet (LX)	WT (lb)	WT (1 mo)	WT (LX)	EG	EG (1 mo)	EG (LX)	KPS	KPS (1 mo)	KPS (LX)	Mo LX
014	Liq*	Reg	Reg	132	129		65	95	95	80	90	90	19
020	C liq	NPO	NPO	141	142		35	24	20	40	40	30	8
024	C obn	Reg	Reg	147	141	145	50	95	95	90	90	90	11
027	Liq	Reg	Liq	120	134		65	95	65	80	80		6
029	Liq	Reg	Reg	169	174		61	91		40	60		3
031	Liq	Reg	Reg	149	172†		61	91	91	60	60		3
036	Liq	Reg	Liq	99	97		64	94	64	80	80	50	10
049	C obn	Liq	Liq	147	152	152	46	61	61	20	20	20	1
055	C obn		Liq	121		128	42		61	30		30	0.6
073	C obn	Liq		184	178		40	55		40	40		4.5
099	Reg	Reg	Reg	178	172	110	100	100	100	90	100	90	25
105	Liq	Reg	Reg	137	125		84	94	91	70	70	40	11
110	Liq	Reg	Reg	149	134		64	94	91	70	80	80	3
132	C liq	Reg	Reg	106	117	116	68	98	86	70	80	80	10
134	C obn		Soft	99		97	46		81	20		20	0.6
138	Reg	Reg	Reg	145	145	135	100	100	100	100	100	90	17
139	BLND	Soft	Liq	184	169	134	64	84	44	80	80	50	9.5
142	C obn	Soft	Soft	150	154	154	46	81	81	20	40	40	1
162	C liq	Liq		123	126		31	39		40	60		1.5
172	BLND	Reg	Soft	233	218	184	59	70	60	80	90	50	6
173	C obn	Liq	C obn	107	103		40	50		50	50		3.5
175	C liq	Soft	BLND	141	135	119	55	65	57	70	80		5
180	Liq	Reg	Soft	132	136	137	51	81	71	80	90	90	5
186	NPO (TEF)	NPO (TEF)	NPO (TEF)	132	124		46	44	25	30	50	30	2.5
188	NPO (TEF)	NPO (TEF)	NPO (TEF)	96	97		55	40	40	20	40	40	2.5

*Liq, liquid diet; C liq, clear liquid diet; C obn, complete obstruction; Reg, regular diet; BLND, blenderized diet; NPO, able to tolerate nothing by mouth; TEF, tracheoesophageal fistula; WT, weight in pounds; WT (LX), weight at last examination; EG, esophageal grade; EG (LX), esophageal grade at last examination; KPS, Karnovsky performance status; Mo LX, months after first treatment to last examination or death.
†Developed ascites.

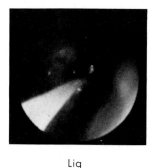

Liq

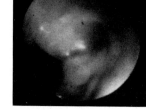

2 months — R.D.

J.B.
Squamous
DOD — 6 months

Fig. 50-1. Patient no. 27. Squamous cell cancer of the esophagus. Patient gained 17 pounds in 2 months. Died of disease *(DOD)* six months after treatment. *Liq,* Liquid diet; *RD,* regular diet.

TABLE 50-3. Clinical effect relative to initial Karnovsky Performance Status

	All (25)			**KPS > 30 (21)**			**KPS ≤ 30 (4)**		
	Weight (lb)	**EG**	**KPS**	**Weight**	**EG**	**KPS**	**Weight**	**EG**	**KPS**
Before treatment	141	58	58	144	59	65	123	48	20
1 month after treatment	142	76	68	144	78	74	134	61	33
Last evaluation	143	70	53	134	72	60	134	66	30
Survival (months)	6.8			7.8			1.3		

Complications

Patient no. 99 required esophageal dilatation and chest tube drainage for posttreatment esophageal edema and sterile pleural effusion. A subsequent stricture required weekly self-dilatations for several months. Twenty-five months after treatment he eats a regular diet, has no evidence of recurrence, and no longer requires dilatation.

One month after treatment, patient no. 138 developed a stricture that required self-dilatation. At 8 months he had recurrence above the treated area and was retreated. Nine months later (17 months from first treatment) he eats a regular diet, but again has recurrent disease.

Within 1 week of treatment, patient no. 139 developed posttreatment edema requiring dilatation. Presently, he eats a soft diet.

Procedure mortality

There were no deaths attributable to the procedure itself.

DISCUSSION

Any technique that can improve the quality of life with a low mortality rate, short hospital stay, and minimal complication rate should be explored further. Photodynamic therapy entails essentially a prolonged flexible esophagoscopy that can be performed as an outpatient procedure with minimal sedation.

Three of our patients who had a KPS of 30 or less never left the hospital. However, they were able to swallow at least liquids until their deaths. Completely obstructed patients who were otherwise active were able, after treatment, to eat popcorn, toast, steak, and so on, until just before their deaths from the ravages of their disease.

One month after the initial treatment of all 25 patients there was an average increase of the esophageal grade of 18 points. The KPS increased an average of 10 points, and weight remained stable. The average minimum opening increased from 5 mm to 11 mm.

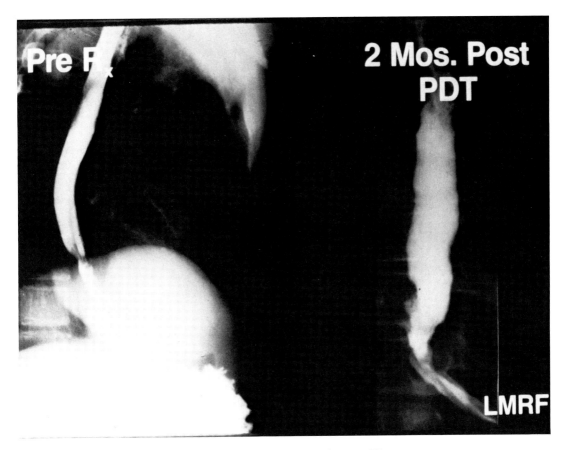

Fig. 50-2. X-ray films of patient no. 27.

The average survival for all patients was 6.8 months. All except two with preexisting tracheoesophageal fistulas and one who received a cervical esophagostomy were able to swallow at least liquids when they died.

Skin photosensitivity to sunlight after injection of hematoporphyrin derivative has not been a serious problem for these patients. They adjust to the sunlight restrictions by using sunscreens, wearing protective clothing, and assuming a nocturnal life-style.

The Nd:YAG laser has been used to create a larger lumen to improve swallowing.[14,15] We have obtained this effect with this technique, but it must be used cautiously since the thermal coagulation can penetrate through the wall of the esophagus and the beam has to be focused directly onto the tumor.

Photodynamic therapy is nonthermal at presently used powers. The light penetrates the tissue a maximum of 1.0 to 1.5 cm to produce its effect. This is an advantage in treating superficial lesions and undetectable mucosal spread. We are now treating large obstructing lesions by first "de-bulking" with the Nd:YAG laser to obtain a larger lumen. Subsequently, we treat the residual tumor with photodynamic therapy.

These techniques appear to be superior to dilatation, since not only is the lumen enlarged, but some of the tumor is destroyed.

While results with the Nd:YAG laser and photodynamic therapy appear to be equal to or better than results with prostheses, a question to be answered is whether increasing the distal lumen will be of any benefit to patients who have esophageal-pulmonary fistulas.

CONCLUSIONS

Photodynamic therapy offers another form of palliation for patients with cancer of the esophagus. Since this therapy essentially entails only a prolonged esophagoscopy under local anesthesia and does not interfere with other types of therapy, it has particular value for patients who have already exhausted other therapy forms or who are not candidates for them.

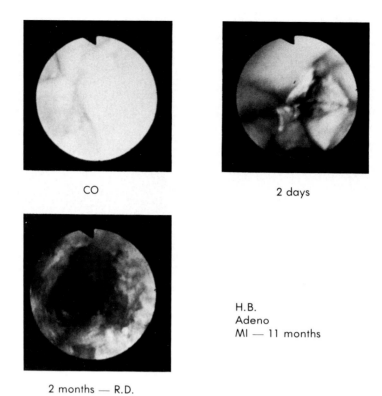

CO

2 days

H.B.
Adeno
MI — 11 months

2 months — R.D.

Fig. 50-3. Patient no. 24. Adenocarcinoma resulting in complete obstruction. The reaction 2 days after treatment is shown in the right upper corner, and its appearance 2 months later is shown in the left lower corner. He died of a myocardial infarction *(MI)* 11 months after his first treatment. He was eating a regular diet at the time of his death. *RD,* Regular diet.

The advantages of photodynamic therapy are as follows:

1. Minimal operative risks
2. Destroys tumor as well as increases the diameter of the lumen
3. No limitations on the number of times that it can be repeated
4. Does not interfere with chemotherapy or x-ray therapy
5. No foreign-body prosthesis
6. Can be performed on an outpatient basis
7. Survival rates appear to be equivalent to those of other forms of palliative therapy
8. Quality of life improved

There have been two main disadvantages:

1. The treatment causes photosensitivity of skin, requiring avoidance of sunlight for 1 to 2 months.
2. Overtreatment can cause esophagitis with pleural effusion, edema, and stricture formation.

REFERENCES

1. Earlam, R., and Cunha-Melo, J.R.: Malignant oesophageal strictures: a review of techniques for palliative intubation, Br. J. Surg. **69:**61, 1982.
2. Finley, R.J., Grace, M., and Duff, J.: Esophagogastrectomy without thoracotomy for carcinoma of the cardia and lower part of the esophagus, Surg. Gynecol. Obstet. **160:**49, 1985.
3. Ellis, F.H., Jr.: Cancer of the esophagus and cardia: role of surgery in palliation, Postgrad. Med. **75:**139, 146, 1984.
4. Dougherty, T.J., Kaufman, J.E., Goldfarb, A., et al.: Photoradiation therapy for the treatment of malignant tumors, Cancer Res. **38:**2628, 1978.
5. Bruce, R.A.: Evaluation of hematoporphyrin photoradiation therapy to treat choroidal melanomas, Lasers Surg. Med. **4:**59, 1984.
6. Schuller, D.E., McCaughan, J.S., and Rock, R.P.: Photodynamic therapy in head and neck cancer, Arch. Otolaryngol. **3:**351, 1985.
7. Benson, R.C., Kinsey, J.H., Cortese, D.A., et al.: Treatment of transitional cell carcinoma of the bladder with hematoporphyrin derivative photothery, J. Urol. **130:**1090, 1983.

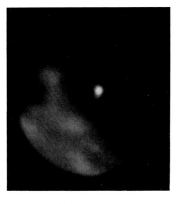
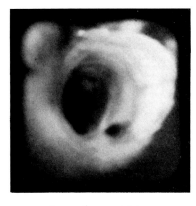

Before   6 months — stricture

J.S.
Melanoma
25 months — RD
NED

Fig. 50-4. Patient no. 99. Melanoma of the esophagus—treated twice. No evidence of disease and patient eating a regular diet 25 months after first treatment. *RD,* Regular diet; *NED,* no evidence of disease.

8. Aida, M., and Kawaguchi, M.: Gastric cancer. In Hayata, Y., and Dougherty, T.J., editors: Lasers and hematoporphyrin derivative in cancer, Tokyo, 1983, Igaku-Shoin, pp. 65-69.

9. McCaughan, J.S., Schelhas, H.F., Lomano, J., and Bethel, B.H.: Photodynamic therapy of gynecologic neoplasms after presensitization with hematoporphyrin derivative, Lasers Surg. Med. **5:**491, 1985.

10. Tokuda, Y.: Primary skin cancer. In Hayata, Y., and Dougherty, T.J., editors: Lasers and hematoporphyrin derivative in cancer, Tokyo, 1983, Igaku-Shoin, pp. 85-96.

11. Hayata, Y., Kato, H., Konaka, C., et al.: Photoradiation therapy with hematoporphyrin derivative in early and stage I lung cancer, Chest **86:**169, 1984.

12. Balchum, O.J., Doiron, D.R., and Huth, G.C.: Photoradiation therapy of endobronchial lung cancers employing the photodynamic action of hematoporphyrin derivative, Lasers Surg. Med. **4:**13, 1984.

13. Gomer, C.J., and Doiron, D.R., editors: Porphyrin localization and treatment of tumors, New York, 1984, Alan R. Liss, Inc.

14. Fleischer, D., and Kessler, F.: Endoscopic Nd:YAG laser therapy for carcinoma of the esophagus: a new form of palliative treatment, Gastroenterology **85:**600, 1983.

15. Krasner, N., and Beard, J.: Laser irradiation of tumors of the oesophagus and gastric cardia, Br. Med. J. **288:**829, 1984.

CHAPTER 51 Endoesophageal intubation for palliation in obstructing esophageal carcinoma

Israel Barnett Angorn and Ariff Ahmed Haffejee

The possibility of a tumor partially or completely obstructing the passage of food down the gullet was first suggested by Galen (131-200 AD). Avicenna, the influential tenth-century Persian physician, accorded the pride of place to esophageal cancer as a cause of dysphagia. John Casaubon, a seventeenth-century British surgeon who died of esophageal carcinoma, suggested that the poor prognosis in this disease could only be improved by early diagnosis. Three major pioneers in the management of esophageal carcinoma were Kussmaul, who passed the first crude esophagoscope in 1868; Torek, who performed the first successful resection in 1913; and Janeway, who introduced a safe esophagoscope in 1918 and contributed greatly to the development of surgical and radiation treatment of esophageal carcinoma.

The 5-year survival for patients with carcinoma of the esophagus varies from less than 1%[1] to 9%[2] no matter what form the initial treatment takes, with 90% of patients dying within 1 year.[3] Because long-term survival is rare, palliation of dysphagia has always been the major consideration in management, with cure being regarded as an added bonus. Resection of the neoplasm, even if this be incomplete, with restoration of alimentary tract continuity, offers the best palliation, and can now be achieved with an acceptable mortality and low morbidity.[4] Approximately 60% of all patients with squamous esophageal cancer presenting with dysphagia have already nonresectable lesions. In this situation, the optimal method of restoring the ability to swallow remains controversial. Bypass procedures using stomach, colon, or jejunum often give unsatisfactory results, with considerable mortality. Limited justification can be found for their preferred use as a means of palliation.[5] Radiotherapy is effective in perhaps half the patients so treated, symptomatic improvement is apparent only after 4 to 6 weeks, and the benefits may be temporary.[6]

Esophageal intubation relieves dysphagia and offers the additional benefits of simple execution and rapid effectiveness.[7] Intubation of malignant strictures of the esophagus, first suggested by Leroy d'Etiolles in 1845,[8] has been practiced successfully since the small series reported by Symonds in 1887.[9] There are two basic techniques: pulsion, whereby the tube is pushed down, usually via the peroral route,[10,11] but occasionally through a cervical[12] or thoracic esophagotomy,[13] and traction, whereby the tube is pulled through the tumor from below, via a high gastrotomy.[14,15]

Carcinoma of the esophagus is extremely common among South African blacks, and annual admissions to King Edward VIII Hospital, our major teaching hospital, have shown a fivefold increase each decade since 1955, when 21 patients were admitted.[16] During the 10-year period from mid-1975 to mid-1985, approximately 5700 patients were admitted to a specialised unit established to deal with this major therapeutic and logistic problem. This report analyzes our experience with intubation in the treatment of carcinoma of the esophagus using both pulsion and traction techniques.

SELECTION OF PATIENTS FOR INTUBATION

For management purposes, the division of the esophagus into cervical, upper thoracic, and lower thoracic/abdominal segments is both useful and practical.[17] All patients with squamous carcinoma of the cervical esophagus are referred for radiotherapy. Tumors of the lower esophagus—that is, from the level of the tracheal bifurcation to the cardia—are considered for resection. Patients with tumors of the upper thoracic esophagus (thoracic inlet to tracheal bifurcation, 20 to 32 cm from incisor teeth) are randomized to curative radiotherapy[18] or to surgery, provided the tumors are less than 6 cm in length, there is no evidence of periesophageal invasion or distant dissemination, and the patients can still swallow solids or semisolids.

Palliative intubation is indicated for patients with any of the following:

1. Medical contraindications to surgery or radiotherapy
2. Irreversible physical debility
3. Clinically detectable invasion of adjacent organs or distant dissemination
4. Dysphagia resulting from recurrence following surgery or radiotherapy
5. Malignant strictures of the upper thoracic esophagus longer than 6 cm
6. Upper thoracic tumors causing complete dysphagia (If the lesion is considered curable, i.e., less than 6 cm, intubation is followed by radiotherapy.)
7. Demonstrable tracheoesophageal or bronchoesophageal fistula
8. Nonresectability established at laparotomy or thoracotomy

MANAGEMENT PROTOCOL

All patients have anteroposterior and lateral x-ray films of the chest following a barium swallow. These demonstrate the level of the tumor, the length of the malignant stricture, and the alignment of the esophageal axis. The indications for intubation are determined on clinical, radiologic, and endoscopic grounds, except for nonresectability established at surgical exploration. All upper-thoracic tumors are intubated using a pulsion technique, since the presence of a normal esophageal segment below the tumor lessens the likelihood of perforation.[19] Traction intubation is reserved for lower-esophageal tumors for which resection is contraindicated or technically not feasible.

PULSION INTUBATION

During the 10-year period from mid-1975 to mid-1985, a total of 2446 patients with a confirmed diagnosis of esophageal carcinoma were

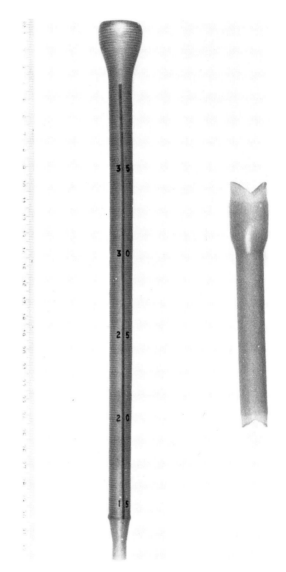

Fig. 51-1. *Left,* Improved version of Celestin tube with nylon spiral in its wall and inkwell-shaped proximal funnel. *Right,* Lateral view of the 15-cm Procter-Livingstone tube, showing expanded proximal end and proximal and distal "fish mouths."

intubated with a pulsion technique.[7] The mean age of the patients was 54.6 years (range, 26 to 80 years), and the male-to-female ratio was 4:1. The mean duration of dysphagia before admission was 6.6 months. The tube used was the Procter-Livingstone tube (Latex Products, Johannesburg, South Africa).[20] This is an armored soft latex rubber tube with an internal diameter of 12 mm and an outer diameter of 18 mm (Fig. 51-1). The proximal end is expanded to an oval of external diameter 3 × 2.5 cm to enable it to fit snugly above the tumor and to prevent the passage of food between the tube and the esophageal wall.

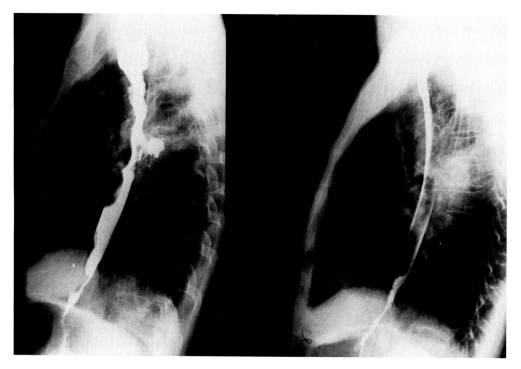

Fig. 51-2. Lateral barium swallow films of a 15-cm malignant esophageal stricture invading the mediastinum, before *(left)* and after *(right)* pulsion intubation.

In lateral view, the ends are "fish-mouthed," while in anteroposterior view, they are curved. This design is determined by the normal resting position of the esophagus, which is collapsed anteroposteriorly.[21] To facilitate insertion and to prevent pressure necrosis of the esophageal wall, both the proximal and distal ends are not armored. The tube is available in three lengths—11 cm, 15 cm, and 19 cm—but because of the length of the tumors in our series, the 11-cm tube was seldom used.

The patient lies supine on the operating table, with the head supported on a grommet ring. The table break permits flexion and extension of the cervical spine. General anesthesia with high-dose fentanyl allows rapid induction and reversal of anesthesia. Bronchoscopy is first performed to identify compression of the tracheobronchial tree, tumor invasion, or the presence of a fistula. Tracheobronchial secretions are aspirated, and an endotracheal tube is inserted. Esophagoscopy is then performed with a large Negus esophagoscope, 17.5 mm in circumference and 45 cm in length. The lubricated esophagoscope is advanced under direct vision as far as the stricture, from which biopsies are taken. Dilatation is achieved by the sequential passage of graduated bougies to 40 Fr gauge. To avoid perforation of the distal esophagus or stomach, the bougie

should traverse only the length of the stricture. Longitudinal rupture of the tumor during dilatation does not increase morbidity, since the tube effectively tamponades any mural defect. A 20 Fr gauge bougie is passed through the dilated stricture and left in situ. A lubricated tube of appropriate length is inserted over the bougie and through the stricture, with the rigid esophagoscope being used as a "pusher." The expanded proximal end of the tube rests on the upper shoulder of the stricture. The bougie and esophagoscope are removed after verification that the tube is correctly sited. Patients must be nursed postoperatively in the semisitting position and carefully observed, particularly for evidence of respiratory obstruction, aspiration pneumonia, or esophageal perforation.[22] Routine contrast studies confirm the position and patency of the tube (Fig. 51-2). In the absence of complications, oral feeding is begun immediately.

TRACTION INTUBATION

During the 10-year period from mid-1975 to mid-1985, 339 patients were intubated with the Celestin tube[15] (Fig. 51-1). Intubation was achieved at laparotomy by means of retrograde passage of the pilot introducer through a limited gastrotomy. The mean age of the patients was 56.4 years and the male-to-female ratio 4:1. The mean duration of dysphagia before admission was 6 months. In 223 patients (66%), intubation was the initial treatment, resection being contraindicated because of local invasion or metastasis in 156 patients (46%), and because of concomitant severe disease, particularly pulmonary, or gross physical debility, in a further 67 patients (20%). In the remaining 116 patients who were explored (34%), intubation was necessary for a nonresectable tumor.

FACTORS INFLUENCING INTUBATION

The following were assessed for significance in regard to their effect on the outcome of the procedure:

1. Nutritional status
2. Length of tumor as determined radiologically, or endoscopically by means of an olive-tipped bougie
3. Presence of total dysphagia or total barium holdup at the tumor site on contrast examination
4. Histopathologic grading (i.e., well differentiated, moderately differentiated, or poorly differentiated)[23]
5. Esophageal axis disturbances on barium examination. These indicate cancerous infiltration into surrounding tissues.[24] Abnormalities may present as proximal esophageal tortuosity, axis angulation, or axis deviation
6. Bronchoscopic evidence of tumor infiltration, deformity of the carina, or the presence of fistula.

Nutritional status

The nutritional status of 15 patients who were intubated using the pulsion technique was determined 1 week before intubation and thereafter up to 3 weeks following intubation, by which time all the patients were restored to positive nitrogen balance. All patients on admission had evidence of protein-calorie malnutrition—that is, a serum albumin level of less than 3.5 g/100 ml, weight loss of more than 9 kg, and decreased food intake for more than 2 weeks.[25] The parameters investigated were preintubation and postintubation weight status, nitrogen balance, serum albumin level, total iron-binding capacity (TIBC), and triceps skinfold thickness. Following intubation, the patients were fed a hospital ward diet providing 2500 calories, supplemented by a chemically for-

mulated diet that boosted the daily energy intake to 3700 calories and nitrogen intake to 200 g/day. Precautions recommended were fine chopping of all meat and removal of bread crusts.

RESULTS

The degree of palliation achieved was measured by a single criterion, namely the ability of the patient to swallow satisfactorily on leaving the hospital.

Mortality and morbidity

All deaths occurring in hospital following intubation were considered to be due to intubation, whether the exact cause of death could be related to the procedure or not. Death most commonly resulted from esophageal perforation with mediastinitis (see Figs. 51-3 and 51-4), from bleeding, or from aspiration pneumonitis.

Table 51-1 compares the results obtained by the pulsion and traction techniques of intubation. Bronchopneumonia was the most common complication in both groups of patients. Wound sepsis, subphrenic abscess, and gastric fistula related to the laparotomy and gastrotomy necessary for traction intubation contributed to the mortality and increased morbidity in this group.

Factors influencing mortality

Several factors that might have adversely affected the results of intubation were analyzed using the chi square test, and the probabilities quoted were significant ($p < 0.05$). Absolute dysphagia or total barium holdup on contrast examination and the degree of histologic differentiation did not influence mortality. Poor nutritional status (Table 51-2), a stricture length greater than 8 cm (Table 51-3), bronchial invasion (either frank fistula or histologic evidence of tumor invasion) (Table 51-4), and severe esophageal axis deviation (Table 51-5) were associated with significantly increased mortality following pulsion intubation. The mortality of traction intubation was not influenced by the factors analyzed.

Success of intubation

Pulsion intubation was attempted in 2446 patients (48% of all admissions for carcinoma of the esophagus) (see Table 51-6). Intubation was not possible in 38 patients (1.5%) because the malignant stricture could not be adequately dilated. Three hundred sixty-six patients died, a mortality of 15%. Intubation failure also resulted from respiratory embarrassment because of tra-

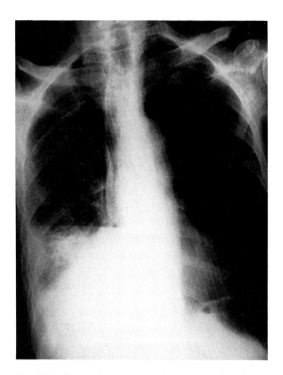

Fig. 51-3. Chest roentgenogram (posteroanterior) showing right hydropneumothorax following Procter-Livingstone intubation for a 10-cm midesophageal carcinoma.

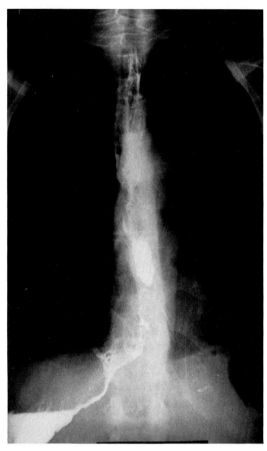

Fig. 51-4. Barium-swallow examination confirming perforation of the esophagus following intubation with a Procter-Livingstone tube for a 10-cm midesophageal carcinoma.

TABLE 51-1. Influence of intubation technique on mortality and morbidity

Intubation technique	No. of patients	Mortality	Complications
Pulsion	2446	366 (15%)	611 (25%)
Traction	339	71 (21%)	122 (36%)
		$p > 0.05$	$p < 0.05$

TABLE 51-2. Nutritional status and mortality

Nutritional status	Pulsion intubation		Traction intubation	
	Patients	Deaths	Patients	Deaths
Moderate	1467	132 (90%)	186	32 (17%)
Poor	979	234 (24%)	153	39 (25%)
TOTAL	2446	366 (15%)	339	71 (21%)
	$p < 0.05$		$p > 0.05$	

TABLE 51-3. Stricture length and mortality

	Pulsion intubation		Traction intubation	
	Patients	Deaths	Patients	Deaths
Stricture <8 cm	1834	164 (9%)	280	44 (16%)
Stricture >8 cm	612	202 (33%)	119	27 (23%)
TOTAL	2446	366 (15%)	399	71 (21%)
		p < 0.001		p > 0.5

TABLE 51-4. Tracheobronchial involvement and mortality

Tracheobronchial involvement	No. of patients	No. of deaths	Percent
Frank fistula	645	148	23
Tumor invasion	271	46	17
TOTAL	916	194	22

TABLE 51-5. Esophageal axis disturbance and mortality

	Pulsion intubation		Traction intubation	
	Patients	Deaths	Patients	Deaths
Slight	807	98 (12%)	104	13 (12%)
Moderate	1217	142 (12%)	125	29 (23%)
Severe	422	126 (30%)*	110	29 (27%)
TOTAL	2446	366 (15%)	339	71 (21%)

*Severe axis deviation significantly increases mortality of pulsion intubation (p < 0.001).

TABLE 51-6. Outcome of intubation

	Pulsion	Traction
No. of patients	2446	339
Deaths	366 (15%)	71 (21%)
Failures	97	15
Respiratory obstruction	48	0
Failed intubation	38	6
Tube migration	0*	7
Refractory blockage	11	2
Successful intubation	1983 (81%)	253 (75%)

*Ninety-two patients successfully reintubated.

TABLE 51-7. Pulsion intubation for esophagorespiratory fistula

Type of fistula	No. of patients	No. of deaths
Esophagotracheal	412 (64%)	65 (16%)
Esophagobronchial	206 (32%)	67 (33%)
Esophagopulmonary	27 (4%)	16 (60%)
TOTAL	645	148 (23%)

TABLE 51-8. Nutritional status following pulsion intubation in 15 patients

	Preintubation	Postintubation
Time	−1 week	+3 weeks
Nitrogen balance (g/day)	−5	+7
Weight (kg)	48	51
Serum albumin (g/100 ml)	3.1	3.8
TIBC (μg/100 ml)	190	270
Skinfold thickness (mm)	4.2	4.6

cheal compression by tumor bulk (48 patients) and tube blockage (11 patients). Proximal migration of the tube occurred in 82 patients and distal migration in 10. Reinsertion was successful in all of these patients. Including reinsertions, successful intubation was achieved in 81% of patients (see Table 51-6), all of whom were swallowing an adequate diet at the time of discharge from the hospital. Most patients could eat a modified soft diet. All food was well masticated; effervescent drinks were recommended at the end of a meal to help clear the tube of food debris. The average hospital stay was 4.5 days. The mean duration of survival was 6.2 months. One patient survived for 21 months.

Traction intubation was attempted in 339 patients, with six technical failures resulting from inability to dilate the malignant stricture. Failure to palliate dysphagia also resulted from tube migration in seven patients and occlusion of the tube in two patients. Seventy-one patients died following intubation, a mortality of 21% (see Table 51-6). Successful intubation was achieved in 75% of patients, all of whom were discharged swallowing satisfactorily. The average hospital stay was 15 days. The mean duration of survival following traction intubation was 5.7 months, the longest survival being 16 months.

Intubation for esophagorespiratory fistula

The presence of an esophagorespiratory fistula was confirmed by bronchoscopy and x-ray examination in 645 patients (12% of all admissions). The communication was with the trachea in 64%, the bronchus in 32%, and a pulmonary abscess in 4% (see Table 51-7). All patients were intubated by means of a pulsion technique, with an overall mortality of 23%. The tube effectively tamponaded the fistula, with palliation of dysphagia as well as respiratory symptoms.

Nutritional status after intubation

The nutritional status of 15 patients assessed prior to intubation and 3 weeks after intubation is shown in Table 51-8. Following intubation and oral feeding, a mean daily positive nitrogen balance of 7 g was achieved at 3 weeks. Other evidence of adequate oral intake was the mean weight increase from 48 kg to 51 kg, a rise in serum albumin to normal levels, and an increase in skinfold thickness. All patients were able to swallow saliva and food, and no incident of tube blockage occurred in the 15 patients studied. The chemically formulated diet supplement was well tolerated, and no gastrointestinal symptoms referable to osmolality or volume were evident.

PULSION INTUBATION VERSUS RETROSTERNAL GASTRIC BYPASS

We reported a randomized prospective study of pulsion intubation versus retrosternal gastric bypass for palliation of nonresectable carcinoma of the upper thoracic esophagus.[26] The mortality and the success of palliation of dysphagia were not significantly different in the two groups of patients (see Table 51-9). Nutritional status improved more rapidly following intubation. Pulsion intubation is now our preferred palliative procedure because of fewer complications, a lesser degree of postoperative catabolism, and a shorter hospital stay.

DISCUSSION

Obstructive symptoms appear relatively late in the natural history of esophageal malignancy and indicate a poor prognosis for cure or even for prolonged survival.

Intubation for the palliation of dysphagia resulting from esophageal carcinoma offers the most satisfactory solution to a difficult problem in the majority of patients. Several historical reviews outline the evolution of intubation as a therapeutic modality and the progressive modifications in the tubes utilized.[15,27,28] Tubes may be pushed through (pulsion)[10,29] or pulled through (traction).[14,15] Traction techniques require laparotomy and gastrotomy, which increase morbidity and prolong hospital stay.[29] These disadvantages are avoided with peroral pulsion techniques.[7]

Pulsion intubation is indicated particularly for lesions of the upper thoracic esophagus, since the presence of an uninvolved segment of esophagus distal to the tumor lessens the hazard of perforation.[19] The Souttar tube has been extensively used, but we believe that the Procter-Livingstone tube has significant advantages. The lumen is larger, blockage appears to be less frequent, and distal migration is less frequent.[7] Traction intubation is preferred for tumors of the lower esophagus, and the later version of the Celestin tube,[30] with an improved proximal funnel, which is a more flexible and resilient tube, appears to be the prosthesis of choice.

Tumors at the gastroesophageal junction pose a particular problem. Pulsion intubation across the cardia into the stomach has been considered hazardous,[27] but the advent of fiberoptic endoscopy has now provided a safer technique of esophagoscopy and has made possible the accurate insertion of devices through tumors of the lower esophagus and cardia. Fiberoptic endoscopy permits dilatation of these tumors by the Eder-Puestow method preparatory to pulsion intubation, which is achieved by sliding the tube over the endoscope itself[31] or over the Puestow wire behind the olive of the dilator.[32] Successful prosthesis insertion depends to a great extent on adequate dilatation of the malignant stenosis.[33] This technique is particularly useful for stricturing lesions that are eccentric, tortuous, or at a right angle to the esophageal lumen, as is frequently encountered after previous radiotherapy or surgery. Den Hartog Jager et al.[34] achieved successful intubation in 193 of 200 consecutive patients with obstructing esophagogastric malignancy. Perforation occurred in 8% of patients, but the overall mortality rate resulting from the procedure itself was 2%. Endoscopic peroral intubation using the Nottingham tube introducer is also a simple and relatively safe procedure for relieving dysphagia in inoperable esophagogastric neoplasms. Intubation using this method was attempted by Atkinson et al.[35] in 63 patients, with a mortality of 19%. The risk of proximal displacement can be overcome by the use of a tube with a shoulder near its distal end.

Solid, stepped, radiopaque dilators, passed

TABLE 51-9. Success of palliation by intubation compared with bypass

	Intubation	Bypass
No. of patients	55	51
Deaths	3 (5.5%)	4 (7.8%)
Failures	1	0
Postoperative hospital stay (days)	5.5	18.7
Successful swallowing	51(93%)	47 (92%)

over a guide wire, have been used with success to dilate malignant esophageal strictures.[36] The shape of the stepped dilator allows the tissues to be stretched to the same degree through the length of the stricture. Prostheses are not used in patients with lesions in the cervical esophagus, because of the lesion's relatively fixed position and the tendency for the prosthesis plus tumor bulk to produce posterior tracheal compression at this level.

Seven percent of our patients died without any procedure being performed, a reflection of the advanced nature of their tumors and their gross physical debility. Taking this into consideration, intubation in a homogeneous patient population was achieved with a hospital mortality of 15% for pulsion technique and 21% for traction technique. This compares favorably with other series.[29,37-39] Girardet et al.,[27] reviewing intubation in patients with esophageal carcinoma, reported a hospital mortality of 14%; the mortality for traction techniques was two to six times greater than that for pulsion techniques. The mortality of intubation should be weighed against that of bypass procedures, which may be as high as 60%.[5,40]

The main cause of operative death is esophageal or gastric perforation. Tumor fracture during dilatation is not a hazard, because the tube effectively tamponades the breach. Bleeding is another frequent cause of death, followed by aspiration pneumonia, particularly with pull-through tubes, since these render the gastroesophageal junction incompetent. In this series the complication rate for traction intubation (36%) was significantly higher than that for pulsion intubation (25%), chiefly because of wound sepsis, gastric fistula, and subphrenic abscess directly related to the technique of traction intubation.[29,38,39] Tube dislodgment was more frequent with pulsion intubation, occurring in 4% of patients. All patients were successfully reintubated. The problem is far greater with Souttar tubes, as illustrated by Mounier-Kuhn et al.,[41] who replaced dislodged tubes in 101 of their 453 patients (22%). Intraoperative perforations are usually related to the technique of dilatation and tube insertion, and the incidence of these should decrease with fiberoptic endoscopic control of intubation.[31,32] Prosthetic erosion into the mediastinum,[38] aorta, and pulmonary artery[29] may occur, but was not observed in any of our patients.

Swallowing after intubation has been reported by various authors as excellent,[37] satisfactory,[29] or "adequate" (i.e., liquids could be swallowed for more than half the survival time).[38] Little objective information is available on the nutritional status of patients before or after intubation. The 15 patients we evaluated all showed evidence of protein-calorie malnutrition. Following intubation and oral feeding, a mean positive nitrogen balance of 7 g was achieved in 3 weeks, with an increase in serum albumin and TIBC levels. The intake of protein and calories was adequate, necessitating minimal dietary modifications. Tube blockage by food was not a problem in this group, but should it occur, it can be easily corrected by using carbonated beverages or by resorting to esophagoscopy.

Mannell et al.[42] compared esophageal intubation with esophageal dilatation plus a 5-day course of intramuscular bleomycin in the treatment of advanced esophageal cancer.[42] Dilatation and chemotherapy was associated with fewer complications. However, only a majority of patients responded symptomatically to bleomycin, and patients with esophagotracheal, esophagobronchial, or esophagopulmonary fistulas were not eligible for this study because they could not be treated by esophageal dilatation plus bleomycin. Substernal gastric bypass of the excluded thoracic esophagus is another option available for palliation of dysphagia resulting from malignant obstruction,[43,44] but it is associated with appreciable morbidity and a hospital mortality of 21%.[45]

In our series, failure to intubate was rare (4%), and in patients in whom intubation was not technically successful on the first occasion, or tube dislodgment occurred, reintubation usually produced a satisfactory result. Following pulsion intubation, 81% of patients were discharged swallowing satisfactorily, and after traction intubation 75%. Those factors which increase mortality and morbidity and which compromise successful intubation are due to advanced disease and should not therefore exclude the patient from palliative treatment. Even in severely ill patients with esophagorespiratory fistulas, intubation relieves dysphagia and minimizes respiratory symptoms. Intubation will achieve reasonable palliation of malignant dysphagia in the majority of patients. Newer techniques should diminish the mortality rate and the incidence of complications.

ACKNOWLEDGEMENTS

The significant contribution of the members of the Esophageal Carcinoma Unit, King George V Hospital, Durban, to the management of the patients in this series is gratefully acknowledged. We would like to thank Miss Vanessa Byrnes and Mrs. N. Ramlall for their secretarial assistance.

REFERENCES

1. Lowe, W.C.: Survival with carcinoma of the esophagus, Ann. Intern. Med. **77:**915, 1972.
2. Gunn Laugsson, G.H., Wychulis, A.R., Roland, C., and Ellis, F.H., Jr.: Analysis of the records of 1657 patients with carcinoma of the esophagus and cardia of the stomach, Surg. Gynecol. Obstet. **130:**997, 1970.
3. Plested, W.G., Tildon, T.T., and Hughes, P.K.: A philosophy of treatment of esophageal cancer, Am. Surg. **34:**650, 1968.
4. McKeown, K.C.: Carcinoma of the esophagus, J.R. Coll. Surg. Edinb. **24:**254, 1979.
5. Postlethwait, R.W., Sealy, W.C., Dillon, M.L., and Young, W.G.: Colon interposition for esophageal substitution, Ann. Thorac. Surg. **12:**89, 1971.
6. Wilson, S.E., Plested, W.G., and Carey, J.S.: Esophagogastrectomy versus radiation therapy for mid-esophageal carcinoma, Ann. Thorac. Surg. **10:**195, 1970.
7. Angorn, I.B., and Hegarty, M.M.: Palliative pulsion intubation in esophageal carcinoma, Ann. R. Coll. Surg. Engl. **61:**212, 1979.
8. d'Etiolles, L.: In de Lavacherie del'Oesophagotomie, Brussels, 1845. Cited by Celestin.
9. Symonds, C.J.: The treatment of malignant stricture of the esophagus by tubaje or permanent catheterism, Br. Med. J. **1:**870, 1887.
10. Souttar, H.S.: A method of intubating the esophagus for malignant stricture, Br. Med. J. **1:**782, 1924.
11. Angorn, I.B., and Haffejee, A.A.: Carcinoma of the esophagus, Continuing Medical Education **2:**61, 1984.
12. Kropff, G.: Intubation oesophagienne par tube en matiere plastique suivie de radiumtherapie dans le traitement du cancer de l'oesophage, Mem. Acad. Chir. [Paris] **80:**628, 1985.
13. Mackler, S.A., and Mayer, R.M.: Palliation of esophageal obstruction due to carcinoma with a permanent tube, J. Thorac. Cardiovasc. Surg. **28:**431, 1954.
14. Mousseau, M., Le Forestier, J., Barbin, J., and Hardy, M.: Place de l'intubation a demeure, dans le traitement palliatif du cancer de l'oesophage, Arch. Fr. Mal. App. Dig. **45:**208, 1956.
15. Celestin, L.R.: Permanent intubation in inoperable cancer of the esophagus and cardia, Ann. R. Coll. Surg. Engl. **25:**165, 1959.
16. Angorn, I.B.: Carcinoma of the esophagus in Natal: a local review. In Silber, W., editor: Carcinoma of the esophagus, Cape Town, 1978, A.A. Balkema, pp. 248-257.

17. Sweet, R.H.: Late results of surgical treatment of carcinoma of the esophagus, JAMA **155:**422, 1954.
18. Pearson, J.G.: The value of radiotherapy in the management of squamous esophageal cancer, Br. J. Surg. **58:**794, 1971.
19. Craddock, D.R., Logan, A., and Maynell, M.: Traumatic rupture of the esophagus and stomach, Thorax **23:**657, 1968.
20. Procter, D.S.C.: Experience with esophageal intubation for esophageal carcinoma, S. Afr. Med. J. **37:**967, 1968.
21. Procter, D.S.C.: Esophageal intubation for carcinoma of the esophagus, World J. Surg. **4:**451, 1980.
22. Angorn, I.B.: Pulsion intubation of the esophagus. In Dudley, H., Pories, W., and Carter, D., editors: Rob and Smiths' Operative surgery: alimentary tract and abdominal wall, 4, London, 1985, Butterworths, pp. 170-173.
23. Meissner, W.A., and Warren, S. In Anderson, W.A.D., editor: Pathology, ed. 6, St. Louis: 1971, The C.V. Mosby Co., p. 539.
24. Akiyama, H., Takashi, K., and Yugi, I.: The esophageal axis and its relationship to the resectability of carcinoma of the esophagus, Ann. Surg. **173:**30, 1972.
25. Law, D.K., Dudrick, S.J., and Abdou, N.I.: Immunocompetence of patients with protein calorie malnutrition, Ann. Intern. Med. **79:**545, 1973.
26. Angorn, I.B., and Haffejee, A.A.: Pulsion intubation v. retrosternal gastric bypass for palliation of unresectable carcinoma of the upper thoracic esophagus, Br. J. Surg. **70:**335, 1983.
27. Girardet, R.E., Randell, H.T., Jr., and Wheat, M.S.: Palliative intubation in the management of esophageal carcinoma, Ann. Thorac. Surg. **18:**417, 1974.
28. Earlam, R., and Cunha-Melo, J.R.: Malignant esophageal strictures: a review of techniques for palliative intubation, Br. J. Surg. **69:**61, 1982.
29. Amman, J.R., and Collis, J.L.: Palliative intubation of the esophagus, J. Thorac. Cardiovasc. Surg. **61:**863, 1971.
30. Celestin, L.R.: Improvements in the Celestin tube for endo-esophageal intubation in carcinoma and strictures, Armamentarium **4:**8, 1965.
31. Tytgat, G.N.J., Den Hartog Jager, F.C.A., and Haverkamp, H.J.: Positioning of a plastic prosthesis under fiber-endoscopic control in the palliative treatment of cardio-esophageal cancer, Endoscopy **8:**180, 1976.
32. Atkinson, M., and Ferguson, R.: Fiberoptic endoscopic palliative intubation of inoperable esophagogastric neoplasms, Br. Med. J. **1:**266, 1977.
33. Boyce, H.W., Jr.: Peroral prosthesis for palliating malignant esophageal and gastric obstruction (editorial), Gastroenterology **77:**1141, 1979.
34. Den Hartog Jager, F.C.A., Bartelsman, J.F.W., and Tytgat, G.N.J.: Palliative treatment of obstructing esophagogastric malignancy by endoscopic positioning of a plastic prosthesis, Gastroenterology **77:**1008, 1979.
35. Atkinson, M., Ferguson, R., and Ogilvie, A.L.: Management of malignant dysphagia by intubation at endoscopy, J. R. Soc. Med. **72:**894, 1979.
36. Celestin, L.R., and Campbell, W.B.: A new and safe system for esophageal dilatation, Lancet **1:**74, 1981.
37. Thomas, A.N.: Endoesophageal intubation for esophageal obstruction, Am. J. Surg. **128:**306, 1974.
38. Duvoisin, G.E., Ellis, F.H., Jr., and Payne, W.S.: The value of palliative prostheses in malignant lesions of the esophagus, Surg. Clin. North Am. **47:**827, 1967.
39. Saunders, N.J.: The Celestin tube in the palliation of carcinoma of the esophagus and cardia, Br. J. Surg. **66:**419, 1979.
40. Stephens, H.B.: Colon bypass of the esophagus, Am. J. Surg. **122:**217, 1971.
41. Mounier-Kuhn, P., Gaillard, J., Haguenauer, J.P., and de Champs, B.: Les indications de l'intubation par voie des cancers de l'oesophage, J. Fr. Otorhinolaryngol. **17:**491, 1968.
42. Mannell, A., Becker, P.J., Mellissas, J., and Diamantes, T.: Intubation v. dilatation plus bleomycin in the treatment of advanced esophageal cancer, S. Afr. J. Surg. **24:**15, 1986.
43. Ong, G.B.: Unresectable carcinoma of the esophagus, Ann. R. Coll. Surg. Engl. **56:**3, 1975.
44. Orringer, M.B., and Sloan, H.: Substernal gastric bypass of the excluded thoracic esophagus for the palliation of esophageal carcinoma, J. Thorac. Cardiovasc. Surg. **70:**836, 1975.
45. Conlan, A.A., Nicolaou, N., Hammond, C.A., de Nobrega, C., and Mistry, B.D.: Retrosternal gastric bypass for inoperable esophageal cancer: a report of 71 patients, Ann. Thorac. Surg. **36:**396, 1983.

Endoesophageal intubation for palliation in obstructing esophageal carcinoma

DISCUSSION

Anthony Watson

This impressive review of the use of intubation as a valuable modality in the palliation of esophagogastric malignancies unsuitable for resection comes from a center with one of the largest experiences in the world. The very high incidence of esophageal carcinoma among South African blacks poses enormous logistical problems in early diagnosis and management, necessitating a greater reliance on palliative measures than is the case in the United States and Europe. The large experience consequently obtained in intubation, along with the careful studies undertaken in Natal, has yielded much valuable data relating to morbidity and mortality, comparison of intubation with other modalities, predisposing factors to morbidity and mortality, and nutritional status following intubation.

The results presented should help dispel the reluctance existing in many American centers to employ intubation as a palliative procedure when resection is inappropriate either because of tumor staging or because of the unfitness of the patient to withstand thoracoabdominal resection. Both of these contraindications to resection are indeed contraindications to any surgical intervention when alternative and safer forms of palliation exist. The authors have shown a considerably lower mortality with intubation than with surgical bypass, as well as a reduced number of complications and a shorter hospital stay. Mortality rates of 40 to 60% are being reported for surgical bypass.[1,2] It surely must be more humane, in a patient whose life span is limited, to avoid prolonged hospitalization with the immunodepressive and emotional effects of major surgery, which at best may slightly increase eating capacity and, at worst, result in deatth.

If one accepts the concept of intubation, it appears logical to employ the method that is least invasive and offers adequate palliation. Traction intubation has the disadvantage of requiring laparotomy, with all its problems in these frail, malnourished patients, and consequently its mortality is higher in most series than with pulsion intubation.[3,4] In some cases the mortality is as high as 45%.[5] Of the pulsion intubation techniques, the Souttar tube, as the authors indicate, has a narrow internal diameter, blocks easily, and has a high incidence of migration. The Procter-Livingstone tube overcomes some of these disadvantages. It has a much larger internal diameter and is associated, in the authors' hands, with a remarkably low incidence of proximal migration, despite the absence of a distal flange. The principal disadvantage is the necessity to introduce it with the rigid esophagoscope and, therefore, the necessity for general anesthesia.

These latter disadvantages have been overcome by the advent of fiberoptic endoscopic intubation, using either a Celestin or an Atkinson tube inserted under sedation with diazepam and an analgesic agent. We prefer the former tube because of its wider internal diameter of approximately 12 mm and the circumferential distal flange, which prevents proximal migration of the tube. The authors give a misleading impression of the mortality associated with this technique by quoting the preliminary Nottingham experience of 19% mortality in 63 patients. More recent experience from the same center has reported a mortality of 11% in 122 patients.[6] Our experience in Lancaster has been similar, with a mortality of 11% between 1974 and 1982,[7] falling to 4% of 45 patients with intubations performed between 1982 and 1985.[8] These trends suggest increasing safety of the technique with experience. Current mortality figures are superior to those of techniques requiring rigid esophagoscopy and general anesthesia. As a result, fiberoptic endoscopic intubation is now the preferred palliative technique in Europe. In contrast to the authors' experience, we have found this form of pulsion intubation applicable to tumors involving the distal esophagus and cardia,[9] thus excluding another group of patients from the need for palliative surgery. We now use traction intubation rarely, either in situations where gross narrowing or tortuosity preclude the endoscopic passage of a guide wire or on the few occasions where nonresectability is discovered at operation. In these circumstances, we find that tube displacement can be prevented by suturing the distal end of the Celestin or Mousseau-Barbin tube to the gastric wall with nonabsorbable sutures.[9] The only other circumstances in which palliation by fiberoptic endoscopic intubation is inappropriate is in cases of radioresistant proximal tumors, in which discomfort and pharyngeal irritation may result from the proximal funnel of the tube. In these circumstances, palliation by laser therapy is superior.

Those opposed to the concept of intubation as a palliative modality cite the poor quality of palliation as a major disadvantage. However, a study in our institution[10] has shown that after fiberoptic endoscopic intubation, all patients could take an adequate diet, comprising solids or semisolids, and 33% of patients reported entirely normal swallowing. The nutritional studies from Natal using a similar-sized tube confirm these observations. However, it should be stated that, of our resected patients, 91% were able to swallow normally and that surgical removal of the tumor, when appropriate, offers the best form of palliation.

Although discussion of the results of surgery is outside the scope of this commentary, the gloomy survival figures following resection, based on references between 1968 and 1972, should not pass without comment. In our institution, the hospital mortality for resection in appropriate cases is 9.7%, similar to that for intubation. The 1-year survival is 51%, and the 5-year survival is 11%.[8] These figures are similar to those in other currently reported series.

The ultimate goal in this distressing disease must, in appropriate circumstances, be an attempt at cure. This can be achieved by resection with an acceptable mortality in a proportion of patients. Even when cure is not achieved, the quality of palliation by resection exceeds that of any other modality. However, such figures are attainable only by careful selection. When so employed in the Western world, where tumors are frequently advanced at the time of presentation and patients often too frail to withstand major surgery, a palliative approach is indicated to prevent an unpleasant demise from starvation. In these circumstances, the humane approach is one that avoids surgery and prolonged hospitalization, and allows the patient to spend the short remaining time with his family. Intubation allows realization of these objectives. It is my belief that fiberoptic endoscopic intubation is not only the least invasive, but currently the safest, means of achieving this palliation.

REFERENCES

1. Postlethwait, R.W.: Surgery of the esophagus, East Norwalk, Conn., 1986, Appleton-Century-Crofts, pp. 416-420.
2. Stephens, H.B.: Bypass of the esophagus, Am. J. Surg. **122:**217, 1971.
3. Watson, A.: A study of the quality and duration of survival following resection, endoscopic intubation and surgical intubation in oesophageal carcinoma, Br. J. Surg. **69:**585, 1982.
4. Johnson, I.R., Balfour, T.W., and Bourke, J.B.: Intubation of malignant oesophageal strictures, J. R. Coll. Surg. Edinb. **21:**225, 1976.
5. Lishman, A.H., Dellipiani, A.W., and Devlin, H.B.: The insertion of esophagogastric tubes in malignant esophageal stricture, endoscopy or surgery? Br. J. Surg. **67:**257, 1980.
6. Ogilvie, A.L., Dromfield, M.W., Ferguson, R. et al.: Palliative intubation of esophagogastric neoplasms at fibreoptic endoscopy, Gut **23:**1060, 1982.
7. Watson, A.: Therapeutic options and patient selection in the management of oesophageal carcinoma. In Watson, A., and Celestin, L.R., editors: Disorders of the oesophagus, London, 1984, Pitman, pp. 167-186.
8. Watson, A.: The current status of resection in the management of oesophageal carcinoma (Hunterian Oration), Ann. R. Coll. Surg. Engl. (In press.)
9. Watson, A.: Palliative intubation in inoperable esophageal neoplasms, Ann. Thorac. Surg. **39:**501, 1985.
10. Watson, A.: Survival following resection, endoscopic intubation and surgical intubation in oesophageal carcinoma. In Proceedings of the Second International Congress, International Society for Diseases of the Esophagus, 1985, pp. 377-386.

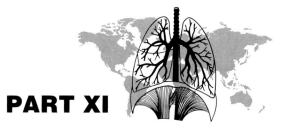

PART XI

AN OVERVIEW OF THE PROBLEM OF ESOPHAGEAL CARCINOMA

52 Update of experience
with esophageal cancer:
now and tomorrow

Aylwyn Mannell

SURVIVAL STATISTICS
The untreated patient

Carcinoma of the esophagus is not only a lethal malignancy but also one of the most distressing. It deprives an individual of the ability to eat, a fundamental pleasure and a basic requirement for life. Without treatment, patients with esophageal cancer die of starvation. But before death occurs, their suffering may be increased by other complications of this terrible disease. These include pneumonia and lung abscess secondary to aspiration of food debris from the obstructed esophagus, fistulization of the cancer into the airway, leading to paroxysms of coughing with every swallow, and the constant pain of malignant invasion into the mediastinum.

It is not surprising, therefore, that the survival of the untreated patient with esophageal cancer can be measured in days or weeks after diagnosis. In the series reported by Adelstein et al.[1] the mean survival of patients not considered candidates for radiotherapy or surgery was 2.8 months; this was reduced to a mean of 10 weeks in those with metastatic disease. Aygun et al.[2] found that untreated patients with tumor spread into the tracheobronchial tree survived 3 weeks. Patients with frank esophago-airway fistulas, receiving supportive care only, die within 14 days of diagnosis.[3]

Given the misery and grim prognosis of the untreated patient, many different methods have been used to relieve dysphagia and improve survival. The large number of techniques applied over the last 5 years is indicative of the fact that no single treatment is appropriate for all patients with esophageal cancer. It also suggests that those treating the disease have had more experience and success with one form of therapy than with others.

Palliative therapy

In most specialist centers managing esophageal cancer patients, feeding gastrostomies or jejunostomies, as a single treatment, are used only as a "last resort" when all other methods have failed. Instillation of food directly into the stomach or jejunum may alleviate hunger but offers no palliation for dysphagia. One out of four patients dies as a result of these procedures.[4,5] When patients with malignant esophago-airway fistulas are managed by gastrostomy alone, a mean survival of 6 weeks can be expected.[3]

A time-honored method of mangement, introduced over 100 years ago[6] and still in use, is aimed at restoring the esophageal lumen by dilatation or intubation, leaving the tumor untreated. Dilatation of malignant strictures can be safely performed at endoscopy with fluoroscopic screening.[7] The initial improvement in swallowing appears greater after simple dilatation than after intubation,[8] and several authors have suggested that chronic peroral dilatation is an effective method of palliating dysphagia.[9-11] But the role of dilatation in the management of esophageal cancer has not been critically evaluated, nor has the survival in cases managed by dilatation alone been documented.

On the other hand, the ability to insert an endoesophageal prosthesis at the time of gastroscopy has led to renewed enthusiasm for intubation. Deaths in hospital after endoscopic intubation vary from 5% to 26% (see Table 52-1), compared with mortality rates of up to 40.8% for tubes that require laparotomy for insertion. Undoubtedly, endoscopic intubation is safer than operative intubation, but survival of patients with a tube in the esophagus is often difficult to ascertain. Many series do not distinguish between sur-

TABLE 52-1. Results of esophageal intubation

Author(s)	No. of cases	Method	Hospital deaths (%)	Mean survival (weeks)
Den Hartog Jager et al.[12] (1979)	161	Endoscopic	16	16
Nullen et al.[4] (1982)	111	Operative	34	—
Watson[13] (1982)	49	Operative	40.8	32
	32	Endoscopic	15.6	43
Pietropaola et al.[14] (1982)	67	Endoscopic	—	24
Ogilvie et al.[15] (1982)	121	Endoscopic	16	12
Rose and Smith[16] (1983)	100	Endoscopic	26	16
Diamantis and Mannell[17] (1983)	325	Operative	25	9
		Endoscopic	31	
Procter[18] (1980)	2000	Endoscopic	36*	11
Sarr et al.[19] (1984)	44	Endoscopic	14	13
Buess et al.[20] (1985)	93	Endoscopic	14	11
Valbuena[21] (1984)	40	Endoscopic	5	—

*Died within 2 weeks of intubation.

vival in cases with squamous carcinoma of the esophagus and those with adenocarcinoma of gastric origin. In addition, patients in these series have often been treated with radiotherapy or surgery before intubation, and, in some cases, adjuvant therapy was given after insertion of the prosthesis. Another difficulty in comparing survival after intubation to that following other palliative treatments is the lack of staging of the disease by the TNM or similar classification before insertion of the tube. Differences in stages of the cancer, the histology of the tumors, and the use of adjuvant therapy may explain fourfold differences in survival reported after intubation (see Table 52-1). But it appears that the median survival, after intubation of gastroesophageal malignancies, is 3 to 4 months. Very few patients live more than 1 year. Watson[13] and Rose and Smith[16] noted that the maximum survival did not exceed 18 months.

Two recent series have documented survival after intubation of primary esophageal squamous carcinomas. The survival figures are even more dismal than those quoted above. In 2000 cases of squamous cancer of the esophagus managed by intubation, Procter[18] reported a mean survival of 11 weeks; in the Baragwanath Hospital series,[17] the median survival after intubation was 2.2 months.

Esophageal intubation is usually reserved for patients with advanced malignancy, so that the short survival times are not unexpected. However, bolus obstruction and dislodgment of the prosthesis are common complications of intubation, and the quality of palliation is less than perfect. About 50% of intubated patients are able to swallow soft foods, and the remainder are restricted to a liquid diet.[19]

To overcome the disadvantages of semirigid tubes, laser technology has been applied to the palliation of esophageal cancer. With this method, the intraluminal component of the cancer is fulgurated to restore esophageal patency. The initial reports are encouraging, but this technique may be hazardous when applied to cervical tumors, those of the desmoplastic-stenosing variety with a large submucous component, and tumors complicated by extensive extraesophageal spread that has distorted the esophageal axis.[22] It appears that laser treatment has to be repeated every 4 to 6 weeks to maintain swallowing capability.[22,23] However, not much is known about survival of patients with primary esophageal malignancies who are receiving maintenance laser therapy. Cello et al.[24] reported a wide range of survival times—between 2 weeks and 7 months (median survival, 3 months)—in patients with squamous carcinoma of the esophagus undergoing endoscopic Nd:YAG laser treatment. McCaughan et al.[23] have used a tunable dye argon laser system after intravenous administration of a hematoporphyrin derivative. These workers noted that sur-

TABLE 52-2. Results of radical radiotherapy

Author(s)	No. of cases	Method of irradiation (dose)	Median survival (mo)	Five-year survival (%)
Beatty et al.[45] (1979)	146	External beam (4000-6000 r)	12	0
Earlam and Cunha-Melo[38] (1980)	8489	External beam (5000-6800 r)	—	6
Newaishy et al.[44] (1982)	444	External beam (5000 r)	13	9
Miao et al.[46] (1982)	203	Intracavitary	<12	8.4
Morita et al.[47] (1985)	119	External beam (5000-7000 r)	—	8
Wilson et al.[50] (1985)	19	External beam (6000 r)	8.3	0

vival during the laser therapy was influenced by the Karnofsky performance rating, which is probably an indirect measure of tumor load. It is evident that more follow-up studies, of accurately staged cases, are necessary before the role of maintenance laser therapy in esophageal cancer palliation can be determined.

The principal disadvantage of palliative techniques such as dilatation, operative or endoscopic intubation, and laser fulguration is their failure to permanently restore swallowing capability. These failures are due to bolus obstruction, prosthesis dislodgment, and tumor regrowth. In addition, short survivals after intubation may be related to constant pressure of the semirigid tube on the thin walls of the esophagus leading to necrosis and erosion into the mediastinum. This unfortunate sequence of events appears to be hastened by the use of adjuvant therapy.[25,26] Laser therapy may also be complicated by perforation of the esophagus at the sites of malignant infiltration. To permanently restore the ability to swallow and to avoid these complications, extraesophageal bypass surgery is an attractive alternative to intubation or laser therapy. However, in earlier series, when long, isolated segments of colon or jejunum were used for the bypass, the operative mortality rates were very high, varying between 30% and 50%.[27-29] But in the last few years, part or all of the stomach has most often been selected as the bypass viscus. In experienced hands the hospital death rate for gastric bypass surgery has been reduced to less than 10%.[30-33] One exception is the large series reported by Wong et al.,[34] in which the overall hospital mortality was 41.5%. However, these workers attribute this unacceptably high mortality, in part, to the inclusion of a large number of high-risk cases. Their findings support the concept that no single technique of palliation is appropriate for all cases of advanced esopha-

geal cancer. When gastric bypass operations are performed for malignant esophago-airway fistulas, mortality rates have varied from 12.5%[35] up to 56%.[36] These variations emphasize the value of experience with, and careful selection of patients for, any particular technique of palliation.

Survival after a successful bypass operation depends on two factors—the extent of disease and the use of adjuvant therapy. In patients with massive tumor loads or when no adjuvant therapy is given, the average survival after operation is 4 to 5 months.[33,34] When esophageal bypass is combined with radiation treatment to a tumor localized to the esophagus, the median survival is 11 months, with 29% of patients surviving at least 1 year.[37] Cases with locally advanced tumors have a median survival of 9 months, and 18% live for a year or more.[37] These results suggest that successful palliation of esophageal cancer is influenced by experience with the methods used, appropriate selection of patients, and combined modalities of treatment.

Radiotherapy

Radiotherapy has been used to treat thousands of patients with esophageal cancer because it is a relatively safe method of treatment that can be stopped when complications occur. When given with curative intent, to tumors apparently localized to the esophagus, the median survival is approximately 12 months, and, on average, 6% of these patients will survive 5 years[38] (see Table 52-2). There is no evidence that the overall results of curative radiotherapy have been influenced by the use of hypoxic cell radiosensitizers,[39] fast neutron teletherapy,[40] or helium charged-particle radiotherapy.[41,42] It would appear that the response to radiation therapy depends on the site, length, radiologic type, and histology of the tumor. Pearson[43] indicated that the results of radiotherapy

TABLE 52-3. Results of esophageal resection for early esophageal cancer

Author(s)	No. of cases	Operative mortality (%)	Five-year survival (%)
Shao et al.[52] (1981)	210 (carcinoma in situ)	2.9	90
Shao et al.[53] (1982)	2099 (stage 0 to II)	4.7	53.5
Xu et al.[54] (1983)	664	10	22
Launois et al.[55] (1983)	41	15.3	23
Pralat et al.[56] (1983)	102	9.4	23.7
Akiyama et al.[57] (1984)	86	1.4	54
Ellis[58] (1984)	Not stated	1.3	43.4*
Huang et al.[59] (1985)	847	4.2	25†

*Includes adenocarcinoma of the cardia.
†May include stage III cases.

TABLE 52-4. Results of esophageal resection for stage III esophageal cancer

Author(s)	No. of cases	Operative mortality (%)	Five-year survival (%)
Akiyama[60] (1981)	121	1.4	15.3
Shao et al.[53] (1982)	NS*	4.7	15
Fu et al.[61] (1982)	69	NS	10.3
Ellis[58] (1984)	NS	1.3	12.8

*Not stated.

for cancers of the cervical esophagus were better than those for intrathoracic esophageal carcinoma. This was confirmed by Newaishy et al.,[44] who reported a 5-year survival rate of 18.9% for tumors confined to the cervical esophagus. In their review of 146 patients treated by radical doses of irradiation at the Princess Margaret Hospital, Beatty et al.[45] noted that all T_1 lesions (of length < 5 cm, incomplete circumferential involvement) responded to treatment, and Newaishy et al.[44] reported 11.9% 5-year survival for patients with tumors less than 5 cm in length. In one study of 203 Chinese patients given intracavitary radiotherapy,[46] the 5-year survival rate for patients with superficial cancers was 26%, compared with a 5-year survival of 5.7% in patients with infiltrative lesions. Morita et al.[47] found that 25% of tumors that had a superficial or proliferative appearance on barium-swallow examination were cured by radiotherapy. This was significantly better than the 2% 5-year survival reported, by the same workers,[47] in patients with radiologic evidence of stenosis before the treatment. Other factors that favored response to treatment in the Princess Margaret Hospital series[45] included well-differentiated squamous cell histology, age of 70 years or more, and female sex. In the Edinburgh series,[44] the 5-year survival

rate in females was twice that of males: in fact, Newaishy et al.[44] suggest that radical radiotherapy in males seems justified only for localized cancers no greater than 5 cm in length.

Radiotherapy for palliation

It is evident that only selected patients with localized esophageal cancers will be cured of this disease by radiation therapy. It is therefore important to consider the quality and duration of palliation achieved by radiotherapy for the majority of patients treated in this way.

Beatty et al.[45] reported that 61% of patients with tumors apparently localized to the esophagus responded to irradiation. Of those who responded, one third had durable palliation for the remainder of their illness but two thirds suffered asymptomatic recurrence in the esophagus. The 1-year survival of nonresponders (39%) and of patients treated with less than radical doses for advanced tumors was 17%. Only 21% of patients with locally advanced disease, and none of those with distant metastases, had a response to radiotherapy. Therefore patients with localized disease failing to respond to irradiation and those with advanced disease require another method of palliation. Beatty[48] has suggested that resection or bypass surgery offers 75% of patients reasonable

TABLE 52-5. Results of "curative" esophageal resections

Author(s)	No. of cases	Operative mortality (%)	Mean survival (mo)	Five-year survival (%)
Anne et al.[62] (1982)	90	16	13.6	10.5
Shao et al.[53] (1982)	2099	4.7	NS‡	42.2
Couraud and Meriot[63] (1982)	256	7	NS	21
Zhang et al.[64] (1982)	2069	6.5	NS	23.5
Fu et al.[61] (1982)	202	NS	NS	10.3
Pralat et al.[56] (1983)	102	14.8	NS	5.6
Skinner[65] (1983)	80	11	NS	18
Forni et al.[66] (1984)	102	8.1†	NS	10.2
Akiyama et al.[57] (1984)	295	1.7	NS	34.7
Ellis[58] (1984)	125*	1.3	17.3	21.6
Keagy et al.[67] (1984)	60	6.7	13.5	5
Hennessy and O'Connell[68] (1984)	62	12.9	12	11.5
Huang et al.[59] (1985)	1164	4.3	NS	25

*Includes adenocarcinoma of the cardia.
†Mortality rate after 1976.
‡Not stated.

palliation and that radiotherapy should be used as the primary method of palliation only for those in whom surgery is contraindicated. This opinion is shared by Kelsen,[49] who reviewed the results of irradiation at the Sloan-Kettering Memorial Cancer Center and concluded that surgery was a more certain method of palliating dysphagia.

When patients with advanced tumors are given palliative irradiation, 50% will have some improvement in swallowing but the other 50% will need additional treatment, such as rigid tube placement, to restore or maintain the ability to swallow.

Esophageal resection

Esophageal resection is the standard method of treatment for esophageal cancer. Like radiotherapy, intubation, or use of the laser, the immediate results are directly related to the judgment and expertise of the physician administering the treatment. Radiotherapy must be given carefully to avoid damage to heart, lungs, and spinal cord; intubation or laser fulguration require skill to avoid the potentially lethal complication of esophageal perforation. Likewise, esophageal resection is best undertaken by those experienced in the technique if morbidity and mortality are to be kept within acceptable limits.

In the collected series published by Earlam and Cunha-Melo,[51] the average hospital mortality after esophagectomy was an alarming 33%. But this review included 36 papers published over 20 years ago, with some dating back to the 1950s, and at least 21 authors reported an experience of less than 30 resections. With advances in anesthesia

and postoperative care, esophageal resection has become less hazardous. It is encouraging to note that, in the last 5 years, operative mortality rates of less than 10% are the rule (see Table 52-3 to 52-5) rather than the exception.

Esophageal resection is commonly performed for three groups of patients:

1. Those in whom cure is likely (stage 0 to II*)
2. Those in whom cure is unlikely (stage III)
3. Those in whom cure is not possible (stage IV or incompletely resected cancers)

For those with cancers limited to the esophagus and no lymph node metastases, the 5-year survival in recent Chinese, Japanese, and Western series varies from 22% to 53.5% (see Table 52-3). The cure rate is even more impressive if esophageal cancer is detected in the preinvasive stage. Shao et al.[52] reported a 5-year survival rate of 90% in 210 patients undergoing esophageal resection for carcinoma in situ. But the results are much less encouraging in cases with positive lymph nodes: 10% to 15% of this group will be alive 5 years after operation (see Table 52-4). Nevertheless, these results still compare favorably with those obtained by resection of stage III gastric and pancreatic carcinomas.

Precise histologic staging is not possible before operation. Table 52-5 documents the overall results in patients undergoing ''curative'' resections. It can be seen that in Western series reporting at least 50 cases and published in the last

*TNM classification of malignant tumors, International Union Against Cancer, 1982.

5 years, the average 5-year survival rate is 10% (range, 5% to 21%). By contrast, the 5-year survival in Japanese and Chinese series, which usually contain a large number of early cancers, is approximately 25% (range, 10.3% to 42.2%). But irrespective of the survival rates, most surgeons report that after "curative" esophageal resection, the ability to swallow is restored for the duration of the life of the patient.

Esophageal resection for palliation

In the attempt to extend the benefits of esophageal reconstruction to larger numbers, many patients have undergone "palliative" or incomplete resections. When the surgical approach included a thoracotomy, the mortality for incomplete resection in earlier reports was often greater than 40%[69-70] and the median survival of those discharged from hospital less than 6 months. More recently, Postlethwait[71] found that "palliative" resection had an operative mortality of 22.7%. The large multicenter study conducted by the European Organization for Research on Treatment of Cancer[72] reported that the operative mortality for "palliative" resection was 31%, compared with 16% for "curative" resection. It also appears that survival after incomplete resection is not improved by the use of adjuvant therapy. Mannell et al.[73] found that the 1-year survival rate after incomplete excision of identifiable tumor tissue was only 21%, despite radical irradiation to the sites of residual cancer.

The technique of "blunt esophagectomy," popularized by Grey Turner[74] 50 years ago, has been reintroduced to allow palliative resection of esophageal cancer without the hazards of thoracotomy. As shown by Grey Turner, this technique can be dangerous when the tumor has invaded the aorta or tracheobronchial tree. But if macroscopic tumor does not extend beyond the esophagus, the operation can be performed with an acceptably low mortality rate.[75-77] However, the results of "blunt esophagectomy" are difficult to assess, because the preoperative TNM staging of tumors removed by this technique is not usually documented. Since mediastinal lymph nodes are not systemically removed by this technique, it is of palliative benefit only to *all* stage III cases, including the 10% to 15% who may be cured if the dissection of tumor and regional lymph nodes is performed under vision. But this operation may have particular value in those cases assessed as stage 0 to II disease in which thoracotomy is contraindicated for medical reasons.

Combination therapy

Surgery will cure the asymptomatic case with preinvasive esophageal cancer. But, by the time of diagnosis, 50% to 60% of patients with dysphagia have advanced disease. Of those who are still suitable for resection, the majority have lymphatic metastases and are incurable. The clinician treating typical cases of carcinoma of the esophagus is therefore faced with two major problems: first, how to make advanced tumors resectable and, second, how to cure disseminated disease.

Combined modalities of therapy have been tried, with many investigators adding irradiation to surgery. But the results are conflicting (see the following) and, at best, suggest that this combined treatment leads to only a small improvement in the cure rate.

Preoperative irradiation

An early nonrandomized study by Akakura et al.[78] found that 5000 to 6000 r, given in standard fractions over 4 to 6 weeks prior to surgery, increased resectability and improved survival. The resection rate in 229 patients treated by surgery alone was 39.7%, the operative mortality 13.2%, and the 5-year survival 13.6%. When preoperative irradiation was combined with surgery in 117 patients, resectability rose to 82.1%, the operative mortality was 20.8%, and the 5-year survival reached 25%. The improved survival came at the expense of increased treatment mortality.

However, three recent *randomized* studies have failed to show any benefit from preoperative radiotherapy. Launois et al.,[79] using a radiation dose of 4000 r administered over 8 to 12 days, found that this did not improve the rate of resection. In fact, this high-dose irradiation appeared to increase acute postoperative mortality and may have contributed to the unusually short median survival time of 4.5 months in the combined treatment modality group. In another trial, involving 192 patients, Gignoux et al.[80] did not find the resectability or operative mortality was altered by the addition of preoperative irradiation: the median survival of both groups in this study was 24 months. The large trial, coordinated by the European Organization for Research on Treatment of Cancer,[72] consisted of 229 patients with operable squamous esophageal cancer who were randomized between a control group and a preoperative radiotherapy group (3300 r given over 12 days). Both treatment groups appeared similar in histopathologic parameters. There was no difference in the postoperative mortality or the late results, median survival being about 12 months.

However, there are three other studies that have demonstrated a survival advantage for this combination therapy. Sasaki et al.,[81] in a prospective randomized trial of 93 patients, showed that survival was improved in stage III or IV disease. These workers reported that the 5-year survival in cases receiving preoperative irradiation was 22%, compared with a 15% 5-year survival for surgery alone. Of particular interest was their observation that response appeared to be influenced by tumor site: 21% of patients with upper- or middle-third cancers survived 5 years, compared with 0% of those with tumors in the lower third of the esophagus. By contrast, Wilson et al.[50] found that the disease-free interval of 13 months after operation in patients with distal esophageal cancers was increased to 24.1 months by preoperative irradiation. This study was, however, nonrandomized and included cases of adenocarcinoma of the cardia. A recent prospective randomized study from China[59] reported that 45.5% of patients given preoperative radiotherapy survived 5 years, compared with 25% of those treated by surgery only (but it is not certain if the two groups were similar with respect to stage of disease).

The results of preoperative irradiation in patients undergoing esophagectomy are conflicting, but there is no survival benefit for radiotherapy in patients whose cancers are found to be *nonresectable*. An early study by Van Andel et al.[82] found that no patient with nonresectable esophageal carcinoma survived 5 years, despite preoperative and postoperative radiotherapy to a total dose of 6600 r. The series reported from the Soviet Union by Mamontov and Simanchev[83] tends to confirm the findings of Van Andel: they had a 17.6% 5-year survival in patients with resectable tumors treated by preoperative irradiation. When preoperative irradiation (dose, 4000 r) was followed by an incomplete resection, no patient survived 3 years. A similar result was reported by Mannell et al.[73]

It is evident that the value of preoperative radiation therapy has not been proved. But, provided the morbidity of rapid, high-dose irradiation is avoided, there appears to be a case for further study of this combination in carefully staged patients. More randomized prospective studies are in order.

Postoperative irradiation

To date, the combination of surgery and postoperative irradiation has not been systematically studied in patients with resectable disease. Kasai et al.[84] suggest that prophylactic postoperative irradiation does benefit those with minimal disease: they found that the 5-year survival rate in patients with negative nodes improved—from 27.3% after surgery only, to 87.5% in those who received 6000 r to the neck and mediastinum. But there was no survival advantage for postoperative irradiation in patients with positive nodes.

In a more recent, but nonrandomized, study[73]

the 3-year actuarial survival in 39 patients with stage III disease evaluated after resection and radiotherapy (dose, 5000 r) was 34%, compared with 0% in 13 patients treated by surgery only for stage III tumors. Of the 39 patients treated with the combined therapy, no survival difference was noted in the 20 patients receiving part of the total dose before operation.

Both series[73,84] suggest that irradiation may be effective treatment for residual microscopic disease. But data from randomized trials of postoperative irradiation, in patients free of gross disease after surgery, are not yet available.

Chemotherapy

Chemotherapeutic agents are currently under investigation for their effect on the resectability of esophageal carcinoma and have the potential of improving survival in patients with disseminated disease.

Preoperative chemotherapy plus irradiation

Following the suggestion that the results of radiotherapy could be improved by using the radiosensitizing effect of bleomycin,[85] two prospective randomized trials were undertaken to investigate this combination. Andersen et al.[86] found that neither resectability nor survival was improved by the addition of bleomycin to preoperative irradiation. Mannell[87] terminated a prospective randomized trial when it became evident that the postoperative mortality in the group receiving combination therapy was significantly higher than in those treated by preoperative irradiation alone. Increased morbidity and mortality rates following the use of preoperative chemotherapy were also reported by Leichman et al.[88] and Parker et al.[89] Both studies included preoperative irradiation. Pulmonary toxicity has been a common problem associated with the preoperative use of many cytotoxic drugs, particularly bleomycin.

Most pilot studies of preoperative chemotherapy and irradiation suffer the disadvantage of using historical controls. But one hopeful finding has been the absence of residual disease in up to 33% of resected specimens.[88] Whether a disease-free operative specimen can be equated with improved long-term survival is not yet known. Parker et al.[89] reported that the 2-year survival of patients given preoperative chemoradiation therapy was identical to that of patients treated by preoperative radiotherapy only, despite an increase in the number of disease-free, resected specimens in the chemoradiation group.

Although the effect of preoperative chemotherapy added to irradiation is uncertain, the me-

TABLE 52-6. Results of preoperative chemotherapy and irradiation

Author(s)	Drugs	Radiation dose	No. of patients	Resect-ability (%)	Treatment mortality (%)	Median survival (mo)
Fujimaki[85] (1975)	Bleomycin	3000 r	76	63	7	NS*
Andersen et al.[86] (1984) (random-ized trial)	Bleomycin	3500 r	63	36	12	6.2
Werner[90] (1979)	Methotrexate	2000 r	55	NS	14.5	26
Leichman et al.[88] (1984)	5-fluorouracil + mitomycin C	3000 r	23	78	30	12
	5-fluorouracil + cisplatin	3000 r	19	71	27	18
Parker et al.[89] (1984)	5-fluorouracil + mitomycin C	3000 r	31	72	6	NS

*Not stated.

TABLE 52-7. Results of preoperative chemotherapy

Author(s)*	Drugs	No. of patients	Resectability (%)	Treatment mortality (%)	Median survival (mo)
Kelsen et al.[91] (1981)	Cisplatin + bleomycin + vindesine	34	76	11	9.7
Bains et al.[92] (1982)	Cisplatin + bleomycin + vindesine	34	82	9	18.5
Ladd et al.[93] (1983)	Cisplatin + mitomycin C + bleomycin	29	37.9	NS†	NS‡
Desai et al.[96] (1985)	Methotrexate + cisplatin	88	10	NS†	NS§

*EDITOR'S NOTE: The first two items listed are both from the Memorial Sloan-Kettering Cancer Center series.
†Not stated.
‡Not stated: 2% survival at 2 years.
§Not stated: 16% alive at 3 years.

dian survival times reported by some investigators are encouraging (see Table 52-6).

Preoperative chemotherapy

Most cytotoxic drugs have only modest activity against esophageal cancer when used alone. But trials of multidrug chemotherapy have now begun, and the results of several preoperative studies have been reported (see Table 52-7). Bleomycin combined with cisplatin was shown to have moderate activity in squamous carcinoma of the esophagus; the response rate is improved by the addition of vindesine.[94] Esophageal cancer can no longer be regarded as resistant to chemotherapy, but the response rate has not been as favorable as in other solid tumors, such as testicular and ovarian carcinomas. Given before surgery, multidrug therapies are not without risk: in the study reported by Kukla et al.,[95] using cisplatin, mitomycin C, bleomycin, and prednisone, the postoperative mortality was 45%, with four out of five deaths drug related. Since there is, as yet, no irrefutable evidence that preoperative che-

motherapy improves either the resectability or the long-term survival rate, multidrug therapy must be regarded as under investigation and studies of its use should be restricted to those centers able to accurately monitor both response and toxicity.

However, promising results have been reported. Desai et al.[96] treated 88 cases of advanced and inoperable esophageal cancer with cisplatin and methotrexate and obtained an overall response rate of 75%. Of particular interest was the observation that nine of these patients, after two cycles of the drug combination, were found to be suitable for resection, and the 3-year survival rate for the group as a whole was significantly better than for the historical controls.

COMBINATION THERAPY FOR ADVANCED ESOPHAGEAL CANCER

The established methods of palliation have little to offer patients with metastatic disease and a large tumor burden. When a tumor is more than

TABLE 52-8. Results of combination therapy for advanced esophageal cancer

Author(s)	Drugs	Irradiation	No. of patients	Response* rate (%)	Median duration of response (mo)
Kolaric et al.[97] (1980)	Bleomycin	3600-4400 r	24	62	9
	Adriamycin	3600-4400 r	15	60	8.6
	Bleomycin + adriamycin	3600-4400 r	15	60	11
Kelsen[98] (1982)	Cisplatin	—	20	40	7.8
	Bleomycin				
	Vindesine				
Vogl et al.[99] (1981)	Cisplatin	—	10	50	6
	Methotrexate				
	Bleomycin				
Le Chevalier et al.[100] (1981)	Vindesine	—	10	10	2
	Nitrosourea				
	Cyclophosphamide				
	Cisplatin				
Gisselbrecht et al.[101] (1982)	5-Fluorouracil	—	21	33	9
	Adriamycin				
	Cisplatin				
Sasaki et al.[102] (1982)	Cisplatin	—	10	40	1.5
	Bleomycin				
Kelsen et al.[103] (1983)	Cisplatin	—	9	33	2-3
	Vindesine				
	Methyl-glyoxal bis				
Coai et al.[104] (1984)	5-Fluorouracil	5000 r	5	80	Not stated
	Mitomycin C				
Kolaric et al.[105] (1984)	5-Fluorouracil	3600-4000 r	28	73	12†
	Bleomycin				
	5-Fluorouracil	3600-4000 r	28	64	6.8†
	Adriamycin				
Dinwoodie et al.[106] (1985)	Cisplatin	—	32	29	"Brief"
	Bleomycin				
	Vindesine				
Resbeut et al.[107] (1985)	Vincristine	Split course	28	75	8
	Methotrexate				
	Cisplatin				

*Complete and partial responses.
†Duration of complete response.

10 cm in length, most surgeons consider it nonresectable, and less than 30% of malignancies this size show any response to radiation therapy. Mechanical restoration of the esophageal lumen by intubation or dilatation provides incomplete palliation of dysphagia for about 3 to 4 months. Bypass surgery in these patients is associated with an increased risk of morbidity and mortality, with mean survivals of not greater than 4 months.

It is for patients with advanced, inoperable carcinoma of the esophagus that combined modalities of therapy offer the greatest hope of relief. However, as the tumor burden increases and the patient's general condition deteriorates, the likelihood of complete or partial response to multi-

drug therapy is reduced. But even a minor (50%) response can result in significant improvement in the ability to swallow. Table 52-8 lists some of the recent studies[97-107] of patients with advanced disease treated by combination chemotherapy with or without irradiation. These cases are incurable, so the principal aim of treatment is to improve the quality of life rather than simply prolonging it. For this group of patients the duration of response to therapy is more important than length of survival.

Kolaric et al.,[97] in a randomized trial using bleomycin and adriamycin, found that these drugs had a very limited effect on esophageal cancer if used as single agents. But when they were combined with radiation therapy, the response rate and duration of response were significantly increased. Combinations of drugs have, in general, an effect greater than the additive effects of those drugs administered separately.[98,101] However, toxicity is increased by multidrug therapy. Le Chevalier et al.[100] reported that the four-drug combination used in their study had severe side effects, and 30% of the patients treated by Vogl et al.[99] suffered severe hematologic toxicity. Drug-related deaths occurred with the combination of bleomycin, cisplatin, and vindesine.[98,106] Toxicity can be reduced as new, safer drugs become available. Kelsen et al.[103] reported that substitution of methyl-glyoxal bis for bleomycin resulted in less toxicity without a reduction in the response rate.

Palliation of dysphagia depends on the response of the tumor to therapy, and it is encouraging to note that, in 8 of the 11 series documented in Table 52-8, more than half of the patients responded to combination treatment, frequently for 6 months or longer. But side effects of cytotoxic agents must also be considered when the palliative value of any drug regimen is assessed. If the therapy is complicated by severe mucositis, retrosternal pain, nausea, and vomiting,[98,105] the quality of life may *not* be improved, irrespective of an increased ability to swallow. At this time, palliative combination therapies must be regarded as promising modalities that are still in the initial phases of investigation. Prospective, randomized studies of larger numbers of patients are necessary before the role of this treatment for advanced esophageal cancer can be accurately evaluated.

FUTURE PROSPECTS IN THE MANAGEMENT OF ESOPHAGEAL CANCER
Detection

The principal aim in the treatment of cancer is to cure the patient, and it is obvious that cure of esophageal cancer depends on diagnosis at an early stage. The 5-year survival after esophagectomy for carcinoma in situ is over 90%[52]; the 5-year survival after resection of invasive cancers that have *not* spread through the wall of the esophagus or to lymph nodes is 61%.[84] But the 5-year survival rate falls to 10% to 15% once lymphatic metastases have occurred. The other advantage of early diagnosis is a technical one: removal of a macroscopically normal esophagus has a mortality of less than 5%.[52]

Substantial progress in the detection of early lesions has been made by workers in the People's Republic of China. Mass screening in areas where the disease is prevalent has shown that blind abrasive cytology (BAC), using a balloon sampling technique, can detect early esophageal cancer in asymptomatic individuals. Detection of early esophageal cancers by cytologic studies appears to be more accurate than either endoscopic or radiologic methods, and it is said that BAC can differentiate between benign and malignant lesions with an accuracy in the range of 90%.[108] Yang et al.[109] found 115 cases of early esophageal cancer in 28,139 people undergoing BAC in Henan, a province in the north of China where the incidence of carcinoma of the esophagus is very high. If these "early" cases had progressed to frank malignancy, the incidence of esophageal cancer in this population would be approximately 400 per 100,000. However, in 1980, Yang[110] reported that the incidence of esophageal cancer in the same area was 130 per 100,000. The threefold discrepancy in prevalence rates is difficult to explain: either differentiation of severe dysphagia from carcinoma in situ on cytologic examination may not always be possible or every case of carcinoma in situ does not necessarily progress to invasive carcinoma. One solution to the difficulties in diagnosis of "early" cancer by BAC is the use of endoscopically guided biopsy after in vivo staining. If severe dysplasia or carcinoma in situ is diagnosed by BAC, a 3% Lugol solution and/or 2% toluidine blue will identify early lesions not visible to the naked eye, and endoscopic biopsy can be performed.[111,112]

There is no doubt that mass screening programs, with BAC, should be introduced wherever esophageal cancer is prevalent. Until this is possible, both the physician and the population in a high-risk area should be alerted to the symptoms of early carcinoma of the esophagus. These include dysphagia, "slight" esophageal pain or "tingling" when swallowing, a foreign-body sensation in the throat, and a feeling of fullness in the distal esophagus after swallowing.[112] In high-risk areas, even minor symptoms connected with the esophagus are an indication for cytologic and endoscopic esophageal examination.

However, in other countries, including the United States, where the incidence of the disease is low, mass screening is hard to justify. But selective screening of patients known to have an increased risk of esophageal cancer is feasible. These patients would include those with long-standing achalasia, caustic strictures, Barrett's esophagus, scleroderma, or a cancer in the head and neck region. If the patient had histologic abnormalities identified by BAC, or minor esophageal symptoms, double-dye staining and guided endoscopic biopsies would be indicated.[113]

Treatment

It is unlikely that any major changes in the techniques of radiotherapy and surgery are imminent. Modifications of the standard methods of esophagectomy, such as "en bloc resection"[65] or extensive lymph node dissection,[57] have not made any marked impact on 5-year survival rates once lymphatic metastases have occurred. However, reduction in the morbidity and mortality of esophageal resection is likely, as soon as recent advances in identifying and correcting risk factors for esophageal surgery are universally appreciated. These recent advances include the definition of cardiorespiratory and renal criteria for safe esophagectomy,[84,114] use of plasma protein levels to identify patients at high risk for postoperative complications,[115] and experimental proof that an atraumatic, bloodless surgical technique is of critical importance in anastomotic healing.[116]

As indicated above, significant advances have already been made in chemotherapy for esophageal cancer. Studies on new cytotoxic agents are being reported at an increasing rate. So it is possible that effective, multidrug chemotherapy, to allow locally advanced tumors to be safely and completely resected, will be available in the not-too-distant future. As new cytotoxics with increased activity against squamous esophageal cancer are developed, cure of patients with disseminated disease may be possible and bypass surgery or esophageal intubation may become largely outmoded techniques for palliation. Laser technology may, however, find a role in palliation: it could be used to restore luminal patency to the esophagus while the patient is undergoing chemoradiation therapy and waiting for remission to occur.

Prevention

One of the most striking features of carcinoma of the esophagus is the extraordinary variation in its geographic distribution. It is not a cancer peculiar to any one racial group but a disease in which most cases occur within certain clearly demarcated regions throughout the world. The latter include the northern provinces in China, the Caspian littoral in Iran, Brittany, Normandy, and Pays de Laire in France, and along the east coast of South Africa.[117]

The cause of esophageal cancer is unknown, but the geographic localization of the disease suggests that environmental factors are important. The list of possible carcinogens is long and varied, many being peculiar to specific endemic areas. They include fungal infestation of corn in Africa,[118] "bush tea" in Curacao,[119] opium pyrolysates in Iran,[120] well water containing petroleum products in Saudi Arabia,[121] nitrosamine precursors in food and water sources contaminated by microorganisms in China,[122] a high concentration of iron in home-brewed beer in South Africa,[123] and the nitrosamine compounds in tobacco smoke[124] and alcoholic beverages.

In addition to ingested carcinogens, recent work has incriminated certain viral infections in the etiology of esophageal cancer. The human papilloma virus (HPV) has been identified in esophageal squamous papillomas,[125,126] and Syrjänen[127] found histologic changes identical to those of condylomatous lesions caused by HPV in 24 of 60 squamous esophageal cancers. The herpesvirus has also been identified by electron microscopy in material from squamous carcinoma of the esophagus.[128]

Of particular interest is the fact that chickens raised in Linxian province, a high-incidence area in China, develop epidermoid cancers of the pharynx and esophagus at a rate that parallels that of their human owners. This has been attributed to a dietary carcinogen, but it is equally likely that a transmissible agent could be involved. Discovery of the etiologic role of the AIDS virus in Kaposi's sarcoma, of hepatitis B virus in hepatoma, and of the Epstein-Barr virus in Burkitt's lymphoma suggests that further research into the viral associations of esophageal cancer is indicated.

Irrespective of the etiology of esophageal cancer, one factor common to all high-incidence areas is the low socioeconomic status of its victims. Carcinoma of the esophagus is a disease of poverty and malnutrition: numerous experimental studies have shown that esophageal carcinogens are potentiated by vitamin and trace element deficiencies.[129-131] Even in Western countries, where cancer of the esophagus occurs sporadically, poor nutritional status is a major risk factor.[132,133] Another factor of epidemiologic importance is that most of the carcinogens implicated appear to act directly on the esophagus. This is unusual, and it suggests that the disease could be prevented by primary means.

Therefore, preventative measures should be twofold. First, the general nutritional status of people in the endemic areas must be improved. Second, risk factors in the diet and habits of these people should be identified and, whenever possible, eliminated.

REFERENCES

1. Adelstein, D.J., Forman, W.B., and Beavers, B. Esophageal carcinoma: a six-year review of the Cleveland Veterans Administration Hospital experience, Cancer **54**(5):918, 1984.

2. Aygun, C, Slawson, R.G., Hankins, J., et al.: Treatment of esophageal carcinoma with tracheobronchial tree involvement: a ten-year experience (meeting abstract), Radiology **53(p):**101, 1984.

3. Symbas, P.N., McKeown, P.P., Blasis, S.E., and Hatcher, C.R., Jr.: Tracheoesophageal fistula from carcinoma of the esophagus, Ann. Thorac. Surg. **38:**382, 1984.

4. Nullen, H., Sailer, R., and Jaeschock, R.: Nonresectable palliative measures in inoperable carcinoma of the esophagus and cardia, Aktuel. Chir. **17**(6):219, 1982.

5. Beck, R., and Kienzle, H.F.: Feeding gastrostomy: last possibility for a palliative operation in malignant stenoses of the esophagus-cardia, Chirurgie **54**(7):484, 1983.

6. Girardet, R.E., Ransdell, H.T., and Wheat, M.N.: Palliative intubation in the management of esophageal carcinoma, Ann. Thorac. Surg. **18**(4):417, 1974.

7. Boyce, H.W., Jr.: Medical management of esophageal obstruction and esophageal pulmonary fistula, Cancer **50**(Suppl 11):2597, 1982.

8. Mannell, A., Becker, P.J., Melissas, J., and Diamantis, T.: Intubation versus dilatation plus bleomycin in the treatment of advanced esophageal cancer: the results of a prospective randomized trial, S. Afr. J. Surg., 1986. (In press.)

9. Moses, F.M., Peura, D.A., Wong, R.H., Johnson, L.F.: Palliative dilatation of esophageal carcinoma, Gastrointest. Endosc. **31**(2):61, 1985.

10. Graham, D.Y., and Smith, J.L. Balloon dilatation of benign and malignant esophageal strictures: blind retrograde balloon dilatation, Gastrointest. Endosc. **31**(3):171, 1985.

11. Aste, H., Munizzi, F., Martinez, H., and Pugliese, V.: Esophageal dilatation in malignant dysphagia, Cancer **56**(11):2713, 1985.

12. Den Hartog Jager, F.C.A., Bartelsman, J.F.W.M., Tytgat, G.N.J.: Palliative treatment of obstructing esophagogastric malignancy by endoscopic positioning of a plastic prosthesis, Gastroenterology **77**(5):1008, 1979.

13. Watson, A.: A study of the quality and duration of survival following resection, endoscopic intubation and surgical intubation in esophageal carcinoma, Br. J. Surg. **69**(10):585, 1982.

14. Pietropaola, V., Bogliolo, G., Vinceconte, G.W., et al.: Endoscopic treatment of neoplasms of the esophagus and cardia (meeting abstract), I Cono Internazionale de Aggiornamento in Diagnostica Chirurgia Endoscopia, December 2 to 4, 1982, Catania, Sicily, 1982, Societa Italian di Endoscopia Digestiva.

15. Ogilvie, A.L., Dronfield, M.W., Ferguson, R., and Atkinson, M.: Palliative intubation of esophagogastric neoplasms at fibreoptic endoscopy, Gut **23**(12):1060, 1982.

16. Rose, J.D., and Smith, P.M.: Fibre endoscopic insertion of palliative esophageal tubes with the Nottingham introducer, J. R. Soc. Med. **76**(4):266, 1983.

17. Diamantis, T., and Mannell, A.: Oesophageal intubation for advanced oesophageal cancer: the Baragwanath experience, 1977-1981, Br. J. Surg. **70**(9):555, 1983.

18. Procter, D.S.C.: Esophageal intubation for carcinoma of the esophagus, World J. Surg. **4:**451, 1980.

19. Sarr, M.G., Harper, P.H., and Kettlewell, M.G.: Peroral pulsion intubation of malignant esophageal strictures using a fibreoptic technique, Am. Surg. **50**(8):437, 1984.

20. Buess, G., Kometz, B., Schellong, H., and Roos, B.: Endotube as a palliative measure in stenosing cancer of the esophagus and cardia, Leber Magen Darm **15**(1):26, 1985.

21. Valbuena, J.: Endoscopic palliative treatment of esophageal and cardial cancer: a new antireflux prosthesis— a study of 40 cases, Cancer **53**(4):993, 1984.

22. Fleisher, D., and Sivak, M.V., Jr.: Endoscopic Nd:YAG laser therapy as palliation for esophagogastric cancer: parameters affecting initial outcome, Gastroenterology **89**(4):827, 1985.

23. McCaughan, J.S., Jr., Williams, T.E., Jr., Bethel, B.H.: Palliation of esophageal malignancy with photodynamic therapy, Ann. Thorac. Surg. **49**(2):113, 1985.

24. Cello, J.P., Gerstenberger, P.D., Wright, T., et al.: Endoscopic neodymium-YAG laser palliation of nonresectable esophageal malignancy, Ann Intern. Med. **102**(5):610, 1985.

25. De Moor, N.G.: Preliminary report on survey conducted by the Johannesburg group of hospitals on cancer of the oesophagus in the African: aims, policies and results, S. Afr. Med. J. **42:**892, 1968.

26. Smit, B.J., Levin, J., McQuaide, J., et al.: Treatment of carcinoma of the oesophagus in Port Elizabeth. In Silber, W., editor: Carcinoma of the Oesophagus, Cape Town, 1978, A.A. Balkema, pp. 263-271.

27. Gordon, W.: Bypass for malignant obstruction of the esophagus, Ann. Surg. **158:**47, 1963.

28. Ong, G.B., Lam, K.H., Wong, J., and Lim, T.K.: Jejunal esophagoplasty for carcinoma of the esophagus, Jpn. J. Surg. **10**(1):15, 1980.

29. Nicks, R.: Colonic replacement of the oesophagus, Br. J. Surg. **54:**124, 1967.

30. Akiyama, H., and Hiyaima, M.: A single esophageal bypass operation by the high gastric division, Surgery **75:**674, 1974.

31. Dzieniszewski, G.P., Gamstatter, G., Klotter, H.J., and Rothmund, M.: Palliative surgical therapy of incurable cancer by stomach bypass and endotube, Zentralbl. Chir. **109**(24):1550, 1984.

32. Angorn, I.B., and Haffejee, A.A. Retrosternal gastric bypass for the palliative treatment of unresectable oesophageal carcinoma: a simple technique, S. Afr. Med. J. **64**(23):901, 1983.

33. Mannell, A.: The palliation of esophageal cancer. In Nyhus, L.C., editor: Surgery annual 1985, Norwalk, Conn., 1985, Appleton-Century-Crofts, pp. 249-270.

34. Wong, J., Lam, K.H., Wei, W.I., and Ong, G.B.: Results of the Kirschner operation, World J. Surg. **5**(4):547, 1981.

35. Mannell, A., and Plant, M.: The management of malignant oesophago-airway fistulae, Aust. N.Z. J. Surg. **53:**31, 1983.

36. Conlan, A.A., Nicolaou, N., Delikaris, P.E., and Pool, R.: Pessimism concerning palliative bypass procedure for established malignant esophagorespiratory fistulae: a report of 18 patients, Ann. Thorac. Surg. **37**(2):108, 1984.

37. Mannell, A.: Palliative surgery for oesophageal cancer (meeting abstract), 6th Biennial Congress of the World Council of Enterostomal Therapists, Perth, Australia, April 14 to 18, 1986.

38. Earlam, R., and Cunha-Melo, J.R.: Oesophageal squamous cell carcinoma: II. A critical review of radiotherapy, Br. J. Surg. **67**:457, 1980.

39. Asakawa, H., Watanari, J., and Hoshino, T.: Clinical evaluation of hypoxic cell sensitizer (misonidazole), Gan To Kagaku Ryoho **11**(6):1225, 1984.

40. Laramore, G.E., Davis, R.B., Olson, M.H., et al.: RTOG phase 1 study on fast neutron teletherapy for squamous cell carcinoma of the esophagus.

41. Castro, J.R., Chen, G.T., Pitluck, S., et al.: Helium charged-particle radiotherapy of locally advanced carcinoma of the esophagus, stomach and biliary tract, Am. J. Clin. Oncol. **6**(6):629, 1983.

42. Hancock, S.L., and Glatstein, E.: Radiation therapy of esophageal cancer, Semin. Oncol. **2**(2):144, 1984.

43. Pearson, J.G.: The present status and future potential of radiotherapy in the management of oesophageal cancer, Cancer **39**:882, 1977.

44. Newaishy, G.A., Read, G.A., Duncan, W., and Kerr, G.E.: Results of radical radiotherapy of squamous cell carcinoma of the oesophagus, Clin. Radiol. **53**:347, 1982.

45. Beatty, J.D., De Boer, G., and Rider, W.D.: Carcinoma of the esophagus: pretreatment assessment, correlation of radiation treatment parameters with survival, and identification and management of radiation treatment failure, Cancer **43**:2254, 1979.

46. Miao, Y., Gu, X., Hu, Y., et al.: Intracavitary radiotherapy of esophageal cancer, Zhonghua Zhongliu Zazhi **4**(1):45, 1982.

47. Morita, K., Takagi, I., Watanabe, M., et al.: Relationship between the radiological features of esophageal cancer and the local control by radiation therapy, Cancer **55**:2668, 1985.

48. Beatty, J.D.: Radiotherapy versus resection for palliation of carcinoma of the esophagus (letter to editor), Can. J. Surg. **28**(2):108, 1985.

49. Kelsen, D.: Current concepts in the treatment of esophageal cancer, Cancer Treat. Res. **18**:124, 1984.

50. Wilson, S.E., Hiatt, J.R., Stabile, B.E., and Williams, R.A.. Cancer of the distal esophagus and cardia: preoperative irradiation prolongs survival, Am. J. Surg. **150**:114, 1985.

51. Earlam, R., and Cunha-Melo, J.R.: Oesophageal squamous cell carcinoma: I. A critical review of surgery, Br. J. Surg. **67**:381, 1980.

52. Shao, L., Li, Z., Liu, S., and Wong, M.: Surgical treatment of 210 cases of early carcinoma of the esophagus and gastric cardia, Zhonghua Waike Zazhi **19**(5):259, 1981.

53. Shao, L., Li, Z., Wong, M., et al.: Results of surgical treatment of 3,155 cases of esophageal and cardiac carcinoma, Zhonghua Waike Zazhi **20**(1):19, 1982.

54. Xu, L.T., Sun, Z.F., Li, Z.J., and Wu, L.H.: Surgical treatment of carcinoma of the esophagus and cardiac portion of the stomach in 850 patients, Ann. Thorac. Surg. **35**(5):542, 1983.

55. Launois, B., Paul, J.L., Lygidakis, W.J., et al.: Results of the surgical treatment of carcinoma of the esophagus, Surg. Gynecol. Obstet. **156**:753, 1983.

56. Pralat, U., Dragovevic, D., Metzer, R, and Borst, H.G.: Long-term results following resection and esophageal reconstruction in esophageal cancer, Langenbecks Arch. Chir. **360**(4):251, 1983.

57. Akiyama, H., Tsurumaru, H., Kawamura, T., et al.: Development of surgery for carcinoma of the esophagus, Am. J. Surg. **147**(1):9, 1984.

58. Ellis, F.H., Jr.: Cancer of the esophagus and cardia: role of surgery in palliation, Postgrad. Med. **75**(3):139, 1984.

59. Huang, G.J., Wong, L.T., Liu, J.S., et al.: Surgery of esophageal carcinoma, Semin. Surg. Oncol. **1**(2):74, 1985.

60. Akiyama, H., Tsurumaru, M., Kawamura, T., and Ono, Y.: Principles of surgical treatment for carcinoma of the esophagus, Ann. Surg. **194**(4):438, 1981.

61. Fu, Y.C., Zhang, Z.T., Liu, F.X., et al.: Surgical treatment of carcinoma of the esophagus and gastric cardia, Kyobu Geka **35**(8):618, 1982.

62. Anne, T., Berwounts, L., Wehlou, M., et al.: Surgical treatment of esophageal carcinoma: experience between 1965 and 1980, Acta Chir. Belg. **92**(4):359, 1982.

63. Couraud, L., and Meriot, S.: The treatment of carcinoma of the lower and middle thirds of the esophagus by resection and isoperistaltic tubular gastroplasty: short and long-term results in a series of 256 cases, Chirurgie **108**(9):703, 1982.

64. Zhang, K., Du, X., Zhang, W., et al.: Surgical treatment of 4,310 cases of carcinoma of the esophagus and gastric cardia, Zhonghua Zhongliu Zazhi **4**(1):1-4, 1982.

65. Skinner, D.B.: En bloc resection for neoplasms of the esophagus and cardia, J. Thorac. Cardiovasc. Surg. **85**(1):59, 1983.

66. Forni, E., Borri, A.M., Zadra, F., et al.: Results of the treatment of carcinoma of the thoracic esophagus with one-stage resection and esophagogastrostomy, Chir. Ital. **36**(4):589, 1984.

67. Keagy, B.A., Loves, M.E., Murray, G.F., et al.: Esophagogastrectomy as palliative treatment for esophageal carcinoma: results obtained in the setting of a thoracic surgery residency program, Ann. Thorac. Surg. **38**:611, 1984.

68. Hennessy, T.P., and O'Connell, R.: Surgical treatment of squamous cell carcinoma of the oesophagus, Br. J. Surg. **71**(10):750, 1984.

69. Ong, G.B., Lam, K.H., Wong, J., and Lim, T.K.: Factors influencing morbidity and mortality in esophageal carcinoma, J. Thorac. Cardiovasc. Surg. **76**(6):745, 1978.

70. Belsey, R., and Hiebert, C.A.: An exclusive right thoracic approach for cancer of the middle third of the esophagus, Ann. Thorac. Surg. **18**(1):1, 1974.

71. Postlethwait, R.W.: Complications and deaths after operations for esophageal carcinoma, J. Thorac. Cardiovasc. Surg. **85**(6):827, 1983.

72. European Organization for Research on Treatment of Cancer, Gastrointestinal Tract Cancer Cooperative Group: Preoperative radiotherapy for carcinoma of the esophagus: results of a prospective multicenter study. In DeMeester, T.R., and Skinner, D.B., editors: Esophageal disorders: pathophysiology and therapy, New York, 1985, Raven Press, pp. 367-371.

73. Mannell, A., Nissenbaum, M., and Plant, M.: Radical treatment for squamous carcinoma of the thoracic oesophagus: the late results in 89 cases, Br. J. Surg., 1986. (Submitted for publication.)

74. Turner, G.G.: The oesophagus, London, 1946, Cassell & Co., pp. 81-82.

75. Orringer, M.B.: Transhiatal esophagectomy without thoracotomy for carcinoma of the thoracic esophagus, Ann. Surg. **200**(3):282, 1984.

76. Kron, I.L., Cantrell, R.W., Johns, M.E., et al.: Computerized axial tomography of the esophagus to determine the suitability for blunt esophagectomy, Ann. Surg. **200**(2):173, 1984.

77. Ulrich, B., Crabitz, K., and Kockel, N.: Results of stomach pull-through operations without thoractomy in the treatment of advanced esophageal cancer, Zentralbl. Chir. **109**(16):1033, 1984.

78. Akakura, I., Nakamura, Y., Kakegawa, T., et al.: Surgery of carcinoma of the esophagus with reoperative radiation, Chest **57**:47, 1970.

79. Launois, B., Delarue, D., Campon, J., et al.: Preoperative radiotherapy for carcinoma of the esophagus, Surg. Gynecol. Obstet. **153**:690, 1981.

80. Gignoux, M., Buyse, M., Segal, P., et al.: EORTC multicenter randomized study comparing preoperative radiotherapy with surgery only in cases of resectable esophageal cancer, Acta Chir. Belg. **82**(4):373, 1982.

81. Sasaki, T., Mitomi, T., Nakasaki, H., et al.: Evaluation of preoperative irradiation therapy for carcinoma of the esophagus, Nippon Geka Gakkai Zasshi, **85**(9):1054, 1984.

82. Van Andel, J.G., Dear, J., Dijkuis, C., et al.: Carcinoma of the esophagus: results of treatment, Ann. Surg. **190**:684, 1979.

83. Mamontov, A.S., and Simanchev, V.N.: Combined treatment of locally advanced esophageal cancer, Sov. Med. **10**:102, 1982.

84. Kasai, M., Mori, S., and Watanabe, T.: Follow-up results after resection of thoracic esophageal cancer, World J. Surg. **2**:543, 1978.

85. Fujimaki, K.: A new chemotherapy as preoperative treatment for esophageal cancer surgery, In Proceedings of the 7th International Congress on Chemotherapy, Prague, 1971, pp. 543-646.

86. Andersen, P., Berdal, P., Edsmyr, F., et al.: Irradiation, chemotherapy and surgery in esophageal cancer: a randomized clinical study—the first Scandinavian trial in esophageal cancer, Radiother. Oncol. **2**(3):179, 1984.

87. Mannell, A.: Oesophagectomy: the lessons learnt from 128 cases, Aust. N.Z. J. Surg., 1986. (Submitted for publication.)

88. Leichman, L., Steiger, Z., and Seydel, H.G.: Preoperative chemotherapy and radiation therapy for patients with cancer of the esophagus: a potentially curative approach, J. Clin. Oncol. **2**(2):75, 1984.

89. Parker, E.F., Marks, R.D. Jr., Kratz, J.M., et al.: Chemoradiation therapy and resection for carcinoma of the esophagus: short-term results, Ann. Thorac. Surg. **40**(2):121, 1984.

90. Werner, I.D.: The multidisciplinary approach in the management of squamous carcinoma of the esophagus: the Groote Schuur Hospital experience, Front. Gastrointest. Res. **5**:130, 1979.

91. Kelsen, D.P., Chapman, R., and Bains, M.: Cisplatin, vindesine and bleomycin combination chemotherapy of esophageal cancer (meeting abstract), Proc. Ann. Assoc. Cancer Res. **22**:454, 1981.

92. Bains, M.S., Kelsen, D.P., Beattie, E.J. Jr., and Martini, N.: Treatment of esophageal carcinoma by combined preoperative chemotherapy, Ann. Thorac. Surg. **34**(5):521, 1982.

93. Ladd T.E., Kukla, L.J., Haas, A.J., et al.: Multimodality treatment of squamous cell carcinoma of the esophagus (meeting abstract), Proc. Ann. Soc. Clin. Oncol. **2**:C-448, 1983.

94. Kelsen, D., Bains, M., Hilaris, B., and Martini, N.: Combined-modality therapy of esophageal cancer, Semin. Oncol. **22**(2):169, 1984.

95. Kukla, L., Ladd, T., McGuire, W., and Thomas, P.: Multimodal therapy of squamous carcinoma of the esophagus (meeting abstract), Proc. ASCO and AACR, **22**:449, 1981.

96. Desai, P.B., Advani, S.H., Dinshaw, K.A., et al.: The long-term impact of front loading chemotherapy in advanced esophageal cancers: a report of 88 patients treated with cisplatin-methotrexate (meeting abstract), Proc. Am. Soc. Clin. Oncol. **4**:93, 1985.

97. Kolaric, K., Maricic, Z., Roth, A., and Dujmovic, I.: Chemotherapy versus chemoradiotherapy in inoperable esophageal cancer, Oncology 37(suppl. 1):78-82, 1980.

98. Kelsen, D.: Treatment of advanced esophageal cancer, Cancer **50**:2576, 1982.

99. Vogl, S.E., Greenwald, L.E., and Kaplan, B.H.: Effective chemotherapy for esophageal cancer with methotrexate, bleomycin and cis-diamminedichloroplatinum II, Cancer **48**(12):2555, 1981.

100. Le Chevalier, T., Rouesse, J., Arrigada, R., et al.: Combination of nitrosourea, vindesine, cyclophosphamide and cisdichlordiammineplatinum in inoperable lung and oesophagus squamous cell carcinoma (meeting abstract), UICC Conference on Clinical Onclogy, October 28 to 31, 1982, Lausanne, Switzerland, 1981, Switzerland Internation Union Against Cancer.

101. Gisselbrecht, C., Calvo, F., Mignot, L., et al.: Treatment of advanced epidermoid carcinoma of the esophagus with combined 5-FU, adriamycin and cis-platinum (FAP), Nouv. Presse Med. **11**(24):1859, 1982.

102. Sasaki, T., Ibuka, T., Imai, K., et al.: Combination chemotherapy with cisplatin and bleomycin in esophageal cancer, Gan To Kagaku Ryoho **9**(8):1442, 1982.

103. Kelsen, D.P., Coonley, C., Bains, M., and Hilaris, B.: Cisplatin, vindesine and methyl-glyoxal bis (Guanylhydrazone) combination chemotherapy of esophageal carcinoma (meeting abstract), Proc. Am. Soc. Clin. Oncol. **2**:C-501, 1983.

104. Coai, L.R., Engstrom, P.F., Paul, A., Gallagher, M.J.: A pilot study of combined radiotherapy and chemotherapy for esophageal carcinoma (meeting abstract), Am. J. Clin. Oncol. **7**(2):116, 1984.

105. Kolaric, K., Roth, A., and Dujmovic, I.: The value of two combined chemoradiotherapy approaches in the treatment of inoperable esophageal cancer, Tumori **70**(1):69, 1984.

106. Dinwoodie, W., Bartolucci, A., and Lyman, G.: Cisplatin, bleomycin and vindesine in advanced squamous cell carcinoma of the esophagus: a Southeastern Cancer Study Group study (meeting abstract), Proc. Am. Soc. Clin. Oncol. **4**:80, 1985.

107. Resbeut, M., Le Prise–Fleury, E., Ben-Hassel, M., et al.: Squamous cell carcinoma of the esophagus: treatment by combined vincristine-methotrexate plus folinic acid rescue and cisplatin before radiotherapy, Cancer **56**(6):1246, 1985.

108. Shu, Y.J.: Cytopathology of the esophagus: an overview of esophageal cytopathology in China, Acta Cytol. (Baltimore), **27**(1):7, 1983.

109. Yang, G., Huang, H., Qui, S., and Chang, Y.: Endoscopic diagnosis of 115 cases of early esophageal carcinoma, Endoscopy **14**(5):157, 1982.

110. Yang, C.S.: Research on esophageal cancer in China: a review, Cancer Res. **40**:2633, 1980.

111. Jessen, K., Paolucci, P., and Classen, M.: Detection of "early" esophageal carcinoma in high-risk patients: role of in vivo staining (meeting abstract), The World Congress in Stockholm, Sweden, June 14 to 19, 1982, Stockholm, 1982, The Swedish Society of Medical Sciences.

112. Endo, M., Yamado, A., Ide, H., et al.: Early cancer of the esophagus: diagnosis and clinical evaluation, Int. Adv. Surg. Oncol. **3**:49, 1980.

113. Lightdate, C.J., and Winawer, S.J.: Screening diagnosis and staging of esophageal cancer, Semin. Oncol. **11**(2):101, 1984.

114. Mannell, A., and Plant, M.: Thoracotomy and lung function. In Jamieson, G.G., editor: The surgery of the oesophagus, Edinburgh, 1986, Churchill Livingstone, Section 4, Ch. 2.

115. Pettigrew, R.A., and Hill, G.L.: Indicators of surgical risk and clinical judgement, Br. J. Surg. **73**:47, 1986.

116. Foster, M.E., Laycock, J.R.D., Silver, I.A., and Leaper, D.J.: Hypovolemia and healing in colonic anastomoses, Br. J. Surg. **72**:831, 1985.

117. Mannell, A.: Carcinoma of the esophagus. In Ravitch, M.M., editor: Current problems in surgery, Chicago, 1982, Year Book Medical Publishers, Inc., vol. 19, no. 10, pp. 558-563.

118. Marasas, W.F., Van Rensburg, S.J., and Mirocha, C.J.: Incidence of *Fusarium* species and the mycotoxins deoxynivalenol and zeatalone in corn produced in esophageal cancer areas in Transkei, J. Agric. Food Chem. **17**:1108, 1979.

119. Freni, S.C.: Long-term trends in the incidence rates of upper digestive tract cancer in the Netherlands Antilles, Cancer **53**:(7):1618, 1984.

120. Ghadirian, P., Stein, G.F., Gorodetzky, C., et al.: Oesophageal cancer studies in the Caspian littoral of Iran: some residual results, including opium use as a risk factor, Int. J. Cancer **35**(5):593, 1985.

121. Amer, M.H., El-Yazigi, A., Hannan, M., et al.: Esophageal cancer at Gassim region, Saudi Arabia (meeting abstract), Proc. Annu. Meet. Am. Assoc. Cancer Res. **26**:297, 1985.

122. Shu, Y.J.: Detection of esophageal carcinoma by the balloon technique in the People's Republic of China, Adv. Clin. Cytol. **2**:67, 1984.

123. Isaacson, C., Bothwell, T.H., MacPhail, A.P., and Simon, M.: The iron status of urban black subjects with carcinoma of the oesophagus, S. Afr. Med. J. **67**(15):591, 1985.

124. Tuyns, A.J., and Estere, J.: Pipe, commercial and hand-rolled cigarette smoking in oesophageal cancer, Int. J. Epidemiol. **12**(1):110, 1983.

125. Lesec, G., Gogusev, J., Fermond, H., et al.: Presence of papilloma group viral antigen in an esophageal condyloma in man, Gastroenterol. Clin. Biol. **9**(2):166, 1985.

126. Ottenjann, R., Kuhner, W., and Weingart, J.: Esophageal papilloma: potential precursor of squamous cell carcinoma? Dtsch. Med. Wochenschr. **109**(16):613, 1985.

127. Syrjänen, K.J.: Histological changes identical to those of condylomatous lesions found in esophageal squamous cell carcinomas, Arch. Geschwulstforsch. **52**(4):283, 1982.

128. Spence, I.M.: Electron microscopic evidence of herpesvirus in asociation with oesophageal carcinoma, S. Afr. Med. J. **68**:103, 1985.

129. Mellow, M.H., Layne, E.A., Lipman, T.O., et al.: Plasma zinc and vitamin A in human squamous carcinoma of the esophagus, Cancer **51**(9):1615, 1983.

130. Van Rensburg, S.J., Hall, J.M., and du Bruyn, D.B.: Effect of various dietary staples on esophageal carcinogenesis induced in rats by subcutaneously administered *N*-nitrosomethylbenzylamine, JNCI **75**(3):561, 1985.

131. Barch, D.H., Kuemmerle, S.C., Hollenberg, P.F., and Iannaccone, P.M.: Esophageal microsome metabolism of *N*-nitrosomethylbenzylamine in the zinc-deficient rat, Cancer Res. **44**(12, part 1):5629, 1984.

132. Ziegler, R.G., Morris, L.E., Blot, W.J., et al.: Esophageal cancer among black men in Washington, D.C. II. Role of nutrition, JNCI **67**(6):1199, 1981.

133. Mettlin, C., Graham, S., Priore, M., et al.: Diet and cancer of the esophagus, Nutr. Cancer **2**(3):143, 1981.

CHAPTER 53 Perspective

Earle W. Wilkins, Jr.

For the practitioner who has spent a professional lifetime dealing with the unfortunate victims of esophageal carcinoma, or for the student who has labored long in perusing the contents of a volume devoted to the status of current therapy for the disease, it is difficult to feel other than real depression. Hints of progress are sufficiently sparse in providing any offsetting enthusiasm. Yet the problem persists, in many world regions to an alarmingly "epidemic" degree. Shunning the challenge it presents would be unexpected and inhuman. Progress in the half-century of surgical and radiotherapeutic techniques has been limited; at this particular point in time, future prospects are specifically few. The one hopeful note, however, resides in the enormous volume of human energy that has already been directed toward alleviating suffering in patients afflicted with the disease and in the unflagging willingness of medical scientists to continue plugging away at the problem and its challenges.

It seems clear that there is a need for a more unified or combined world effort in this enterprise. The triennial International Symposium on Esophageal Disorders (Rome, 1980; Chicago, 1983; Munich, 1986) is a step in this direction, but carcinoma is just one of the esophageal topics on which information and learning are shared at these meetings. And, thus far, surgeons have dominated the subjects and discussions. In an era in which multimodal therapy is the apparent wave of interest, more evidence of conjoint enterprise in combined surgery, radiotherapy, and chemotherapy is desperately needed. Reports with statistically insignificant numbers of patients frequent the oncologic literature. Almost nowhere is the scientific paragon of randomized, prospective trial exercised. Esophageal therapists, of differing specialties and of differing nations, need to get together to combine not only their statistics but their thoughts and theories. Finally, basic scientific investigation in the areas of etiology and prevention merits encouragement, financial support, and improved sharing of information. It is here that the needed breakthrough would have the greatest impact.

THE MANNELL OVERVIEW

In Chapter 52 Dr. Aylwyn Mannell has presented a balanced overview of the "current situation," with eight helpful review tables summarizing results of specific therapeutics modalities. These include esophageal intubation, radical radiotherapy, esophageal resection (early, stage III, and "curative"), preoperative adjuvant therapy (chemotherapy-irradiation and chemotherapy alone), and combination therapy for advanced esophageal cancer. This overview has been developed from a representative reference list of 133 reports, largely European, North American, South African, and East Asian. It is unfortunate that Iran has been relatively shut off from the medical worlds, east and west, and that its studies of esophageal carcinoma in the Caspian littoral are not more available and better understood.

AN ALGORITHM FOR THERAPY

As a corollary to Mannell's analysis of the current situation, it may be helpful to develop a therapeutic algorithm (Fig. 53-1) summarizing the present status of accepted treatment. To maintain a certain "purity" of approach, it will be limited to squamous carcinoma of the esophagus. It is intended only as an example of guidelines for the practitioner, and is actually a summary of presently accepted practice at the Massachusetts General Hospital.

In general, the more aggressive, multimodal forms of therapy are directed toward early and possibly curable lesions. When palliation is clearly the only possible goal, unimodal treatment is more appropriate (bypass, irradiation, intubation, laser therapy). In actual practice, the majority of patients fall between these extremes of management. When the "advanced" nature of a carcinoma is not clinically appreciated by preoperative staging and imaging techniques, becoming obvious only at surgery, the physician must decide between continuing the multimodal

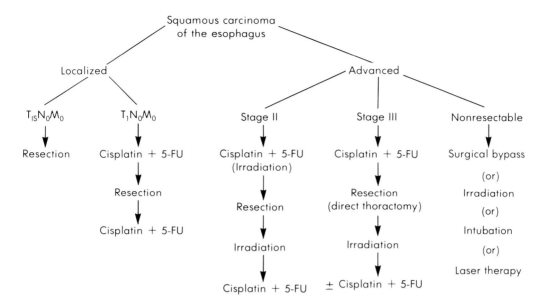

Fig. 53-1. A schema for choosing options in the treatment of squamous esophageal carcinoma as of 1987. The physiologic status of the patient may preclude resection at any point and shift the therapy to that for surgical nonresectability *(right)*. There is a potential role for combination chemotherapy with irradiation in nonresectable cases.

aggressive effort and providing truly palliative, unidirectional treatment.

Combination therapy for advanced carcinoma of the esophagus is, as Mannell points out, one possible change in such a pattern of treatment.

Localized carcinoma

1. Carcinoma in situ ($T_{is}N_0M_0$ by the accepted clinical staging system for carcinoma of the esophagus). These tumors are invariably detected by mass screening techniques or incidentally by the careful, experienced esophagogastroscopist who detects a mucosal abnormality while assessing some other problem in the upper gastrointestinal tract. Computed tomography shows no enlarged periesophageal draining lymph nodes. Systemic imaging techniques reveal no suggested metastatic foci. Here, aggressive extirpational therapy (see Chapter 19) is in order *without* adjuvant therapy, either before or after surgery. Depending upon mucosal evaluation by direct staining techniques, a high intrathoracic or cervical esophagogastric anastomosis is carried out. The resection is possible by either the standard direct thoracotomy or by a transhiatal-transcervical dissection.

2. Limited frank carcinoma ($T_1N_0M_0$). By definition a nonobstructing tumor of less than 5 cm without evidence of extraesophageal extent, this is best treated by combined chemotherapy and surgical extirpation (see Chapter 40). The chemotherapy is multi-agent and given both before

and after surgery. A typical protocol, for example, would be preoperative cisplatin and 5-fluorouracil for two cycles and the same combination of agents for four to six cycles postoperatively. Irradiation is not necessary in the absence of involved lymph nodes. The surgical options are as with carcinoma in situ.

Advanced carcinoma

The term "advanced carcinoma" refers to any tumor that is not in situ or stage I. Such carcinoma involves length greater than 5 cm, invasion through the full thickness of the esophageal wall, lymph node involvement, or distant metastases. Thorough patient evaluation is in order and proof is essential before a patient is assigned to this category. General principles of management include multimodal therapy with surgical removal as long as total tumor resection is possible or seems likely in the preoperative assessment.

1. Stage II ($T_1N_{1-2}M_0$ or $T_2N_{0-2}M_0$). A number of protocols are under evaluation; preliminary assessment of the results indicates a leading approach may be preoperative chemotherapy, surgery, and postoperative radiation and chemotherapy.[1] There has, incidentally, been little consistent, reproducible evidence that *pre*operative irradiation improves survival in patients with esophageal carcinoma. Again, early evidence suggests a spectrum of response to preoperative chemotherapy, almost irrespective of the agents employed, as long as the combinations are ration-

al. This response, in approximation, may be arithmetically reduced to one third showing full response, one third partial response, and one third no response. There is little reason to use chemotherapy after an operation if there has been no response before.

2. Stage III (T_3N_{0-3}). The guiding principle here should be that surgical extirpation is indicated or attemptable only (1) if there has been a response to preoperative chemotherapy or (2) if there is no preoperative evidence that complete resection is not possible. There seems to be no justifiable reason for esophagectomy if there are distant metastases. The decision to attempt resection hinges, therefore, on the status of the primary tumor and mediastinal nodes. Conclusive evidence for resectability is often difficult to come by, but assessment should include bronchoscopic evaluation along with esophagoscopy, mediastinal computed tomography, or magnetic resonance imaging, and occasionally angiographic studies (azygography, superior cava venography. aortography). Mediastinoscopy is an avenue for assessment of mediastinal tumor involvement, either by direct tumor extension or lymph node metastasis, that has not been extensively evaluated. The presence of an esophageal-airway fistula, bronchoscopic evidence of an incipient fistula or tracheobronchial invasion itself, and vascular invasion or obstruction are good evidence of nonresectability (except in the very unusual circumstance where combined resection of trachea or aorta is possible, as presented in Chapter 32).

If an attempt is made to resect a stage III carcinoma, it is preferable to do so by a procedure under direct vision—that is, a standard thoracotomy approach. The transhiatal method both diminishes the likelihood of totality of tumor removal and increases the risk of life-threatening complications such as azygos vein laceration, tracheal membranous wall tear, recurrent nerve avulsion, or thoracic duct injury. Postoperative irradiation will almost always be in order following resection of stage III tumors; postoperative chemotherapy is usually in order, although once again, nonresponse in advance of the operation may indicate the fruitlessness of such therapy.

Nonresectability

Nonresectability may be determined by certain of the stage III findings above, or by a physiologic status that does not permit conduct of a nonfatal procedure. Earlam and Cunha-Melo,[2] in their literature analysis (1980) of worldwide treatment for esophageal carcinoma (122 reports) found a hospital mortality of 29% following resection. A large proportion of these were the result of predisposing bad-risk medical or physiologic factors. Resection of a stage III esophageal carcinoma in the presence of a prohibitive medical risk is not justified. The esophageal surgeon must assume the responsibility for decision-making in the risk of the operation to the patient. Medical factors that are particularly threatening include limited respiratory capability (such as a forced expiratory volume in 1 second of less than 1 liter), recent myocardial infarction (within 6 months), current congestive heart failure, evidence of hepatic decompensation, age in excess of 80, and morbid obesity. A dead patient cannot be cured of esophageal carcinoma.

What then are the palliative procedures to be entertained in the management of nonresectable carcinomas, and in what order of consideration? The options include (1) surgical bypass, usually gastric or colonic, (2) irradiation, (3) intubation, (4) laser therapy, and (5) chemotherapy.

The gastric or colonic bypass, accomplished by the anterior mediastinal, retrosternal route, may be used for (1) the respiratory poor-risk patient in whom a transthoracic approach is likely to be poorly tolerated and in whom a full combined chemotherapy-irradiation approach is possible (for the primary tumor) or (2) the patient, otherwise in good condition, with an esophago-airway fistula. Orringer (Chapter 25) would utilize the transhiatal approach for resection in the first of these.

Irradiation may be well tolerated for palliation, but the duration of therapy (four weeks or more) is lengthy and reduces the interval of possible palliative success. The greater the obstruction, unfortunately the less likely a satisfactory response to irradiation. It is in this method of therapy only that a feeding gastrostomy is justified and then just to permit nourishment *during* the phase of treatment. In frank or incipient esophago-airway fistula, irradiation is not indicated without a prior bypass procedure (see Chapter 48), perhaps not at all.

Endoscopic intraluminal intubation is often an effective means of palliation (see Chapter 51). Successful utilization requires experience on the part of the operator[3]; the list of possible complications is virtually endless.[4] Pulsion techniques seem preferable to traction.

Esophagoscopic application of the laser (see Chapter 49) to provide an effective esophageal lumen offers promise but along with it a potential for complications. This technique may require repeated sessions for continued palliation. The advantage of both intubation and laser therapy is that palliation is obtained in the shortest interval.

Chemotherapy is a hope of the future.

TABLE 53-1. Three-year survival after esophagectomy

Technique	Author	Year	No. of resections	Survival at 3 years (%)
Transhiatal	Orringer	1986	147	23
Conventional	Katlic[6]	1982	142	24
Radical	Skinner	1986	80	24
Historical	Sweet[5]	1952	254	22*

*The Sweet survival rate is computed for those patients who survived the operation; it is therefore not valid for exact statistical comparison with the other listed techniques, but not wholly unreasonable in that these figures record the experience of the pioneering decade of the 1940s, before the cuffed endotracheal tube, modern anesthetic agents and methods, broad-spectrum antibiotics, respiratory therapy, and intensive care units.

RESECTIONAL METHODS

A great deal of emphasis has been placed, both in the thoracic surgical literature and in the popular continuing surgical education courses, on the methodology of resection of the esophagus. A convenient classification is to describe the techniques as radical (Skinner, Chapter 24), conventional, or transhiatal (Orringer, Chapter 25). No one has compared the outcomes for these approaches. An attempt is made here, therefore, to look at patient survival for these techniques and indeed to compare them with more historical methods. The example utilized for the latter are the Sweet statistics[5] from the Massachusetts General Hospital (MGH) in 1952. Statistics for the conventional resection, defined as direct transthoracic resection of the esophagus with lymph node dissection, are taken from the Katlic and Grillo MGH study[6] of 1982.

The comparison is presented in Table 53-1, which shows numbers of resections, author and year of reporting, and the cumulative survival estimates at 3 years.

It appears that methodology, perhaps, is a less important variable in survival following esophagectomy than surgeons have thought. In fact, during 35 years, resectional progress, when measured in 3-year survivals, has been very limited. Therefore, a surgeon should choose the technique that provides the lowest complication rate for him or her. For most surgeons, this is the standard transthoracic approach.[7] Future gains in patient survival are likely to come from application of adjuvant therapy.[1]

Too much emphasis cannot be placed on the safety of the method. This in particular involves the details of performance of the anastomosis. The goal must always be a zero leakage rate; the MGH series, in which 90% of operations were performed by senior thoracic residents under attending-level supervision, has achieved this record in 104 resections in the period from 1980 to 1986.[7] Mathisen et al. in this comparative report found that the two-layer interrupted or the stapled anastomosis produced the lowest leakage rates.

A leakage rate is no longer acceptable only because it is less than 10%. Churchill and Sweet[8] defined the requisite technical care 45 years ago (1942): the "mucous membrane sutures are placed with the exactitude and with the degree of tension that we would use in the fine plastic procedure on the lip" and "we have paid unusual attention to the detail of the anastomosis [in explaining the absence of strictures]."

A SURGICAL SUMMARY

Specific principles are clear for the surgeon in considering the form of therapy:

1. Resection has little to offer in long-term salvage unless it involves total removal of the carcinoma.
2. Extreme care must be taken to avoid resectional therapy in the medically compromised patient who cannot make the grade following this physiologically massive procedure.
3. When surgery is possible and indicated, it is essential that every effort be made to avoid life-threatening complications, especially the leaking anastomosis.
4. Adjuvant therapy is advisable in all but the earliest lesions. This should involve preoperative chemotherapy plus postoperative irradiation if lymph node metastases are detected, mediastinal invasion is encountered, or resection margins are positive, and then postoperative chemotherapy too if the preoperative response has been total or partial.
5. Esophageal resection is not for the casual surgeon.
6. The esophageal surgeon must be expert in a variety of surgical techniques and willing to apply them both appropriately and thoughtfully.

DeMeester's four questions (see p. 102) should always be kept in mind.

THE FUTURE

Where do we go from here? Dr. Mannell has covered the prospects thoroughly under her three headings of detection, treatment, and prevention.

Detection

It is clear that early diagnosis diminishes hospital mortality following esophagectomy and improves long-term survival: 90% at 5 years following resection for carcinoma in situ, 60% for invasive carcinoma limited to the esophagus, and 10% when lymphatic invasion is present. This supports the use, in endemic areas, of screening efforts with techniques such as blind abrasive cytology (see Chapter 4) and endoscopic double-dye staining (see Chapter 6). Do we know the other side of this coin? How many patients diagnosed by cytology as having carcinoma (accuracy of 90%) had esophagectomy, after which only inflammatory lesions were found in the pathologic specimens? Was the morbidity significant in the 10% noncarcinoma patients who may have had unnecessary esophagectomy? And, most important, would any patient die as the result of an erroneous diagnosis?

In nonendemic areas, blind abrasive cytology and double-dye staining seem worthwhile in the presence of conditions that are considered to predispose to the development of carcinoma: achalasia, Barrett's esophagus, caustic stricture, scleroderma, heavy combined alcohol and tobacco usage, Plummer-Vinson (Paterson's) syndrome, and mucosal carcinomas of the head, neck, and airways regions.

Treatment

Despite the various surgical advances in the management of squamous esophageal carcinoma, it seems unlikely that further technical advances will produce more surviving patients. Surgeons cannot do wider dissections. Better patient selection and lowered operative morbidity, though applaudable achievements, will not alter overall survival, especially if all carcinoma patients are considered and not just those who are resectable. The addition of irradiation prior to surgery has not improved results. The verdict on postoperative radiotherapy is not yet in. Improved results from treatment, therefore, hinge on chemotherapy with or without radiation, or other as yet unproved modalities, such as hyperthermia (Chapter 42) or immunochemotherapy (Chapter 43). Chemotherapy does offer promise. It is hoped that improved application of the techniques, including newer multidrug combinations, will further enhance patient survival. Therapy for adenocarcinoma involving the esophagus has not been studied to the extent that squamous carcinoma has.

Prevention

It is in the area of prevention that the greatest potential for progress in the management of esophageal carcinoma lies. Prevention in turn depends on understanding possible etiologies. The various theories have been listed in Chapter 1. Considering the remarkable geographic localization of the disease, with endemic incidences in China, South Africa, Iran, the Caspian areas of the Soviet Union, and parts of France, the most likely causative agents would seem to be nitrosamine precursors in the diet, particular soil characteristics (alkalinity, nitrates, low molybdenum level, and mold aflatoxin), or a viral agent, such as the human papilloma virus or the herpesvirus. In addition, the avoidance of alcohol, tobacco, and opium agents is desirable and the maintenance of adequate nutritional status essential.

• • •

Carcinoma of the esophagus is not just a surgical disease. In fact, surgeons have gone as far as they can go, provided one accepts the premise that esophageal surgery is not for the beginner or for the casual surgeon. The radiotherapist has long been involved. The chemotherapist is already on the scene and assuming a more important role. The basic scientist is eagerly awaited for what he or she can teach us concerning the etiology, and ultimately the prevention, of this disease.

REFERENCES

1. Hilgenberg, A.D., Carey, R.W., Choi, N.C., Wilkins, E.W., Jr., et al.: Preoperative chemotherapy and resection for esophageal squamous cell carcinoma, Ann. Thorac. Surg., 1988. (In press.)
2. Earlam, R., and Cunha-Melo, J.R.: Oesophageal squamous carcinoma. I. A critical review of surgery, Br. J. Surg. **67**:381, 1980.
3. Boyce, H.W.: Non-surgical measures to relieve distress of late esophageal carcinoma, Geriatrics **28**:97, 1973.
4. Adams, C.L.: The complications of endoesophageal tubes, J. Thorac. Cardiovasc. Surg. **51**:685, 1966.
5. Sweet, R.H.: The results of radical surgical extirpation in the treatment of carcinoma of the esophagus and cardia with five-year survival statistics, Surg. Gynecol. Obstet. **94**:46, 1952.
6. Katlic, M.R., and Grillo, H.C.: Carcinoma of the esophagus: a current perspective. In Choi, N.C., and Grillo, H.C., editors: Thoracic oncology, New York, 1983, Raven Press, pp. 279-301.
7. Mathisen, D.J., Grillo, H.C., Wilkins, E.W., Jr., et al.: Transthoracic esophagectomy: a safe approach to carcinoma of the esophagus, Ann. Thorac. Surg. **45**:137, 1988. (In press.)
8. Churchill, E.D., and Sweet, R.H.: Transthoracic resection of tumors of the stomach and esophagus, Ann. Surg. **115**:897, 1942.

Index

Italicized page numbers indicate illustration; t following page number indicates table.

445